Children and young people with cancer

Guidance for occupational therapists

Edited by Catriona Ogilvy

TEENAGE CANCER TRUST
HELPING YOUNG PEOPLE FIGHT CANCER

College of Occupational Therapists

Specialist Section
Children, Young People & Families

This edition published in 2010
by the College of Occupational Therapists
106–114 Borough High Street
London SE1 1LB
www.cot.org.uk

Edited by: Catriona Ogilvy on behalf of the College of Occupational Therapists Specialist Section – Children, Young People and Families.
Category: Guidance

Other enquiries about this document should be addressed to the Practice department at the above address.

British Library Cataloguing in Publication Data
A catalogue record for this book is available from the British Library.

ISBN 978-1-905944-17-0

Typeset by Servis Filmsetting Ltd, Stockport, Cheshire
Digitally printed on demand in Great Britain by The Lavenham Press, Suffolk

FSC
Mixed Sources
Product group from well-managed forests and other controlled sources
www.fsc.org Cert no. SGS-COC-004865
© 1996 Forest Stewardship Council

Contents

Acknowledgements **iv**
Foreword: a parent's view **v**
1 Key recommendations **1**
2 Occupational therapy **2**
3 Guidance development **3**
4 Introduction to cancer in children and young people **8**
5 A holistic and family-centred approach to care **12**
6 Occupational therapy assessment **14**
7 Standardised assessments **17**
8 Occupational therapy intervention **20**
8.1 Self-care 20
8.2 Play and leisure 22
8.3 Life skills and productivity 23
9 Occupational therapy intervention in symptom management **27**
9.1 Management of cancer-related fatigue 27
9.2 Pain management 30
9.3 Management of breathlessness 31
9.4 Management of anxiety 33
9.5 Multiprofessional management of symptoms 35
10 The needs of children with cancer **37**
11 The needs of adolescents and young adults with cancer **39**
12 Palliative care in paediatric oncology **41**
13 Multiprofessional working, communication and collaboration **46**
14 Equipment provision **48**
15 Outcome measures **50**
16 Caring for oneself as a professional **52**
17 Implications for future practice **53**
18 Summary **54**
Glossary **56**
Appendixes **57**
1 Levels of research evidence 57
2 Distribution of childhood cancers in the UK (2003) 59
3 Types of childhood cancers 60
4 Anti-cancer treatments 62
5 Side effects of common chemotherapy drugs 64
6a Surgical procedures and post-operative precautions for bone tumours 66
6b Occupational therapy intervention for children and young people with bone tumours 68
Further resources **70**
References **72**

Acknowledgements

The guidance development group would like to thank all those who have contributed to the guidance and who have made publication of this document possible.

In particular the development group would like to thank the College of Occupational Therapists for their ongoing support, advice and belief in the importance of producing guidance in this specialised area. A special thank you is extended to the family members co-opted onto the group, for the invaluable insight they gave into the real needs of children, young people and their families.

Our thanks are extended also to all those involved in the consultation over the document who have offered their valuable feedback.

The guidance has taken two years to develop and all those involved in its writing have worked hard in bringing the document to fruition. The group would finally like to thank all those around them who have supported them during this process.

Foreword

A parent's view

Our son Ben was a very healthy, intelligent and sporty young man when he was diagnosed with a spinal cord tumour at the age of 11. At school he was in all the top groups and was a very promising student. He participated in many sports, including tennis, cricket, swimming and skiing with his main love being rugby. As you can imagine his diagnosis of a highly malignant tumour, with an extremely poor likely outcome, was a complete shock. He underwent major surgery three times, and required radiotherapy and several different courses of chemotherapy. Throughout his treatment, there was very little good news but we always managed to remain positive, taking any sign of encouragement and moving forward to the next stage of treatment.

Throughout his 18 months of treatment, Ben became increasingly disabled, finally requiring surgery that left him paraplegic and permanently in a wheelchair. During this time we needed input from a number of occupational therapists.

Initially the occupational therapists helped by arranging a wheelchair from our local wheelchair service. We were also given a bath lift at this stage. Although he didn't use it immediately, the bath lift became an important piece of equipment in the months that followed when Ben couldn't manage to get in or out of the bath unaided. He really enjoyed a good soak, often emerging like a prune!

Over the following months, we acquired more equipment to help Ben in his daily activities, including a ramp for getting in and out of the house (fortunately we lived in a bungalow, so we did not have stairs to worry about); a transfer board to aid movement from one chair to another without falling into the gap; a standing frame to help Ben's posture; an armchair raiser to help with transfers; a back raiser and bars on his bed to help him manoeuvre; a pressure mattress; and a commode (primarily used to help Ben get into our very small bathroom). Alterations were made to the bathroom to promote his independence.

The equipment was readily available to us and normally delivered swiftly and without delay, but I sometimes found it difficult to accept, and often found myself being defensive towards the occupational therapists who were trying to help us. I'm not sure whether the therapists understood why I was being like this, but when presented with a commode that looked like it would be suitable for Ben's Gran, or a chair that probably would have helped Ben, but looked as though it was only fit for an extremely disabled child, I hope you can see where I was coming from. Ben's dad didn't have these feelings and simply saw the equipment as a way to help us manage in this terrible situation. He found it difficult to understand why I was finding this aspect of Ben's care so difficult. I wanted to help Ben, but I guess I wasn't ready to let my sporty little boy go. I sometimes wished I could have been given more time to 'get my head around things', before being presented with the next item of equipment.

We were allocated an occupational therapist for Ben at his school. We were very fortunate in that the school was already well adapted, with lifts, ramps and disabled toilets, and a school move was not necessary. The school also had a very well established Special Educational Needs Co-ordinator (SENCO) team with experience of meeting the needs of other wheelchair users. The teachers allowed Ben to move between classrooms a few minutes before the lesson finished, with a friend, so that he had more time and could avoid the rush. Although as it turned out we didn't have much contact with the school occupational therapist, it was a real support to know that there was someone trained in this area to assess Ben's needs as and when they might arise.

Over the course of Ben's treatment, we were involved with at least four occupational therapists, as well as with a number of physiotherapists. We made daily visits to the hospital for treatment. Ben had to have frequent blood tests. We were kept very busy looking after Ben and his many needs – trying to keep some schooling going, to maintain a relatively normal life for his younger brother, running the house, and trying to get to work when Ben had better periods. Making appointments for home visits was sometimes necessary, but difficult to arrange because of all these commitments. In the midst of all this we tried to make space for some special family time. We were grateful that all the occupational therapists communicated well with each other and with us so that we didn't have to repeat conversations. They also talked to Ben respectfully, not as a child who didn't have an opinion. They took the time to develop a relationship with him and to understand his needs.

One of the most valuable skills we received from an occupational therapist was relaxation techniques. During Ben's final course of chemotherapy, the drugs used were extremely nasty and made Ben feel rotten. Ben often experienced panicky periods during chemotherapy, because of his fear of the side effects. By using techniques taught to us by the occupational therapist, we were able to help Ben relax: the exercises often left Ben fast asleep – and sometimes us as well! This made a huge difference to the whole experience and I'm not sure we would have got through it without this help.

Ben coped well with adapting to being paraplegic. He learned to cook in the kitchen and to shop in the supermarket using the trolley for wheelchair users. We started looking into sports for disabled users, including basketball, archery and skiing. Ben even talked about entering the 2012 Olympics. He was told he could learn to drive at the age of 16 and he looked forward to driving in an adapted car and charging his friends for journeys! Sadly, despite all the interventions and the hard work of the multidisciplinary teams involved with Ben, he died at home, peacefully, after a short period of being disease free. Ultimately, even if there were times I didn't appear to be, we were extremely grateful for all the time and resources that the occupational therapists gave to Ben's care throughout his treatment.

Caroline Cross – Ben's Mother

1 Key recommendations

1. Occupational therapy intervention must be flexible, in accordance with the fluctuating nature and presentation of cancer and its treatment, and should focus upon need rather than diagnosis or prognosis.
2. Occupational therapists working with children and young people with cancer should have a clear understanding of anti-cancer treatments, their side effects, and implications for clinical practice.
3. Communication between occupational therapists must be effective and timely to prevent duplication of assessments or delay in equipment provision.
4. Research into the effectiveness of specific occupational therapy interventions used within paediatric oncology needs to be conducted urgently, in order to develop a robust evidence base for this area of practice.

2 Occupational therapy

Through the practice of meaningful activity, occupational therapists aim to promote and facilitate independence in all aspects of daily life. For children and young people, everyday activities or 'occupations' are seen as self-care, life skills, play, leisure and education (Case-Smith 2001). Adopting a holistic approach, occupational therapists assess and treat the physical, cognitive, perceptual, sensory and psychological components of a person that may affect ability and success in engaging in everyday activities. Research demonstrates that the practice of purposeful activity improves the performance of activities of daily living (Lin et al 1997) and that through the adaption of task or environment, independence can be maximised and quality of life enhanced.

As will be demonstrated throughout the guidance, cancer and its treatment impacts upon the physical, cognitive, sensory, social and emotional wellbeing of the child or young person. It can dramatically affect a child or young person's ability to engage in any or all aspects of daily living. Occupational therapists are trained to understand the interaction between physical, cognitive and psychological needs, the environment and occupation, and are therefore highly suited to the holistic approach to care required in oncology practice.

3 Guidance development

Background

Following a paediatric brain tumour study day for allied health professionals (AHPs) in May 2007, an email-based clinical network was created for occupational therapists working in the area of paediatric oncology. Of particular concern to those involved in this network was the lack of robust research evidence, literature and guidance relating to this specialist area of occupational therapy practice. Consequently, a clinical guidance development group was established, consisting of senior and specialist occupational therapists from across the United Kingdom with extensive experience in paediatric oncology and/or palliative care.

The aim of the group was to produce a guidance resource for this specialist area of occupational therapy practice. The group planned to draw together research evidence, guidance and literature relevant to the area, and to supplement any gaps with their expert knowledge and understanding.

Guidance development group

Catriona Ogilvy	Highly Specialist Occupational Therapist The Royal Marsden NHS Foundation Trust, Sutton
Elizabeth Rowen	Highly Specialist Occupational Therapist Children's Services, Newcastle General Hospital
Elizabeth Smith	Highly Specialist Occupational Therapist Birmingham Children's Hospital
Annabelle Jones	Highly Specialist Occupational Therapist Great Ormond Street Hospital for Children, London
Claire Tester	AHP Lead, Professional Practice Development, NHS Quality Improvement Scotland – formerly AHP Consultant in Cancer For Scotland (2005–2008)
Paula Galloway	Highly Specialist Occupational Therapist Royal Manchester Children's Hospital, Central Manchester University Hospitals NHS Foundation Trust

Co-opted members

Caroline Cross	Parent
Janet Appleton	Highly Specialist Occupational Therapist Teenage Cancer Trust Unit University College Hospital, London

Objectives

- To provide an evidence-based resource for occupational therapists working with children and young people with cancer.
- To support and facilitate clinical decision-making.

- To promote a consistent, best-practice approach to occupational therapy intervention for children and young people with cancer across the UK.
- To highlight the role of occupational therapists working with children and young people with cancer and to demonstrate their contribution in this area of practice.

Why develop practice guidance?

Children's oncology is a specialised area of paediatric occupational therapy and the number of occupational therapists working specifically in this area is very small. However, occupational therapists from other clinical settings may encounter and/or work with children and young people diagnosed with cancer during their clinical career. This guidance has therefore been developed to support occupational therapists in what can often be a demanding and challenging area of occupational therapy practice.

Treating a child or young person with cancer can seem a daunting task for an occupational therapist with little or no previous experience of paediatric oncology, but this guidance will show how all paediatric occupational therapists have the transferable clinical skills required for working with children and young people with cancer, and the ability to apply these skills to practice.

As will be discussed throughout this document, the presentation and nature of cancer is diverse and multifaceted. For this reason, the guidance does not, neither could it, propose a set formula for treating every child or young person with cancer. Instead the guidance is seen as a tool for informing and facilitating clinical reasoning and guiding evidence-based occupational therapy intervention.

The guidance development group recognises that the word 'cancer' can provoke a range of emotions for the therapist, who may even have had a previous personal or professional connection with cancer. As in any area of clinical practice, it is important for occupational therapists to have regular supervision and support in place. Caring for yourself as a professional and developing self-awareness will be discussed later in the document.

Intended audience

The guidance is intended for all occupational therapists working with a child or young person with a diagnosis of cancer. Primarily targeted at occupational therapists with little or no past experience in children's oncology, the guidance may nevertheless be beneficial to occupational therapists with experience in this area. This will be the case particularly for those wishing to further develop their clinical skills or, in accordance with good clinical governance, compare their service against recommended best practice.

This guidance document may also be useful to service managers, commissioners or purchasing managers, as well as to a general readership.

Place of service provision

The number of children or young people an occupational therapist will see with a diagnosis of cancer will vary according to the setting in which they work. Children and young people with cancer can be referred to or seen by occupational therapists in a number of settings. These settings may include the following, although this list is not exhaustive:

- Children's Cancer and Leukaemia Group (CCLG) Centre.

- Teenage Cancer Trust Centre.
- Acute neuro-surgical and orthopaedic centres.
- Acute shared-care trust or district general hospitals.
- Local authority services.
- Child development centres.
- Wheelchair services.
- Schools.
- Child and Adolescent Mental Health Services.
- Hospices.
- Voluntary settings.

Who will be covered by the guidance?

The guidance will cover children (from birth) and young people into their late teens and early twenties who present with malignant disease. There is no upper age limit specified in the document. This is in keeping with the National Institute for Health and Clinical Excellence's *Guidance on cancer services: improving outcomes in children and young people with cancer* (NICE 2005), which found during its consultation period that setting an arbitrary upper age limit was inappropriate.

The guidance will not cover the role of occupational therapy in the management of the long-term effects of cancer or its treatment, nor does it cover children and young people with benign tumours or benign haematological conditions.

Dissemination and implementation

It is planned that the publication of the guidance will be brought to the attention of occupational therapists through a number of channels:

- An article in *Occupational Therapy News*.
- Promotion on the College of Occupational Therapists' (COT) website.
- Presentation at the COT Specialist Section – Children, Young People and Families Annual Conference.
- Presentation at the COT Annual Conference.
- An article in the COT Specialist Section – Children, Young People and Families Journal.
- An announcement in the COT Specialist Section – HIV, Oncology and Palliative Care newsletter.
- Promotion at COT Specialist Section – Children, Young People and Families regional group meetings.
- Promotion at the COT Specialist Section – Children, Young People and Families Acute Clinical Forum.

Review of guidance

In accordance with maintaining up-to-date clinical evidence, the guidance will be subject to ongoing review. Reviews will be undertaken by a working party assembled by the COT Specialist Section – Children, Young People and Families. The relevance and effectiveness of the guidance will be evaluated and amendments to the guidance made accordingly. Following publication of revised and updated guidance, this new information will be disseminated to interested parties through the channels noted above.

Methodology

An extensive literature search was initially conducted by the COT librarian on behalf of the development group.

The following search engines were used: AMED, CINAHL, HMIC, PsycINFO, Medline, COT catalogue, NLH, Guidelines, DARE database and Metasearch Engines.

As the guidance covers a wide range of diagnoses, symptoms and occupational therapy interventions, each member of the practice development group conducted further searches focusing on specific topics and areas of the document. The engines outlined above were searched with wider terms detailed below. References listed in the retrieved articles were reviewed. The internet was searched, using Google, for published guidance or guidelines on cancer-related symptom management, paediatric palliative care and paediatric oncology.

Inclusion criteria

The literature search focused upon articles relating to:

- Occupational therapy intervention in oncology.
- Rehabilitation in oncology.
- Rehabilitation in palliative care.
- All aspects of paediatric oncology that include transferable evidence to underpin occupational therapy practice.
- Symptom management in adult oncology.

Exclusion criteria

- Research articles published prior to 1995.
- Articles not written in the English language.

Search terms

- Paediatric(s), pediatric(s), child, childhood, children, teenager, adolescence, adolescent, family.
- Cancer, tumour, oncology, neoplasm, malignancy, neuro-oncology, brain tumour, bone marrow transplant, amputation, limb-salvaging.
- Occupational therapy, therapy, rehabilitation, outcome measures.
- Development, neuro-development, developmental milestones, play.
- Leisure, independence, advocacy, education, school, pre-school, employment.

- Fatigue, pain, breathlessness, dyspnoea, anxiety, symptom clusters, non-pharmaceutical intervention, peripheral neuropathy.
- Self-care, body image, self-image, self-esteem.
- Palliative care, palliative rehabilitation, symptom control, end of life, quality of life, supportive care.

Finally, a 'top up' search was performed prior to publication of this guidance to ensure the latest evidence was included. No further searches took place after 5 June 2009 and for this reason articles published after this date will not have been included in the guidance.

Levels of evidence

As the group had expected, the search found only a small number of documents and articles that might relate to paediatric occupational therapy in this area (see Appendix 1). Currently, there is no robust research evidence demonstrating the effectiveness and value of occupational therapy for children and young people with cancer – thus highlighting the importance of producing practice guidelines for this specialist area. This means that our first objective, to provide an evidence-based resource for occupational therapists working with children and young people with cancer, cannot fully be met at present. This document therefore draws together the evidence that is available from the literature, including that from other practice areas and disciplines deemed relevant and transferable. As is the case in other aspects of paediatric oncology, much of the literature underpinning the guidance has come from an adult oncology background or from a paediatric nursing perspective. Where there are gaps, the expert opinion of members of the guidance development group is given and clearly indicated as such. The group acknowledges that expert opinion is positioned at the bottom of the hierarchy of research evidence; however, in the absence of other evidence, in such instances it was felt to be a valid alternative. It should be noted that opinion within the group was firm and unanimous on all topics discussed.

Peer review

Prior to publication, the guidance was reviewed by peers working in the field of, or with a special interest in, paediatric oncology. The occupational therapy paediatric oncology email network group was consulted on the guidance.

To gain the views of the guidance's main readership, the document was also reviewed by occupational therapists with little or no experience of paediatric oncology. Occupational therapists consulted in this review came from a cross-section of clinical settings. These included:

- The National Executive Committee (NEC) members of the COT Specialist Section – Children, Young People and Families.
- The COT Specialist Section – Children, Young People and Families clinical advisors.
- NEC members of the COT Specialist Section – HIV, Oncology and Palliative Care.

All suggestions and comments were welcomed. Amendments and/or inclusions were made to the document as appropriate in the view of the guidance development group.

4 Introduction to cancer in children and young people

Incidence

Cancer in children, thankfully, is rare, with the chance of developing cancer before the age of fifteen approximately 1 in 600. There are roughly 1,700 new cases of childhood cancer diagnosed each year in the UK, of which almost half occur in children under the age of five, and boys are universally more affected than girls (Tobias and Eaton 2001). Appendix 2 details the distribution of types of childhood cancers.

Survival

Although the total number of children developing cancer has changed little in the last 40 years, advances in treatment have dramatically improved survival outcomes. On average, 75 per cent of children (aged 0–15) with cancer in the UK today are still alive five years after their initial diagnosis, compared to 25 per cent in 1962–1971 (Tobias and Eaton 2001).

Cancer diagnosis

Childhood cancers are uniquely different from cancers found in the adult population. They occur in different parts of the body, look different under the microscope, and respond differently to treatment. For adults, cancer incidence data can be classified largely in terms of the site of the disease; for children the cell type (histology) also needs to be taken into account (Tobias and Eaton 2001). Appendix 3 has further details of specific childhood cancers.

Childhood cancer has lifelong consequences and the course of both disease and treatment can be unpredictable. For example, acute episodes of illness due to reactions to medications, surgery or disease progression, which result in a sudden deterioration of physical and psychological wellbeing, may occur. With increasing survival rates, the difficulties faced by long-term survivors of childhood cancer, such as impaired cognitive function, chronic fatigue, behavioural changes and reduced self-esteem, become more prevalent. Timely therapeutic intervention is therefore essential.

Treatment

All children diagnosed with cancer will be treated in one of the UK's 22 Children's Cancer and Leukaemia Group (CCLG) centres. These centres have large multidisciplinary teams and follow national protocols for children's cancer treatment. In accordance with NICE guidance (2005), young people aged 15–18 should be referred to principal centres with teenage facilities, and those aged 18–24 years should have unhindered access to specialist teams skilled in treating young people.

The treatment of cancer in children and young people will vary according to the tumour type, its site and the age of the child. It will involve single use, or a combination, of chemotherapy, radiotherapy, surgery, stem-cell transplant or bone-marrow transplant.

- *Chemotherapy* is the use of cytotoxic drugs, which act to interfere with the growth of rapidly dividing cancer cells. As chemotherapy directly targets rapidly dividing cells, other healthy tissues with high proliferation rates, such as hair follicles, bone marrow and mucous membranes in the mouth and bowel, are often also affected. Chemotherapy drugs may be given orally or intravenously via a central line, PICC line or port (Tobias and Eaton 2001).
- *Radiotherapy* is the use of ionising radiation to damage and destroy cancer cells. As chemotherapy has become more effective, the use of radiotherapy in children has declined. Radiotherapy does remain the main modality of treatment for brain tumours in children, however. Fractions of radiotherapy are given daily for a period of 4 to 6 weeks. For young children this may require the use of a daily general anaesthetic (Dixon-Woods et al 2005, Tobias and Eaton 2001).
- *Surgery* is the surgical removal or debulking of tumour cells.
- *Stem-cell and/or bone-marrow transplants* enable high-dose chemotherapy and/or total body irradiation to be used. Such transplants are used for children with high-risk disease, in situations in which standard chemotherapy alone would not be sufficient (Dixon-Woods et al 2005, Miller et al 2008).

Implications and precautions for occupational therapy intervention

Risk of infection

Precautions to protect children and young people with cancer from infection are paramount due to their lowered immunity levels as a result of treatment. Children should not be seen by therapists who are displaying symptoms of infection (such as cough, cold, sore throat, vomiting or diarrhoea), and stringent cleaning of toys and equipment should be adopted. In a community setting, some parents may prefer their child to be seen at home to reduce risk of infection when their white blood-cell count is low (neutropenic) and/or if they are feeling unwell.

Anti-cancer treatment

When considering intervention, careful thought should be given to the implications of line care, for example when positioning children or when attending to self-care needs. Consideration should also be given to the side effects of current medication and to treatment regimes. For instance, appointments for ongoing community intervention should be arranged at certain points in the intervals between chemotherapy cycles, when children are most likely to be medically well and able to tolerate intervention. Conversely, some families may wish to make the most of the time when their child is feeling well, is medically stable and out of hospital, and as a result may be reluctant to attend occupational therapy appointments during this time. This should be discussed with families individually and the wishes of each respected.

Disease progression

Occupational therapists should be aware of, and able to notice, clinical signs of disease progression. Assessing and treating physical, cognitive and sensory deficits, occupational therapists may notice changes over the course of intervention. Following sensitive discussion with the family, the principle treatment centre should be notified of any concerns.

Signs of disease progression will be dependent upon tumour type, but may include pain over the site of the tumour, swelling, breathlessness, fatigue, headaches, nausea, vomiting, visual disturbances, ataxia, hemiplegia, reduced mobility, sensory changes, decreased bladder/bowel function, facial palsy, language difficulties, and altered behaviour.

Side effects of anti-cancer treatments

It is important for occupational therapists working with children and young people with cancer to have an awareness of potential treatment-related side effects that may impact functional performance and/or have implications for intervention and therapy.

Common side effects include:

- Increased risk of bruising and bleeding (due to low platelet counts)
- Increased risk of infection
- Loss of appetite
- Weight loss or weight gain
- Nausea, vomiting and diarrhoea
- Constipation
- Fatigue
- Mouth ulcers (mucositis)
- Taste changes
- Skin changes
- Hair loss
- Chemotherapy-induced peripheral neuropathy

(Tobias and Eaton 2001)

Long-term side effects include:

- Heart and lung complications
- Affected intellectual development
- Affected physical growth and development
- Infertility
- Endocrine problems
- Second malignancies

(Tobias and Eaton 2001)

For full details of anti-cancer treatments and their specific side effects see Appendix 4.

Appendix 5 highlights specific side effects of key chemotherapy drugs.

Duration of treatment

The overall length of treatment will vary depending on the treatment protocol and will be based upon diagnosis, as well as response to treatment. Some protocols may be mainly out-patient based, whereas others will require extended periods of hospital admissions. Disruption to family life during this time should not be underestimated. Practical considerations such as the effects of travelling often long distances between home and hospital (sometimes daily), arranging alternative childcare for siblings, and the uncertainty of sudden unplanned hospital admissions, should also be taken into account when planning occupational therapy intervention (Dudgeon 2001, Slade 2000).

5 A holistic and family-centred approach to care

The impact of cancer

The impact of cancer treatment and the debilitation it can cause may affect a child's ability to cope with the life-changes that follow diagnosis. These may include being in hospital for a prolonged period of time and the suspension of normal life at home and school. In addition a child's sense of self, body image or self-esteem may be affected. For some children these factors result in a regression of skills or emotional maturity. This can be reinforced, often unwittingly, by parents being protective and wanting to be as active as possible in the care of their child. This can result in the child's own independence being thwarted. It is understandable for parents to be anxious or fearful for the wellbeing of their child; however, these emotions can unconsciously be transferred to the child. Young children are particularly sensitive to their parents' emotions when in close proximity. Frequent visits to clinic, life on a ward, indeed having cancer, are not normal, which can be easy to forget for a therapist working in oncology (Tester 2006).

A family-centred approach

Taking a family-centred approach involves understanding the child as part of a family. The occupational therapist should always be aware that the parent is a client too, actively involving them as a part of the therapeutic intervention, and supporting them in recognising their own needs when these impact upon the child. Each family is different. The role of the grandparent may be overlooked by hospital and community staff, though grandparents often fulfil the role of a main carer. The support and relationship of siblings is often particularly important to a child or young person with cancer, who may feel 'cut off' from the family unit. There are few opportunities in a child's cancer treatment when family members can be actively involved: involving family members in occupational therapy sessions is one way of engaging and supporting different family members.

The parent or main guardian provides 'emotional containment' for a child or young person (Bion 1984). Emotional containment may be understood as unconditional understanding and support. This may be unspoken, but is nevertheless critical at times of distress. If such unconditional understanding and support is unavailable to a child or young person, he or she may experience a sense that their distress will not end, which then becomes more acute as a consequence.

Often a family pet has an important role. Although animals cannot be brought to clinic or onto a ward, children or young people may be encouraged to keep a photograph, or the animal may be brought to the window. These gestures, showing understanding of the family context, may seem small but can be very helpful. A hospital setting can begin an institutionalising process, and the resulting detachment and despair which Bowlby (1997) describes can be difficult to reverse in the event of a prolonged stay.

To support a child or young person and their family, occupational therapists must remember that:

- Children need reassurance and a sense that they are safe at all times if they are to develop confidence.
- At times children and young people with cancer feel particularly vulnerable and wish to withdraw; at other times, conversely, they feel angry and frustrated. All of these are normal reactions to cancer and its treatment.
- It is important to gain a sense of the child's behaviour and personality before the cancer was diagnosed in order to develop an understanding of their coping strategies.
- It is important to discover what the child enjoys doing and what is important and meaningful to him/her.
- It is important to ask parents about their child too. This contributes to them sharing their experience and concerns and it acknowledges their role as a parent in an active way.
- Supportive discussions with the child, and also separately with the parent(s), provide the occupational therapist with information on the usual behaviour and normal life of the child.
- It is important to ask parents how the child or young person reacts to stressful situations and if there are any examples in the past which they can share, such as being separated or the experience of stress at exams, which may indicate coping behaviours.
- The cultural diversity and differences of families need to be acknowledged and respected, which includes religious practices. Assumptions can easily be made on what is acceptable for a family and child, and without sensitive discussion upset may be caused inadvertently.

This information can act as a baseline for a holistic view of the child as a member of a family.

These considerations serve to highlight the importance of the family and the need to understand different families' different, but nonetheless normal, ways of coping with stress and of supporting the child or young person.

Note that any information received by the occupational therapist should be shared with other health colleagues only with the permission of the parent of the child or young person who is providing this information.

6 Occupational therapy assessment

Occupational therapy assessment may take place at any time during the cancer journey and can take place in a variety of clinical or community settings. All occupational therapy practice should be in accordance with current guidance and standards set out by the professional body. In all cases, the occupational therapy process of information gathering, initial interview, assessment, intervention and evaluation should be followed (Creek 2003). However, the way in which the process is implemented will vary according to the setting, and of course the needs of the child and family, at any given time (Cooper 2006a).

It should be noted that to date there is no published evidence supporting this approach to assessment recommended by the guidance development group. Rather, it is based on the experience and expert opinion of group members and others who have written of their experience in this field.

First, it is important to remember that each child is an individual and will be experiencing a number of changes in their daily life. How children respond and react to these changes should be taken into account during any assessment. Children with cancer have varying degrees of understanding about their illness, depending on their age and on what they have been told. It is important to establish through parents or other members of the multiprofessional team what degree of understanding children and young people have of their illness. Their experiences, particularly those at the time of diagnosis and during initial treatment often affect their emotional wellbeing and some children may appear vulnerable and immature for their age. Conversely other children may appear mature with a great deal of knowledge about their disease. This knowledge may not, however, always be fully understood by the child.

Initial assessment

The majority of children and young people are fit and well prior to a diagnosis of cancer. A sensitive approach to initial assessment is therefore required. Asking detailed questions about previous levels of functional ability can be frustrating, upsetting and often inappropriate for parents and young people. Rather, it is more appropriate briefly to confirm that there were no functional difficulties prior to diagnosis. Alternatively, this can often be confirmed by speaking with another member of the medical staff who has already taken a full history, or by contacting the referring therapist. When treating a child or young person with a diagnosis of cancer, building a therapeutic relationship and establishing trust between therapist, child and parent is paramount before any formal assessment is undertaken. In an acute setting there may be pressure to conduct formal assessments and to begin intervention within a short space of time. However, taking the time to establish a trusting relationship and adopting an informal approach in getting to know the child and family lends itself well to the future care and treatment of that child (Wavrek 2001). Parents may need emotional support before taking part in any initial interview, and it should be remembered that questions about the home environment and functional ability may either seem far removed from their current circumstances, or irrelevant at a time when they are coming to terms with a cancer diagnosis and the uncertainty that surrounds it. The needs of the children and their families will often change over the course of the occupational therapy process and will therefore require regular review and attention in maintaining an effective therapeutic relationship (Dudgeon 2001).

Functional assessment

This guidance will look at areas of daily life affected by cancer and/or its treatment. In every instance occupational therapy assessment should be guided by the child, young person and their family, with the focus of intervention on addressing those areas of greatest significance to the child, young person and/or their parents.

As in all areas of occupational therapy, when addressing aspects of self-care, life skills, productivity, play and leisure, functional ability will be assessed taking into account:

- Physical skills.
- Sensorimotor skills.
- Cognitive skills.
- Psycho-social skills.

Difficulties in any one of these areas can impact upon a child or young person's functional ability and should be assessed in conjunction with environmental factors to ensure safety, optimise function and maintain quality of life.

Ability to participate in any activity of daily living may also be influenced by:

- The age and developmental stage of the child or young person.
- Their motivation to participate.
- The involvement of parents and members of the wider family.
- Cultural and social expectations.
- Sick role identification.
- Diagnosis, medical status and treatment regime.

Diagnosis

A child's diagnosis may provide indicators of potential difficulties that may affect function. Potential difficulties associated with specific tumour types, and/or their treatment, are listed below. It must be noted, however, that while diagnosis may offer an indication of potential functional difficulty, each child will present differently. A holistic approach to assessment and intervention, one that focuses on need rather than diagnosis or prognosis, is therefore required in each instance.

Central nervous system tumours:

- Cognitive difficulties
- Perceptual difficulties
- Personality/behavioural changes
- Sensory changes
- Visual disturbances
- Hearing loss
- Altered body image
- Upper limb weakness
- Spinal cord compression
- Hemiparesis
- Hemiplegia
- Dyspraxia
- Ataxia
- Communication difficulties
- Posterior Fossa syndrome
- Somnolence
- Fatigue

(Carr et al 2008)

Bone tumours

- Reduced upper limb function
- Reduced range of movement
- Restricted mobility
- Pain
- Breathlessness (as a result of lung metastases)
- Amputation
- Limb salvaging surgery
- Altered body image
- Fatigue

Complications of bone tumours may also include avascular necrosis and osteomyelitis.

(Richards et al 2008)

Appendix 6 details surgical interventions used for bone tumours and the post-surgical precautions that occupational therapists may need to consider in their intervention.

Leukaemia

- Chemotherapy-induced peripheral neuropathy
- Fatigue (particularly following bone-marrow transplant)
- Developmental delay

Lymphomas

- Breathlessness (as a result of mediastinal masses)
- Fatigue

Models of occupational therapy practice

Treatment approaches and models of practice that guide occupational therapy intervention will be discussed in context throughout the document with regard to specific areas of intervention. As with all aspects of occupational therapy intervention in paediatric oncology, the treatment approaches and models of practice employed should continually be evaluated as the needs of children and young people with cancer fluctuate over time.

7 Standardised assessments

Standardised assessments are routinely used within paediatric occupational therapy as a way of supplementing informal methods of information gathering and assessment. They can be an effective way of evaluating outcome measures and can be useful in directing intervention. Traditionally, standardised assessments have measured a child or young person's ability in comparison to other children to identify impairment in function. However, as the World Health Organisation's International Classification of Functioning, Disability, and Health (WHO 2001) shifts the focus towards participation for people with disability, occupational therapists will increasingly use tools available to them to assess the wider issues that influence participation, such as motivation, roles/habits and the environment. These tools will offer the opportunity of capturing a child or young person's strengths and values as well as areas of difficulty (Kramer et al 2009).

It is important that care is taken when implementing standardised assessments, as the reliability of the information gathered and the interpretation of results will directly relate to the competence of the assessor (Richardson 2001). When using standardised assessments occupational therapists need to be confident of selecting the right standardised assessment tools and that they know when and when not to administer a test. It is also important to ensure that the child or young person has the prerequisite skills to complete the standardised assessment. This will require the therapist to have knowledge of other factors such as sight, hearing, language, cognitive and physical abilities. Specific factors relevant to children or young people with cancer should also be considered and are discussed here further.

Timing of assessment

As highlighted within this guidance, the abilities and therapeutic needs of children and young people with cancer are likely to shift during and according to the course of the disease and its treatment. As symptoms or functional difficulties are often transient in their nature, care should be taken over administering standardised assessments during times of active treatment. Assessments under these circumstances may lead to erroneous and misleading results; therefore it may be appropriate to refrain from administering standardised assessments until the child or young person's condition has stabilised. Some specialist cancer centres carry out developmental screening assessments prior to bone-marrow transplant in order to identify those children at greatest risk of developmental delay as a result of their treatment. It should be noted, however, that there is currently no evidence to support this approach and therapists should consider exploring its effectiveness in future research.

Children and young people with central nervous tumours are a particularly vulnerable group, often experiencing complex long-term physical, cognitive, social and emotional difficulties as a result of their treatment. Some symptoms, however, are not always immediately obvious and for this reason these children and young people should be closely monitored. Those with residual neurological deficits following treatment should be referred to community occupational therapists for follow-up and ongoing assessment. In these instances, standardised assessments can help therapists set specific goals and target treatment. The results will also provide useful information that can define the difficulties experienced by children and young people and may be beneficial for colleagues and teachers to facilitate a return to school and ensure that appropriate help or assistance is provided.

Considerations

There must be a clear goal or objective whenever performing standardised assessments and, before administering such tests, it is important to consider the benefits versus the adverse implications for children and young people with cancer (Tester 2006). For example, consideration should be given to the psychological effects of using standardised assessments with children and young people who have insight into their performance if this is poor in comparison to peers of a similar age, or when compared to their previous level of ability. Some parents may have difficulty understanding the purpose of particularly lengthy tests when their child is facing a potentially life-limiting illness. The prognosis and likely long-term outcome may therefore affect the decision to carry out a standardised test. Conversely, where assessments are positively valued by a family and child, results may be used to develop goals and a therapeutic plan, and active co-operation may be facilitated (Diamantis 2008).

Checklist for standardised assessments

- Is there a clear objective to administering a standardised test?
- Will the test provide information that could not otherwise be gained, i.e. through observation or functional assessment?
- How will the results be used to the benefit of the child/young person?
- Have the psychological implications been considered?
- Does the child/young person have the prerequisite skills to complete a test?
- Have influencing factors such as fatigue and pain been considered?
- Is treatment still in the acute phase, where ability is likely to change rapidly?
- Do the parents and young person understand why the test is being used?

(Richardson 2001)

Assessment choice

Choosing an appropriate assessment will depend upon the age and specific needs of the child or young person, the resources available, and the occupational therapist's clinical experience and reasoning. The occupational therapist must be familiar with the administering and scoring of the assessments chosen, be able to clinically justify their use, and to explain the evidence that supports the use and reliability of the assessments. Standardised assessments used by occupational therapists in paediatric oncology can be found in Appendix 7. Please note that this list is not exhaustive; nor does it promote the use of one assessment over another.

Assessment choice checklist

- How old is the child or young person?
- Have you considered the length of the test versus factors affecting the child's ability to attend to the task (e.g. fatigue, concentration and/or pain)?
- What component areas require assessment?
- Does the child possess the prerequisite skills (e.g. language or cognition) to complete the test?
- Does the assessor possess the knowledge and has he/she received the appropriate training in administering the chosen test?
- Is the assessor competent in interpreting and utilising the test results?

(Richardson 2001)

Interpretation of results

The results of standardised assessments enable the therapist to build upon the clinical picture. Informal observations of the child's behaviour, concentration and general demeanour during testing also provide valuable information and should be taken into consideration when reviewing results. Following standardised assessments, occupational therapists must be confident that they are able to interpret test results accurately in order to advise on remedies for any difficulties identified, to set treatment goals and/or to signpost families to other agencies for further help.

8 Occupational therapy intervention

The aim of intervention in cancer care should be no different from the aim in other conditions such as cerebral palsy or traumatic brain injury: to achieve the highest possible functional level within the limits of disease, treatment and the environment (De Lisa 2001). However, specific factors make intervention in cancer care unique and sometimes challenging.

Cancer and the course of its treatment are often unpredictable. Children and young people may experience side effects such as episodes of fatigue and reduced physical or cognitive ability, which in turn may affect functional independence (Tester 2006). Unlike, for example, traumatic brain injury – a single event, following which rehabilitation continually seeks to improve function – intervention in cancer often fluctuates according to treatment protocols and disease trajectory. Occupational therapy intervention must therefore be flexible, taking into account children and young people's fluctuating needs. In particular, where a need is indicated the rehabilitation of children and young people with cancer should begin at diagnosis, or as soon as needs become apparent, and should take into account all potential implications for the future, no matter what the diagnosis or prognosis is (Bradwell and Hawkings 2000).

8.1 Self-care

Self-care is part of daily life and normal routine for all children and young people and should be viewed in accordance with a child's developmental age. It incorporates many aspects of daily living, from grooming tasks such as brushing hair or applying make-up, to showering, bathing, eating and drinking.

Shepherd (2001) identifies four treatment approaches that are used by occupational therapists to facilitate improvement in children and young people's self-care skills, namely: *developmental*, *remedial*, *compensatory*, and *educational* approaches. These approaches are outlined further below. They may be used individually or can be combined when treating children or young people with cancer, depending upon their needs and age.

Developmental approach

Self-care tasks encompass many essential skills that children learn as part of normal development (Shepherd 2001). Due to episodes of illness and prolonged hospital admissions, children diagnosed with cancer before mastering these skills are at risk of falling behind their peers in terms of their overall development and independence in self-care. Children who have recently developed skills in this area are at risk of regressing and losing skills they have learned, as parents adopt a carer's role in helping their child during episodes of illness. Educating parents in the developmental needs of children is therefore an important aspect of any intervention. Occupational therapists may encourage and facilitate the development of skills in areas such as cutlery use, and dressing and undressing.

Mouth care

Good mouth care for children and young people with cancer is essential because of the mouth ulcers caused by chemotherapy, known as mucositis, and the increased risk of infection. From experience, the group has found that parents often wish to attend to their child's mouth care themselves, rather than encouraging independent teeth brushing. This should be discussed with each family.

Remedial approach

Self-care tasks are a significant area of occupational performance. They utilise physical skills, such as gross and fine motor skills, and address generalised weakness and co-ordination, as well as involving cognitive, perceptual and sensory aspects of function. Through the use of self-care activities, areas of deficit can be assessed and a remedial approach to intervention employed.

Compensatory approach

Equipment may be provided to compensate for functional loss due to physical deficits, but may also be provided in the treatment of cancer-related symptoms such as breathlessness or pain. Equipment may be required for long- or short-term use, but in any case should be provided in a timely and sensitive manner to facilitate independence, maintain quality of life and ensure safety.

In other incidences an adaptive approach to intervention may be used, such as teaching of alternative ways of getting dressed to compensate for decreased range of movement, hemiparesis or pain.

Educational approach

For older children, an educational approach to self-care may be taken in teaching self-management strategies. For example, to address cancer-related fatigue, older children and young people may be taught to conserve energy by sitting down while dressing, bathing at a time of day when energy levels are higher, and by advising good sleep hygiene.

Family life and routine

Some aspects of self-care take place in a social context and are part of everyday family life. Children and young people are often used to eating with others, for example with siblings or as a whole family, and bathing for young children is an activity often shared with siblings. Encouraging self-care in the family context helps reinstate routine and structure to daily life which may have been lost or disrupted during hospital admission. As with all aspects of daily living, self-care routines differ from family to family and may be culturally sensitive. They should therefore be respected at all times.

Body image

Body image is important to both boys and girls of all ages. Changes in appearance are commonly seen in children and young people with cancer as a result of their tumour or anti-cancer treatments and can give rise to negative feelings about the body and, as a consequence, low self-esteem. Occupational therapists must be sensitive to these changes of appearance and may address body image during self-care activities.

Line care

Within self-care, attention should be paid to central lines (sometimes known as Hickman lines or 'wigglies'). Most lines will have a waterproof cover to accommodate showering and bathing. If bathing, shallow baths are recommended since lines should not be submerged because of the risk of infection from the bath water. However, each treatment centre may have different policies for the care of lines, so it is advisable to seek information from a child's principal treatment centre with regard to showering or bathing with lines. This may impact upon equipment provision.

8.2 Play and leisure

Play and leisure are important aspects of the lives of children and adolescents alike. For younger children play is their primary occupation and is an integral part of development, providing opportunities to explore, create and develop physical, cognitive and social skills (Tester 2008). Anti-cancer treatments and their side effects often hinder development in these areas, as opportunities for play, social interaction and leisure activities are restricted. For some children and young people, tumours that cause physical or cognitive deficits can also restrict participation in play or leisure activities.

Occupational therapists who work with children have knowledge of developmental play and understand that a child's age, culture, environment, family and motivation, as well as medical, physical, cognitive, social and sensory factors, all influence participation in play. Occupational therapists may seek to improve or adapt any area that limits access to or hinders participation in play, for example provision of a static seating system that facilitates optimum positioning for play. Alternatively, play may be used as a therapeutic tool in intervention when addressing specific skills such as problem-solving, sitting balance, or fine motor movement. Care should be taken, in every case, to create environments where the child will feel safe to engage and explore. This includes establishing trust between child and therapist.

For teenagers and young people, developing independence in leisure activities, such as shopping, going to the cinema and spending time with friends, are part of adolescent development and provide the context in which social and self-management skills are learned. Adapting and modifying these activities will be discussed in greater focus in Section 11 of the guidance, along with alternative ways of 'keeping up with' friends, for example via email, webcam, and social networking sites.

As previously stated, children and young people with cancer are usually fit and well prior to diagnosis. By facilitating and enabling play and leisure, occupational therapists can assist with maintaining or re-establishing normal routines and relationships within a family. This may be particularly important during and following long hospital admissions when family life is often disrupted and siblings may become isolated.

8.3 Life skills and productivity

Life skills and productivity for children and young people encompass education, work (paid or voluntary), and household chores such as laying the table, preparing snacks, doing the laundry and going to the shops. As with self-care, cancer and/or its treatment often impacts upon a child's ability to participate in or learn life skills. Occupational therapists may work to facilitate children and young people in mastering such skills and to enable them to engage in such activities to their full potential.

Life skills

The development of life and household skills is often overshadowed by the medical, physical and educational needs of children with cancer (Shepherd 2001). However, mastering household skills such as cooking, cleaning and laundry is integral to normal child development and crucial in achieving successful maturation. At an early age, children imitate housework, copying parents while they carry out domestic tasks. Throughout childhood, children develop independence through engaging in household activities such as putting away toys, making their beds and answering the telephone. During adolescence young people continue to develop independence through engaging in more complex tasks such laundry, cooking and shopping. Not only is each stage and each skill important in itself, but each life skill also facilitates the ongoing development of motor, cognitive, psycho-social and self-management skills. Furthermore, participation in household chores is part of normal family life and everyday routine. As with education, a diagnosis of cancer should not prevent or restrict a child or young person from taking part and developing such skills.

Discussions with parents may include highlighting the importance of maintaining roles within family life and re-establishing routine. For example, helping siblings to lay the table or taking turns to dry the dishes may represent 'normal' family life for some children with cancer. In other instances, life skills such as cooking may be used as part of intervention, to aid sensory integration, improve upper-limb strength and regain stamina and exercise tolerance. Activities such as shopping and managing money may also be used in the functional assessment and treatment of cognitive and executive functioning difficulties. It should be noted, however, that the level to which children and young people engage in household chores and develop life skills will depend upon their age, culture, environment, family make-up, and in some instances gender. Therefore, taking time to understand and get to know the family is imperative in providing quality care and effective intervention (Trapp 1998).

Productivity

School and college

Schooling is a legal requirement for all children and those with medical needs should have access to as much education as their medical condition will allow (Department for Education and Skills (DfES) 2001). Education not only involves learning but also supports the development of social skills, such as boundaries and self-awareness, as well as preparing young people to make choices about their future. Children and young people with cancer are no different, and opportunities for these experiences should not be limited because of their diagnosis or treatment. This is also true for children whose prognosis is poor and life expectancy limited (DfES 2001, Petersen-Broyd et al 2006).

Return to school

Dixon-Woods et al (2005) explain how adults and children differ when returning to the social and productive world following cancer. The option available to many adults with cancer is to return to familiar territories of work and stable friendships. Conversely, for children and young people peers may have moved ahead into different year groups as well as friendship circles in childhood frequently changing.

For children and young people with cancer, participation in school or college will be influenced by their motor performance, perceptual processing, and psycho-social and cognitive abilities (Case-Smith et al 2001). Each should be taken into account, along with environmental and medical factors, when assessing children and young people in school. Where appropriate, the views of the child or young person should be actively sought. As highlighted by Egilson and Hemmingsson (2009), involving young people in decisions concerning their schooling and those which influence their everyday lives offers them the opportunity to express choice and thus reduces feelings of dependency.

Re-entry to school is a challenge for some children and young people with cancer, however, and occupational therapists can play an important role in supporting this process.

Barriers to Return to School

- Fatigue
- Pain
- Reduced attention
- Cognitive difficulties
- Perceptual difficulties
- Language difficulties
- Visual or hearing disturbances
- Bullying
- Co-ordination difficulties
- School environment
- Difficulty with handwriting skills
- Anxiety
- Altered body image
- Reduced self-esteem

Assessment and liaison

As the ability of children and young people with cancer fluctuates according to and throughout treatment, in-depth assessment during active treatment may not be appropriate. Rather, ensuring access to school environments and access to learning must take priority. Environmental assessment visits conducted by occupational therapists will facilitate a safe return to school and enable participation in the classroom. Visits may include assessment of access, bathroom facilities and classroom layout, as well as advising teachers of a child's particular needs. In some instances occupational therapists may advocate on behalf of children and young people, liaising with the Special Educational Needs Co-Ordinator (SENCO) to ensure that necessary changes are made to the school or college environment to enable a return to school or continuation of learning (Egilson and Hemmingsson 2009). Effective communication between the occupational therapist, the family, healthcare professionals and school is paramount to ensure that children and young people's needs are addressed in a timely and appropriate manner. Effective collaboration between all parties will enable continuity of education and make sure that pupils are successfully re-integrated into school (DfES 2001, Prevatt et al 2000).

Time of school return

Return to school should take place as soon as it is safe to do so following diagnosis (Petersen-Broyd et al 2008). Indeed returning to school or college as soon as possible following diagnosis has been shown to enhance the school performance of children and young people with cancer as well as fostering a sense of hope and positive self-concept that in turn relates to overall school achievement and psycho-social development (Moore et al 2009, Vance and Eiser 2002). For this reason continued attendance at school or college should be encouraged during treatment wherever possible. This may not be possible on a full-time basis. However, even when part-time attendance, for example mornings only, is not possible, visiting the school and friends during a break time will help ensure the success of later re-integration to school. Following treatment, a gradual, graded return to school may be recommended to re-establish tolerance and stamina.

If the occupational therapist or parents are unsure whether the child or young person is medically well enough to attend school, advice should be sought from medical staff at the child's treating hospital. When children are unable to attend school, home tuition can be arranged. During hospital stays attendance at the hospital school, as provision allows, is encouraged if children and young people are well enough to do so. Many hospital teachers will be experienced in facilitating the return to school and may liaise directly with school teachers or home tutors. In some areas, outreach nurses will also visit a child's school to give medical advice and offer support (Moore et al 2009, Petersen-Broyd et al 2008). In these instances, communication between the occupational therapist, hospital teacher and outreach nurse is important to ensure that no conflicting advice is given nor work duplicated.

Following treatment

Following treatment, when symptoms and functional levels have stabilised, a thorough review of a child's ability in all performance areas will ensure all aspects are considered and therefore that all needs may be met. The use of standardised assessments has been discussed. However assessments such as the Developmental Test of Visual Perception (DVPT) and the Test of Everyday Attention for Children (TEA-Ch) may be used to good effect by community occupational therapists in assessing the long-term needs of survivors of childhood cancer.

Cancer's impact upon higher education and employment for young people will be discussed later in the guidance in Section 11.

Case study:[1] acute occupational therapy intervention

Charlie is a 3½-year-old boy who was admitted for emergency debulking of a posterior fossa tumour following a two-week history of headaches, vomiting and increasing difficulties in co-ordination. Histology later confirmed the tumour to be a medulloblastoma. Charlie was seen by the occupational therapist (OT) at the regional neurosurgical centre two days after his surgery. He was displaying signs of posterior fossa syndrome; he was frightened, irritable, and difficult to comfort. His parents were worried that he had not spoken since the operation.

During his inpatient stay, which lasted just under two weeks, Charlie remained irritable and disliked being touched. The OT explained the role of occupational therapy to Charlie's parents and listened to their concerns. His mother was worried about hurting Charlie when she moved him and she was upset that she was unable to comfort him. The OT reassured both parents and discussed strategies as to how they could support Charlie, for example by creating a safe environment, with no sudden noises or bright lights, and by providing positive feedback. The OT introduced a recliner buggy to the room so that Charlie could get used to it before being seated out. Strategies such as putting toys in the seat were tried before Charlie was sat into it. When Charlie did sit out for the first time, he did so with just his parents and the OT in the room, with the OT supporting his parents to help him into the new buggy. Charlie was seen by the OT twice a day, for just a few moments, until he got used to the OT, so that trust could be built up between Charlie, his parents and the OT. As the time of discharge got closer, Charlie remained irritable and disliked being touched. He had not regained any speech, had poor sitting balance and global ataxia. The OT had been unable to conduct any direct intervention with Charlie, but had made positive steps towards encouraging and facilitating his parents in all other aspects of his care. His mother was now confident in handling him and both parents were able to attend to his needs and soothe him when he became distressed. A referral was made to the local authority OTs for provision of a bath seat, and to the local wheelchair service for provision of a suitable buggy. A referral was also made to the local community OTs and a report sent to the OT at the regional cancer centre. The referral and report documented Charlie's current needs, indicating that his needs were likely to improve once he began anti-cancer treatments and had spent time at home – as had been found through experience.

Charlie was admitted to his regional children's cancer centre two weeks after his discharge from the neuro-surgical centre. Before carrying out any formal assessments or intervention, a relationship was built with his parents, discussing how they had managed at home following surgery, any progress Charlie had made and what was most important to them as a family. At this time, their main priority was beginning anti-cancer treatment and their concerns surrounded the potential side effects of chemotherapy. However, once chemotherapy began, and following discussions with the OT, the physiotherapist and the speech and language therapist, their attention turned to rehabilitation. All intervention was based within play and was provided in a safe environment. Intervention sought to improve sitting balance and co-ordination, and informally assess cognition.

During his in-patient treatment, Charlie was actively seen by the hospital OT. On his first discharge home he did not see the community OT as his parents felt that time spent as a family and a short spell at home with no hospital appointments was vital for them. On subsequent discharges, Charlie was seen by his community OT and following close communication with the hospital OT a programme of intervention was agreed.

[1] Please note that in the interests of confidentiality, names and any other identifying features have been removed or replaced in all case studies.

9 Occupational therapy intervention in symptom management

Occupational therapy intervention is often led by symptoms and their impact on functional performance rather than the disease or diagnosis itself (Cooper 2006a). Evidence tells us that children and young people experience a wide variety of symptoms, from nausea and constipation to pain and anxiety. These symptoms are often complex, occur both during and following anti-cancer treatments, and vary in intensity (Ruland et al 2009). Effective management of cancer-related symptoms can significantly improve quality of life and as such is seen as integral to cancer care throughout disease trajectory (Berde et al 2005, Lacasse and Beck 2007).

Until recently, researchers have focused upon single symptoms; however, in reality symptoms rarely occur in isolation (Hockenberry and Hooke 2007, Kirkova and Walsh 2007). Most recent studies have therefore focused upon and demonstrated the notion of symptom clusters. Ruland et al (2009) implore healthcare professionals to fully understand the complexity of cancer-related symptoms before a truly tailored approach to individual management can be offered. For that reason, symptoms and their management will be discussed here separately, but with the intention of demonstrating how each one is multifaceted and how they are inextricably interlinked. As a result, a holistic approach to occupational therapy assessment and intervention, which considers all symptoms, is necessary in the management of cancer-related symptoms.

9.1 Management of cancer-related fatigue

> *Cancer-related fatigue is a distressing persistent subjective sense of physical, emotional and/or cognitive tiredness or exhaustion related to cancer or cancer treatment that is not proportional to recent activity and interferes with usual functioning.*
>
> (The National Comprehensive Cancer Network (NCCN) 2009, p. 6)

Cancer-related fatigue is widely recognised in the adult population as one of the most reported and pervasive symptoms experienced by patients during and following anti-cancer therapies. Recent studies have shown that children and young people also experience cancer-related fatigue, which impacts significantly on their everyday lives and meaningful activity (Erickson 2004, Mooney-Doyle 2006). Indeed, young people have identified fatigue to be the most distressing or troubling treatment-related symptom that they experience, indicating that it is the reason that they are unable to return to normal activities (Hinds et al 2000). In a study by Hockenberry et al (2003), children described fatigue as 'a sense of physical tiredness', including having difficulty with moving their legs, using their arms, and/or opening their eyes. Young people, however, describe a more multidimensional sensation of fatigue, one that encompasses not only physical feelings, but also cognitive and emotional tiredness.

Cancer-related fatigue can be the result of a number of factors, including anti-cancer treatments such as chemotherapy, radiotherapy or surgery, prolonged periods of time in hospital, reduced nutritional intake, the emotional impact of a cancer diagnosis, or indeed may be caused by the cancer itself (NCCN 2009). Often there is no one single contributory factor, but rather a number of factors that collectively contribute to an overall picture of fatigue. For this reason, assessment and treatment of cancer-related fatigue should reflect this and be addressed on multiple levels (Mooney-Doyle 2006).

A holistic approach to intervention is imperative to consider the physical, cognitive, social and emotional aspects of fatigue; a notion that sits well within the framework of occupational therapy (Lowrie 2006) and is conceptualised by the framework proposed by Purcell et al (2009). Children and young people's experiences of fatigue will be unique in every case. Occupational therapy intervention must therefore adopt a tailored approach to address the multifaceted nature of fatigue at any given time (Ogilvy et al 2008).

The NCCN guidelines (2009) recommend that fatigue management be provided by a multiprofessional team. As Ogilvy et al (2008) describe, areas of cancer-related fatigue treatment overlap and although each discipline has a set of core competencies, professional boundaries may become blurred. As a result, effective communication, collaboration and understanding between clinicians is paramount.

A number of non-pharmacological strategies based upon current research, which are routinely employed by occupational therapists in the treatment of cancer-related fatigue, are shown in the box below.

Cancer-related fatigue management strategies

- Education
- Graded activity
- Energy conservation strategies
- Routine and set rest times
- Relaxation training
- Sleep hygiene promotion
- Exercise

(Barsevick 2002, Davidson et al 2002, Erickson 2004, Jakel 2002, Lowrie 2006, Ogilvy et al 2008, Ream et al 2003)

Education

A young person's need for information about their treatment and its side effects should not be underestimated (Hollis and Morgan 2001). Studies have shown that, through information-giving and effective education, young people are better equipped to manage treatment-related symptoms (Hedstrom et al 2004). Indeed, timely information given before the likely onset of fatigue, providing management strategies such as those highlighted here, have been shown to reduce negative experiences of fatigue (Ream et al 2003). However, as Lowrie (2006) discusses, occupational therapists should take care to provide information in a sensitive and measured manner in order not to place young people under undue stress or worry.

Energy conservation and graded activity

Practical energy conservation strategies taught by occupational therapists can be employed by young people in everyday life and have been shown to reduce the effects of fatigue (Barsevick et al 2004). Strategies may include sitting down while dressing, restricting climbing the stairs to once a day at bedtime, and attending school for mornings only. A compensatory approach to energy conservation may be adopted at any stage of disease or treatment, but will be particularly valuable towards the end of life. Examples of this approach include the provision of bathing equipment and/or a wheelchair. It should be noted that wheelchairs or buggies are often required even if children and young people are able to mobilise independently. This is to facilitate engagement in activities such as shopping or going to school, which would otherwise be restricted by fatigue. Where the need for equipment is indicated, its provision should be made in a timely manner, particularly where prognosis is time-limited (NICE 2005).

Pacing, planning and prioritising, as identified by Barsevick (2002), also play an important role in managing and reducing cancer-related fatigue. For example, spreading activities out over a week, rather than concentrating them into one or two consecutive days, or planning to see friends at a place that requires minimum amount of energy to get to will reduce fatigue. Keeping up with friends and peers is an integral part of adolescence and prioritising activities can be difficult for young people. However, by removing or limiting activities a young person deems less essential, energy can be conserved for those activities he or she finds most meaningful. Skilled and trained in the therapeutic use of meaningful activities, occupational therapists are well suited to facilitating young people in planning and prioritising in their daily lives.

For younger children, a creative approach to explaining energy conservation may be required. For example, analogies such as an energy tank, engine or battery can be useful. The tank is usually full, but when you are unwell some energy is lost. When there is less energy in the tank, the energy left has to be divided up or saved for the important things. This can sometimes be depicted in drawings or through the use of building blocks.

Relaxation in the management of fatigue

The NCCN cancer-related fatigue guidelines (2009) recommend the use of relaxation strategies such as guided imagery and progressive muscular relaxation in the non-pharmacological treatment of fatigue. Studies continue to highlight the effectiveness of relaxation in cancer care (Miller and Hopkinson 2008), with a randomised control trial by Dimeo et al (2004) concluding a programme of relaxation to be effective in reducing the symptoms of cancer-related fatigue. No research is available that promotes one relaxation strategy over another in the management of fatigue; however, the potential implications of particular strategies (such as using progressive muscular relaxation techniques, which may exacerbate pain), and factors such as the age of the child should be considered. For younger children guided imagery is recommended and can be used successfully in the form of story-telling (Boog 2008).

It should be noted that the use of relaxation techniques is not a skill specific to occupational therapy and that other professionals working with young people with cancer may use relaxation as part of their work.

Sleep hygiene promotion in the management of fatigue

Sleep disturbance is a commonly reported occurrence for young people with cancer (Davidson et al 2002, Gerald and Rosen 2007). Lowrie (2006) describes how disruption of sleep at night-time can lead to increased feelings of fatigue during the day and in turn behaviours that perpetuate insomnia, such as daytime napping. Educating parents on the importance of routine, particularly with regard to bedtimes and rest periods during the day, may also help to reduce symptoms of fatigue for younger children.

Sleep hygiene

Good sleep hygiene helps alleviate symptoms of fatigue. This may involve:

- Going to bed and rising at the same time each day.
- Avoiding daytime naps where possible.
- Ensuring that bedroom environments are conducive to sleep; not too hot or cold, with levels of light and noise reduced as far as possible.
- Not eating prior to bedtime and avoiding caffeine in the hours before sleep.

(Lowrie 2006)

Exercise in the management of fatigue

Research continues to demonstrate that graded exercise is effective in managing cancer-related fatigue (Lowrie 2006, Mock 2004). Occupational therapists are able to recommend a graded and gradual increase in a child or young person's activity levels, which is particularly appropriate following treatment or hospital admission. During what can often be lengthy hospital admissions, advice can be given by occupational therapists on how to maintain levels of activity. Going to the playroom, walking to the canteen, spending time in the adolescent room, and attending the hospital school should be encouraged when a child or young person is medically able to do so.

9.2 Pain management

Pain is not simply a physical experience. It is the sum of the physical experience and the patient's interpretation of that experience, taking into account personality, mood, understanding, past experiences and social relations.

(Sugden 2001, p. 2)

It is estimated that more than half of children with cancer experience moderate to severe cancer-related pain (Hockenberry and Hooke 2007). Pain in childhood cancer can be acute, either because of the site of the tumour(s) or as a result of treatment; or chronic, as a result of the lasting effects of cancer treatment.

Cancer pain is a complex phenomenon affected by physical and psychological factors. The first to use the term 'total pain', Dame Cicely Saunders' (1967) description of cancer-related pain takes into account the emotional, cognitive, behavioural, social and spiritual aspects of a person. Robb and Ewer-Smith (2008) went on to describe how pain impacts upon concentration, appetite and sleep, and may cause irritability, low mood, low self-esteem, lack of interest and reduced ability to problem-solve or make decisions. Comprehensive, multidimensional programmes are therefore required in addressing the complexities of cancer-related pain (Dixon-Woods et al 2005).

There is a growing role for occupational therapists in the management of pain in children's cancer care because, like fatigue, pain impacts upon the ability to participate in meaningful activities of daily living. The role of the occupational therapist is to enable a child or young person to adapt tasks or adopt strategies to overcome difficulties caused by pain. This should lead to an increase in quality of life and fuller engagement in the activities of daily living.

Relaxation in pain management

Strategies such as guided visualisation relaxation training have been shown to be effective in managing cancer-related pain (Syrjala et al 1995, Thomas and Weiss 2000), as well as reducing other symptoms such as nausea (Luebbert et al 2001, Walker et al 1999). Recent research demonstrates how education and teaching relaxation techniques prior to surgical intervention and bone-marrow transplants reduces both anxiety and pain levels for young people. This evidence supports the view that it ought to be standard practice to teach young people relaxation techniques prior to such medical interventions (Luebbert et al 2001, Sahler et al 2003).

Graded activity

Grading activities that exacerbate pain, or those which pain restricts, enables young people to continue to engage in meaningful activities (Robb and Ewer-Smith 2008). A compensatory approach in equipment provision may be indicated, and/or a behavioural approach involving energy conservation and lifestyle management such as those discussed in the management of cancer-related fatigue.

9.3 Management of breathlessness

Breathlessness is 'a term used to characterise a subjective experience of breathing discomfort that consists of qualitatively distinct sensations that vary in intensity. The experience derives from interactions among multiple physiological, psychological, social and environmental factors, and may induce secondary physiological and behavioural responses.'

(American Thoracic Society 1999, p. 321)

Breathlessness, also known as dyspnoea, can occur at any stage during cancer treatment. Often associated with lung cancer in adult patients, the physiological causes of breathlessness in children are more commonly related to mediastinal masses, lung metastases, graft-versus-host disease (GvHD) of the lung, cardiac complications, or brain stem involvement. However, breathlessness is often multidimensional, arising from a combination of physiological, psychological, social and environmental factors (Fisher and Lowrie 2008). As a result, and in keeping with the management of other cancer-related symptoms, the treatment and management of breathlessness must be holistic, addressing the emotional, physiological and environmental aspects of the symptom.

The physiological and psychological responses to episodes of breathlessness will vary from person to person; therefore strategies for managing breathlessness must be tailored to each young person. The goal of occupational therapy intervention, to minimise the impact of breathlessness on the young person's ability to engage in meaningful activities, can be achieved via a number of non-pharmacological strategies.

Behavioural approaches

Breathlessness is a highly subjective symptom, the experience of which varies according to the individual. The link between intensity of symptoms and anxiety is widely reported in the literature (Fisher and Lowrie 2008, Payne 2000) Exploring and addressing factors such as fear and anxiety which are so often associated with breathlessness is vital. Anxiety or fear can exacerbate feelings of breathlessness, which consequently result in further exacerbation of anxiety and feelings of being unable to cope with the symptom (Cooper 2006b). An educational approach providing strategies, such as breathing techniques and relaxation, which enable young people to take control of feelings and symptoms, is recommended.

Positioning

When breathlessness occurs, an individual may automatically adopt a position or posture that relives the sensation of breathlessness. Occupational therapists can help children and parents to identify these positions, or suggest and trial other positions known to alleviate breathlessness.

Positioning relating to breathlessness

- High side lying supported by pillows.
- Leaning with the back against a wall, legs slightly apart and arms hanging by the sides.
- Leaning forward in a standing position, with arms resting on a surface such as a windowsill, worktop, or table that best suits the height of the young person.
- Leaning forward in a sitting position, with arms resting on a surface such as a table top.

(Cooper 2006b, Fisher and Lowrie 2008)

Provision of equipment, such as a pillow lift or wedge, can be beneficial in attempting to reduce breathlessness through positioning.

Lifestyle management

Once again, occupational therapists' skills in activity analysis lend themselves well to the management of cancer-related symptoms. Through graded activity and modification of tasks, ventilatory requirements can be reduced, in turn minimising breathlessness and enabling independence (Fisher and Lowrie 2008). Changes may involve modification of particular tasks, for example using equipment such as shower stools, or planning and pacing, for example climbing the stairs only when necessary, or having someone else carry a child's books for them at school.

To be effective, the interventions employed by occupational therapists in the management of cancer-related breathlessness may have to change over time, according to diagnosis, the stage of the illness and the child's emotional state (Fisher and Lowrie 2008). Regular assessment and re-evaluation of the success of intervention is therefore required.

9.4 Management of anxiety

Anxiety is a multi-system response to a perceived threat or danger that is triggered by the brain to keep us safe; a fight or flight response.

(Cooper 2006c)

Anxiety is a normal biological reaction to stress that all of us will have experienced at some time. For example, we experience anxiety when sitting an exam, when we get lost, are running late or when we lose something. For children and young people however, cancer and its treatment will inevitably provoke higher levels of anxiety. If left unchecked, high levels of anxiety can, for people of all ages, reduce quality of life, reduce the ability to engage meaningfully in daily activities, and hinder future development (Dixon-Woods et al 2005; Ramini et al 2008).

Signs of anxiety

Anxiety may induce both physical and cognitive effects in children and young people.

Physical signs include:

- Sweating
- Increased heart beat
- Increased respiration rate
- Tightness across the chest
- Muscular tension
- Nausea
- Dry mouth
- Feeling faint or light headed

Cognitive signs include:

- Poor concentration
- Irritability
- Reduced ability to engage
- Negative thoughts such as:
  - feeling out of control
  - feelings of 'I can't do this'
- Aggression

(Cooper 2000c)

It is important that occupational therapists are able to recognise signs of anxiety or stress so that the effect on daily life may be minimised and potential triggers are reduced.

In order first to identify triggers of anxiety, the causes of stress must be understood. For children and young people with cancer, the triggers will differ according to their age, understanding and situation. Once triggers are identified and understood, occupational therapists may employ strategies such as modifying environments, the use of distraction, relaxation or breathing techniques, educating parents and carers as to how to support their child, and using effective communication.

Causes of stress include:

- Unfamiliar environments/surroundings
- Separation from parents and other family members
- Being looked after by unfamiliar people
- Painful procedures
- Lack of understanding
- Worries about side effects of treatment
- Side effects of treatment
- Worries about response to treatment
- Concern for other family members
- Fear of the unknown
- Uncertainty
- Loss of privacy/dignity

(Cooper 2006c, Harding 2000, Nadeane-McCaffrey 2006)

Modifying environment

The strange and unfamiliar environment of a hospital can be a frightening place, with unusual sounds, unknown people and the association of being unwell and of painful procedures. Environments can be modified and parents may be asked to bring in toys, bed clothes, and photographs from home. Hospital staff can help also by keeping noise to a minimum and by ensuring that privacy and dignity is always respected.

Distraction

Play may be used to distract young children from their worries. Other meaningful activity can be used to good effect in reducing anxiety in young people. Occupational therapists are able to facilitate children and young people's participation in play and leisure activities, ensuring that neither diagnosis nor treatment restricts access or the ability to engage. In a hospital setting, play specialists trained in the use of distraction techniques will work with children and young people when they undergo painful or stressful procedures.

Communication

It is widely documented that the way in which professionals communicate with patients bears strongly on their experience of treatment (DH 2005). Fear of the unknown and feelings of uncertainty are common in cancer care. Occupational therapists should be aware of the language that they use and be clear in explaining the role of occupational therapy intervention to both child and family so as not to cause anxiety or apprehension. When working with pre-school and school-age children, play may be used as a valuable intervention through which to communicate and to gain trust, thus reducing fear and anxiety (Sepion 2009).

Education and coping strategies

Understanding and enhancing the coping strategies employed by a child or young person is important to aid adjustment to cancer (Jackson et al 2009, Palmer et al 2000). Occupational therapists can help children and young people, and their parents, to recognise strategies that have been adopted since diagnosis, as well as to identify those which they have used to good effect in the past. Parents can then facilitate their children in the use of these strategies when they are required or in situations in which triggers of stress or anxiety may be present. In a study by McCaffrey (2006) the teaching of new coping strategies and self-control techniques to children is also highlighted as an effective method for reducing the effects of stresses related to cancer and its treatment. Strategies may include the use of relaxation or breathing techniques. Educating and giving children and young people the skills with which to manage cancer-related stresses is an important aspect of cancer care. This is because how well young people cope with and adapt to a diagnosis of cancer can determine the extent of long-term difficulties or successful development (Ramini et al 2008).

Anxiety can also be caused by, or be the result of, the cancer-related symptoms discussed above: fatigue, pain and breathlessness. It should therefore not be treated as a symptom alone, but regarded in the context of a total approach to assessment and care.

9.5 Multiprofessional management of symptoms

Outlined above are evidence-based non-pharmacological strategies employed by occupational therapists in the management of cancer-related symptoms. However, as has been clearly illustrated here, cancer-related symptoms and their causes are multidimensional and interlinked. A multiprofessional approach to care which includes both pharmacological and non-pharmacological interventions is therefore recommended. Such an approach has been shown to offer the potential for the most effective relief of symptoms, when compared to offering individual therapies alone (Barsevick 2002, Ogilvy et al 2008).

Case study: symptom management

Daniel, who is 13 years old, is seven months on from having had a bone-marrow transplant for multiple-relapsed leukaemia.

On assessment, Daniel reported the presence of pain and fatigue to be the most troubling symptoms affecting his everyday life. Prior to assessment, the occupational therapist ensured that possible medical explanations for the symptoms had been explored and ruled out. The occupational therapist then discussed with Daniel all his activities of daily living and adopted a problem-solving and educational approach to intervention.

Daniel was attending school on an ad hoc basis and had difficulty sleeping at night due to generalised pain. Exploring further, it became apparent that Daniel was attending school for one or two full days and would then struggle to get in on the following days. Liaising with school it was agreed that Daniel would attend for mornings only while his exercise tolerance was restored. It was also agreed that Daniel would leave lessons a few minutes earlier than his peers, so that he did not have to rush between classes. General fatigue management strategies, such as planning and prioritising, were taught to Daniel, giving him the ability to manage fatigue levels himself.

Sleep hygiene was promoted. Daniel was encouraged to go to bed and rise in the morning at the same time each day. Napping during the day was discouraged. A release-only relaxation technique was taught to Daniel over the course of four relaxation training sessions, which he then used before going to bed to reduce pain and aid sleep.

A thorough review of Daniel's daily and weekly routine and the employment of appropriate strategies and techniques led to fatigue and pain levels being reduced. This in turn enabled a gradual increase in exercise tolerance and greater participation in the activities of daily living. Daniel learned valuable self-management skills, and his motivation and self-esteem increased.

10 The needs of children with cancer

The individual needs of children with cancer will vary according to their age, diagnosis and the mode of treatment. This section discusses the common areas of need associated with children and should be taken in the context of offering intervention within a holistic, family-centred approach to care.

Development

Chronic illnesses, such as cancer, do not themselves alone cause developmental delay. Instead developmental delay in children with cancer is often the combined result of a number of factors (Wray and Sensky 1999).

Improved survival rates for children with cancer are the result of ever more effective treatments. Anti-cancer treatments are often intensive and aggressive, however, and may require prolonged hospital admissions with periods of being acutely unwell (Dixon-Woods et al 2005). Global weakness and general de-conditioning is commonly seen following hospital stays and anti-cancer treatments. Inactivity, side effects of chemotherapy such as peripheral neuropathy, and/or reduced nutritional intake in turn affect a child's ability to interact physically with his or her environment, restricting play and consequently hindering the development of motor, cognitive and exploratory skills.

The restrictive nature of a hospital environment and rigid treatment regimes can also exacerbate developmental regression or delay (Townley and Welton 2000, Wavrek 2001). Occupational therapists working in a hospital setting need to be creative in adapting the environment. They may also work with play specialists to provide play activities beside the bed. Development of social skills can also be affected by cancer and its treatment, as regular social interaction is disrupted during long hospital stays, which sometimes require a child to be in isolation, as well as being away from siblings and spending time out of nursery or school.

Occupational therapists understand the importance of play and have knowledge of age-appropriate developmental tasks. Using this knowledge, occupational therapists can support and provide advice to parents as to how best to maintain and facilitate their child's development during and following anti-cancer treatments.

Sensory processing

Development of sensory integration occurs during the early years of life, with children mastering, with increasing levels of complexity, the ability to organise sensory information (Ayres 1979). Adaptive responses, which are goal-directed responses to sensory experiences, facilitate development as responses become increasingly complex. Young children who are acutely unwell can become deprived of sensory stimulation. Particularly during long hospital stays, opportunities to organise and act upon sensory input may be limited. Occupational therapists working in paediatrics will be aware of the important relationship between the ability to organise and process sensory information, and development and functional ability, and should therefore seek to provide opportunities for sensory experiences, especially during acute phases of treatment.

Understanding of illness

Children will have varying degrees of knowledge and understanding of their diagnosis and its treatment. Families may use different words to describe tumours, medicines, and lines. Occupational therapists should be aware of these terms used by families, and adopt them wherever possible when communicating with children. This can often be done by listening to the way in which parents interact with and talk to their child.

Wheelchairs and buggies

Children with cancer are often referred to their local wheelchair and specialist seating services for provision of wheelchairs and buggies. For young children (depending upon their age and size), a decision will be made as whether to prescribe a buggy or a wheelchair. Factors influencing this decision, such as the need, duration and frequency of use and parent choice should be considered.

In terms of need, the reasons for referral vary, but often include:

- fatigue
- weakness
- ataxia
- poor trunk control
- hemiplegia
- peripheral neuropathy
- breathlessness
- pain

In terms of duration and frequency of use:

- Some children may require a wheelchair for the foreseeable future; for example, a child who has motor difficulties as a result of a brain tumour, or a child who becomes breathless due to graft-versus-host disease (GvHD) of the lung following bone-marrow transplant.
- Other children may require a wheelchair for outdoor use for a number of years following treatment, as a result of side effects such as fatigue or pain.
- Others require a chair during certain periods of their treatment, for example, following chemotherapy or radiotherapy, when mobility may be restricted due to pain in the legs, weakness, and/or fatigue. Use of chairs in these instances may be continuous over a period of many months, or may be intermittent due to side effects experienced following regular cycles of chemotherapy.

The guidance development group recommends the provision of standard buggies for young children requiring seating for infrequent or short-term outdoor use. Provision of a wheelchair should be considered for young children thought to have long-term mobility needs and who will require a wheelchair in the future. However, all decisions should be made in consultation with parents, taking into account their needs and preferences. Introducing wheelchairs should be done sensitively as, for some, a wheelchair may be seen as a symbol of disability. Environmental factors should also be taken into account, including whether there is adequate space for storage, appropriate access and transport.

This section has highlighted key considerations for occupational therapists treating a child with cancer. However, all children have unique needs. An individual approach to assessment and intervention is therefore essential in each case.

11 The needs of adolescents and young adults with cancer

It is now widely recognised that young people with cancer have distinct needs, which differ significantly from either adults or children with cancer (DH 2007, Grinyer 2007, NICE 2005, Whelan et al 2007). It is for this reason that NICE guidance (2005) stipulates that staff looking after young people with cancer must be knowledgeable in adolescent development, with understanding of how cancer and its treatment may disrupt successful maturation.

Adolescence development

Adolescence itself is a complex life stage during which young people negotiate the transitional process from childhood to adulthood, developing physically, psychologically and socially. It is a multifaceted and critical period in the life of a young person, during which identify is formed, independence gained and where preparation for adult life begins (Hollis and Morgan 2001, Kelly 2008, Neville 2000, Palmer et al 2007).

Independence

Establishing independence and autonomy in decision-making is part of 'adolescence' and is integral to maturation. However, by their nature, cancer and its treatment often hinder independence, autonomy and control. Independence is lost on a number of levels – from going out with friends, learning to drive and going to the shops, to smaller everyday tasks such as being able to wash, dress and even eat. Although cancer's impact on independence at any age can be devastating, in adolescence independence is particularly fragile as it is not fully established and remains in the framework of a degree of dependence upon parents (Grinyer 2002, Dixon-Woods et al 2005). The role of occupational therapists is ideally suited to maintaining or re-establishing independence in young people, whether through education (for example, managing fatigue so that energy is available to spend time with friends), or through adaption (for example, providing bathing equipment so that a young person can bathe independently rather than have to rely on a parent).

Identity

Creating and establishing an identity is another key part of the transitional process from childhood to adulthood. However, at the same time as discovering independence and an identity, young people also develop a strong desire to 'fit in' and belong. A crisis of identity is normal and expected during adolescence; however, adverse effects on identity, including body image, increase significantly as a result of cancer (Dixon-Woods et al 2005, Neville 2000).

Peer relations, a major source of influence upon identity formation, are described by young people with cancer as difficult to maintain. This is largely due to practical factors such as spending long periods of time away from school or college, but also due to changes within the dynamics of a peer group and the stigma that sometimes surrounds cancer (Grinyer 2007, Neville 2000). Occupational therapists can facilitate young people in keeping up with peer relationships, educating and helping them to manage symptoms that sometimes restrict activities and time spent with friends. During prolonged periods of time in hospital, keeping in contact with friends via email, webcams, chat-rooms and social networking sites should be encouraged. Where possible, and taking into account hospital policy, distance from home, and medical status, friends may be encouraged to visit.

Body image

Undeniably, body image and appearance becomes an increasing preoccupation for young people during adolescence.

The potential physical effects of cancer and anti-cancer therapies on appearance are many and can be short-term or long-lasting.

Changes to appearance

- Hair loss
- Skin changes
- Weight loss
- Weight gain
- External influences such as NG tubes, gastrostomy, central lines
- Muscle wasting
- Loss of limbs
- Facial palsy
- Hemiparesis

Body image is intrinsic to identity and it is easy to see how changes in appearance can lead to a negative view of self, loss of confidence and low self-esteem (Abrams et al 2007). For this reason, it is vital that issues relating to body image are tackled, particularly as developing a positive self-image is pivotal to achieving successful adolescent development and maturation (Lewis 2005). Occupational therapists are ideally positioned to address issues relating to body image in young people in the course of discussing and attending to self-care needs.

Although body image is discussed here in terms of its importance for young people, it should be noted that effects of cancer and its treatment on body image is significant and can be distressing for all age groups.

Higher education and employment

As has been shown in Section 8, disrupted school attendance, the long-term physical and psycho-social side effects of treatment and ongoing uncertainty can all affect a young person's future prospects of further training, education or employment (Neville 2000). Plans that have been made may have to be postponed (for example deferral of a university place) and choices that have yet to be made, such as which A-level subjects to take, may be considered irrelevant during such uncertain times. Occupational therapists can work to facilitate independence in life skills such as self-management, which are required for succeeding in higher education or employment. Occupational therapists are also well suited to provide support and advice when young people are making career choices, and can suggest any alterations or adaptions to task or environment that may be required.

12 Palliative care in paediatric oncology

Palliative care for children and young people with cancer should be an active, total approach to care embracing physical, emotional, social and spiritual elements. It should focus on enhancing quality of life for the child, support for the family, which should include the management of distressing symptoms, provision of respite and care through death and bereavement.

(Association for Children with Life-threatening and Terminal Conditions and their Families (ACT) and the Royal College of Paediatrics and Child Health (RCPCH) 2003)

Although survival rates have dramatically improved in paediatric oncology, some children cannot be cured of their disease. On average 300 children die of cancer each year in the UK (Cancer Research 2005). Occupational therapists play a key role in supporting and facilitating a child or young person at this time to enable and enhance quality of life. It is recognised that working with children who are dying and their families can be challenging and will test occupational therapists' own emotions; this is particularly true when having worked with a family for a long time or having had personal experience of bereavement. Caring for yourself as a professional is an important aspect of working with children and young people with cancer and is discussed later within the guidance.

Palliative care, still regarded as an emerging specialty within paediatrics (Boog 2008), takes into account the physical, psychological and social needs of a child or young person. With a holistic approach to care and core skills that address the physical, psychological and social wellbeing of a child, occupational therapists, alongside professional colleagues, may provide input that allows children and their families to function at an optimum level despite disease or prognosis.

When does palliative care begin?

Palliative care should begin as soon as the disease is no longer deemed curable, not when it is at its end stage. In reality, however, the point at which curative care ceases and palliative care begins is often blurred and will differ from child to child (ACT 2003, Tester 2006). Indeed, it is not uncommon for children with non-curable disease to receive palliative care and symptom control alongside further life-extending anti-cancer treatments such as surgery, chemotherapy and radiotherapy. Indeed the time-span and length of many children's treatment may mean that palliative care extends over many years. Moreover, children may continue to develop physically, emotionally and cognitively throughout the course of their condition, which in turn may affect their health and social needs, as well as their understanding of disease and death (DH 2008, Tester 2008).

Understanding of death

It is important for occupational therapists to be conscious of a child or young person's awareness and understanding of death. This will include and may be depend on what the child has been told by their parents. This knowledge is important because a child or young person's understanding of death or prognosis may impact the direction of intervention and goal-setting.

Developmental understanding of death

- Aged 1–3 years: no understanding of death itself. However, children of this age will be sensitive to the behaviours of others and may sense changes in the moods or routines of parents or caregivers.
- Aged 3–5 years: death is viewed as temporary notion, reversible and impersonal.
- Aged 6–9 years: a child begins to realise that death is final. However, death is still not perceived as being personal, rather something that happens to others.
- Aged from 9 years to adolescence: thinking and understanding becomes increasingly abstract and intellectual; not only is there now knowledge that death is irreversible, but there is greater understanding of how death and grief will affect others around them.

(Tester 2006)

Family-centred care

As is the case in all aspects of occupational therapy intervention, a family's cultural and spiritual beliefs must always be respected, and the importance of family-centred care is discussed in Section 5 of the guidance. With regard to palliative care, it should be noted that a family's spiritual beliefs may become heightened and more important as the prospect of death triggers changes in values, priorities and understanding (Boog 2008). Conversely, families may struggle with feelings of anger and question their faith. A sensitive approach in this area is therefore vital.

Working with a family from diagnosis, as recommended by the International Children's Palliative Care Network (2008) and the World Health Organisation (2007), trust and professional relationships may be built up prior to the family entering difficult periods. The treating occupational therapist will have gained previous insight into the needs and wishes of the child and family. With this foundation future needs may be better anticipated and as a result intervention may be planned and acted upon more effectively. The guidance development group acknowledges that in practice this is not always possible because referral to an occupational therapist may only occur following deterioration in function as a result of progressive disease. In this instance, advice and information may be sought from professionals, or indeed other occupational therapists who are better acquainted with the family. Information such as the family's understanding of the disease and potential future treatment; their response to difficult news; the child or young person's goals and aspirations; and the goals and aspirations of parents or carers all will help to shape the treatment and intervention offered by the occupational therapist.

Rehabilitation in paediatric palliative care

Although rehabilitation in cancer care is not a new concept, it is still often reserved for those with a more favourable prognosis or outcome (NICE 2005). Rehabilitation should, however, be seen as a continuous process appropriate at any stage of the disease trajectory, and one that is not dependent upon prognosis.

Rehabilitation in palliative care recognises the importance of enabling those with limited time to live as fully and independently as possible. This may not be in the traditional rehabilitative sense of restoring them to previous levels of function; rather, palliative rehabilitation will focus upon support and maximising potential. It should be remembered that although children may deteriorate and lose skills over the course of palliative care, they will also continue to develop physically and cognitively during this time. These changes must be taken into account when planning intervention (Tester 2008).

Aims of rehabilitation in palliative care:

- To maintain or enhance quality of life
- To enable participation in family life
- To enable function and independence in activities of daily living
- To reduce dependency
- To maintain and facilitate access to everyday activities, including school
- To reduce symptoms affecting function or quality of life
- To prevent complications, for example pressure sores or contractures

Fluctuating needs

By the nature of palliative care, the overall direction will be one of deterioration and increasing dependence. This shift will not always be one of gradual decline, however, but rather it will be one of ups and downs as treatments and medications are altered. This is particularly true of children and young people who receive life-extending treatment alongside palliative care. A flexible approach to intervention and continual assessment and re-assessment will ensure that needs are met in a timely manner. Goals of rehabilitation may be re-negotiated or put 'on hold' during episodes of deterioration. The treating therapist must, however, take into account that recovery and return of function may occur following such episodes during the palliative care phase.

End-of-life care

The main focus of occupational therapy intervention at end of life will be comfort, ease of care and enhancing quality of life. Intervention will include management of symptoms and provision of equipment.

Symptom management at end of life

There is a role for occupational therapists in the management of cancer-related symptoms at all stages of disease progression, including end of life. Strategies to alleviate symptoms such as pain and fatigue have been discussed in Section 9 of the guidance. However, at end of life it is more likely that a compensatory approach to intervention will be adopted. This will include timely provision of equipment and assistance given by others when attending to self-care needs. Relaxation strategies and breathing techniques may also be used alongside pharmacological agents to reduce pain, and ease fatigue, anxiety and breathlessness experienced at end of life. Breathing techniques are best taught and established before breathing becomes difficult. This applies particularly to those likely to experience breathing difficulties (for example, those with lung metastasis or brain stem tumours).

Equipment provision at end of life

The needs of children and young people may change rapidly during end-of-life care. Timely provision of equipment to facilitate activities of daily living, wheelchairs and buggies can help maintain quality of life and ensure safely. As stated, some needs may be anticipated: many children with brain tumours, for example, require specialist seating at end of life due to a loss of trunk and/or head control. Due to rapid deterioration, however, specialist seating often cannot be provided in time. It is therefore recommended that, where possible, seating needs are anticipated and considered in advance so that appropriate seating is available when it is needed at end of life.

Providing equipment during palliative care or at end of life should be done in a sensitive manner. In the Foreword, Ben's mother describes how she found some equipment difficult to accept as it represented the loss of Ben's independence. As a profession, occupational therapy is about helping to address difficulties and solve problems, yet it is not just the physical needs of the child that must be considered: emotional and psychological impacts have to be considered also. In some instances it may be necessary to provide just one piece of equipment at a time as families adjust. On the other hand, some family members, such as Ben's father, may view provision of equipment more straightforwardly as a practical way to overcome basic needs and as such will find provision of any equipment invaluable. Open and honest discussions with the child or young person and the family will ensure that any equipment deemed necessary is issued in a manner appropriate to the family's needs.

Following death, equipment loaned to a child must be collected in a timely and yet sensitive manner. In some instances equipment and/or wheelchairs may have been loaned by a hospital occupational therapist to ensure timely equipment provision. When family members do not wish to return to the hospital after the death of a child, it may be possible for a member of the hospital outreach team to collect items. Equipment should be loaned, collected and cleaned in accordance with local policies and procedure, taking into account health and safety aspects of moving and handling and infection-control considerations. Alternatively, the occupational therapist may arrange for equipment to be collected by community stores, so that bereaved family members may avoid taking or having to make unnecessary and difficult telephone calls.

Co-ordination of care

The need for a co-ordinated approach to palliative care, with effective collaboration between the NHS, children's hospices, the voluntary sector, social care and education is widely recognised (DH 2005, DH 2008). Indeed effective palliative care requires a multiagency and multiprofessional approach, which also includes the whole family. Multiprofessional working, communication, and collaboration are discussed in full in Section 13 of the guidance. However, it should be noted that proper co-ordination of care and effective communication is of particular importance at end of life because of children and young people's rapidly changing needs and the high level of responsiveness required of occupational therapists in the event of a rapid decline.

Case study: palliative care

Nina, a nine-year-old girl diagnosed with a medulloblastoma, underwent surgical debulking at a neuro-surgical centre before proceeding with radiotherapy as an outpatient at a regional oncology centre. In her third week of radiotherapy Nina's neurological signs deteriorated significantly and she was admitted to the oncology centre. Her parents were informed that the tumour had grown and that there was no longer any chance of cure.

Nina continued with radiotherapy while the multiprofessional team and her family made plans for safe discharge home. With continued radiotherapy and steroids some of the neurological symptoms dissipated. Nina began to regain her sitting balance and movement returned to her right arm.

Working jointly with the physiotherapist, the occupational therapist taught Nina's parents safe moving and handling strategies that enabled them to facilitate safe transfers from bed to commode or wheelchair. Encouraged by her parents, intervention looked at improving sitting balance and use of her right arm.

All intervention was based around games and included her younger brother. Nina fatigued quickly so sessions did not last for more than 10 minutes a day. These sessions, however, gave her parents a focus and allowed Nina's brother to be part of what was happening. It created a safe environment and an opportunity for brother and sister to play together.

Although Nina's sitting balance improved and at the time of discharge she could sit in a standard wheelchair, she was only able to do so for short periods and it was anticipated her sitting balance would deteriorate again in the near future. Working with the wheelchair service, a tilt-in-space wheelchair was ordered while she was discharged home with a 9L chair. A home visit was conducted with the hospital outreach nurse and community nursing team. The home environment was assessed and a hospital bed and commode were ordered for downstairs living.

Nina was discharged from hospital; her parents were confident in aspects of moving and handling and could continue with games taught in hospital that Nina could engage with. As her neurological symptoms increased, the tilt-in-space wheelchair was provided, offering Nina the opportunity to sit out safely and comfortably until end of life.

13 Multiprofessional working, communication and collaboration

Multiprofessional working

The care of a child or young person with cancer should be provided by a team of professionals adopting a multiprofessional approach to intervention (DH 2005, DH 2007, Michaud et al 2005, NICE 2005). Effective communication between professionals will ensure a co-ordinated, holistic approach to care, in the course of which all the needs of a child, young person and their family can be addressed. In addition, the quality of communication between professional and patient is widely believed to have a significant impact upon a patient's experience: effective communication with patient and family is therefore key in providing optimal client-centred care (Cooper 2006a, DH 2005, NICE 2005).

Children and young people diagnosed with cancer meet a large number of professional staff across hospital and community settings from diagnosis to treatment and supportive care or follow-up. Members of the multiprofessional team will vary according to the setting, but will include:

Multiprofessional team

- Oncologist
- Radiologist
- Surgeon (neuro, orthopaedic or general)
- Dietitian (hospital or community)
- Physiotherapist (hospital or community)
- Speech and Language Therapist (hospital or community)
- Occupational Therapist (hospital, community or local authority)
- CLIC Sargent Social Worker
- Clinical Psychologist
- Clinical Psychiatrist
- Play Specialist
- Palliative Care Consultant (hospital or community)
- Paediatric Oncology Outreach Nurse
- Nursing Staff (hospital or community)
- Chaplin (hospital or community)
- Hospital teacher
- Neurologist
- Endocrinologist

Communication and collaboration

Not only will children and young people meet a large number of different professionals, they may also meet a number of different occupational therapists working across different settings. For example, it is possible for a child or young person diagnosed with a bone tumour to see up to five occupational therapists during the initial stages of their treatment.

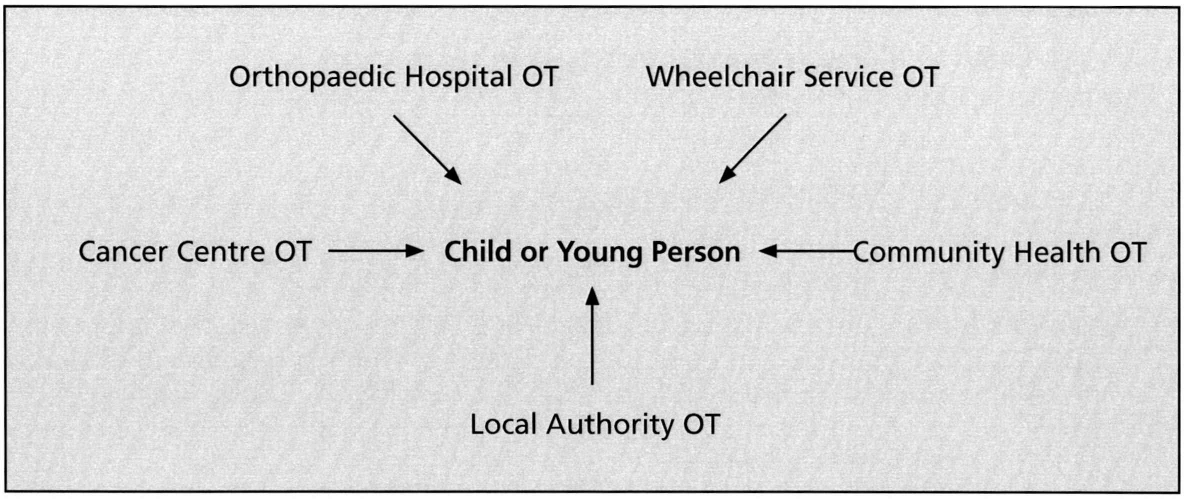

Effective communication therefore is not only imperative between professional groups, but also between occupational therapists themselves. Consent must be gained from parents or a young person prior to any sharing of information between services.

Occupational therapists working in a hospital setting should ensure that community colleagues are kept informed of any changes in a child or young person's treatment or condition. This may include updates of latest scan results, their response to treatment, or information about any sudden and unexpected changes. Due to the immunosuppressant nature of anti-cancer treatments, sudden unplanned admissions to hospital are a frequent occurrence. For this reason communication is not always possible between family and therapists, and therapists may need to adopt a flexible approach to appointments. It is helpful to make telephone contact 24 hours before appointments or equipment deliveries.

14 Equipment provision

Provision of occupational therapy equipment is an important part of therapy, providing practical assistance in facilitating independence and ensuring safety (DH and Department for Education and Skills 2004, NICE 2005). The provision of equipment has been discussed in context throughout the guidance, whether it be to aid rehabilitation (for example, in the provision of a static seating system); to conserve energy (such as in the provision of a wheelchair); or to overcome functional difficulties (for example, by providing bathroom equipment).

Being able to access and make use of bathroom facilities is important for children and young people with cancer due to the side effects of treatment. Some side effects will be short lived, whereas others may be long lasting. Occupational therapists who work in an oncology setting will be able to provide information with regard to the likely duration of needs in this area, which in turn may affect the need for housing adaptations.

Provision of activity of daily living (ADL) equipment

ADL equipment may be provided for a functional need, but side effects of anti-cancer treatments may also require consideration and may indicate a heightened need. For example:

- Increased risk of infection
- Loose stools (which may be caused by chemotherapy, radiotherapy to the abdomen area or GvHD of the gut following transplant)
- GvHD of the skin

Functional difficulties can often occur rapidly and without warning. They can occur at initial presentation, during treatment or towards end of life. Where possible, a flexible approach should be adopted by occupational therapists to ensure that needs are met through the timely provision of equipment. Other aspects of occupational therapy intervention, such as managing fatigue or reducing exacerbation of pain, may be assisted by provision of equipment, and although perhaps not seen initially as a priority, the effect on quality of life should not be underestimated and therefore such provision should be championed by occupational therapists.

Duration and frequency of equipment use

Duration and frequency of equipment use will vary from child to child. In some instances, equipment will be required for a long-term need caused by the tumour itself; in other cases, equipment may be required for a decrease in functional ability caused by treatment. Although a child or young person's functional ability would be expected to increase after treatment has finished, it should be noted that anti-cancer treatment can last months, or even years, and its effects can take many months following the end of treatment to dissipate. For this reason, the majority of equipment provided to children and young people with cancer should be seen as a long-term requirement. Over the course of treatment, needs may fluctuate according to the intensity, stage and modality of treatment. This may mean issued equipment is used constantly, for example following a cycle of chemotherapy, and then only infrequently towards the start of the next cycle. Fluctuation in functional ability according to treatment should be taken into account during any assessment for equipment, particularly when a child is assessed during a period of wellness.

Assessment and provision of equipment

In 2007, an independent review by the Association for Children's Palliative Care (ACT) found that children receiving palliative care often face difficulties in accessing services, most commonly due to local disagreements over how provision of equipment or adaptions should be funded. Parents also reported problems and frustration with multiple assessments. ACT (2007) and NICE (2005) recommend close liaison between agencies and the sharing of information to avoid unnecessary repetition of assessments, prevent delays in equipment provision, and minimise disruption for the family. The guidance development group concludes that all occupational therapists are skilled in the assessment of and prescription of equipment to facilitate activities of daily living and wheelchairs. Wherever possible, therefore, advice should be sought from the assessing occupational therapist, irrespective of their clinical setting, to prevent delay in provision or duplication of assessments.

15 Outcome measures

Measuring the effectiveness of intervention is integral to the occupational therapy process. Within cancer care, regular evaluation and re-assessment ensures that strategies employed and intervention techniques used continue to be appropriate within times of change, fluctuation and uncertainty.

Outcome measures during and following anti-cancer treatments

The guidance development group recognises that there are difficulties associated with the use of outcome measures to determine the success of occupational therapy intervention in paediatric oncology. Outcome measures used within occupational therapy practice, such as the Functional Independence Measure (FIM) or the Canadian Occupational Performance Measure (COPM), are directly linked to functional ability. However, most noticeably in paediatric palliative care or where prognosis is uncertain, functional ability itself is expected to decline. Furthermore, during anti-cancer treatments functional ability may fluctuate, making measurement of improvement difficult. Therefore, measures which assess the extent to which the goals of occupational therapy intervention are met (which may or may not relate directly to functional independence), such as the Goal Attainment Scale (GAS), may be more appropriate and should be considered.

Following active anti-cancer treatments, outcome measures that are based on functional ability and the goals of children, young people and their families may be employed to good effect. Measures employed by occupational therapists within the practice development group include the School Function Assessment (SFA), the Functional Disability Index (FDI) and the Short Child Occupational Profile (SCOPE). Some members of the group were not currently using standardised outcome measures in their settings, preferring instead to rely on their own clinical evaluation skills of observation and reflection, and feedback from parents and the child or young person.

Outcome measures at end of life

Outcome measures at end of life should reflect the aims of palliative care, which will include maintaining quality of life, controlling symptoms and supporting families (Hearn and Higginson 1997). Thought should be given, however, to the appropriateness of implementing outcome measure tools, particularly those that take time to administer and require energy or concentration towards end of life. Although a subjective assessment, the use of self-rating Likert scales is a quick way of measuring symptoms such as pain, and can be effective in evaluating interventions. It should be noted, however, that a child or young person will require the necessary cognitive skills to participate in any self-rating assessment.

A multiprofessional approach to caring for a child or young person with cancer, particularly at end of life, is recommended. Consideration should therefore be given to any outcome measures that have already been adopted by other professionals within the occupational therapist's setting.

Considerations for the future

There is currently no literature to support the use of any one particular outcome measure in the evaluation of occupational therapy practice in paediatric oncology or palliative care. As the brief discussion here indicates, there is a gap in the research. This subject requires further thought and investigation to determine the appropriateness of specific measures that could be employed by occupational therapists for the benefit of their patients and families in this field.

16 Caring for oneself as a professional

Caring for oneself is not always acknowledged as being necessary for a health professional, because the focus, rightly, is always on the child and the family. Occupational therapists do their best to support and provide professional therapeutic intervention, but understandings vary as to what constitutes a professional approach. Some occupational therapists believe they should try to hide their own feelings and sensitivity and be as matter of fact as possible; others are more confident in taking a more obviously compassionate approach and in showing sensitivity to a child, young person or parent. As caring individuals, healthcare professionals cannot fail to be affected by the trauma that surrounds everyday practice within oncology. Staff sickness is, and should be recognised as, an indicator of the stressful work situation (Obholzer and Zagier -Roberts 2002).

There are ways of coping which are healthy and others that are unhealthy. Bottling one's feelings creates a tension that finds its release at some point. Fatigue and burnout are common in oncology. This needs to be identified and recognised by professionals and mutual support encouraged. Reflection on one's work at the end of each day is important. Keeping a confidential, or shared, reflective diary can be helpful (Boog and Tester 2008). Grief among staff is real but not always acknowledged in the work place. It is important that time is taken to consider and reflect upon the child's and family's experience and one's own feelings.

To care for oneself is to recognise the impact of one's own health and wellbeing on the children or young people and families one works with, as well as that of one's professional colleagues. This includes physical health as well as psychological and emotional wellbeing. If professionals do not care for themselves properly, the quality of their work may become compromised.

17 Implications for future practice

Research

Paediatric oncology is a specialist area of children's occupational therapy and one which has grown in recent years. As with any growing area of practice, occupational therapists in this field must establish themselves as integral to the multiprofessional team caring for children and young people with cancer. Evidence supporting occupational therapy intervention within this guidance has been taken from a nursing perspective or from research conducted within an adult population. Consequently, as stated within the guidance, the objective of providing an evidence-based resource for occupational therapists could not fully be met. Therefore urgent research into this area of practice should be seen as a priority.

This guidance recommends that occupational therapists working within paediatric oncology should take a lead in conducting research to establish the effectiveness of specific occupational therapy interventions in order to provide a robust evidence-base from which to inform best clinical practice.

Transitional care

As with all aspects of child health, the debate continues about how best to support young people as they reach adulthood. Transition into, rather than transfer to, adult services is recommended, taking a multiagency approach that considers the full range of health, social, educational and employment needs of young people (DH 2006). Children and young people with cancer are no exception, requiring support during this process in order to achieve optimal outcomes in all areas of daily living. Occupational therapists may play an important role in the transitional process, particularly in the case of young survivors of cancer with long-term and sometimes complex needs.

Survivorship

The long-term side effects of cancer and its treatment have been highlighted in the guidance. However, in accordance with the remit for the guidance, these effects and their implications on independent living have not been discussed in depth.

The cancer reform strategy (DH 2007) recognises that the needs of children and young people who survive cancer are unique and differ from the needs of those who survive cancer in adulthood. There are currently 28,000 survivors of cancer under the age of 24 in the UK; with ever-increasing survival rates, the importance of addressing the long-term needs of survivors of childhood cancer becomes more pressing (Easton 2009).

Occupational therapists are uniquely suited to addressing some of the long-term difficulties faced by survivors of childhood cancer. The guidance group recommends the promotion of occupational therapy in this area.

18 Summary

Occupational therapists have a valuable contribution to make in the area of paediatric oncology, with unique core skills, a holistic training and a philosophy of practice that sits well within the multidimensional and family-centred framework of paediatric oncology. Perceiving and treating the child or young person as developing within the context of their family, their school and wider community is vital for a successful outcome to intervention.

The guidance has focused upon aspects of occupational therapy practice with children and young people with cancer. These include:

- Considerations for use of standardised assessments with children and young people with cancer.
- Addressing the developmental needs of children with cancer including the use of play, sensory processing, and educating and supporting parents/carers.
- Addressing the developmental needs of adolescents and young people with cancer, focusing upon issues relating to independence, self-esteem, body image and access to education.
- The management of cancer-related symptoms that may affect the function, independence and quality of life of children and young people.
- Using self-care and leisure activities and life skills to promote function and aid recovery in independence.
- Using educational and/or compensatory approaches to aid independence in self-care, leisure activities and the development of life skills.
- Ensuring and enabling access to education, whatever the prognosis.

All these aspects of occupational therapy intervention, in seeking to facilitate and enhance independence and quality of life, are relevant at any stage of a child or young person's disease, from initial diagnosis through to completion of treatment or end-of-life care.

The guidance has also set out considerations for the future of occupational therapy practice in this area. These include addressing the long-term needs of survivors of childhood cancer; identifying suitable instruments for the measurement of outcomes of occupational therapy intervention; and especially the need for research to be undertaken into occupational therapy practice for children and young people with cancer. Such research would seek to provide an evidence-base of occupational therapy intervention, which in turn would be of great benefit to children and young people with cancer and their families.

The guidance has not, neither could it, set out a treatment programme for children and young people with cancer. Rather, it has set out some of the specific needs and challenges faced by children, young people and their families that may affect conventional occupational therapy process and intervention. The importance of a flexible approach to intervention has been emphasised throughout the guidance, taking into account the ever-changing needs of children and young people with cancer in accordance with the side effects of treatment and disease progression. Knowledge of tumour type and anti-cancer therapies allows the treating occupational therapist to judge the course of their intervention. Above all, treating the specific needs of a child or young person is paramount when working with young people with cancer, rather than focusing upon their disease or prognosis.

Glossary

Allogeneic transplant	Transplant involving donor stem cells.
Autologous transplant	Transplant using your own stem cells.
Central line	A catheter inserted directly into the central vein above the heart.
Febrile neutropenia	Temperature with reduced levels of neutrophils that will require hospital admission and prophylactic anti-biotics.
Graft-versus-host disease (GvHD)	Following a bone-marrow transplant donor cells may react with and attack the patient's own cells.
Hickman line	A make of central line.
Neutropenic	Low levels of neutrophils, which puts the patient at high risk of infection.
Neutrophils	White blood cells (which fight infection).
PICC line (Peripherally inserted central catheter)	A long, flexible catheter inserted into a peripheral vein in the arm and threaded up into the vena cava central vein.
Posterior fossa syndrome	A combination of motor, sensory, cognitive and language difficulties following surgery to the posterior fossa region.
Port/Portacath	A catheter is inserted underneath the skin into a vein. The end of the catheter is a 'port' which lies beneath the skin and can be accessed via a needle.
Somnolence	Extreme fatigue and lethargy following radiotherapy to the head.
Stem cell	An immature blood cell.
Venous occlusive disease	Occurs when blood vessels in the liver become swollen and blocked.

Appendixes

Appendix 1: Levels of research evidence

Area of practice	Research	Levels of evidence
Fatigue management	Barsevick et al (2004) A randomised clinical trial of energy conservation for patients with cancer-related fatigue.	A randomised controlled study
	Dimeo et al (2004) Effect of aerobic exercise and relaxation training on fatigue and physical performance of cancer patients after surgery.	A randomised controlled study
	Ream et al (2003) Quality and efficiency of educational materials on cancer-related fatigue, including views of patients from two European countries.	A qualitative study using focus groups
Relaxation	Dimeo et al (2004) Effect of aerobic exercise and relaxation training on fatigue and physical performance of cancer patients after surgery.	A randomised controlled study
	Luebbert et al (2001) The effectiveness of relaxation training in reducing treatment-related symptoms and improving emotional adjustment in acute non-surgical cancer treatment.	Meta-analytical review
	Miller and Hopkinson (2008) A retrospective audit exploring the use of relaxation as an intervention in oncology and palliative care.	Retrospective audit
	Sahler et al (2003) The effect of using music therapy with relaxation therapy in the management of patients undergoing bone-marrow transplantation.	A pilot feasibility study
	Syrjala et al (1995) Use of relaxation and imagery and cognitive-behavioural training to reduce pain during cancer treatment.	A controlled clinical study
	Walker et al (1999) Psychological, clinical and pathological effects of relaxation training and guided imagery during primary chemotherapy.	A randomised controlled study

Area of practice	Research	Levels of evidence
Pain management	Syrjala et al (1995) Use of relaxation and imagery and cognitive-behavioural training to reduce pain during cancer treatment.	A controlled clinical study
	Thomas and Weiss (2000) Non-pharmacological interventions with adults in chronic cancer pain.	A randomised clinical study
Anxiety management	Hinds et al (2000) An evaluation of the impact of a self-care coping intervention on psychological and clinical outcomes in adolescents with newly diagnosed cancer.	A randomised controlled longitudinal study
	McCaffrey (2006) Major stressors and their effects on the wellbeing of children with cancer.	A qualitative study making use of focus groups and individual interviews
School and education	Moore et al (2009) School re-entry for children with cancer: perceptions of nurses, school personnel and parents.	A qualitative study
	Vance and Eiser (2002) The school experience of the child with cancer.	A literature review
Occupational therapy	Lin et al (1997) Enhancing occupational performance through occupationally embedded exercise.	A meta-analytic review

Appendix 2: Distribution of childhood cancers in the UK (2003)

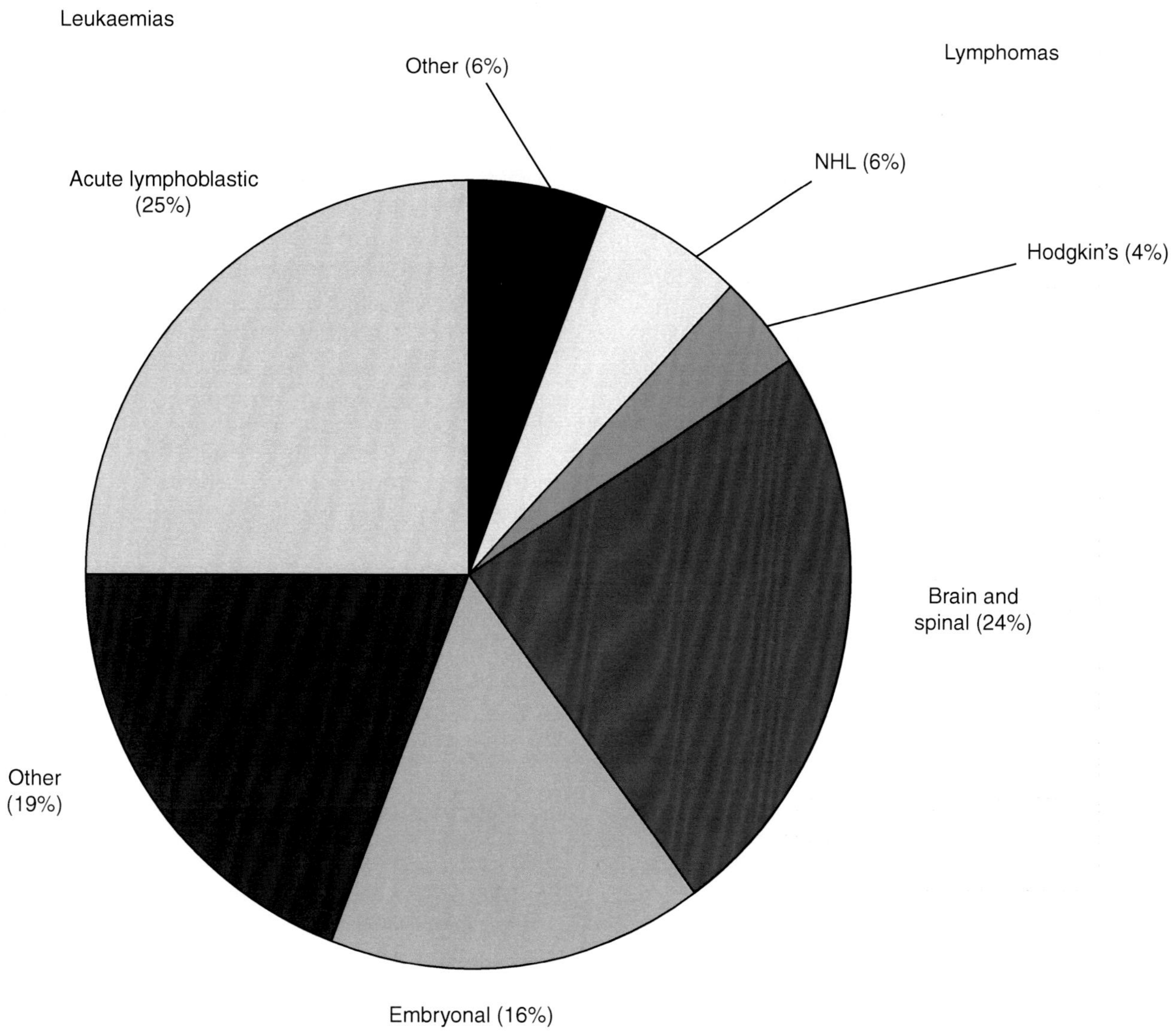

Reproduced with the kind permission from the Office of National Statistics (*http://www.statistics.gov.uk/cci/nugget.asp?id=681* Accessed on 08.02.10)

PSI Licence number: C2008002718

Appendix 3: Types of childhood cancers

Cancer	Specification	Explanation
Leukaemia	Acute lymphoblastic leukaemia (ALL)	Cancer of the white blood cells, where the cells continue to divide within the bone marrow, but do not mature. In ALL white blood cells, called lymphocytes, are affected. In AML monocytes and granulocytes are affected. Cells can get into the blood stream, travel around the body and build up in a different part of the body such as the lymph nodes, bone marrow, spleen, liver, brain, or spinal cord.
	Acute myeloid leukaemia (AML)	
Lymphomas	Hodgkin's lymphomas	Cancers of the lymphatic system, mainly affecting teenagers. Hodgkin's lymphoma has Reed Steinberg cells.
	Non-Hodgkin's lymphomas (T-cell NHL and B-cell NHL)	
Neuroblastomas	Stage 1–4	Cancer of specialist nerve cells called neural crest cells. Most commonly occurs in the adrenal gland, but can occur in the neck, chest and around the spinal cord. Classified into different stages according to severity. (Stage 4 is the most serious.)
Central nervous system tumours	Medullablastomas	Usually develops in the cerebellum, but can spread to other areas of the brain. Primitive neuroectodermal tumours (PNETs) develop from cells which are left over from the earliest stages of a baby's development in the womb.
	Gliomas	Develop from the supporting cells of the brain. They can be subdivided into two main types in children: astrocytomas and ependymomas. Symptoms they cause vary according to the function of the underlying brain tissue they are invading or compressing.
	Spinal tumours	Occur in different places in the spine and can arise from either a primary tumour or from secondary tumours, in particular bone tumours.

Cancer	Specification	Explanation
Embryonic tumours	Neuroblastomas of sympathetic nervous system	Embryonal tumours can occur in many different parts of the body. Characterised by the proliferation of tissue that is normally seen only in the developing embryo, they are rare after childhood and occur most commonly in the first few years of life. Some types are occasionally found to be present at birth.
	Medullablastomas (brain)	
	Retinoblastomas (eye)	
	Wilm's tumour (kidney)	
	Rhabdomyosarcoma (soft tissue tumour)	
	Hepatoblastoma (liver)	
Bone tumours	Ewing's sarcoma	Ewing's sarcoma develops in bones or soft tissues, but normally in the thighs, trunk or pelvis. Highly malignant and prone to spread.
	Osteosarcoma	Osteosarcoma is a cancer that normally develops at the ends of the bones. It usually begins in the legs or arms. Develops in osteoblasts (cells that make growing bone).
Soft-tissue sarcomas	Rhabomyosarcomas (see embryonal section for details)	More than half of soft-tissue sarcomas in childhood are classified as rhabdomyosarcomas, which derive from primitive striated muscle cells. Most childhood rhabdomyosarcomas are of the embryonal type, with the highest incidence in the first few years of life.
Germ cell or gonadal tumours		Germ cell tumours develop from cells that produce eggs or sperm. They mostly affect ovaries or testes. However, during pregnancy the cells that develop into these can develop elsewhere and later on develop into a germ cell tumour in other parts of the body such as the spine, brain, chest or abdomen.

Appendix 4: Anti-cancer treatments

Treatment	Side effects
Chemotherapy	**Short-term side effects** *Effects on the bone marrow, causing:* • Lowered immunity • Tiredness and/or breathlessness • Bruising and bleeding *Effects on digestive system:* • Nausea • Loss of appetite • Diarrhoea or constipation • Mucositis • Taste changes *Effects on the skin or hair:* • Rashes, changes to skin colour, increased sensitivity to sunlight or chlorine in a swimming pool • Hair loss *Other effects:* • Kidney, liver or heart damage • Behavioural changes **Long-term side effects** • Delayed puberty • Infertility • Alterations to workings of lung and heart • Certain types of chemotherapy can affect the kidneys • Secondary cancer • Possible delayed cognitive development with some drugs

<table>
<tr><th>Treatment</th><th colspan="2">Side effects</th></tr>
<tr><td rowspan="23">Radiotherapy</td><td colspan="2">Short-term side effects</td></tr>
<tr><td>• Tiredness</td><td>• Possible change in appetite</td></tr>
<tr><td>• Skin sensitive to sun</td><td>• Altered blood counts</td></tr>
<tr><td colspan="2">• Possible skin changes (soreness and redness)</td></tr>
<tr><td colspan="2">Specific side effects vary according to the site of radiotherapy:</td></tr>
<tr><td colspan="2">Abdomen:</td></tr>
<tr><td>• Diarrhoea</td><td>• Weight loss</td></tr>
<tr><td>• Nausea</td><td>• Pain while passing urine</td></tr>
<tr><td>• Poor appetite</td><td>• Infertility</td></tr>
<tr><td colspan="2">Chest area:</td></tr>
<tr><td>• Swallowing difficulties</td><td>• Nausea</td></tr>
<tr><td colspan="2">• Breathlessness</td></tr>
<tr><td colspan="2">• Affected growth and development</td></tr>
<tr><td colspan="2">Head and neck:</td></tr>
<tr><td>• Hair loss</td><td>• Drowsiness</td></tr>
<tr><td>• Tooth decay</td><td>• Taste changes</td></tr>
<tr><td>• Swallowing difficulties</td><td>• Endocrine difficulties</td></tr>
<tr><td colspan="2">• Possible asymmetrical development of neck muscles or asymmetry face</td></tr>
<tr><td colspan="2">Brain:</td></tr>
<tr><td colspan="2">• Cognitive and learning difficulties</td></tr>
<tr><td>• Somnolence</td><td>• Endocrine difficulties</td></tr>
<tr><td colspan="2">Long-term side effects</td></tr>
<tr><td>• Physical difficulties
• Delayed or early puberty
• Learning difficulties</td><td>• Growth problems
• Infertility</td></tr>
<tr><td>Surgery</td><td colspan="2">Side effects will vary according to the position of the cancer and the amount of tissue that needs to be removed.</td></tr>
<tr><td rowspan="5">Bone-marrow transplant (BMT)</td><td colspan="2">• Graft-versus-host disease (GvHD)</td></tr>
<tr><td>• High risk of infection</td><td>• Anaemia</td></tr>
<tr><td>• Increased risk of bleeding</td><td>• Graft-failure</td></tr>
<tr><td>• Venous occlusive disease</td><td>• Fatigue</td></tr>
<tr><td colspan="2">• Weight loss due to reduced appetite, sore mouth and diarrhoea</td></tr>
</table>

Appendix 5: Side effects of common chemotherapy drugs

This table highlights the many different side effects, some commonly seen, some less so, as a result of various chemotherapy drugs.

Drug name	Used to treat	Possible side effects
Amsacrine	Leukaemia	Tiredness, weakness, abdominal pain, cardiac dysfunction.
Busulfan	Chronic myeloid leukaemia	Raised levels of uric acid in the blood, changes to lungs, bladder irritation, temporary changes to liver, dizziness, blurred vision, confusion, secondary cancer, cataracts, fever, chills, fits or seizures.
Carboplatin	Non-Hodgkin's and Hodgkin's lymphoma and Chronic lymphoblastic leukaemia	Numbness/tingling in hands and feet, changes in hearing, kidneys temporarily effected.
Chlorambusil	Chronic lymphoblastic leukaemia, and Non-Hodgkin's and Hodgkin's lymphoma	Changes to lungs, skin changes, seizures, temporary effect on liver.
Cisplatin	Various	Kidneys may be affected, peripheral neuropathy, hearing changes.
Chlorafabine	Acute lymphoblastic leukaemia	Raised levels of uric acid in the blood, liver and kidney function temporarily affected, soreness and redness to the palms of the hands and soles of the feet, acute inflammatory response, headaches.
Crisantaspase	Acute lymphoblastic leukaemia	Changes in blood clotting, liver temporarily affected, allergic reaction, increase in blood-sugar level, reduced energy, fever/chills.
Cyclophosphamide	Chronic lymphoblastic leukaemia	Irritation of bladder lining, temporary changes to the liver, changes to nails.

Drug name	Used to treat	Possible side effects
Cytarabine	Acute myeloid leukaemia	Gritty eyes due to inflammation in the lining of the eyelids, lethargy, confusion, reduced balance, adverse effects on the nervous system (fits/ mood changes), flu-like symptoms, changes to lungs, sore palms of hands and soles of feet, temporary effect on liver function.
Dacarzabine	Hodgkin's lymphoma, soft-tissue sarcomas and melanoma	Flu-like effect, temporary changes to liver function, allergic reaction, sensitivity to sunlight.
Dactinomycine	Various	Dysphagia, fevers/chills, skin changes.
Daunorubicin	Acute lymphoblastic leukaemia and acute myeloid leukaemia	Sensitivity to sun, bruising, sore mouth, fatigue, weakness, taste changes.
Etoposide	Various	Long-term risk of secondary leukaemia.
Ifosomide	Various	Irritation to the bladder, changes in nails. Less common side effects include confusion, lethargy, and loss of balance.
Mercaptopurine	Acute leukaemias	Liver function temporarily affected, tiredness, weakness.
Methotrexate	Various	Gritty eyes, blurred vision, breathlessness, neuropsychological difficulties.
Mitomycin	Various	Possible breathlessness.
Teniposide	Leukaemias, lymphomas, neuroblastomas	Low blood pressure, dizziness, Long-term risk of secondary cancer.
Vinblastine	Leukaemias and lymphomas	Peripheral neuropathy.
Vincristine	Leukaemias and lymphomas	Peripheral neuropathy, abdominal cramps.

Please note that this list is not exhaustive and represents only commonly used chemotherapy drugs. New chemotherapy drugs may become available; however, more commonly it is the treatment protocols (rather than chemotherapy agents themselves) that are adapted following further research. Online resources outlined in the next section have up-to-date information about chemotherapy drugs used within paediatric oncology.

Appendix 6a: Surgical procedures and post-operative precautions for bone tumours[2]

Surgical procedures	Post-operative precautions
Proximal femoral replacements (PFR) Proximal third of femur is excised and replaced with a prosthesis	The following must be adhered to for at least three months: • No flexion > 80/90°. • No hip adduction beyond midline. • Avoid excessive hip rotation. • No anti-gravity abduction. • Full weight bearing (unless otherwise stated) with brace in situ. • Brace must be worn whenever out of bed (put on while in bed) unless otherwise stated.
Proximal tibial replacement (PTR) Proximal one-third to two-thirds of the tibia is excised and replaced with a massive prothesis. The patella tendon is attached to the prosthesis with a small amount of bone graft and clamped with a plate and screw.	For six weeks: • No active dynamic quadriceps (i.e. knee extension). • Full weight bearing (unless otherwise stated) with splint in situ. For a further six weeks: • No twisting of knee or kneeling.
Total femoral replacements (TFR) Entire femur is excised and replaced with massive prosthesis.	Must be adhered to for at least three months: • No flexion > 80/90°. • No hip adduction beyond midline. • No hip rotation. • No twisting the knee or kneeling. • No anti-gravity abduction. • Full weight bearing (unless otherwise stated) with brace in situ. • Brace must be worn whenever out of bed (put on while in bed) unless otherwise stated.

2 Adapted from and reproduced with kind thanks from the Royal National Orthopaedic Hospital NHS Trust Occupational Therapy Department.

Surgical procedures	Post-operative precautions
Hemipelvic replacements (HPR) Up to half the distal hemipelvis is excised and replaced with a prosthesis, incorporating an acetabular component which is secured into the remaining ilium, and a standard hip replacement or proximal femoral component.	Must be adhered to for at least three months: • No flexion $> 80/90^{\circ}$. • No hip adduction beyond midline. • No hip rotation. • No anti-gravity abduction. • Full weight bearing (unless otherwise stated) with brace in situ. • Brace must be worn whenever out of bed (put on while in bed) unless otherwise stated.
Excision of tumour of the ilium with strut bone grafting Up to half of the ilium is excised and replaced with two struts of bone taken from the fibula.	• No hip flexion $> 90^{\circ}$ for three months. • Mobilise shadow weight bearing for first six weeks, then partial weight bearing for the following six weeks (unless otherwise stated).
Massive proximal humeral replacement Proximal third of humerus is excised and replaced with a prosthesis.	• Polysling to support the arm for six weeks. • No external rotation beyond neutral for the first six weeks. • Assisted shoulder movements from day five. • Active shoulder movements from week three.

Appendix 6b: Occupational therapy intervention for children and young people with bone tumours[3]

Acute occupational therapy intervention following surgery:

Occupational therapy aims:

- Enhance outcome of surgical intervention.
- Where indicated as a risk, to reduce the risk of dislocation.
- To optimise function, independence and quality of life.
- In instances where independence is not achieved, to ensure that there is adequate support to optimise safety in the home during post-operative period.

Surgical aims:

- To excise tumour in order to prevent or slow the spread of disease.
- To spare the limb, rather than proceed to amputation.
- To restore or maintain mobility and function.

Potential post-operative complications to be aware of:

- Dislocation.
- Infection.
- Nerve damage.
- Reduced range of movement.
- Oedema/haematoma.
- Leg length discrepancy.
- Deep vein thrombosis.
- Recurrence of tumour.

Occupational therapy intervention will include:

- Initial interview (pre-operative where appropriate).
- Functional assessment of ADL (activities of daily living) needs and transfers following surgery.
- Advice to child, young person and their carers with regard to post-surgical precautions and impact upon daily activities.
- Referral to outside agencies, i.e. local authority occupational therapists, for provision of ADL equipment or wheelchair services for provision of wheelchairs or major buggies.
- Risk assessment for safety in home and school environments and within the community.
- Liaison with interested parties such as school teachers, principal oncology centre occupational therapists, etc.

[3] Adapted from and reproduced with kind thanks from the Royal National Orthopaedic Hospital NHS Trust Occupational Therapy Department.

Occupational therapy outcome measures:

- Child or young person will be independent in appropriate personal care activities (with or without adaptive equipment) or provision made for assistance with personal care needs on discharge from hospital.
- Child or young person will be independent and safe in all relevant functional transfers (with or without adaptive equipment) or provision made for assistance with this on discharge from hospital.
- The child or young person and their carers will receive relevant advice sheets and have a good understanding of post-operative precautions.
- Risks will have been identified, assessed and managed as far as is reasonably practicable.
- Where indicated, referrals to outside agencies will be made in a timely manner.

Evaluation of service:
The acute occupational therapy service to children and young people with bone tumours following surgery will be evaluated through staff supervision and regular audit in line with trust and department clinical governance policies and procedures.

Further resources

Online resources

Association of Children's Hospices: http://www.childhospice.org.uk

Cancer Back Up: http://www.macmillan.org.uk

Cancer Research UK: http://www.cancerresearch.org.uk

Children's Cancer and Leukemia Group: http://www.cclg.org.uk

CLIC Sargent: http://www.clicsargent.org.uk

Institute of Cancer Research: http://www.icr.ac.uk

International Children's Palliative Care Network: http://www.icpcn.org.uk

National Cancer Institute: http://www.cancer.gov

Teenage Cancer Trust: http://www.teenagecancertrust.org

Teenagers and Young Adults with Cancer: http://www.tyac.org.uk

TIC (Teen Info on Cancer): http://www.click4tic.org.uk

(All websites accessed on 08.02.10.)

Policies, guidelines and guidance

Department of Health

Department of Health (2008) *Better care: better lives: improving outcomes and experiences for children, young people and their living with life-limiting and life threatening conditions*. London: DH. Available at: *http://www.dh.gov.uk/en/Publicationsandstatistics/Publications/PublicationsPolicyAndGuidance/DH_083106* Accessed on 08.02.10.

Department of Health (2007) *Cancer reform strategy*. London: DH.

Department of Health (2005) *Commissioning children and young people's palliative care services: a practical guide for the NHS commissioners*. London: DH.

Department of Health and Department for Education and Skills (2004) *National service framework for children, young people and maternity services: core standards.* London: DH.

National Institute for Health and Clinical Excellence

National Institute for Health and Clinical Excellence (2005) *Guidance on cancer services: improving outcomes in children and young people with cancer*. London: NICE.

Scottish Intercollegiate Guidelines Network

Scottish Intercollegiate Guidelines Network (2008) *Control of pain in adults with cancer: a national clinical guideline.* Edinburgh: SIGN. Available at: *http://www.sign.ac.uk/pdf/SIGN106.pdf* Accessed on 08.02.10.

The National Comprehensive Cancer Network

The National Comprehensive Cancer Network (2009) *Clinical practice guidelines in oncology: cancer-related fatigue*. Fort Washington, PA: NCCN. Available at: *http://www.nccn.org/professionals/physician_gls/PDF/fatigue.pdf* Accessed on 08.02.10.

The National Comprehensive Cancer Network (2007) *Clinical practice guidelines in oncology: pediatric cancer pain.* Fort Washington, PA: NCCN. Available at: *http://www.nccn.org/professionals/physician_gls/PDF/pediatric_pain.pdf* Accessed on 08.02.10.

International Children's Palliative Care Network

International Children's Palliative Care Network (2008) *The ICPCN charter of rights for life limited and life threatened children*. Pinelands, SA: International Children's Palliative Care Network. Available at: *http://www.icpcn.org.uk/page.asp?section=0001000100014&sectionTitle=Charter* Accessed on 08.02.10.

References

American Thoracic Society (1999) Dyspnea: mechanisms, assessment and management: a consensus statement. *American Journal of Respiratory Critical Care Medicine, 159(1),* 321–340.

Association for Children with Life-threatening and Terminal Conditions and their Families (ACT) and the Royal College of Paediatrics and Child Health (RCPCH) (2003) *A guide to the development of children's palliative care services.* 2nd ed. Bristol and London: ACT.

Association for Children's Palliative Care (ACT) (2007) *Palliative care services for children and young people in England: an independent review for the Secretary of State for Health.* London: Department of Health.

Ayres AJ (1979) *Sensory integration and the child.* Los Angeles: Western Psychological Services.

Barsevick AM (2002) Energy conservation and cancer-related fatigue. *Rehabilitation Oncology, 20(3),* 14–17.

Barsevick AM, Dudley W, Beck S, Sweeney C, Whitmer K, Nail L (2004) A randomised clinical trial of energy conservation for patients with cancer-related fatigue. *Cancer, 100(6),* 1302–1310.

Berde CB, Billett AL, Collins JJ (2005) Symptom management in supportive care. In: PA Pizzo, DG Poplack, eds. *Principles and practice of pediatric oncology.* 5th ed. Philadelphia, PA: Lippincott Williams & Wilkins. 1348–1379.

Bion W (1984) *Second thoughts: selected papers on psycho-analysis.* London: Karnac Books.

Boog K (2008) Using guided imagery as a relaxation technique for self-help. In: K Boog, CY Tester, eds. *Palliative care: a practical guide for the health professional.* London: Elsevier. 121–134.

Boog K, Tester CY (2008) *Palliative care: a practical guide for the health professional.* London: Elsevier.

Bowlby J (1997) *Attachment and loss.* 2nd ed. London: Pimlico.

Cancer Research (2005) Childhood cancer statistics: mortality. Available at: http://info.cancerresearchuk.org/cancerstats/childhoodcancer/mortality/index.htm. Accessed on 27.04.09.

Carr J, Finlay P, Pearson D, Thompson K, White H (2008) Multi-professional management of patients with neurological tumours and associated conditions. In: J Rankin, K Robb, N Murtagh, J Cooper, S Lewis, eds. *Rehabilitation in cancer care.* London: Blackwell Publishing. 88–112.

Case-Smith J (2001) An overview of occupational therapy for children. In: J Case-Smith, ed. *Occupational therapy for children.* St Louis, MO: Mosby. 2–20.

Case-Smith J, Rogers J, Johnson JH (2001) School-based occupational therapy. In: J Case-Smith. *Occupational therapy for children*. St Louis, MO: Mosby. 757–779.

Cooper J (2006a) Occupational therapy approach in symptom control. In: J Cooper, ed. *Occupational therapy in oncology and palliative care*. 2nd ed. Chichester: Wiley. 27–39.

Cooper J (2006b) Occupational therapy approach in the management of breathlessness. In: J Cooper, ed. *Occupational therapy in oncology and palliative care*. 2nd ed. Chichester: Wiley. 52–60.

Cooper J (2006c) Occupational therapy in anxiety management and relaxation. In: J Cooper, ed. *Occupational therapy in oncology and palliative care.* 2nd ed. Chichester: Wiley. 41–50.

Creek J (2003) *Occupational therapy defined as a complex intervention.* London: College of Occupational Therapists.

Davidson JR, Maclean AW, Brundage MD, Schulze K (2002) Sleep disturbance in cancer patients. *Social Science and Medicine, 54(9),* 1309–1321.

De Lisa JA (2001) A history of cancer rehabilitation. *Cancer, 92(4),* 970–974.

Department for Education and Skills (2001) *Access to education for children and young people with medical needs.* London: DfES. Available at: *http://publications.dcsf.gov.uk/eOrderingDownload/DFES-0732-2001.pdf* Accessed on 08.02.10.

Department of Health (2005) *Commissioning children and young people's palliative care services: a practical guide for the NHS commissioners*. London: DH.

Department of Health (2006) *Transition: getting it right for young people. Improving the transition of young people with long term conditions from children's to adult health services.* London: Department of Health. Available at: *http://www.dh.gov.uk/en/Publicationsandstatistics/Publications/PublicationsPolicyAndGuidance/DH_4132145* Accessed on 08.02.10.

Department of Health (2007) *Cancer reform strategy*. London: DH.

Department of Health (2008) *Better care: better lives: improving outcomes and experiences for children, young people and their living with life-limiting and life threatening conditions*. London: DH. Available at: *http://www.dh.gov.uk/en/Publicationsandstatistics/Publications/PublicationsPolicyAndGuidance/DH_083106* Accessed on 08.02.10

Department of Health and Department for Education and Skills (2004) *National service framework for children, young people and maternity services: core standards.* London: DH.

Diamantis AD (2008) Use of assessment methods in paediatrics: the practice of private occupational therapists. *British Journal of Occupational Therapy, 71(12),* 524–530.

Dimeo FC, Thomas F, Raabe-Menssen C, Pröpper F, Mathias M (2004) Effect of aerobic exercise and relaxation training on fatigue and physical performance of cancer patients after surgery: a randomised controlled trial. *Supportive Care in Cancer, 11(12),* 774–778.

Dixon-Woods M, Young B, Heney D (2005) *Rethinking experiences of childhood cancer: a multidisciplinary approach to chronic childhood illness*. London: Open University Press.

Dudgeon B (2001) Pediatric rehabilitation. In: J Case-Smith, ed. *Occupational therapy for children.* St Louis, MO: Mosby. 843–863.

Easton C (2009) Living beyond cancer. *Contact, 42,*10.

Egilson S, Hemmingsson S (2009) School participation of pupils with physical and psychosocial limitations: a comparison. *British Journal of Occupational Therapy, 72(4),* 144–152.

Erickson JM (2004) Fatigue in adolescents with cancer: a review of the literature. *Clinical Journal of Oncology Nursing, 8(2),* 139–145.

Fisher S, Lowrie D (2008) Dyspnoea/ breathlessness management. In: J Rankin, K Robb, N Murtagh, J Cooper, S Lewis, eds. *Rehabilitation in cancer care*. London: Blackwell Publishing. 302–318.

Gerald M, Rosen MD (2007) Sleep in children who have cancer. *Sleep Medicine Clinics, 2(3),* 491–500.

Grinyer A (2002) *Cancer in young adults: through parents' eyes*. Buckinghamshire: Open University Press.

Grinyer A (2007) *Young people living with cancer: implications for policy and practice.* London: Open University Press.

Harding R (2000) The impact of diagnosis. In: H Langton, ed. *The child with cancer: family-centred care in practice*. Edinburgh: Bailliere Tindall. 37–78.

Hearn L, Higginson IJ (1997) Outcome measures in palliative care for advanced cancer patients: a review. *Journal of Public Health Medicine, 19(2),* 193–199.

Hedstrom M, Skolin I, Essen L (2004) Distressing and positive experiences and important aspects for adolescents treated for cancer: adolescent and nurse perceptions. *European Journal of Oncology Nursing, 8(1),* 6–17.

Hinds PS, Quargnenti A, Bush AJ, Pratt CB, Fairclough D, Rissmiller G, Betcher D, Gilchrist GS (2000) An evaluation of the impact of a self-care coping intervention on psychological and clinical outcomes in adolescents with newly diagnosed cancer. *European Journal of Oncology Nursing, 4(1),* 6–17.

Hockenberry M, Hooke MC (2007) Symptom clusters in children with cancer. *Seminars in Oncology Nursing, 23(2),* 152–157.

Hollis R, Morgan S (2001) The adolescent with cancer: at the edge of no-man's land. *The Lancet Oncology, 2(1),* 43–48.

International Children's Palliative Care Network (2008) *The ICPCN charter of rights for life limited and life threatened children*. Pinelands, SA: International Children's Palliative Care Network. Available at: *http://www.icpcn.org.uk/page.asp?section=000100010014&sectionTitle=Charter* Accessed on 08.02.10.

Jackson AC, Enderby K, O'Toole M, Thomas S, Ashley D, Rosenfield JV, Simos E, Tokatlian N, Gedye R (2009) The role of social support in families coping with childhood brain tumour. *Journal of Psychological Oncology, 27(1),* 1–24.

Jakel P (2002) Patient communication and strategies for managing fatigue. *Oncology, 16(9),* 141–145.

Kelly D (2008) The physical and emotional impact of cancer in adolescents and young adults. In: D Kelly, F Gibson, eds. *Cancer care for adolescents and young adults: care and policy issues*. London: Blackwell Publishing. 3–12.

Kirkova J, Walsh D (2007) Cancer symptom clusters: a dynamic construct. *Support Care Cancer, 15(9),* 1011–1013.

Kramer J, Bowyer P, O'Brien J, Kielhofner G, Maziero-Barbosa V (2009) How interdisciplinary pediatric practitioners choose assessments. *Canadian Journal of Occupational Therapy, 76(1),* 56–64.

Lacasse C, Beck SL (2007) Clinical assessment of symptom clusters. *Seminars in Oncology Nursing, 23(2),* 106–112.

Lewis I (2005) Patterns of care for teenagers and young people with cancer: is there a single blueprint of care? In: TOB Eden, RD Barr, A Bleyer, M Whiteson, eds. *Cancer and the adolescent*. Oxford: Blackwell. 241–258.

Lin KC, Wu CY, Tickle-Degnen L, Coster W (1997) Enhancing occupational performance through occupationally embedded exercise: a meta-analytic review. *Occupational Therapy Journal of Research, 17(1),* 25–47.

Lowrie D (2006) Occupational therapy and cancer-related fatigue. In: J Cooper, ed. *Occupational therapy in oncology and palliative care.* 2nd ed. Chichester: Wiley. 61–81.

Luebbert K, Dahme B, Hasenbring M (2001) The effectiveness of relaxation training in reducing treatment related symptoms and improving emotional adjustment in acute non-surgical cancer treatment: a meta-analytical review. *Psycho-Oncology,10(6),* 490–502.

McCaffrey CN (2006) Major stressors and their effects on the wellbeing of children with cancer. *Journal of Pediatric Nursing, 21(1),* 59–66.

Michaud LJ, Ried SR, McMahon MA, Pruitt DW (2005) Rehabilitation of the child with cancer. In: PA Pizzo, DG Poplack, eds. *Principles and practice of pediatric oncology*. 5th ed. Philadelphia, PA: Lippincott Williams & Wilkins. 1399–1413.

Miller J, Barrett R, Canning P, Taggart S, Young V (2008) Multi-professional management within haemato-oncology. In: J Rankin, K Robb, N Murtagh, J Cooper, S Lewis, eds. *Rehabilitation in cancer care.* London: Blackwell Publishing. 113–131.

Miller J, Hopkinson C (2008) A retrospective audit exploring the use of relaxation as an intervention in oncology and palliative care. *European Journal of Cancer Care, 17(5),* 488–491.

Mock V (2004) Evidence-based treatment for cancer-related fatigue. *Journal of National Cancer Institute Monographs, 32,* 112–118.

Mooney-Doyle K (2006) An examination of fatigue in advanced childhood cancer. *Journal of Pediatric Oncology Nursing, 23(6),* 305–310.

Moore JB, Kaffenberger C, Goldberg P, Oh KM, Hudspeth R (2009) School reentry for children with cancer: perceptions of nurses, school personnel and parents. *Journal of Pediatric Oncology Nursing, 26(2),* 86–99.

National Comprehensive Cancer Network (2009) *Clinical practice guidelines in oncology: cancer-related fatigue*. Fort Washington, PA: NCCN. Available at: *http://www.nccn.org/professionals/physician_gls/PDF/fatigue.pdf* Accessed on 08.02.10.

National Institute for Health and Clinical Excellence (2005) *Guidance on cancer services: improving outcomes in children and young people with cancer*. London: NICE.

Neville KL (2000) *Mature beyond their years: the impact of cancer on adolescent development.* Pittsburgh, PA: Oncology Nursing Press.

Obholzer A, Zagier-Roberts V (2002) *The unconscious at work*. London: Routledge.

Ogilvy C, Livingstone K, Prue G (2008) Management of cancer related fatigue. In: J Rankin, K Robb, N Murtagh, J Cooper, S Lewis, eds. *Rehabilitation in cancer care.* London: Blackwell Publishing. 264–279.

Palmer L, Erickson S, Shaffer T, Koopman C, Amylon M, Steiner H (2000) Themes arising in group therapy for adolescents with cancer and their parents. *International Journal of Rehabilitation and Health, 1(5),* 43–54.

Palmer S, Mitchell A, Thompson K, Sexton M (2007) Unmet needs among adolescent cancer patients: a pilot study. *Palliative and Supportive Care, 5(2),* 127–134.

Payne RA (2000) *Relaxation techniques: a practical handbook for the health care professional.* London: Churchill Livingstone.

Petersen-Broyd B, DeJong M, Peacock S, Hargrave D (2006) *Returning to school: a teacher's guide for pupils with brain tumours.* Carmarthen: Cerebra; Sutton: Royal Marsden Hospital NHS Trust. Available at: *http://www.royalmarsden.org.uk/NR/rdonlyres/AE5D4366-80F7-454F-83C0-AE3FD4FC103D/0/ReturningtoSchool.pdf* Accessed on 08.02.10.

Petersen-Broyd B, Pritchard-Jones K, Edwards L (2008) *Pupils with cancer: a guide for teachers.* Carmarthen: Cerebra. Available at: *http://www.royalmarsden.nhs.uk/NR/rdonlyres/64E8B14B-5E7E-4025-BF64-476898A5B211/3251/RMHSSATbrochureAW.pdf* Accessed on 23.04.09.

Prevatt FF, Heffer RW, Lowe PA (2000) A review of school reintegration programs for children with cancer. *Journal of School Psychology, 38(5),* 447–467.

Purcell A, Fleming J, Haines T, Bennett S (2009) Cancer-related fatigue: a review and a conceptual framework to guide therapists' understanding. *British Journal of Occupational Therapy, 77(2),* 79–86.

Ramini SK, Brown R, Buckner E (2008) Embracing changes: adaptation by adolescents with cancer. *Pediatric Nursing, 34(1),* 72–79.

Ream E, Browne N, Glaus A, Knipping C, Frei IA (2003) Quality and efficiency of educational materials on cancer-related fatigue: views of patients from two European countries. *European Journal of Oncology Nursing, 7(2),* 99–109.

Richards L, Denning M, Lindsell G (2008) Multi-professional management of musculoskeletal tumours. In: J Rankin, K Robb, N Murtagh, J Cooper, S Lewis, eds. *Rehabilitation in cancer care*. London: Blackwell Publishing. 158–183.

Richardson P (2001) Use of standardized tests in pediatric practice. In: J Case-Smith, ed. *Occupational therapy for children*. St Louis, MO: Mosby. 217–245.

Robb K, Ewer-Smith C (2008) Cancer pain. In: J Rankin, K Robb, N Murtagh, J Cooper, S Lewis, eds. *Rehabilitation in cancer care*. London: Blackwell Publishing. 280–301.

Ruland CM, Hamilton RN, Schjodt-Osmo B (2009) The complexity of symptoms and problems experienced in children with cancer: a review of the literature. *Journal of Pain and Symptom Management, 37(3),* 403–418.

Sahler OJZ, Hunter MBC, Liesvel JL (2003) The effect of using music therapy with relaxation therapy in the management of patients undergoing bone marrow transplantation: a pilot feasibility study. *Alternative Therapies in Health and Medicine, 9(6),* 70–74.

Saunders C (1967) *The management of terminal illness.* London: Hospital Medical Publication.

Scottish Intercollegiate Guidelines Network (2008) *Control of pain in adults with cancer: a national clinical guideline.* Edinburgh: SIGN. Available at: *http://www.sign.ac.uk/pdf/SIGN106.pdf* Accessed on 08.02.10.

Sepion B (2009) Communication with children and young people. In: L Coles, LL Childs, BA Marjoram, eds. *Essential skills clusters for nurses: theory for practice*. London: Blackwell Publishing. 19–28.

Shepherd J (2001) Self-care and adaptations for independent living. In: J Case-Smith, ed. *Occupational therapy for children.* St Louis. MO: Mosby. 489–527.

Slade A (2000) Impact of treatment on the family. In: H Langton, ed. *The child with cancer: family-centred care in practice*. Edinburgh: Bailliere Tindall. 105–139.

Sugden C (2001) Total pain: a multidisciplinary approach. *Scottish Journal of Healthcare Chaplaincy, 4(2),* 2–7.

Syrjala KL, Donaldson GW, Davis MW, Kippes ME, Carr JE (1995) Relaxation and imagery and cognitive-behavioral training reduce pain during cancer treatment: a controlled clinical trial. *Pain, 63(2),* 189–198.

Tester C (2006) Occupational therapy in paediatric oncology and palliative care. In: J Cooper, ed. *Occupational therapy in oncology and palliative care*. 2nd ed. Chichester: Wiley. 107–124.

Tester C (2008) Play and leisure. In: KM Boog, CY Tester, eds. *Palliative care: a practical guide for the health professional.* Edinburgh: Churchill Livingstone. 105–120.

Thomas E, Weiss S (2000) Non-pharmacological interventions with chronic cancer pain in adults. *Cancer Control, 7(2),* 157–164.

Tobias J, Eaton K (2001) *Living with cancer*. London: Bloomsbury.

Townley M, Welton S (2000) Coping mechanisms. In: H Langton, ed. *The child with cancer: family-centred care in practice*. Edinburgh: Bailliere Tindall. 179–209.

Trapp A (1998) Support for the family. In: A Goldman, ed. *Care of the dying child.* Oxford: Oxford University Press. 76–92.

Vance YH, Eiser C (2002) The school experience of the child with cancer. *Child: Care, Health and Development, 28(1),* 5–19.

Walker LG, Walker MB, Ogston K, Heys SD, Ah-See AK, Miller ID, Hutcheon AW, Sarkar TK, Eremin O (1999) Psychological, clinical and pathological effects of relaxation training and guided imagery during primary chemotherapy. *British Journal of Cancer, 80(1/2),* 262–268.

Wavrek BM (2001) Hospital services. In: J Case-Smith, ed. *Occupational therapy for children.* St Louis, MO: Mosby. 807–822.

Whelan J, Dolbear C, Mak V, Moller H, Davies E (2007) Where do teenagers and young adults receive treatment for cancer? *Journal of Public Health, 29(2),* 178–182.

World Health Organization (2001) *International classification of functioning, disability and health (ICF)*. Geneva: WHO.

World Health Organization (2007) *Cancer control knowledge into action: palliative care*. Geneva: WHO. Available at: *http://whqlibdoc.who.int/publications/2007/9789241547345_eng.pdf* Accessed on 08.02.10.

Wray J, Sensky T (1999) Controlled study of pre-school development after surgery for congenital heart disease. *Archives of Disease in Childhood, 80(6),* 511–516.

其二

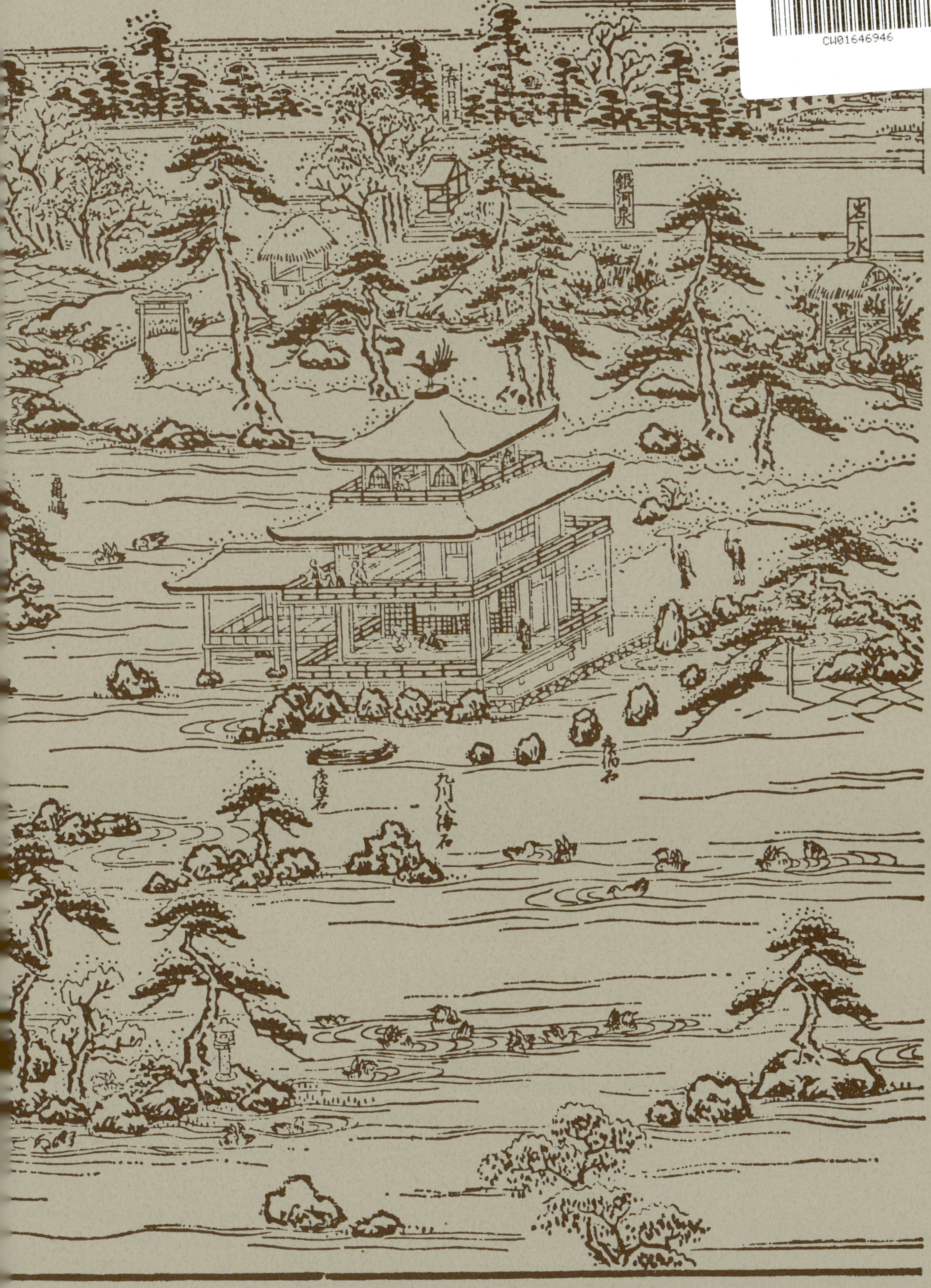

THE GARDEN AS ARCHITECTURE

THE GARDEN AS ARCHITECTURE

Form and Spirit in the Gardens of Japan, China, and Korea

Toshirō Inaji

Translated and adapted by
Pamela Virgilio

KODANSHA INTERNATIONAL
Tokyo • New York • London

NOTE: Names are given in the traditional manner, surname preceding given name. Macrons are used on all Japanese terms except place names.

JACKET PHOTOGRAPHS

Front
JAPAN—Shisendō, Kyoto.

Back (above)
CHINA—Ge yuan, Yangzhou.

Back (below)
KOREA—Kyŏngbokkung, Seoul.

Originally published as *Teien to jūkyo no ariyō to misekata, miekata: nihon, chūgoku, kankoku.* Tokyo: Sankaidō, 1990.

Distributed in the United States by Kodansha America, Inc., 114 Fifth Avenue, New York, New York 10011, and in the United Kingdom and continental Europe by Kodansha Europe Ltd., 95 Aldwych, London WC2B 4JF.

Published by Kodansha International, Ltd., 17–14 Otowa 1-chome, Bunkyo-ku, Tokyo 112-8652, and Kodansha America, Inc.

First edition, 1998
98 99 00 01 02 10 9 8 7 6 5 4 3 2 1

ISBN 4-7700-1712-X

Library of Congress CIP data available

Contents

Preface viii

JAPAN

1 Early Prototypes and Interpretive Approaches 3

City Plan Prototype and Interpretation: Changan and Heian-kyō 6

Shinden-Zukuri Architecture: Symmetrical Prototype, Simplified Interpretations 10

The Abandonment of Symmetry 10

Architectural Design Solutions That Address Spatial Constraints 12

Prototypes and Interpretations in *Shinden-Zukuri* Gardens 13

The Six Basic Elements of Garden Composition 17

The Design Process: Stylized Forms (*Yō*) and Modeling After (*Manabi*) 22

Garden Design Solutions That Address Spatial Constraints 25

The Garden As Architecture 29

2 *Shinden-Zukuri* As Prototype, and Two Divergent Interpretations 32

From Abbreviation to Abstraction 34

Ke and the North Garden 34

Hare and the South Garden 38

Decorative Arrangement of the *Shoin-Zukuri Jōdan Zashiki* 49

Shoin-Zukuri Gardens and Kanō-School Wall Paintings 55

The Threshold of the Garden As Architecture 58

3 Kinetic, Multifaceted Gardens and *Miegakure* 61

Miegakure Linking Qualitatively Similar Garden Areas 62

Combined *Shoin*/*Sukiya*/*Sōan* Structures: *Miegakure* Linking Qualitatively Distinct Buildings and Gardens 68

The Stroll Garden: *Miegakure* Linking Qualitatively Different Garden Areas 74

CHINA

4 Coexisting "Unworldly" and "Mundane" Worlds 83

Traditional Chinese Dwellings 83

Hall and Courtyard Composition 83

Climatic Influences 90

Lifestyle: Hierarchal Private/Communal Composition 91

Contemporary Housing: Single-Family Style 100

Courtyards (*Ting*) Versus Gardens 100

5 Spatial Composition of the Unworldly 103

Ting Yuan, Prototype of the *Yuanlin* 103

Garden-Related Terminology 106

An Outline of the History of Chinese Gardens 106

The Garden Treatise *Yuan Ye* 108

Private *Yuanlin*: Compositional Techniques 110

6 Ideology and Prototypes 119

Confucian Thought and Social Structure 119

Prototype of *Ting Yuan* and *Yuanlin*—Chinese Landscape Painting Theory 120

Hierarchical Dwelling Composition 127

The "Mundane" and the "Unworldly" 127

KOREA

7 Traditional Korean Residences and Their Gardens 131

Influences on the Composition of Traditional Korean Residences 132

Location: Factors Based on the Geomantic Principles of *P'ungsu* 132

Social Status: Factors Based on the Traditional Hierarchical Class System 134
Social Mores: Factors Based on Confucian Principles 137
Function: Factors Based on the *Ondol* System of Heating 143
Locality: Factors Related to the Dwelling's Locale (Urban Versus Rural) 149
Ch'ae and *Madang*: Combined Interior and Exterior Spaces 150
Comparison of Korean with Chinese and Japanese Residences 158

8 The "Uncultivated" Garden 160

Defining the Korean Approach to Garden Making 160
Borrowed Scenery Versus Prospect 163
Prospect and Borrowed Scenery in the Composition of Residences 164
Twitmadang (Rear Garden)—A Private Exterior Space 166
Outer Gardens—The Traditional Form Presented to the Outside World 173
The *Pyŏlsŏ* Environment 178
Korean Garden Forms 184

Notes 186
Chronology of Historical Periods in Japan, China, and Korea 188
Glossary 189
Selected References 196
Acknowledgments 199
Index 200

Preface

I have been studying traditional Japanese dwellings (*minka*) since 1962, particularly in the Kansai, Chūbu, and Tōhoku regions, and have continued to follow the transformations in these homes with great interest over the years. My motivation was very simple—I was interested in the question of why these buildings had survived in Japan. Were *minka* the only example of buildings that had retained their original wood-frame skeletal structure from their construction in the Edo period, through the Meiji and Taishō eras and the turbulent Shōwa period into postwar, modern Japan? And if so, why? My interest stemmed from a fundamental doubt about modern methods of designing and building homes, especially the methods used in multi-storied housing complexes, which are not designed with a mechanism to allow for later renovation.

While conducting successive field surveys of Japanese *minka* dwellings, I also began to look into the history of housing. The method which I used, of searching not only for the underlying structural framework but also its origins, inevitably led me to adopt another methodology—investigation of the historical background to the design of residences. It occurred to me that, by combining the results of these two different paths of investigation, I might be able to spark an "awareness about housing conditions."

My design survey initially focused on the "interactions and correlations between people, their possessions, and their homes." This inevitably resulted in my conducting thorough unit surveys of homes. The home is something that exists on the basis of the relationships between a person and the people around him, as well as the many others beyond them. Thus, it goes without saying that each home exists on the basis of its relationship with its immediate neighbors on either side and its more distant neighbors on either side of them.

In 1977, Tokyo University of Fine Arts and Music's Department of Design instituted a new course in environmental design, and I was chosen to be in charge of the lectures. One day, during the process of gathering materials for the course, it struck me that I was unaware of any research published on the relationship between interior design and exterior design—between, for example, a rural home and its garden, or a row of houses in a town and the street outside, or an abbot's quarters in a Zen temple and the garden adjacent. I hurriedly searched through my own limited library, but the books on architecture were concerned solely with buildings, and the books on gardens solely with gardens. I could not find a single plan or photo depicting the nature of the relationship between buildings and gardens.

With this, I decided to revisit the many residences and temples I had visited in the past. In spring, I was overwhelmed by the profusion of blossoms, and in summer everything was swathed in lush green. The season when the form of the gardens was revealed at its most distinct was in the depth of winter, when ice formed on ponds and the Zen temples extended an especially warm welcome to the unexpected early morning visitor. I went from place to place to see how gardens had been juxtaposed with *shoin* audience halls and abbot's quarters—both the rooms inside and their verandas—to try to understand the relation between the way the garden was seen and the way it was displayed.

Perhaps it is best to say a word here about an aspect of the Japanese design process—prototypes and their interpretations—that is critical to understanding the composition of Japanese gardens, so critical, in fact, that it is the basis upon which I have structured my research.

In general, creation is based on individual originality that is not subject to external constraints. But in the historical development of the Japanese arts, and particularly in the development of garden design, the existence of an "ideal form" takes precedence, thus originality and individuality manifest within a predetermined framework. The ideal form is a "conceptual prototype" that is divorced from a real, physical form.

The process that leads to the creator's "interpretation," or design solution, involves observing and recreating a model, regulated by site conditions and the intended functions of the space. Over time an endless variety of interpretations develop for a single prototype.

The prototype and corresponding interpretations found in the relationship between gardens and architecture also evolved with tremendous variety. Throughout most of Japanese garden history, gardens were intended purely for contemplation, to be viewed from a fixed vantage point seated at floor-level inside an adjoining building. (The stroll garden, which the viewer physically enters and moves through the space, is a relatively late development in the art.) Accordingly, the relationship between the seated view and garden composition are integrally linked, and changed in accordance with changes in the building's attributes, function and site conditions through the ages. This relationship is unparalleled in the history of gardens of other countries and perhaps the most important characteristic in the evolution of Japanese garden forms.

Differing ideological, political and economic conditions from period to period in Japanese history imposed new constraints on these interpretations, while the prototype remained essentially unchanged. Functional aspects of the architecture and garden along with site conditions and other constraints of a given period gave rise to "period" interpretations and led to the formation of "period garden types." When the techniques created to express these interpretations outlived the periods in which they first appeared, they came to be termed characteristically Japanese garden-making techniques.

The Japanese garden, which for the most part is not a place to stroll but a living picture to be viewed by people sitting inside a building, occupies a special place in the annals of world gardens. Indeed, its true significance is best understood if we consider it as part of a whole that also includes any paintings, pottery, flower arrangements, and other crafts displayed in the room from which the garden is viewed. Together they form a unified space. This is a unique characteristic without analogy anywhere else in the world.

The many papers which I wrote on these topics came to form the basis for the first section of this book, on Japan.

In 1984 and 1985, as a member of a group from the architecture and design departments of Tokyo National University of Fine Arts and Music, I participated in research trips to China to conduct surveys of housing mainly in Anhui and Jiangsu provinces, and of *ting yuan* and *yuanlin* gardens in Jiangsu and Zhejiang provinces. I returned in 1986 to survey the circular communal housing of the Hakka people centered in Fujian.

However as the saying goes, you can't say you've seen China until you go to Beijing, and without visiting the *siheyuan* residences which are the prototype for Chinese housing, or the magnificent gardens of the Imperial palaces, we felt we were missing a vital part of our survey. By complete coincidence, in June 1988, I was invited to lecture at the Beijing Central Polytechnic Institute of Fine Art, and spent forty days in Beijing. During that period, with the cooperation of the Institute, I was able to gather material on housing and gardens in and around Beijing, Chengde and Xian.

In the beginning, I had intended to study the relationship between Chinese gardens and buildings from the same perspective as I had applied to my earlier study in Japan, but my simplistic expectations were quickly thwarted. I discovered that, in China, the home and the garden are unrelated, and that the guiding rule is that a *yuanlin* garden is seen as a world apart, completely untouched by the "Confucian order" and the highly regimented form of the home. The *yuanlin*, on the other hand, is a world similar to the circumstances and spirit of Chinese landscape painting in which eternal time and infinite space are condensed. The various papers that I wrote during this period form the second section of this book, on China.

In 1986, I began a study of traditional Korean residences and gardens.

At first I was bewildered by what I saw in the site and floor plans of Korean dwellings. I think now that this was because I did not understand the unique "conditions" of Korean architectural environments and was, therefore, unable to read the plans in a meaningful way. So once again I started from the basics—that is, extracting the cultural factors that took on architectural form—in this case Korean geomantic beliefs, the hierarchical system of premodern Korean society, the social customs rooted in Confucianism, the functional constraints of the *ondol* system of floor heating, and the cross-influences between urban and rural customs, as well as the historical background surrounding these factors.

Armed with this understanding I made another visit to Korea, and this time I was made powerfully aware that these five basic factors, apart from the rapidly disappearing traditional class system and the Confucian mores of Chosŏn society, continue to hold great meaning in many situations today.

The composition of the main spaces of a traditional Korean residence—both home and garden— is extremely pure and simple. Some people say there are no real gardens in Korea, at least not as we understand the term. Nevertheless, there are, and for a long time have been, spaces that are structured—if vaguely—and that seek somehow to unify the inside and outside of a building with the world around it. I had been expecting to find a strong influence from the Chinese tradition of *yuanlin*, so it was refreshing to find something completely different. In Korea I experienced the joy of discovery. Comparing what I saw there with my many years of observing Japanese gardens, I simultaneously felt skeptical about what it means to cultivate a garden, and sorry that I had not studied Korea in greater depth earlier. Though close neighbors, we remain far apart in many ways. In the third section, on Korea, I outline four types of traditional Korean gardens.

Each of the three sections mentioned above merely sets out the relationship of homes to gardens in Japan, China, and Korea, respectively. They do not purport to be a comparative study.

I have taken the viewpoint that the relationship between Japan and China in the early period of import of ideas and objects from the continent was very much one of a weaker country borrowing the forms of a more powerful and developed one, and adapting those forms to a smaller space to produce something "native." In general, Korean culture seems closer to that of Japan, there being a sense that the two countries are separated by only a narrow strip of water, while the culture of China seems more removed, as if it came from the far western reaches of the continent. However, I still find it remarkable just how much the relationship between homes and gardens in each of these three neighboring countries differs according to their separate customs, histories, and lifestyles.

The design surveys I have conducted were intended to seek out new values and approaches to design through direct field research, and not through methodology alone. I believe that I always had some key antithesis at the root of my design surveys.

I carry out all my design surveys with design concepts as the starting point. By going out into the field, I am able to expand the horizons of my own limited experiences, and by objectifying my thoughts, I can construct design concepts. This is my method of concept formation. I approach each design survey as an "awareness activity" that forms the basis of "creative activity" in design work. This awareness comes from experience, observation, and deliberation, and is the springboard for creativity. We sometimes have a tendency to try to turn design survey results into design techniques. However, I am convinced that although the formation of concepts through improved awareness does not always lead directly to creative design, the best planning and design activity springs from concept formation based on such heightened awareness.

To me, design surveys are an extremely valuable means of concept development, since they are the springboard to posing a question and starting to form a hypothesis. The value of the research described in this publication as I see it, is to seek answers to the questions related to high-density urban housing in the modern world and how to create a more pleasant environment for urban residents.

My colleagues have given me great support in the preparation of this publication. I am indebted to Professors Mogi and Katayama for their advice and cooperation, and to the members of their respective laboratories, and the members of my own research lab at Tokyo National University of Fine Arts and Music, for their assistance in executing the many drawings for this publication, and for the additional assistance of the Chinese and Korean exchange students in my department in compiling materials—particularly Ms. Kim Hyonson and Ms. Shin Julee. I would like to take this opportunity to thank them all.

In conducting surveys and collecting research material I received invaluable assistance from many members of the Chinese Society of Architects in various regions, and from the staff of the Beijing Central Polytechnic Institute of Fine Arts, particularly Zhang Qi-man and Qi Ai-guo, associate professor and lecturer respectively at the same institution, with research and interpretation. I am grateful to the staff of the Graduate School of Environmental Studies at Seoul National University for making available many valuable materials, and for their kind guidance. I am also indebted to the Office of Cultural Properties for its cooperation in my visits to several important sites. My warmest thanks go out to the numerous people in China and Korea who cooperated in my research.

For their expertise and invaluable advice over the course of preparing the English text, I would like to thank Hugh Wylie and Wonyoung Koh of the Royal Ontario Museum, Lee Chi Woo of the Korea Cultural Service at the Embassy of the Republic of Korea in Tokyo, Alain Coulon, Kim Hyo Keun, Kirstin McIvor, and Edwin Whenmouth. I would also like to pay tribute to my editors Shigeyoshi Suzuki and Elizabeth Ogata at Kodansha International. And finally I would like to express my gratitude to Pamela Virgilio for her painstaking work in the translation and adaption of the Japanese text for the English-speaking reader—I trust her understanding of the material completely.

Japan

1

Early Prototypes and Interpretive Approaches

Mount Miwa in Yamato (present-day Nara Prefecture) is a sacred mountain, thought to be manifested spirit according to the indigenous animistic religious beliefs of Shintō. Pre-Nara–period Shintō (pre-645) focused on nature worship in sacred sites—roped-off clearings surrounding unusually-shaped mountains, trees, rocks, waterfalls and other natural phenomena. The present Ōmiwa Shrine at the base of Mount Miwa consists of only a *torii* gate marking the entrance to the sacred grounds and a *haiden*, or worship hall, reminiscent of the early Shintō sites which lacked an architectural structure to enshrine *kami*, or spirit (Figure 1).

Mount Miwa is covered with primeval forest, revered and untouched from protohistoric times. Roped-off areas of old cryptomeria trees and clusters of rocks designated as *himorogi* and *iwakura* respectively—trees and rocks inhabited by divine spirit—have the appearance of playgrounds or "gardens" for *kami*. These *iwakura* megaliths, whether left untouched as nature set them or artificially clustered to create ritual spaces, cannot really be called gardens, but their playful grouping is in close accord with the guidelines for "setting stones" in *Sakuteiki* (Notes on garden making), the earliest known written document on Japanese garden making:

> In the work of stone arrangement, you should first complete the placing of the principal stone having a distinct character, and then proceed to set other stones complying with the "requesting" mood of the principal stone ...
>
> The stones placed at the foot of the hill or in the hillside plain should resemble a pack of dogs crouching on the ground, or a running and scattering group of pigs, or else a calf playing nearby the seated mother cow.
>
> In general, for one or two "running away" stones there should be placed seven or eight "chasing" stones. Stones thus placed may resemble, for example, children playing tag.[1]

The arrangement of rocks on sacred Mount Miwa is not, of course, the rock composition of a garden. However, with the gradual rearrangement of natural clusters of stones, the ancestral form of the Japanese garden began to emerge (Figures 2.1–2.3). This concept of natural order had developed more than four hundred years before it was expressed in the mid–eleventh-century *Sakuteiki* as "... set[ting] other stones complying with the 'requesting' mood of the principal stone." Among the unique characteristics of

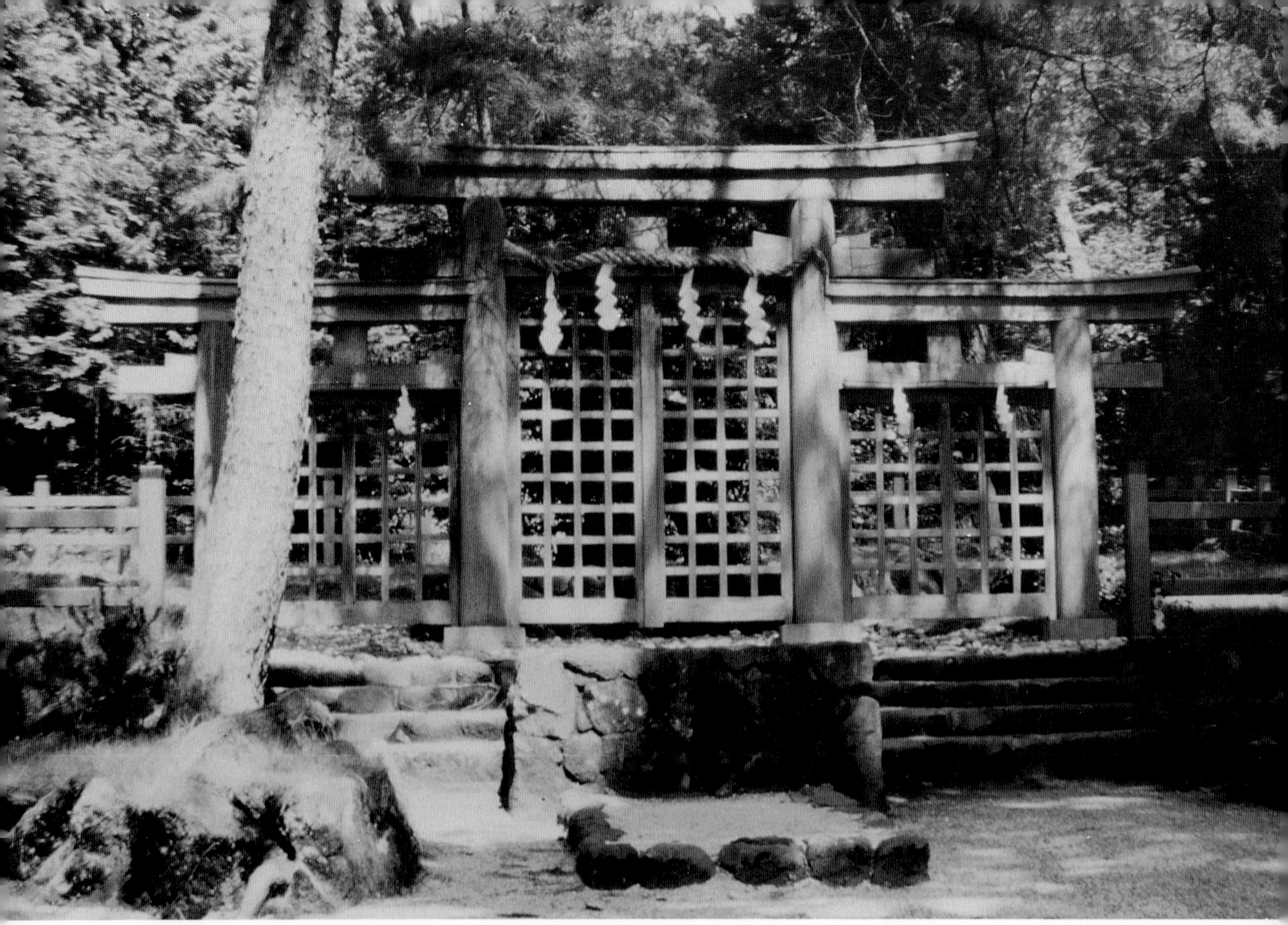

1 *Torii* gate at Ōmiwa Shrine, Mount Miwa, Nara Prefecture.

Japanese gardens, which this book will attempt to define, this concept forms the foundation of and is seminally linked to the historic development of garden making in Japan through the present day.

Attributed to Tachibana no Toshitsuna (A.D. 1028–1094), a Heian-period aristocrat accomplished in landscape garden design, *Sakuteiki* has long been regarded as a classic on the art of garden making. It is cited in virtually all studies of Japanese gardens written in Japan or abroad, and is itself the subject of numerous scholarly works. It is described in the introduction of one such book, by twentieth-century garden historian Tamura Tsuyoshi, as "... contain[ing] profoundly significant material, even when read today, regarding the basic structural techniques of Japanese gardens. One might even say it reveals the mysteries of the art of garden making."

Sakuteiki was written at the height of the first phase of refinement in the developmental process of the Japanese garden. Tamura describes this historical phase:

> There is no doubt that Japanese gardens broke away stylistically from Chinese gardens. From the late Nara period (A.D. 710–794) through the early Heian period (794–898) that which needed to be learned from Chinese gardens was ingested, and its nutritive value fully absorbed. In the late Heian period (898–1185) this was successfully developed into the Japanese garden.[2]

The assimilation phase in the process of adopting and then assimilating foreign elements, often cited as a basic factor in the formation of Japanese gardens, is documented in *Sakuteiki*. Most books fail to deal with the question of just what was acquired from the palaces and gardens created for China's vast open spaces and climate, which differ completely from the conditions in Japan. Neither do they describe in any detail how these imported forms were absorbed and transformed into the Japanese garden.

This chapter will examine the images inherited from

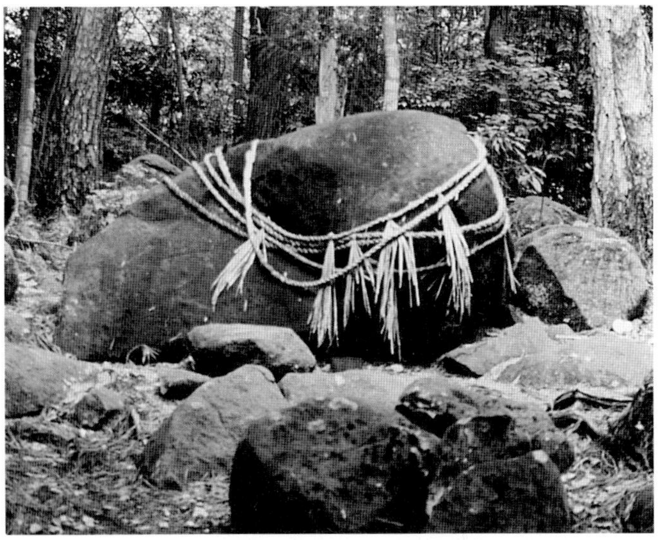

2.1 *Iwakura* on Mount Miwa.

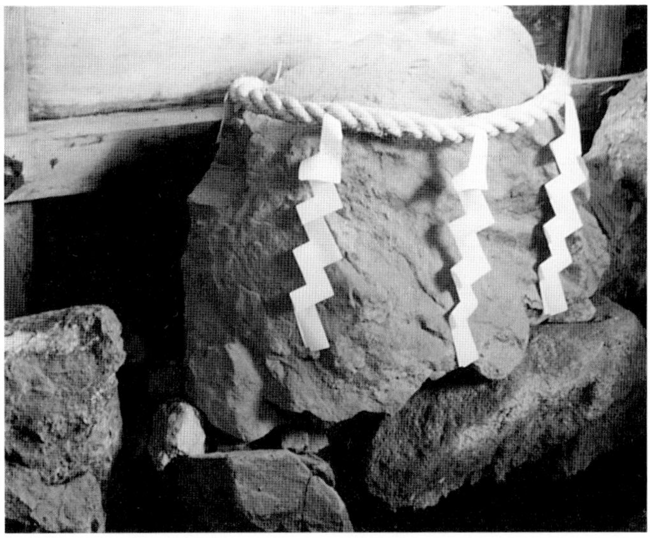

2.2 Stone arrangement at Onjōji Akai, Shiga Prefecture.

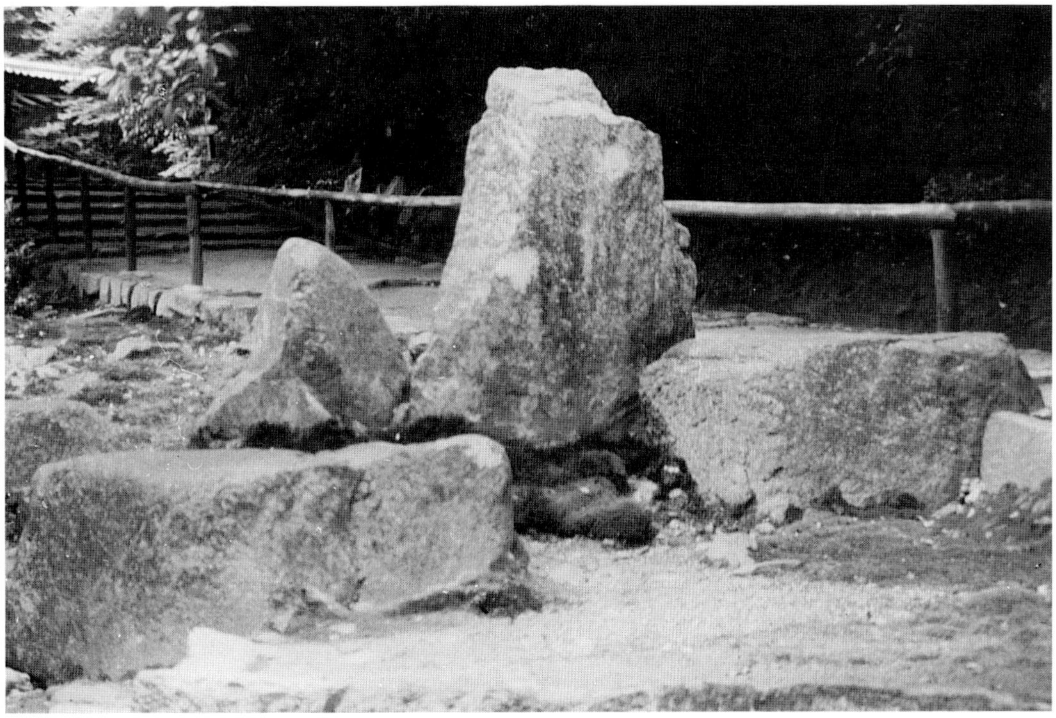

2.3 Stone arrangement near Onjōji Akai.

the Chinese cities, palaces, and gardens that gave rise to conceptual prototypes, as well as the relationship between the palatial buildings and gardens designed for a totally different space and climate—the interpretation at the ancient capital of Heian-kyō (present-day Kyoto).

Between the years A.D. 630 and 838, Japanese envoys made a total of fifteen trips to the Tang dynasty (A.D. 618–907) capital of Changan (present-day Xian). Each mission comprised 250 to 600 monks and aristocrats traveling on two to four ships. From the vast accumulation of information brought back by these envoys in the form of books, plans, paintings, and sundry documents, a capital was first constructed at Heijō-kyō (present-day Nara) on the model of Changan; it was later reconstructed at Heian-kyō.

An idealized configuration of the Chinese cities, palaces, and gardens was distilled into a design formula; thus an "ideal" original forms the prototype. Unlike a real, physical form, a conceptual prototype is not subject to scale. This prototype implemented in the context of Japanese spatial and climatic conditions gave rise to a variety of simplified interpretations. These interpretations are in no way a rejection of the formula, since in essence they adhere to the formula's framework, which is in part responsible for the tremendous degree of variety. Examination of these interpretations should make it possible to identify any uniquely Japanese methods of expression.

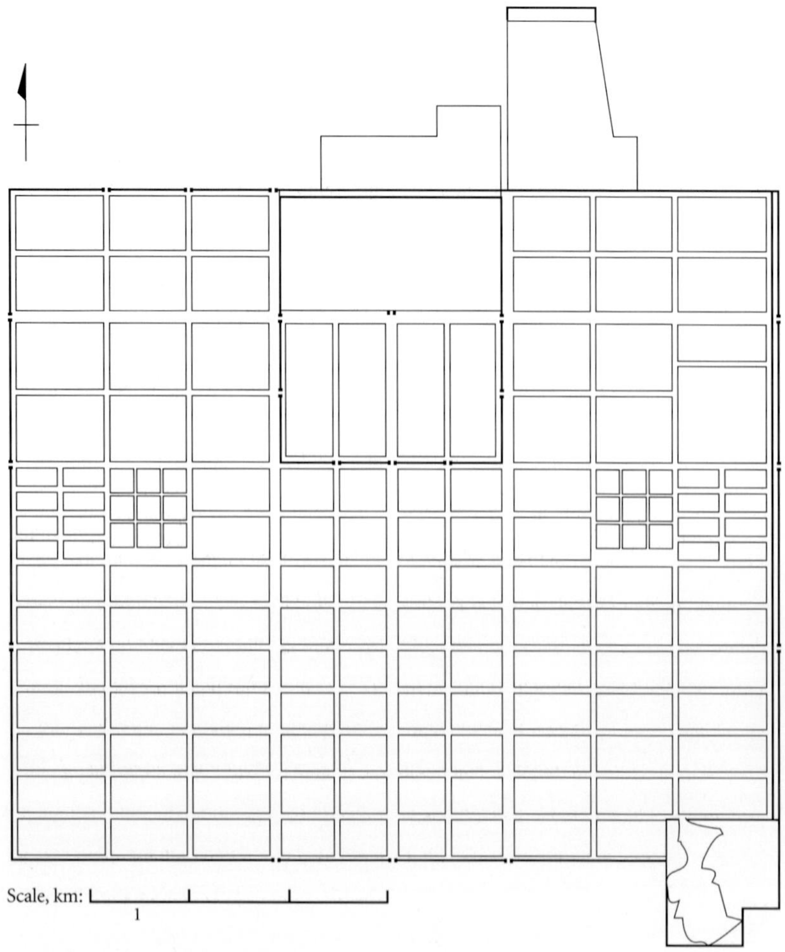

3.1 Changan city plan. Reproduced from *Chūgoku kodai kenchiku-shi* (The history of ancient Chinese architecture).

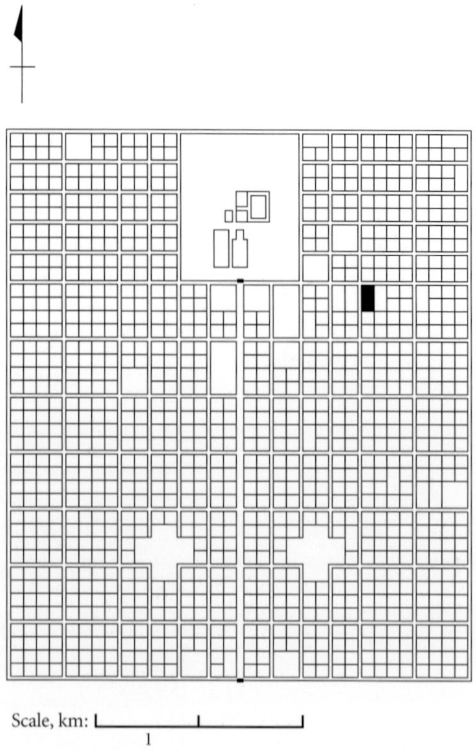

3.2 Heian-kyō city plan indicating the site of Higashisanjō Palace.

City Plan Prototype and Interpretation: Changan and Heian-kyō

The two Japanese cities that were built in a space and climate vastly different from China's, at approximately "one-quarter the scale of Changan, should probably be called scale-reduction models. The main avenues of Heijō-kyō measured 85 meters [279 feet] in width, in comparison to Changan's, which were 150 meters [492 feet] … Japan's many early capitals, from Naniwa-kyō [present-day Osaka] to Heian-kyō, were modeled after Changan, and although Heian-kyō was modeled on Heijō-kyō, it emerged as a superior piece of city planning."[3]

Changan was about four times the area of Heian-kyō. Changan's largest blocks measured 650 *bu* (roughly 975 meters, or 3,200 feet) on the east-west axis, and 550 *bu* (approximately 825 meters, or 2,700 feet) on the north-south axis. Blocks subdivided by narrow crossroads were 320 by 270 *bu* (roughly 480 by 405 meters, or 1,570 by 1,320 feet), which gives an idea of the unit size of Changan's grid plan. (The *bu* is an ancient Chinese unit of measure, converted at about 1.5 meters/4.9 feet to 1 *bu*.)[4]

All Heian-kyō city blocks measured one *chō*, approximately 120 meters (394 feet) square. There were thirty-eight such blocks on the north-south axis and thirty-two on the east-west axis. The same block units continued through the Imperial Palace grounds, although at those locations where various buildings of state occupied larger multiblock sites, the smaller crossroads were omitted. One *chō* was the standard lot size for an aristocrat's residence. These one-*chō* units were sometimes combined into two- or four-*chō* blocks for the estates of high-ranking nobles (Figures 3.1–3.2). For medium-sized and smaller com-

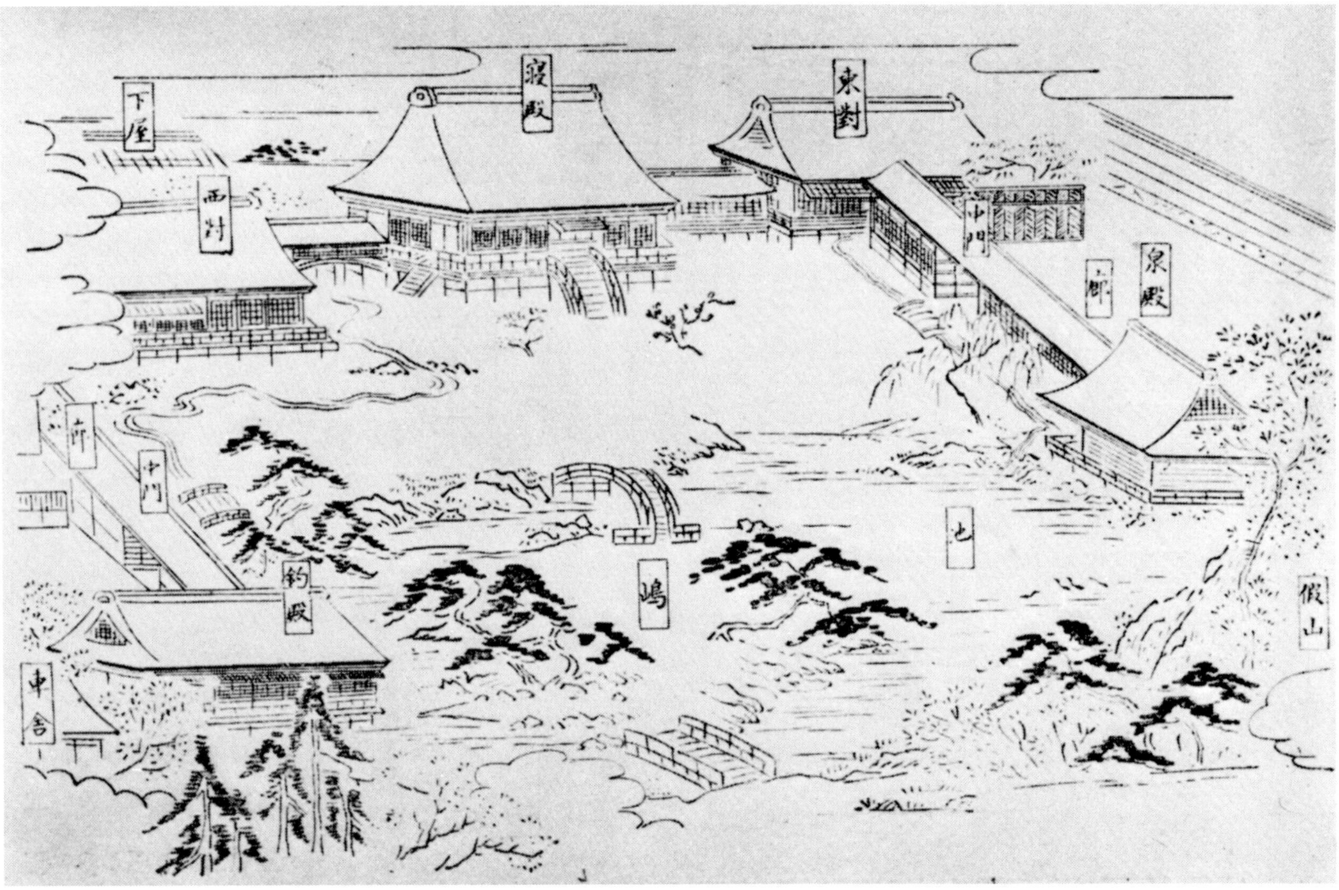

4.1 Rendering of a prototypical *shinden-zukuri* residence and garden from *Kaoku zakkō*.

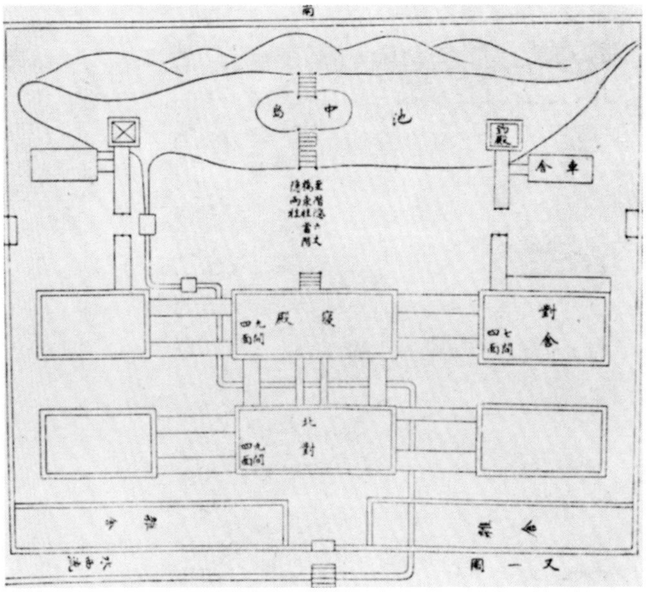

4.2 Plan view.

mon residences, narrow lanes were cut through the center of the one-*chō* blocks, subdividing them into as many as thirty-two lots.[5]

A hypothetical plan view and rendering of a Heian aristocrat's residence, showing an idealized layout of the buildings and garden on a one-*chō* site, are illustrated in *Kaoku zakkō*, a five-volume miscellany on residential architecture written in 1842. This style of architecture and garden is known as *shinden-zukuri*, which comprises a central *shinden* (or main hall, in which the master resided) facing the garden to the south, flanked by opposing annexes known as *tainoya*, which served as the family's residential quarters, to the north, east and west, interconnected by open *sukirō* corridors (Figures 4.1– 4.2).

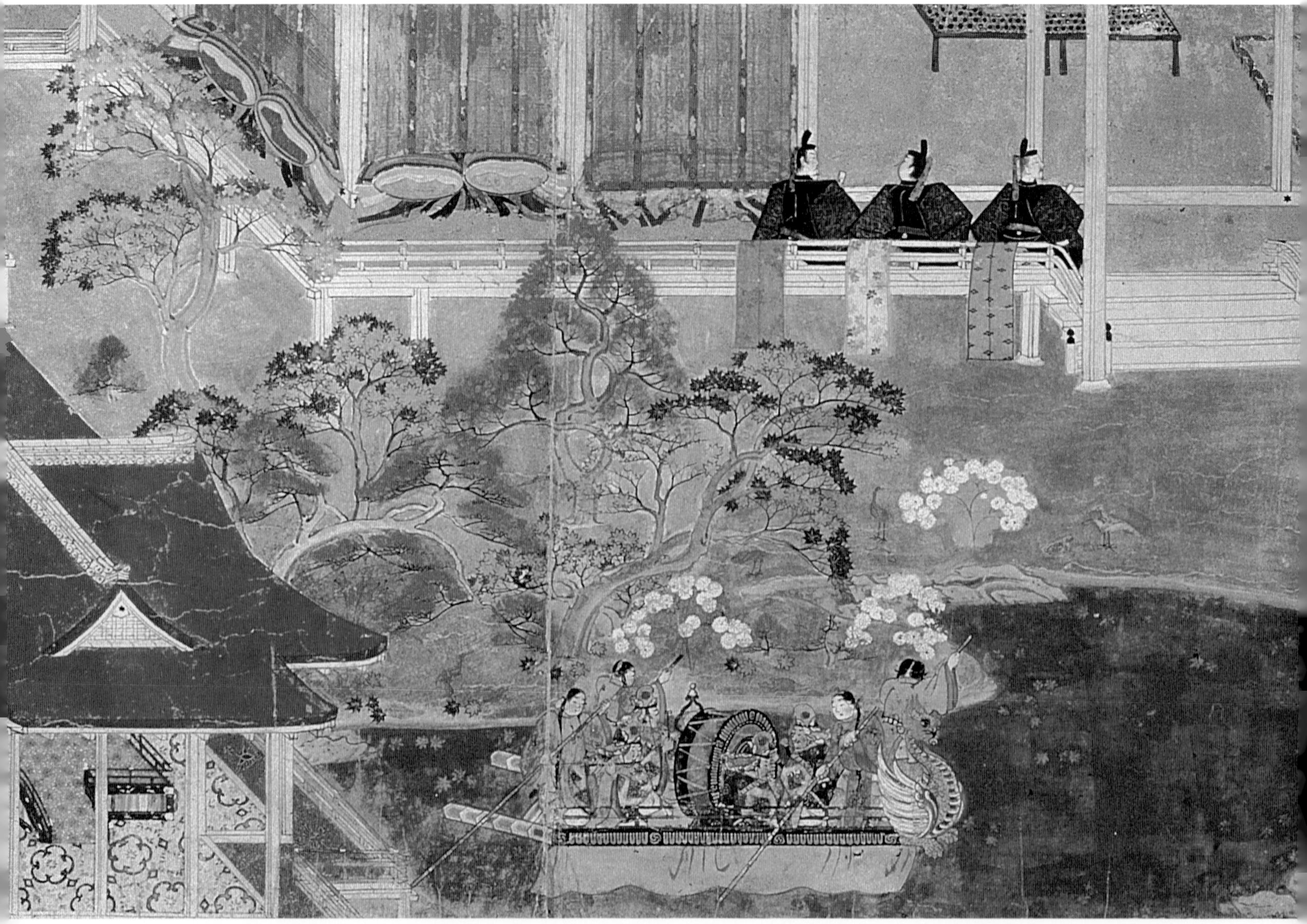

5 A view of the *shinden* and south garden in a depiction of an Imperial visit to a villa, from a late-thirteenth/early-fourteenth–century handscroll. *Komakurabe gyōkō emaki*, Kuboso Memorial Museum of Arts, Izumi, Osaka. Important Cultural Asset.

On the east-west axis the plan view shows a nine-*ken* (bay, or span between pillars)/four-*men* (*hisashi*, or outer aisles on four sides) *shinden* with seven-*ken*/four-*men* *tainoya* to the east and west, connected by five-*ken sukirō*—a total of thirty-three *ken*. Although the length of one *ken* varies regionally, excavations of Heian-kyō ruins revealed a three-meter (9.8–foot) span between pillars, which makes the overall width of the buildings ninety-nine meters, or 325 feet.[6] With the inclusion of *zatsuden* auxiliary buildings, the architecture barely fit the width of the site.

On the north-south axis, the palace (*shinden*, north *tainoya*, and *sukirō*) totaling fifteen *ken*, together with the north *zatsuden*, occupied almost the entire northern half of the site. Regarding the required components of the south garden to be fitted within the remaining approximately sixty meters, or 197 feet, *Sakuteiki* specifies:

Concerning the layout of the South Garden (*nantei*), the distance of sixty to seventy feet will be required from the outer pillars supporting the roof of the staircase southward to the shoreline of the pond. For the Imperial Palace, the distance should extend even to eighty or ninety feet to provide space for the Imperial ceremonies.[7]

[P]rovide space for the Musician's Stage toward the far side of the island. Since the musician's stage extends seventy to eighty feet across …[8]

When temples and palaces are built, their surroundings are landscaped [with artificial hills] to embellish the architecture. This was mentioned early in such a book as the Illustrated Scripture of Jeta Vana (*Gion zukyō*).[9]

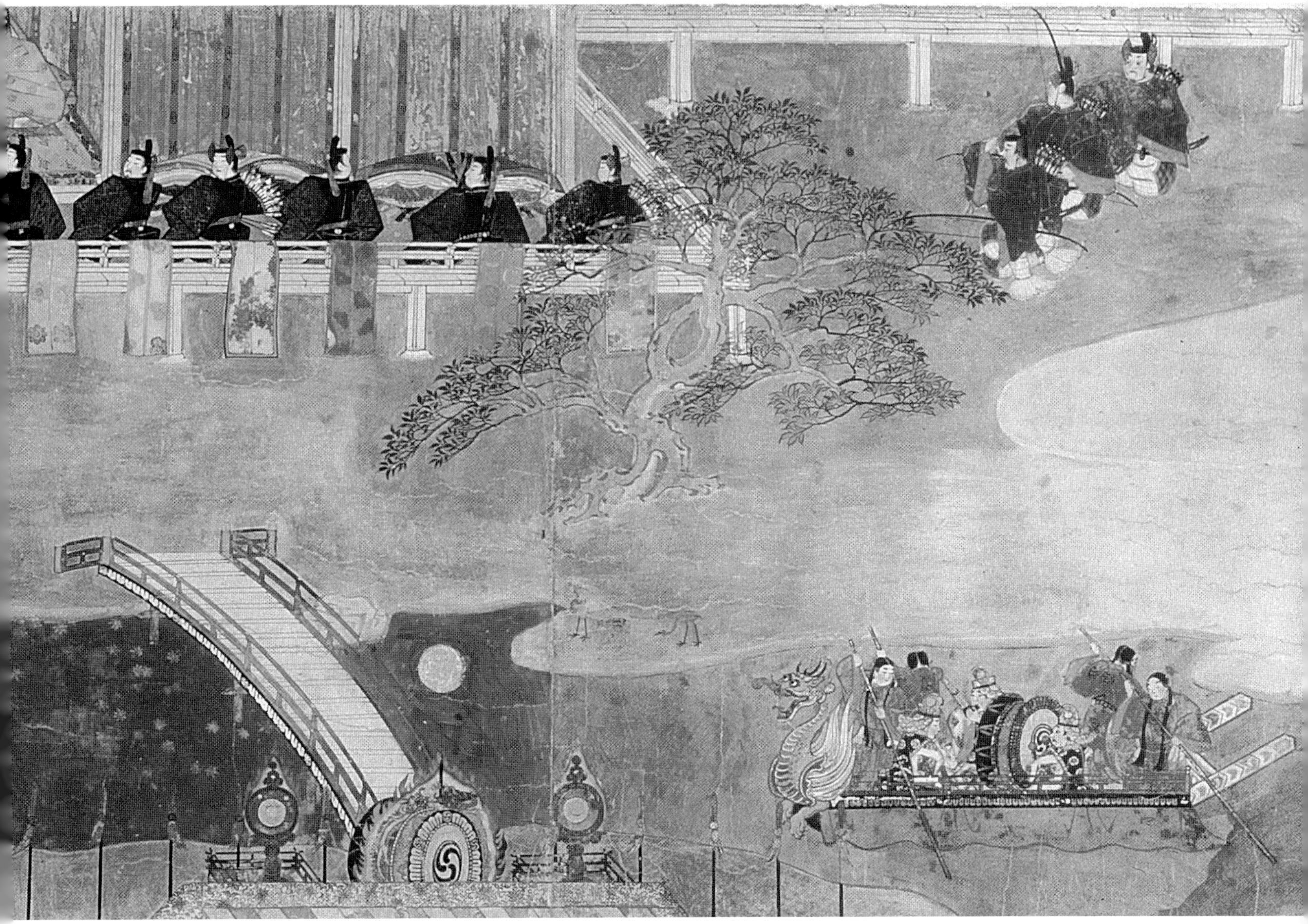

The south garden was to "provide space for the imperial ceremonies"; it comprised a ceremonial area measuring twenty-one to twenty-seven meters (70 to 90 feet) north-south, and beyond this, a pond "in the ocean style," on which Chinese-style boats with dragon-head prows could float to and fro, and containing an island upon which a musician's stage "extend[ing] seventy to eighty feet across" was built (Figure 5). Furthermore, artificial hills were to be created to the south of the pond, to "embellish the architecture." Painstaking effort must have been made to fit all the requisite elements of the prototype for the south garden—the ceremonial area, the pond, the islands, and the artificial hills—within the approximately sixty-meter (197-foot) southern half of the site.

Toshitsuna immediately qualifies this list of criteria for *shinden-zukuri* gardens by asking, "However, you must consider that if the pond is to be dug at the south side of a city estate whose area is only one *chō* square, and the courtyard alone took up a space of eighty or ninety feet there, how much would be left for the pond?"[10] This question is rhetorical, and indicates that the prototype is not something to be followed literally, but calls for a subjective judgment in creating an interpretation that will accommodate the palace, garden, and pond along the north-south axis. It is clearly the advice of a designer.

The city plan shows both the east and west sides of the city to contain more than twenty sites measuring two *chō* each, including that of Higashisanjō Palace. Judging from the scale of the sites of Heian-kyō's main palaces, it is probably safe to assume that two *chō* was the standard site size for these residences.

Shinden-Zukuri Architecture: Symmetrical Prototype, Simplified Interpretations

"As a rule, a one-*chō* site contains east and west *tai* and east and west *chūmon.*" According to this excerpt from *Chūyūki,* the diary of Heian-period courtier Fujiwara no Munetada (1062–1141), the *shinden-zukuri* style for a one-*chō* site has a central *shinden* hall, with east and west *tainoya* opposing annexes and *chūmon* corridors with inner gates. In other words, a one-*chō,* bilaterally-symmetrical palace was the rule. It was the accepted concept, the "formula" for the prototype of *shinden-zukuri.*

Although the *Kaoku zakkō*'s accuracy is sometimes questioned, it does offer a description of the salient features of *shinden-zukuri* as the architectural style was understood in the mid-nineteenth century:

> Starting with Heian-kyō, all aristocratic residential architecture followed continental palatial style in the Tang tradition, known as *azumaya* construction. Thus palace architecture thereafter differed stylistically from the architectural traditions of previous Japanese capitals.
>
> A *shinden-zukuri* residence has a central *seiden* facing south, with buildings called *tainoya* to the east, west, and north. The *seiden* is the master's quarters, and the *tainoya* are the quarters for family and dependents. Some tens of feet in front of the *seiden* there is a pond with an island connected [to the shore] by a bridge. There are also corridors that run southward from the east and west *tainoya.* These corridors end at the edge of the pond, where a fishing pavilion and fountain pavilion are built. An open gateway cuts through each corridor at the approximate center. These gateways are called *chūmon.*[11]
>
> Formula *shinden-zukuri* must be complete with *tainoya,* east and west corridors, *chūmon,* a pond with an island, a fishing pavilion, etc., in order to fulfill the old [Heian] system.[12]

The pattern for *shinden-zukuri* did not originate in ancient Imperial Japan, but was adopted from the architectural style used for palatial buildings in Tang China. These buildings had hipped roofs (in Japanese, known as *azuma-zukuri* or, more commonly, *yosemune*), which the Chinese thought added monumentality and dignity. More importantly, they were completely symmetrical, in plan and structure of the individual buildings as well as in arrangement of the buildings on the site. The *shinden-zukuri* "formula" required furnishing a *seiden,* or *shinden,* with east and west *tainoya,* east and west *sukirō,* east and west *chūmon,* a pond, an island, a fishing pavilion, etc. It is essential to remember that the formula for *shinden-zukuri* emerged from an existing symmetrical pattern.

The Abandonment of Symmetry

Higashisanjō Palace, for generations home to the powerful aristocratic Fujiwara family, was a representative piece of Heian-period residential architecture. Yet even this classic palace lacked many of the requisite components that defined *shinden-zukuri.* The palace had no west *tainoya* proper. The east *chūmon* served as the main entrance and the east fishing pavilion was omitted. The west fishing pavilion was positioned at the edge of the pond and was linked to the *shinden* by a west *sukirō* corridor. Higashisanjō Palace was built on a two-*chō* site in an asymmetrical layout (Figure 6).

The *shinden* was located slightly west of the center of the site. The building that should have, according to the formula, been the west opposing annex was positioned vertically to the northwest, while the east opposing annex

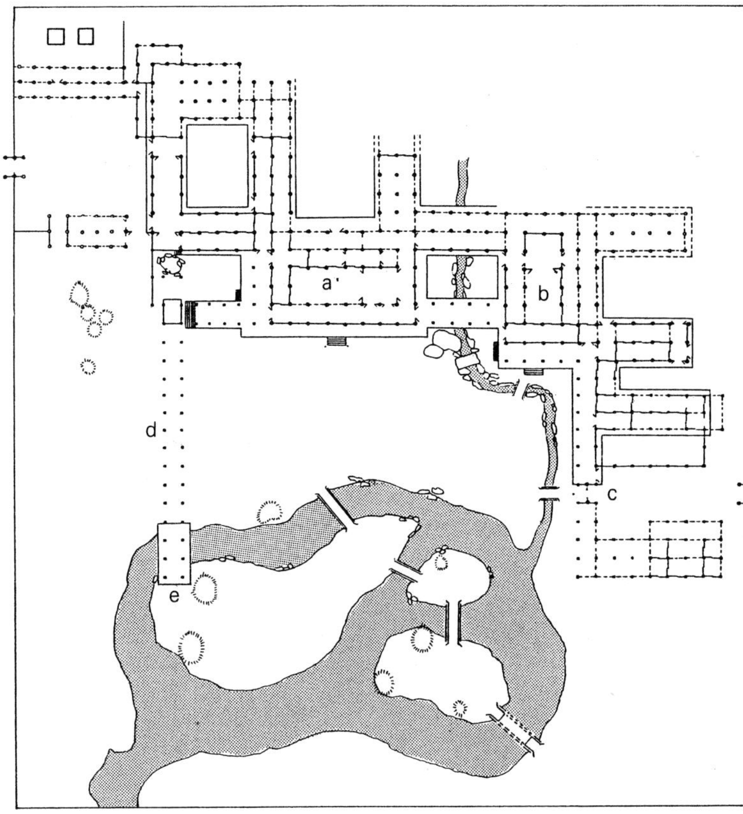

6 *Shinden-zukuri* abbreviated interpretation—reconstructed plan of Higashisanjō Palace by Ōta Seiroku.

a. *shinden.*
b. east *tainoya.*
c. east *chūmon.*
d. west *sukirō.*
e. fishing pavilion.

extended southward. In ground plan, the buildings had a diagonally-stepped, or zigzag, *gankōkei* "geese-in-flight" form. The design emphasizes the main entrance east *chūmon,* imparting to it a sense of impressiveness. Upon entering the *chūmon,* one faced the wide-open west side of the site. Unconstrained by architectural structures, the garden looks quite imposing. By excluding the west *tainoya,* this simplification of the symmetrical formula created an interpretation with a greater sense of grandeur than could be achieved with a symmetrical layout.

Even Heian-kyō's most representative residence, Higashisanjō Palace, abandoned the symmetrical formula adopted from Tang China, and in reality was asymmetrically formed. It is thought, therefore, that the majority of palaces built on one- and two-*chō* sites may also have been asymmetrical in form.

Architect and historian Horiguchi Sutemi explains that the residences of most public officials were not symmetrical:

> The old plan view drawing of the *shinden-zukuri* [residence] included in *Kaoku zakkō* and the drawing entitled *Kujō ke honkaimon* can both be thought of as rough concept sketches of an ideal. This layout defined the *shinden-zukuri* formula, and yet most of the architecture actually built in this period was not true to the formula.[13]

The extent to which the Japanese intentionally replaced symmetry with asymmetry merits consideration. Architects and historians repeatedly attribute the abandonment of symmetry to Japanese aesthetic taste—an aversion to symmetry, or a preference for asymmetry. Architecture historian Ōta Hirotarō cites economic concerns, the asymmetrical use of the *shinden,* and Japanese aesthetic taste, in descending order, as influences.

> If by definition *shinden-zukuri* has a symmetrical arrangement, then any form that is not symmetrical cannot be considered *shinden-zukuri.* However, if symmetry is posited simply as "fundamental," asymmetry becomes justifiable. [The ostensible contradiction] is easier to understand if [asymmetry] is thought of as a schematic or simplification, in which case variety in appearance is to be expected … one [form, i.e., symmetry] is considered the standard, and all others variations.[14]

While the formula for Heian-kyō's *shinden-zukuri* was bilaterally symmetrical, "formula" *shinden-zukuri* architecture was never realized; it existed only prototypically. Site restrictions and other considerations gave rise to simplified interpretations of the prototype, and the birth of a myriad of asymmetrical forms.

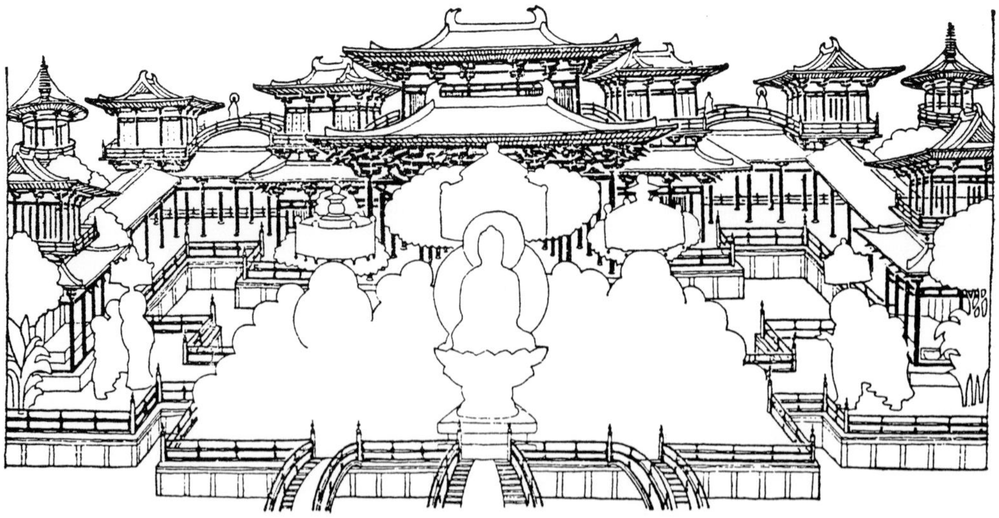

7.1 Xian cave painting no. 148, *Chūgoku kodai kenchiku shi* (The history of ancient Chinese architecture).

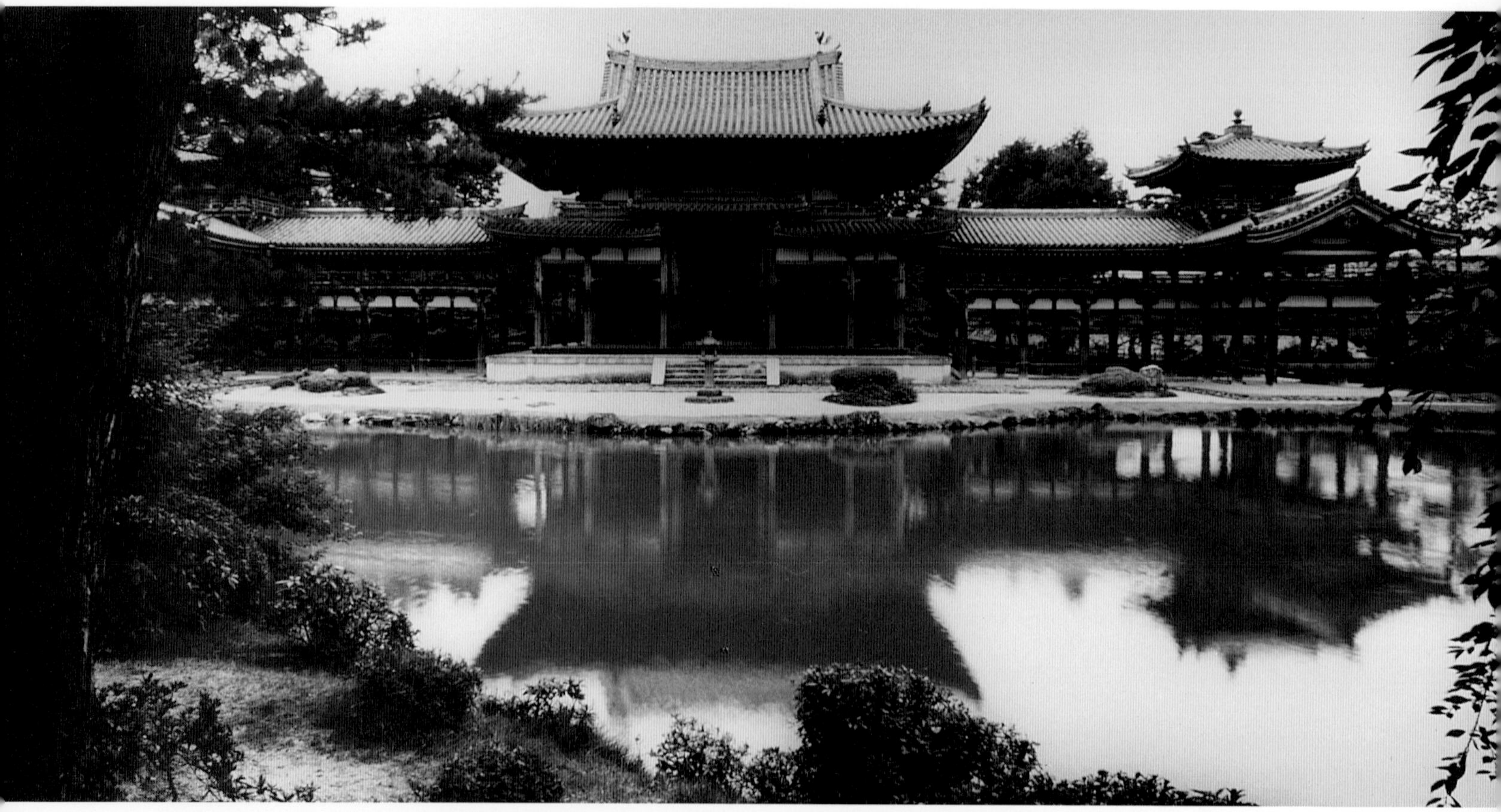

7.2 Byōdō-in Hōōdō (Phoenix Hall), Uji, Kyoto Prefecture. National Treasure.

Architectural Design Solutions That Address Spatial Constraints

Given the limited space available on the east-west axis of a one-*chō* site, it was probably not possible to execute the formal arrangement on the north-south axis either. Two different approaches were employed as means of adapting buildings to sites that were limited in size:

Scale Reduction

This method involves reducing the size of all the various structural components to make them fit.

The scale-reduction method was used primarily for villa-temple architecture built by Heian aristocrats during the eleventh and twelfth centuries. Pure Land Buddhism, or *Jōdo*, which offered believers hope of transport after death to the "Pure Land," or Western Paradise, of the Amida

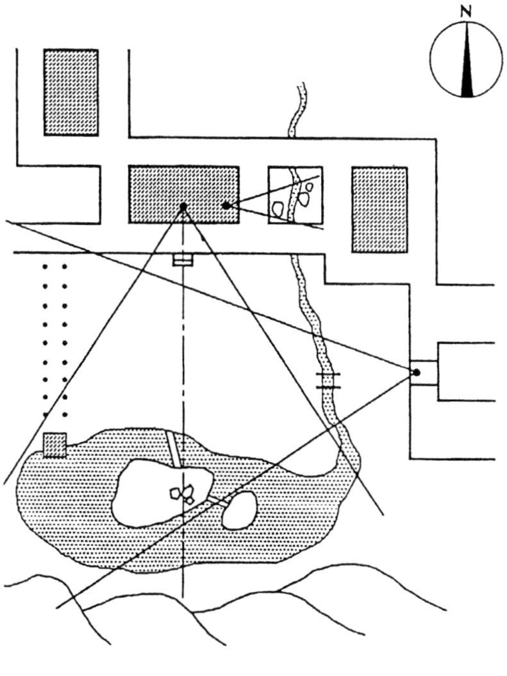

8 Schematic of asymmetrical *shinden-zukuri* architecture and corresponding garden views.

Buddha, appealed to the Heian aristocracy, who attempted to create architectural renditions of Western Paradise. The finest remaining example of these Pure Land villa-temples is Byōdō-in at Uji, south of Kyoto. The Hōōdō, or Phoenix Hall, of Byōdō-in was patterned after the palaces depicted in paintings of Amida's Pure Land (*jōdo hensō*); these illustrative depictions of the paradise dwellings described in sutras were themselves modeled on existing Chinese palaces (Figure 7.1). The central hall of Byōdō-in was scaled to house the temple's main statue of Amida Nyorai, and the flanking *yokurō* "wing" corridors, *birō* "tail" corridor, and *rōkaku* pavilions were all built in proportion to this image as well, and not on a human scale. Set on the west bank of a lotus pond that represents the ocean, the Phoenix Hall is reflected in and appears to be floating on the water, giving a sense of otherworldliness (Figure 7.2). In this way, it is an expression of the inherited Chinese prototype, realized on a reduced scale.

Abbreviation

This method seeks to convey the essence of the model by emphasizing the most important structural components and abbreviating the others—i.e., retaining the essence of the formula while seeking to imbue limited space with a sense of limitlessness.

Shinden-zukuri residential architecture used abbreviation as its means of adapting the Chinese prototype to a different set of circumstances. This style honored the symmetrical formula as the ideal, while also giving high priority to the need to conform to site conditions and the building's intended function. Architectural interpretations of the prototype shifted to the diagonally-stepped "geese-in-flight" pattern and a myriad of other asymmetrical forms of *shinden-zukuri* (Figure 8).

Prototypes and Interpretations in *Shinden-Zukuri* Gardens

Shinden-zukuri gardens, which were integrally linked to the structure and composition of the corresponding architecture, developed with as much variety as did palatial buildings in the same style. Like palace architecture, gardens too had requisite prototypes. The opening line of *Sakuteiki* in fact refers to the inextricable correlation between prototype and interpretation:

> In making the garden, you should first understand the overall principles.[15]

Sakuteiki then outlines three overall principles which together form the prototype for all garden making, and which epitomize all the garden styles described later in the document.

> 1. According to the lay of the land, and depending upon the aspect of the water landscape, you should design each part of the garden tastefully, recalling your memories of how nature presented itself for each feature.[16]

This first principle cites "the natural landscape" as one of the prototypes for garden making. Design is governed by site conditions and must respect and highlight the natural features of a location. This guideline instructs the designer to recall his own direct experiences and observations of nature, and to use them in interpreting the prototype. A similar line appearing later in the text—"the stones placed and the sceneries made by man can never excel the landscape in nature"—reinforces this principle.[17]

> 2. Study the examples of works left by the past masters and, considering the desires of the owner of the garden, you should create a work of your own by exercising your tasteful senses.[18]

The second principle designates "works left by the past masters" as prototypes, and urges caution in the exercise of creative impulses. This focus on masterful work helped to ensure the continuation of tradition and was an important factor in turning garden masterpieces into prototypes themselves.

Descriptions of early Japanese gardens—such as Soga Umako's "*Shima no Ōomi no niwa*" in the historical chronicle *Nihon shoki* (comprising thirty volumes, compiled in the seventh and eighth centuries), and Prince Kusakabe's "*Tachibanajima no Miya no niwa*" in *Manyōshū* (the seventh- and eighth-century collection of Japanese poetry)—along with vestiges of the gardens of Heijō-kyō excavated in 1975, suggest that all were natural landscape–style gardens. During the mid- through the late Heian period, when *Sakuteiki* author Toshitsuna was active, the development of the *shinden-zukuri* garden had nearly reached maturity. Surrounded by mountains on three sides, the Kyoto basin's natural environment supplied an abundance of the finest varieties of garden materials—rocks, plants, sand, clear streams and natural springs—and was as beautiful as it was rich in resources. Heian-period gardens making ingenious use of the terrain developed as an extension of the natural landscape–style gardens of the Nara period. Today the only remaining natural spring–fed ponds that reflect Heian-period methods are those of the former emperors' villas, Shinsen'en and Saga Betsu-in. Both are traditional natural landscape–style gardens with nature itself as their prototype.

Since the *shinden-zukuri* garden was designed primarily for viewing from inside the palace, the "owner's tastes" as reflected in the room interior would necessarily have had a strong impact on people's perceptions of the garden. Thus "considering the desires of the owner of the garden" was fundamental, and served as the basis upon which the designer should finally "create a work of his own," or bring into play his own creativity and subjective judgment.

> 3. Think over the famous places of scenic beauty throughout the land, and by making your own that which appeals to you most, design your garden with the mood of harmony, modelling it after the general air of such places.[19]

The third principle specifies "famous places of scenic beauty" as a prototype, which relates to the thematic subjects of gardens.

Poetry pervaded all aspects of Heian court life and gardens too bore evidence of literary influence. Gardens were one means of displaying *miyabi*—court elegance and refined aesthetic taste—and served as the setting for formal poetry composition matches. As such, the garden itself should be a "poetic" expression as well as a source of poetic inspiration. As a theme, "the natural landscape" was too broad a topic to express succinctly, and so articulating it metaphorically, in the form of commonly understood poetic images, made it easier for the viewer to grasp and for the designer to narrow down the focus of his expression. Thematically, famous places of scenic beauty such as Wakaura, Suma, Akashi, Amanohashidate, and Shiogama carried specific literary connotations; simply

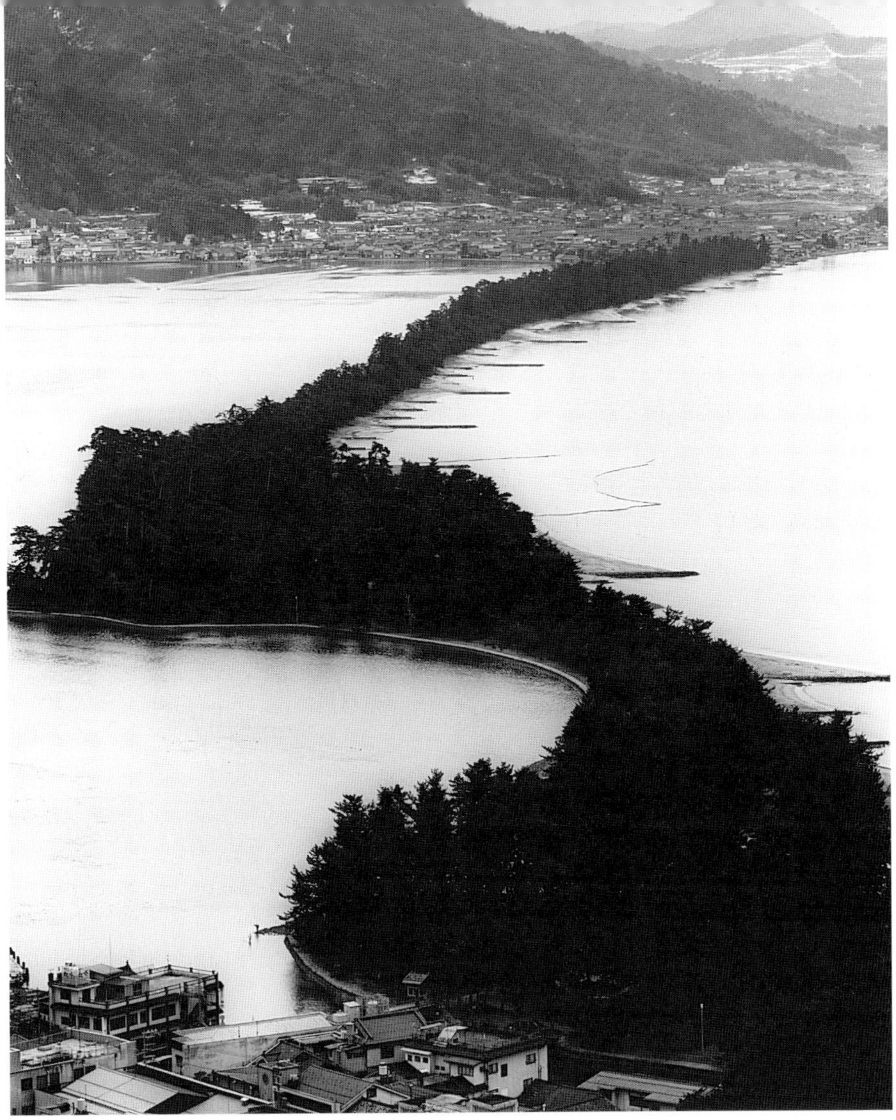

9.1 The famous pine tree–covered sandbar Amanohashidate, Kyoto Prefecture.

9.2 An island recreating the scenery of Amanohashidate in the garden of Katsura Rikyū, Kyoto.

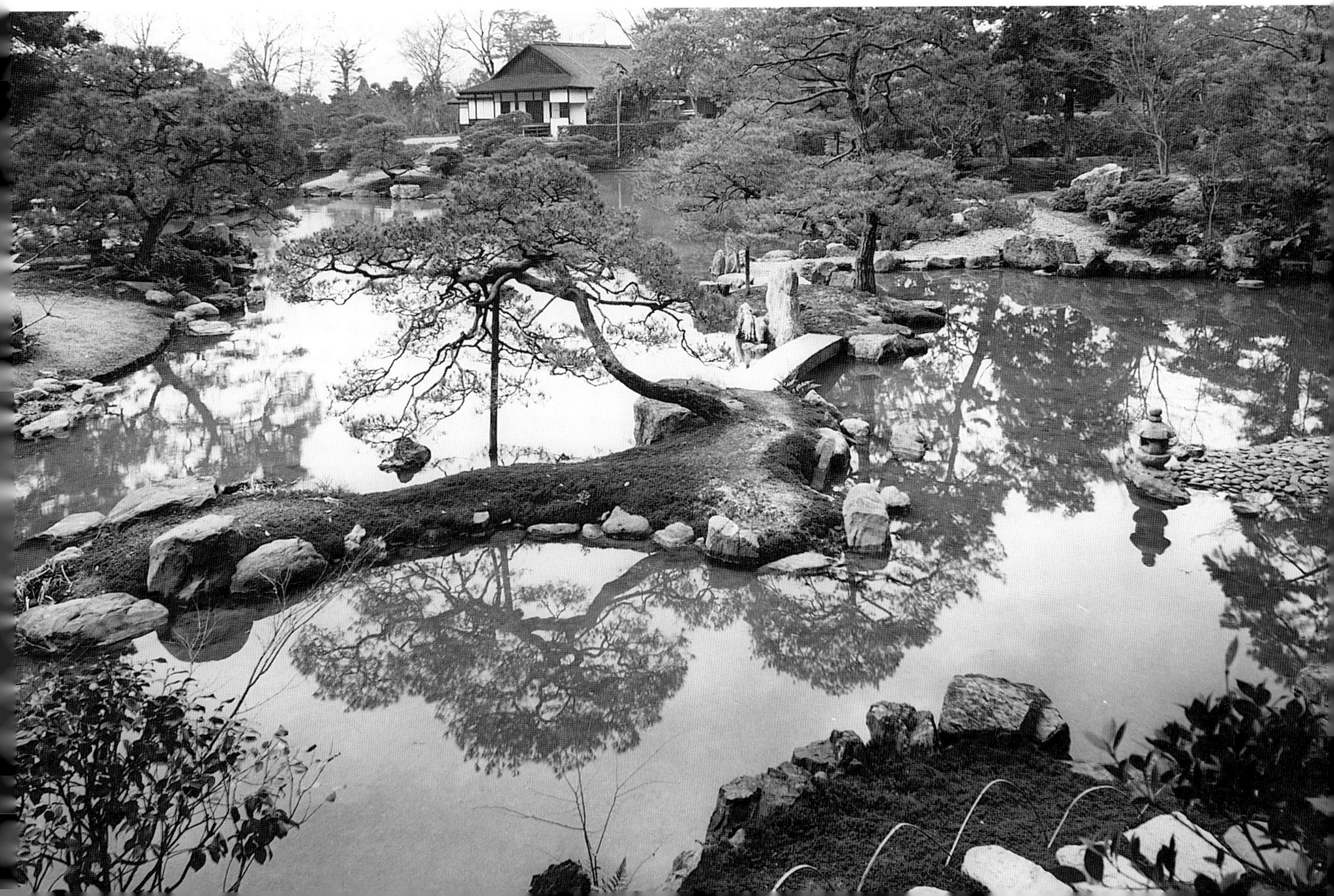

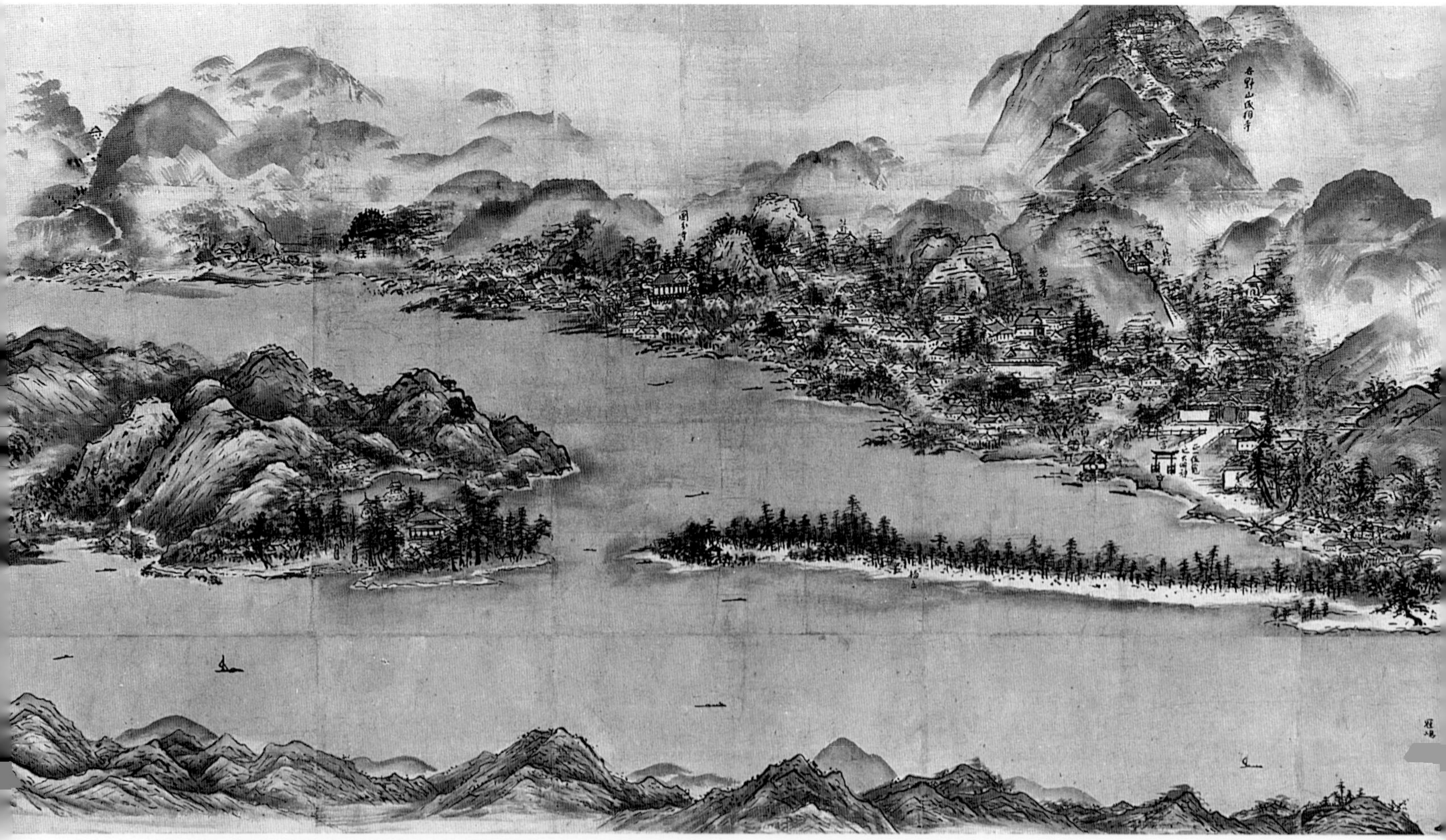

9.3 *Amanohashidate*, a landscape scroll by Sesshū Tōyō depicting the famous scenic spot, ca. 1501, Kyoto National Museum. National Treasure.

alluding to these places evoked particular phrases, moods, or images. "Famous places of scenic beauty" were extracted from the prototype of "the natural landscape." At this point in Japanese garden history, the recreation of famous sights had been established as an appropriate metaphor for "the natural landscape"; it has maintained this same status through the present day (Figures 9.1–9.3).

An excerpt from *Jikkinshō* (also known as *Jikkunshō*), a Kamakura-period collection of tales based on stories dating from the Heian period, describes one such Heian garden recreation of the famous pine tree–covered sandbar called Amanohashidate (literally, "bridge of heaven"), located on Tango Peninsula in the Japan Sea:

> At the southeast corner of Nanajō and Muromachi is the one-*chō* Sukechika residence. Modeled after Amanohashidate in Tango, the island in the center of the pond is elongated and planted with young pines.

The three overall principles in the opening paragraphs of *Sakuteiki* are related to the famous Chinese treatise on art that transcends formal representation—Xie He's Six Laws (*liu-fa*) of painting. First defined in the preface to his *Gu hua-pin-lu*, or Classification of painters (ca. 535), they were continually referred to by Chinese theorists thereafter, and are debated by scholars worldwide to this day.

> Long ago Xie He said that painting has Six Elements [or Laws]. The first is called "engender [a sense of] movement [through] spirit consonance." The second is called "use the brush [with] the 'bone method.'" The third is called "responding to things, image [depict] their forms." The fourth is called "according [adapting?] to kind, set forth [describe] colors [appearances]." The fifth is called "dividing and planning, positioning and arranging." The sixth is called "transmitting and conveying [earlier models, through] copying and transcribing."[20]

The second half of *Sakuteiki*'s third general principle—"by making your own that which appeals to you most, design your garden with the mood of harmony, modelling after the general air of such places"—is analogous to Xie He's second law. The "bone method" is the "depiction of a likeness, while respecting bone spirit"; in other words, it requires seeing through to the skeletal structure, or the very essence of a subject. It is a process of extracting the most characteristic forms and eliminating anything superfluous. The "mood of harmony" mentioned in *Sakuteiki's* third principle is akin to the process of "depicting" or "describing" the extracted abstract form which is the subject of Xie He's third and fourth laws. Further, Toshitsuna's injunction to "study the examples of works left by past masters" is equivalent to Xie He's sixth law, on "copying and transcribing."

The prototype outlined in *Sakuteiki*'s three general principles calls not for a faithful, realistic portrayal of nature, but an evocation of its spirit. That which was acquired by studying nature was to be conveyed figuratively—with for instance a depiction of Amanohashidate. Portraying intrinsic quality has been the most fundamental point in Japanese garden design throughout the ages. By changing the degree and style of "description" added, the Japanese garden developed into the abstract gardens of the Muromachi period (1333–1568) on the one hand, and the condensed gardens of the Azuchi-Momoyama period (1568–1603) on the other. Japanese abstract (Zen) gardens and representational (*shoin-zukuri*) gardens are not at all antithetical styles, since the point of departure for both is "modelling after the general air of such places."

The Six Basic Elements of Garden Composition

The prototype of garden design is described in the opening paragraphs of *Sakuteiki*, while the remainder of the text presents the Japanese garden's six basic compositional elements—the artificial hills, the pond, the island, the white sand south garden, the garden stream, and the waterfall—and also notes that plants and springs may be used as garden accents where appropriate (Figures 10.1–10.6). Through the historical periods—even when later abstracted or condensed—the skeletal structure of the Japanese garden is composed using these six elements to portray the natural landscape in accordance with the prototype. Having defined and documented these alone makes *Sakuteiki* a classic.

Sakuteiki outlines the six basic compositional elements of the garden as:

Artificial Hills

> ... [T]heir surroundings are landscaped [with artificial hills] to embellish the architecture. This was mentioned early in such a book as the Illustrated Scripture of Jeta Vana (*gion zukyō*).[21]

Pond

> Since the stones in the pond landscape are placed to simulate a seascape, be sure to install the "deep-rooted rock" and the "wave-repelling stone" in the scenery.[22]

> In [the Ocean Style], first construct the scene of a rough seashore ...[23]

> [The River Style] should resemble a meandering tract of a dragon or a snake.[24]

Islands

> About the various types of the pond island landscape. They are: the Hill Island, the Field Island, the Forest Island, the Rocky-Shore Island, the Cloud Shape, the Running Stream Type, the Ebb-tide Beach Style, the Pine-bark Pattern, and so on.[25]

South Garden

> Concerning the layout of the South Garden (*nantei*), the distance of sixty to seventy feet will be required from the outer pillars supporting the roof of the

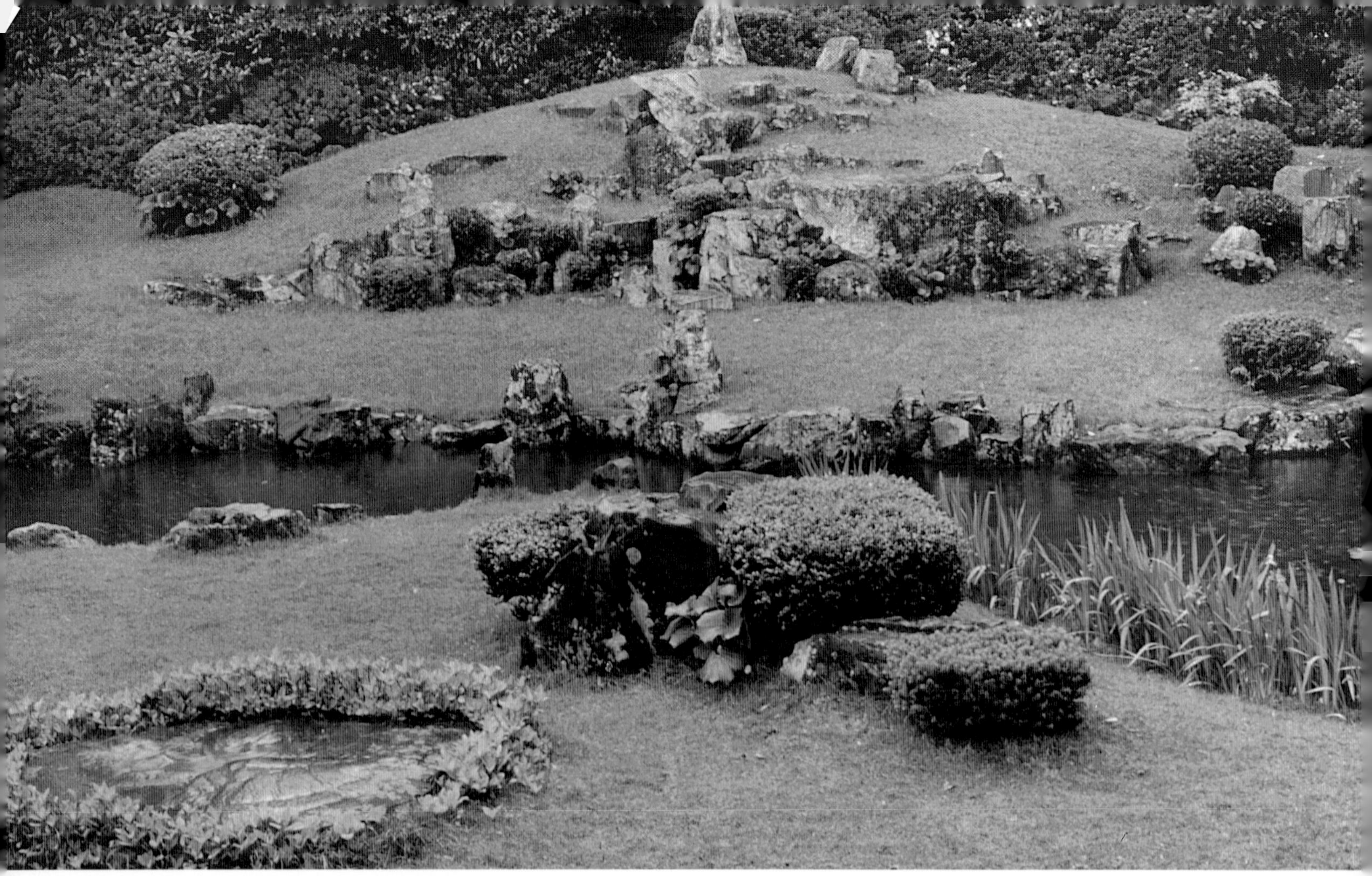

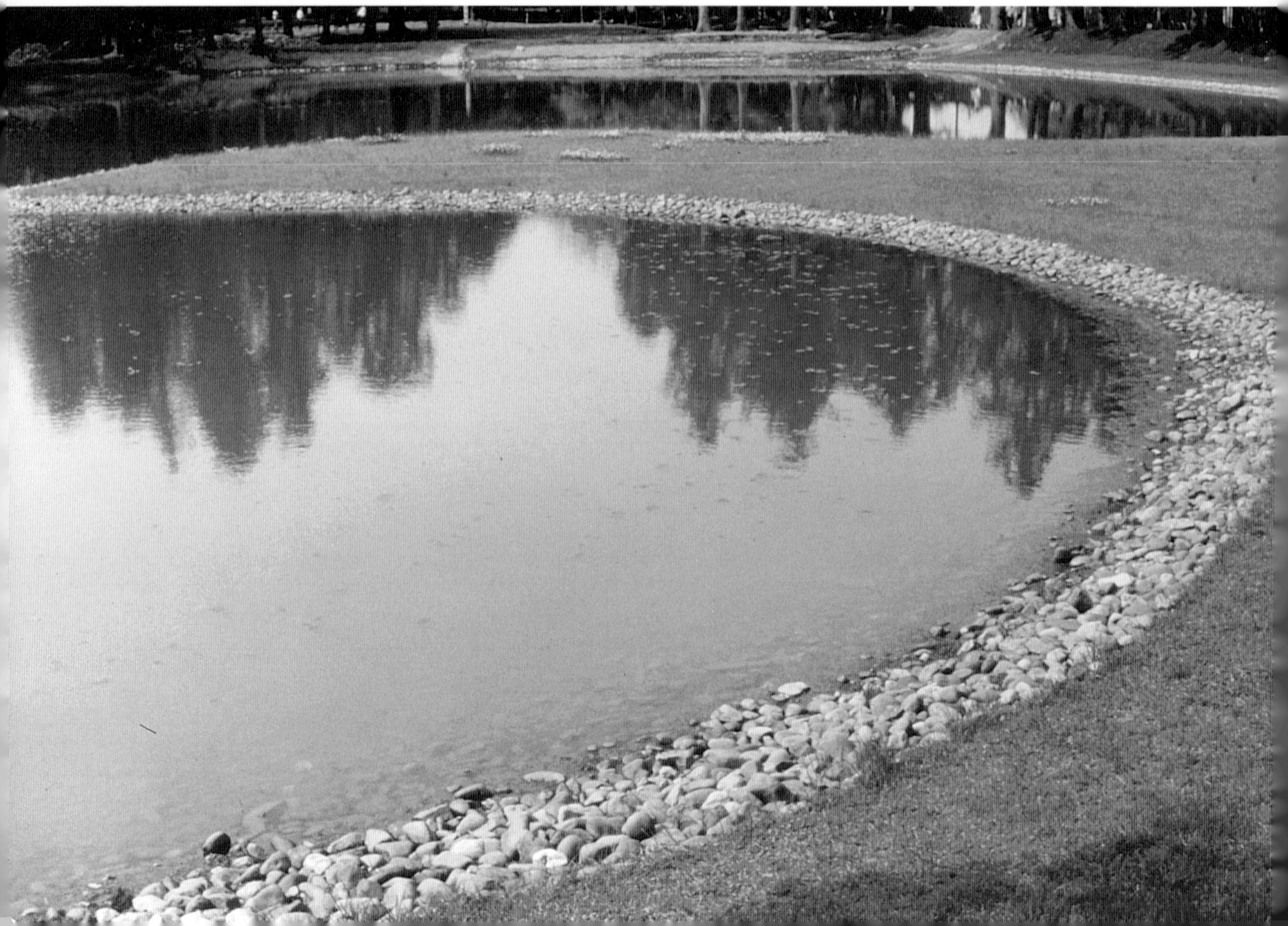

◀ 10.1 Artificial hill garden landscape from the Muromachi period. Manpukuji, Shimane Prefecture.

◀ 10.2 Pond simulating the shoreline of a sandy beach, Mōtsūji, Iwate Prefecture.

> staircase southward to the shoreline of the pond. For the Imperial Palace, the distance should extend even to eighty or ninety feet in order to provide space for the imperial ceremonies.[26]

Garden Stream

> Someone remarked that there is a deeper meaning in designing a landscape and placing stones therein. It is said that the earth signifies the king, whereas water represents his retainers. Water, therefore, proceeds when the earth allows it, and stops when the earth arrests it. Another theory says that the mountain symbolizes the king, and water, his subjects, whereas the stones represent the king's counsellors. According to this theory, water runs at the command of the mountain, the king.[27]

> The mountain rapids style of the garden stream should present the scene of rapids gushing out from the ravine formed by two mountains.[28]

Waterfall

> When we observe natural waterfalls we notice that tall falls are not necessarily wide, nor low falls always narrow in breadth.[29]

The prototypes and interpretations of the garden stream and the waterfall are treated in great detail in individual chapters titled "About the Garden Stream" and "The Procedure for Making the Waterfall." This is an indication of *Sakuteiki*'s recognition of their relative importance among the compositional elements. As time passed and site conditions became more restricted, these two elements were increasingly emphasized.

The prototypes of garden composition—"the natural landscape," "famous places of scenic beauty," and "portraying the essence of scenes from nature"—and the prototypes of the six compositional elements exist as general concepts unaffected by the actual one-*chō* space.

Trees and Shrubs

The majority of *Sakuteiki*'s contents focuses on stones and water. The work's longest chapters are on stones, the stream, and the waterfall, in that order. The subject of trees is touched upon relatively lightly, while mountains, hillside fields and shrubbery are not even treated in independent sections. A chapter entitled "About Tree Planting" focuses mostly on the geomantic significance of the placement of trees in relation to the dwelling, and on various taboos, or warnings which are couched in highly superstitious language but provide very practical, aesthetically pleasing garden-making advice. Garden historian Tamura Tsuyoshi gives the following explanations of the scarcity of discussion of trees and shrubs in his critical work on *Sakuteiki*:

> As the various techniques regarding the placement of stones are applicable *en toto* to trees and shrubs, [their explanation in *Sakuteiki*] was abbreviated to avoid redundancy.
>
> … As the craft of tree planting falls within the domain of farming and gardening, it was, and for the most part still is, considered the work of the garden supplier, only rarely to be handled by a designer. Although [*Sakuteiki*] covers construction to some extent, the text is devoted primarily to the aspect of design. The placement of stones was considered to be the most taxing area of study [in garden design], and planting a less worthwhile pursuit. Since plants must for the most part, conform to the laws of nature, they have severe limitations as design elements, which are difficult to overcome. It was probably for these reasons that lengthy coverage was not provided.[30]

Stone setting is the essential point of *Sakuteiki*. The placement of stones was the basis of garden design in the Heian

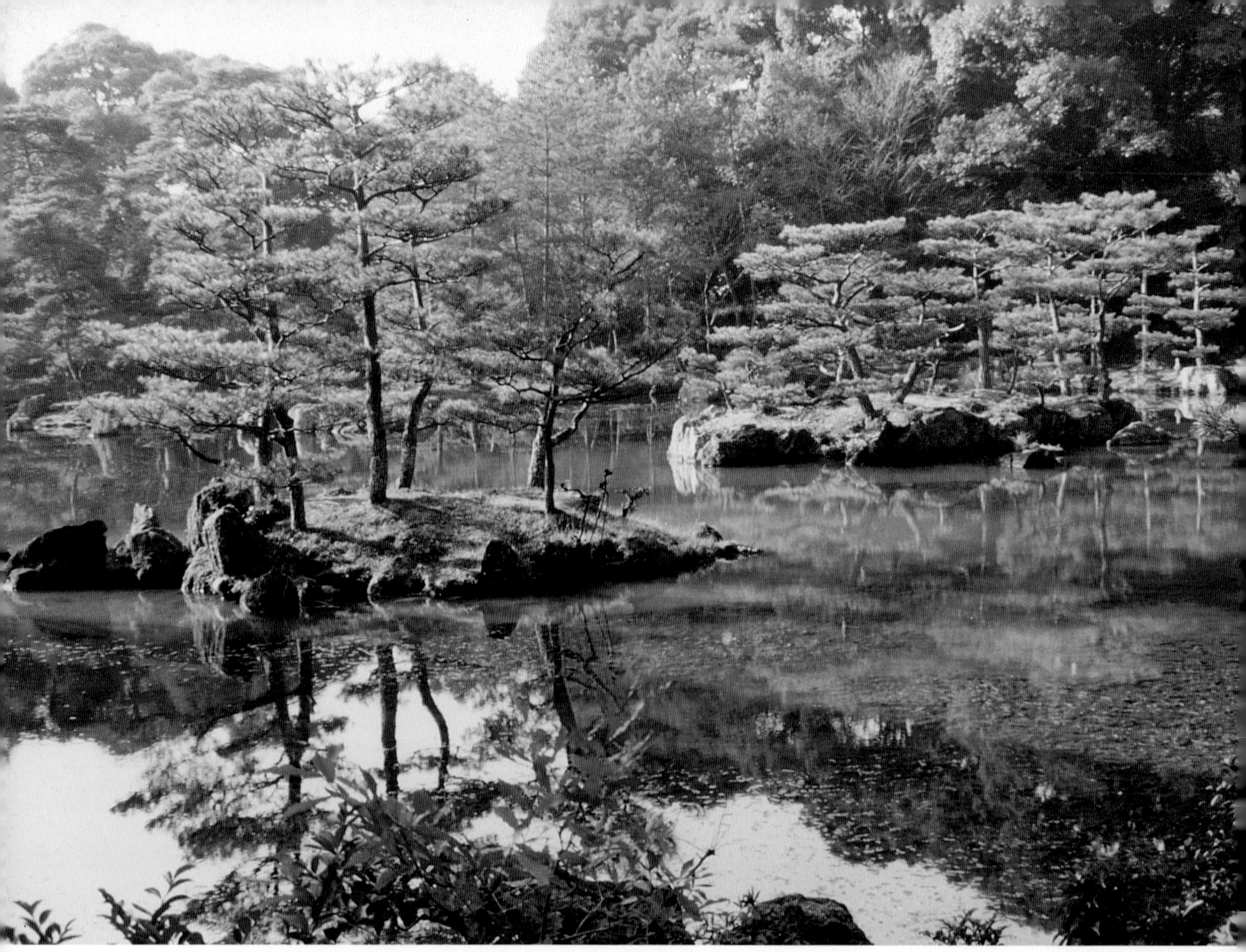

10.3 Pond island landscape of *Kokyō no ike* (Mirror pond) at Kinkakuji, Kyoto.

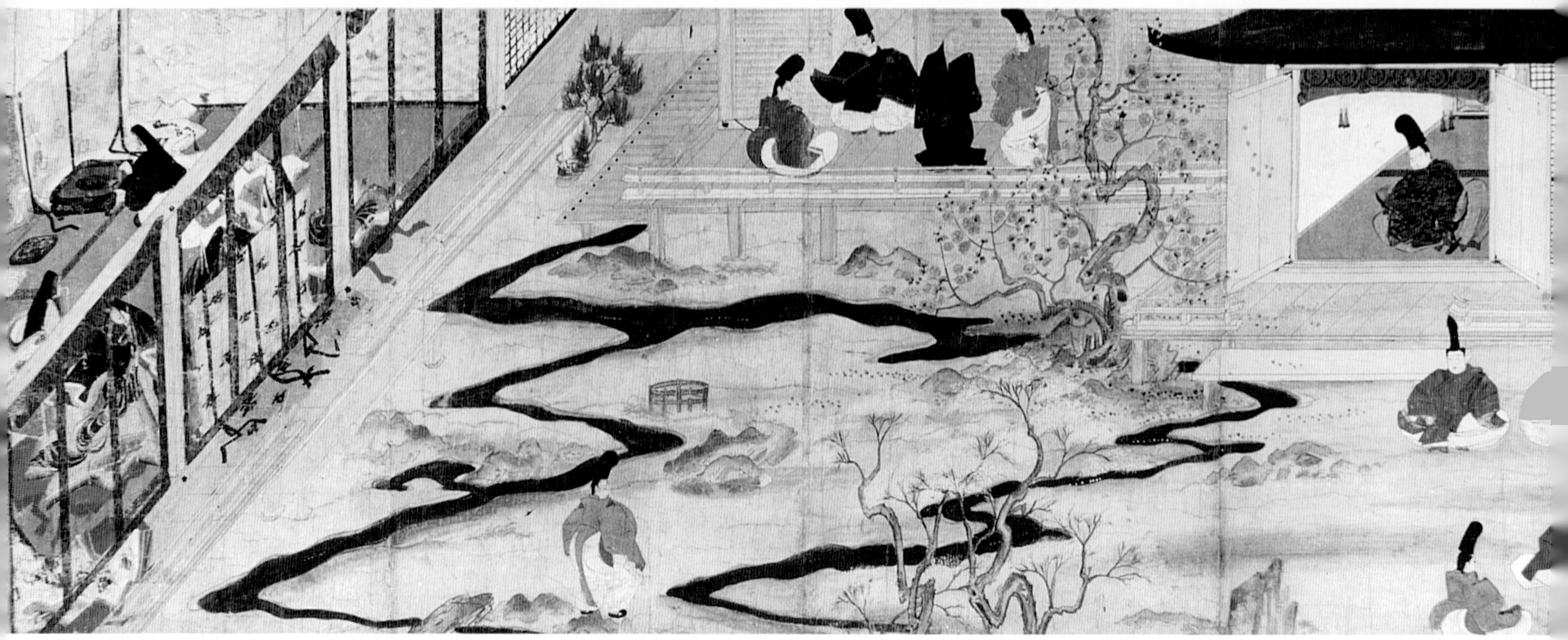

10.4 View of the garden stream in relation to the *shinden* from the early–thirteenth-century handscroll *Kitano tenjin engi* (Legends of Kitano Shrine), Kitano Shrine, Kyoto. National Treasure.

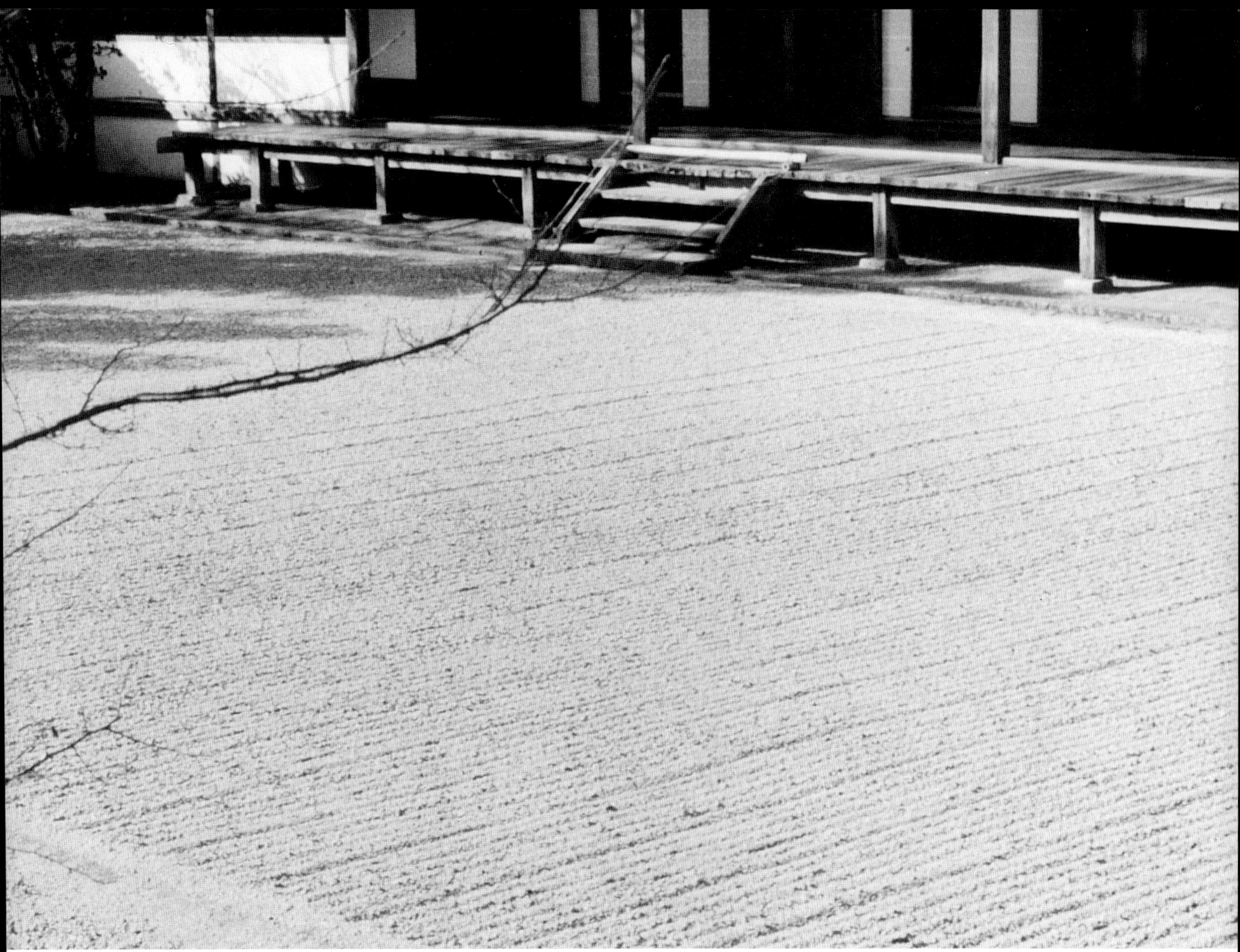

10.5 The south garden white sand area, Nin'naji, Kyoto.

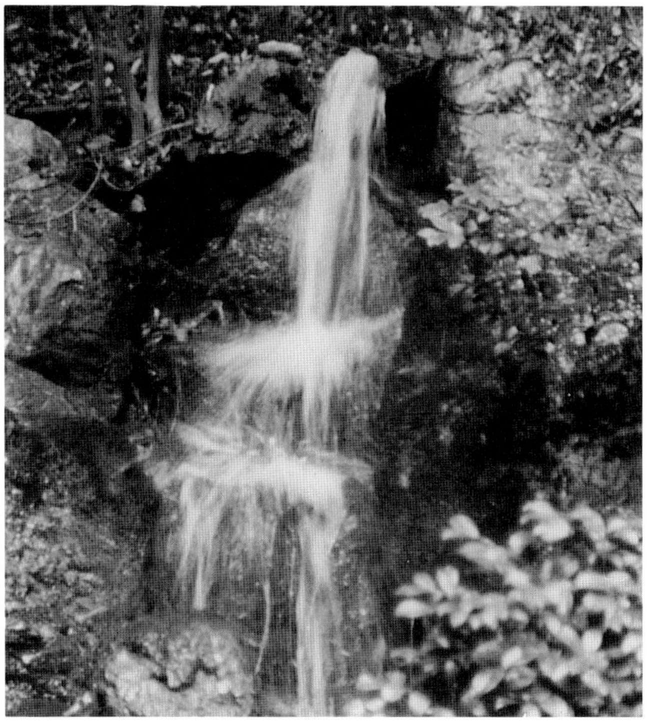

10.6 Waterfall with "water-hitting stones" set at descending stepped elevations, Nanzen'in, Kyoto.

period and for centuries afterward. In fact the term "stone setting" (*ishidate*) is synonymous with "garden making."

In spring, flowers distract the eye, and in summer, foliage envelopes and conceals the garden. It is only in the dead of winter, when the trees lose their leaves, that the skeletal structure of the garden is revealed. In winter it becomes clear that the placement of stones forms the framework of the garden plan, and that stones are the single expressive element that remains unchanged. Trees and plants, by contrast, change constantly. They reflect more the will of the many hands to which they have been subject over the years than the original garden design.

Implicit in *Sakuteiki*'s advice to designers to consider "how much [space] would be left for the pond" is the understanding that stone setting forms the skeletal structure of the garden plan, while trees and plants serve as decorative accents. By the Edo period (1603–1867), however, both plants and stones were used to create the compositional structure of the garden, as is evidenced by the clipped shrub formations found in these gardens. In landscape composition of the garden beginning at this time, a balance was sought between structural elements and changing elements, or accent planting; thus plants began to be used as part of the unchanging structural plan. Shrub clipping at the temple Daichiji in Minakuchi, Shiga Prefecture—its garden comprised solely of clipped shrubs—is traditionally performed by the head priest, as an "inherited duty" (Figure 11).

The Design Process: Stylized Forms (*Yō*) and Modeling After (*Manabi*)

The term "*yō*" appears repeatedly throughout the text of *Sakuteiki*, referring to stylized forms in which each of the six compositional elements can be rendered to express "the natural landscape." "*Yō*" has a broad range of nuances and is used in *Sakuteiki* to indicate form or shape (sometimes also indicated by the term "*kata*"), definitive style, and/or appearance, air, or state. Examples of the key uses of "*yō*" and "*kata*" are shown in boldface in the excerpts below:

> The dry landscape [**form**] ...[31]

> ... some charming mood **such as of** a mountain village ...[32]

> Various **Styles** for Landscape Gardens. The Ocean **Style**, the River **Style**, the Mountain Stream **Style**, the Pond **Style**, the "Reed-hand" **Style**, and so on.[33]

> That there are various **styles** of landscape designs by the placement of stones does not mean all such **styles** should be applied in one garden work. However, depending on the aspect of the pond and the lay of the ground, at times different **styles** may be combined in making one water landscape ... Thus it all depends on each circumstance. Uninformed persons often speak about the specific **style** by which this or that garden was made, but such talk is quite odd.[34]

> About the **Various** Shorelines of Ponds and Rivers. The Spade and Hoe **Shapes** ...[35]

> About the **Various Types** of the Pond Island Landscape. They are: the Hill Island, the Field Island, the Forest Island, the Rocky-Shore Island, the Cloud **Shape**, the Running Stream **Type**, the Ebb-tide Beach **Style**, the Pine-bark **Pattern**, and so on.[36]

> About the **Various Manners** of Falling. Facing Falling, One Way Falling, Running Falling, Leaping Falling, Corner Falling, Linen Falling, Compound Falling, Left and Right Falling, Side Falling.[37]

> There are various **forms** of waterfalls ...[38]

> [Y]ou should use **such** wild-flower plants as the Chinese Bellflower, the Patrinia, the Burnet, Plantain Lily, and the like.[39]

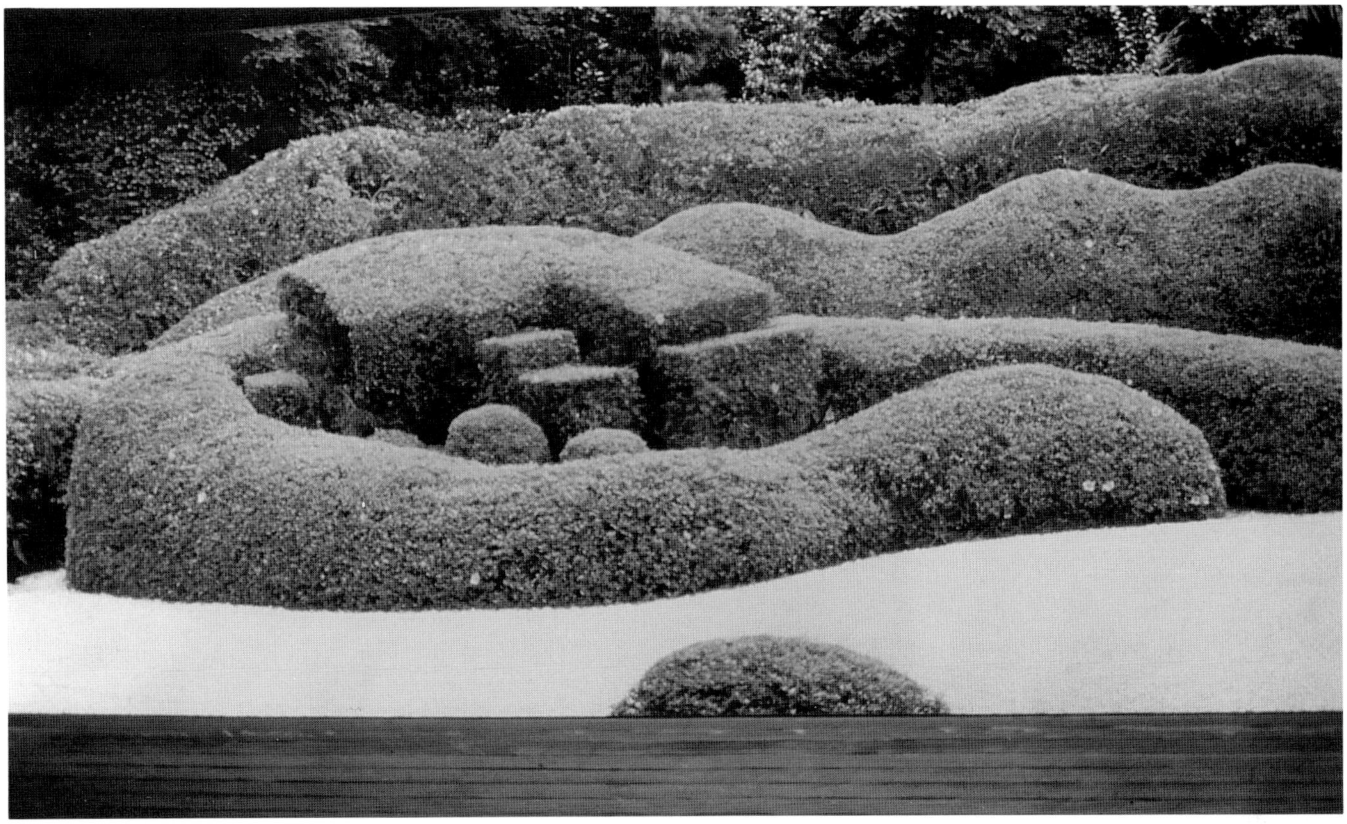

11 A garden landscape composed solely of clipped shrubs, Daichiji, Shiga Prefecture.

> In the stone setting work there are also **such** methods as the Lapping Joints, the Tilted Hat Wearing [**Form**], the Table **Form** and the Tub Setting.[40]

> In [the Ocean Style], first construct **the scene** of a rough seashore ...[41]

> ... This makes the waterfall **appear**, when seen from a distance, **as though** it were falling out of the mountain rocks.[42]

> ... [T]he falls will **look like** a hanging sheet of cloth.[43]

> ... thus presenting a view that **looks as though** a number of threads were hanging.[44]

> ... but when seen from some distance it **looks like** a meaningless pile of stones ... [Y]ou should place the stones [**so as**] **not to** present a poor view when seen from some distance.[45]

All uses of "*yō*" in the *Sakuteiki* relate to visual garden making techniques. The use of "*yō*" or "*kata*" establishes a stylized form of a compositional element as a definitive style.

Intermediating between stylized forms (*yō*) and the act of "design[ing] your garden with the mood of harmony," (that is, implementing the design), is a learning/ideation stage—the process of "studying and modeling after" a subject. The practical aspect of learning (*manabi*) the art of garden making, or any of the traditional Japanese arts, requires repeated simulation of existing models; thus "studying" and "modeling after" are by Japanese terms inextricably linked.

> For the widened portions of the pond and the island shores, the ocean style **is** [**studied and**] **used** [*manabi*], while the aforementioned "reed-hand" style **may be** [**studied and**] **applied** [*manabi*] to the soft landscape of hillside fields.[46]

> In the case of a man-made landscape garden, since only the best parts of the places **are studied and modelled after** [*manabi*], meaningless stones and features are seldom provided along with man's work.[47]

> ... [T]he people of China always build artificial fountains, and place the stand **simulating** (*manabi*) the Isle of Eternal Youth ...[48]

Based on *yō*, or stylistic forms, "studying and modeling after" calls for a profound understanding that facilitates transposition from nature's existing form to the garden form to be implemented.

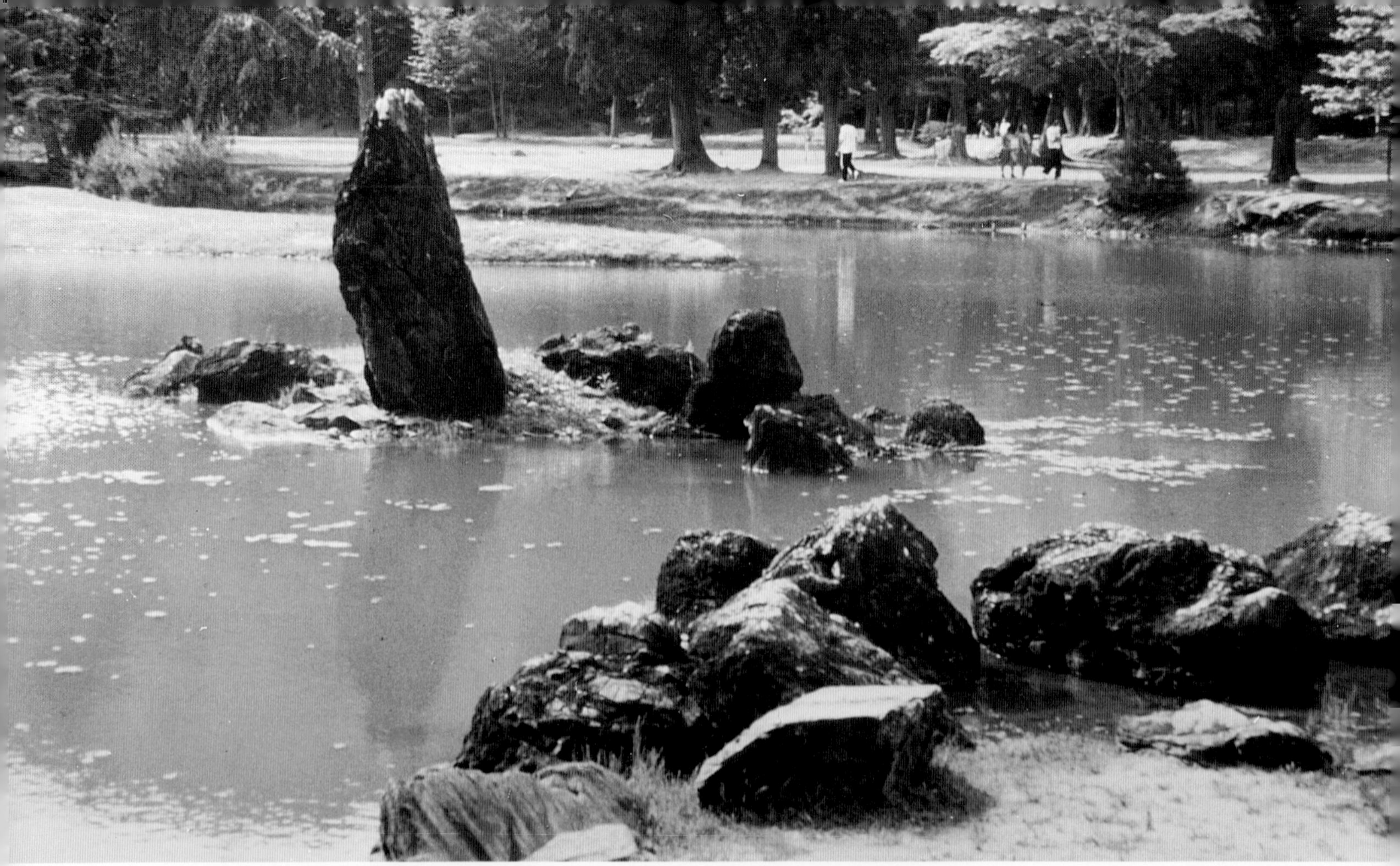

12 Stones placed in a pond landscape to simulate a rough seashore, Mōtsūji, Iwate Prefecture.

> Since the stones in the pond landscape are placed to simulate a seascape, be sure to install the "deep-rooted rock" and the "wave-repelling stone" in the scenery.[49]

Here the prototype of the pond is the sea, and the most essential aspect in implementing the *yō* is indicated as providing a "deep-rooted rock" and a "wave-repelling stone." These two elements are key to expressing the essence of the scene. Likewise, the proper means of expressing a scene of a rough seashore (Figure 12) is prescribed as:

> ... placing there some pointed rocks in a casual-looking manner. Then place a sequence of rocks from the shore toward the offing, making them appear as though the rocks had grown out of the same bedrock extending from the shore. There should be a few rocks isolated from the rest.[50]

The stylized forms (*yō*) were based on existing forms of nature, which—according to the third overall principle—the designer should "make his own" and "model after the general air of," that is acquire an internalized understanding of them and express them in essence. The implementation should be "design[ed] with the mood of harmony." Above all, however, the prototype being expressed must be evident.

None of these stylized forms (*yō*) faithfully reproduces nature in its existing form; instead, each extracts a certain form or air that can be said to exist within nature and, in re-creating it, intensifies and transposes it. Fundamentally abstract in character, this stylization became a primary factor in the development of Japanese gardens thereafter, remaining at the core of the various garden styles that later emerged.

The commonly recognized prototypes of these stylized forms (*yō*) are not contingent upon scale. In the process of implementing these styles, where scale comes into play, a variety of interpretations emerge to accommodate different existing conditions. Thus, for each stylized form there are a myriad of interpretations. Creativity and individuality manifest in the design process, albeit within the confines of the prototype.

The styles and forms passed down from master to apprentice, known as *denshō* (transmitted traditions), *kuden* (oral transmissions), and *hiden* (secret transmissions), were also created within the framework of the prototype. It is precisely because all design refinements are implemented within the format of a stylized form (*yō*) that the prototype is commonly recognizable. The designer's interpretation will ultimately be subject to the viewer's ability to comprehend it; thus it must clearly reflect the prototype.

"Recalling," "thinking over," and "studying/modeling after" are steps in the design process that lead from prototype to interpretation, and from stylized form to implemented form. *Sakuteiki* summarizes the prototype of the Heian garden as "the natural landscape" and "famous places of scenic beauty" and outlines the design process as "recalling your memories of how nature presented itself for each feature" and "think[ing] over the famous places of scenic beauty throughout the land, and by making your own that which appeals to you most, design your garden with the mood of harmony, modeling after the general air of such places." More specific comments such as "[T]he ocean style is used," or "the 'reed-hand' style may be applied" are suggestions of design solutions. The term "modeling after," as seen for instance in *Jikkinshō's* description of the Sukechika residence, "[m]odeled after Amanohashidate in Tango, the island in the center of the pond is elongated and planted with young pines," refers not to a totally realistic depiction of nature, but rather to a process of conveying its essence by extracting a stylized form, or what *Sakuteiki* refers to as "modeling after the general air of such places." "Designing with the mood of harmony" calls for imbuing an interpretation with originality and creativity. The reference to the model—for instance, Amanohashidate—must however be manifestly clear.

The terms "recalling," "modeling after," and "being manifestly clear," in fact describe successive steps in the Japanese garden-making process—a process in which stylized forms are extracted from nature in its existing form and then transposed to create interpretations that also fulfill the functional criteria of specific architectural forms and gardens.

Garden Design Solutions That Address Spatial Constraints

Japanese gardens do not exist as independent entities. Until the Edo period, they were generally designed to be viewed from a seated position in the building interior, and so were directly correlated to the function and style of the architecture. There are no other known examples of this kind of correlation; it is apparently unique to the Japanese garden. *Sakuteiki* offers numerous suggestions for design solutions intended to accommodate particular site conditions and building functions.

The style of the *shinden-zukuri* garden was determined by the function and decorative style of the *shinden* main hall itself, and was subject to the various constraints inherent in the standard one-*chō* site. Specifically, the prescribed stylized forms (*yō*) for expressing each of the six basic compositional elements—artificial hills, pond, island, flat and open white sand space, garden stream, and waterfall—were affected by the standard division of land allotted for the different areas of the garden. In a typical *shinden-zukuri* estate, the buildings occupied the northern half of the site, and the *shinden* was positioned at the center of the southern border. The southern half of the site, approximately 60 meters (197 feet) on the north-south axis by 120 meters (394 feet) on the east-west, was set aside for the garden. Thirty meters (80 to 98 feet) of that area (north-south) was to be set aside for the white sand area, leaving free 30 by 120 meters (98 by 394 feet) to house a pond that imitates the ocean with an island containing a musician's stage of 30 by 120 meters (70 by 80 feet), and artificial hills for embellishment. As we have seen, *Sakuteiki* acknowledges the difficulty of achieving this

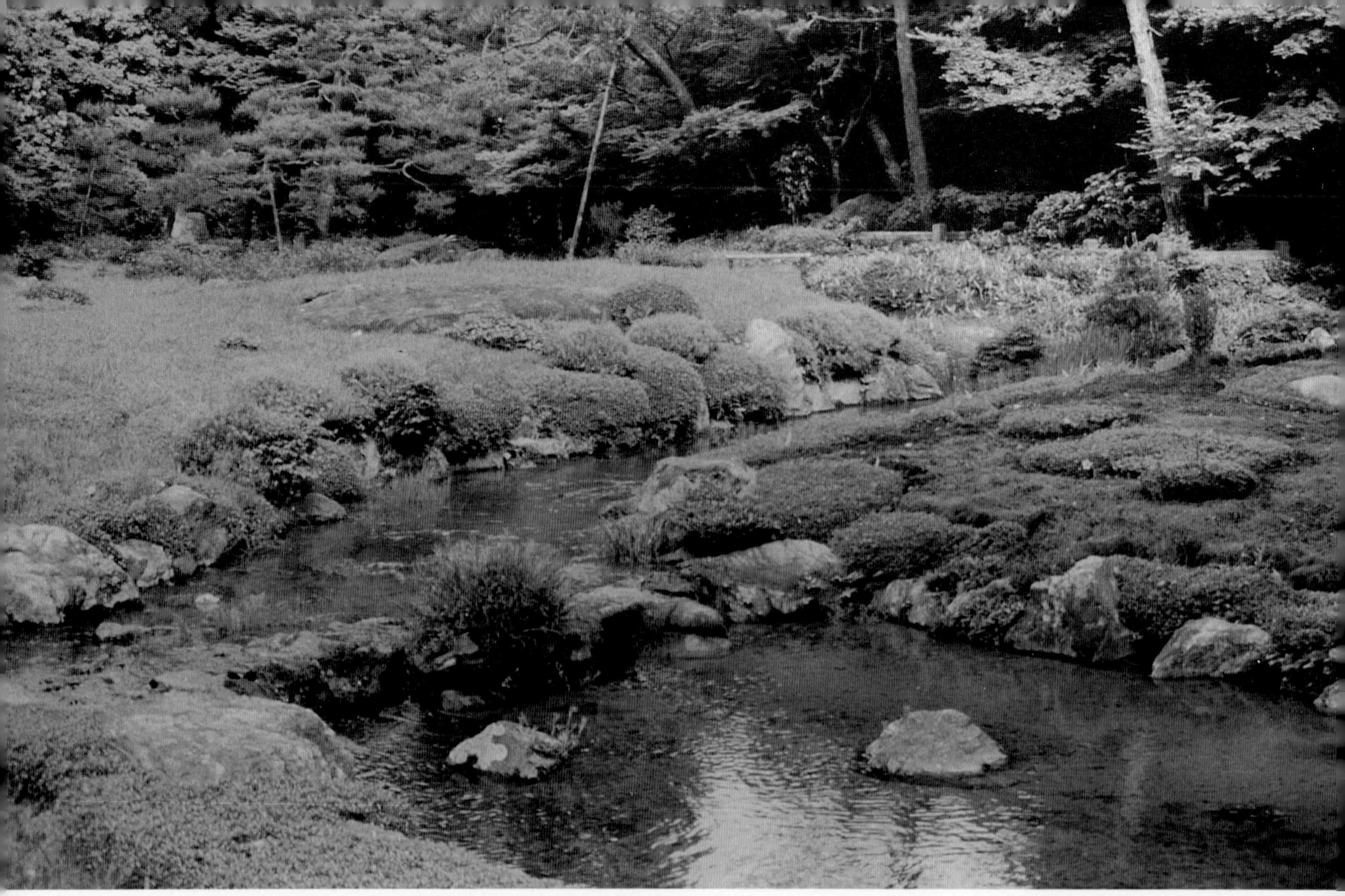

13 A garden stream broadened in the absence of a pond, Murin'an, Kyoto.

feat, and offers various techniques for implementing the stylized forms (*yō*) under specific limiting circumstances.

The myriad of interpretations seen in *shinden-zukuri* gardens corresponds to the simplified arrangement of the palace buildings which developed in response to the limitations posed by the one-*chō* site. There were two main approaches taken in garden design as means of addressing spatial constraints:

Abbreviation

> Whether the island is provided or not will depend on the aspect of the place as well as on the size of the pond. If the place is suitable for making the island, the usual arrangement is to bring the edge of the island toward the front center of the Main Hall (*shinden*), and to provide space for the Musician's Stage toward the far side of the island. Since the musician's stage extends seventy to eighty feet across … when the island lacks in space, there should be a device such as constructing a minor island behind, and extending a temporary wooden-board floor from there over the pond water toward the main island. This device will relieve the narrowness of the island, and will make the front of the Musician's Stage look wider by showing much of the island. Thus it is understood that the temporary wooden floor is provided where there is lack of space, yet keeping the front of the island normal in appearance.[51]

This item provides a good example of an interpretation that addresses the contradiction between the prototype and its implemented form. It proposes to fulfill the requirement for a seventy-to-eighty–foot musician's stage in a creative way, by extending a platform from the rear of the island, thus preserving the frontal view of the island from the *shinden* without inordinately increasing the size of the island in relation to that of the pond. It is an interpretation that reconciles aesthetic and practical concerns, and was passed down as a transmitted tradition (*denshō*).

When there is the garden stream but no pond, you

> should provide in the South Garden such a feature as the Hillside Field and place stones which conform to such a feature. It is also a normal practice to place stones and make the garden on a flat ground where there is no hill or pond. Where the pond is absent, however, the garden stream should be made especially broad, and the knobbed portions of the ground should be levelled off in order to make the view of the running stream visible from the palace hall floor. Along the skirt of the hillside field scene of the garden stream, planting of tall-growing trees and shrubs should be avoided. Instead, you should use such wild-flower plants as the Chinese Bellflower, the Patrinia, the Burnet, Plantain Lily, and the like …
>
> The width of the garden stream should depend on the scale of the estate ground as well as on the available volume of water. The widths of two feet, three feet, four or five feet, are all practicable. If the house and estate are in large scale, and voluminous water is available, the running stream may be made as wide as six or even seven feet.[52]

This description of the small garden "abbreviates" the pond, leaving only the garden stream. Theoretically, it does not "omit" the pond, but provides it by widening the garden stream to the extreme (Figure 13). The combination of techniques used here, which includes also leveling the ground, creates an interpretation that gives an appearance of depth to a viewer seated on the palace floor. Restricting the planting of trees and shrubs near the stream shows that subtle and careful attention is being paid the task of maintaining a unified sense of scale while making a small garden appear as spacious as possible.

On the one hand, the idea that "the garden stream should be made especially broad" in the absence of a pond calls for a subjective judgment as to what size stream would create the illusion of a pond in the context of a particular site. However, one very refined technique is offered for scaling specific details to the overall spatial illusion:

> Sometimes stones are placed where there is no pond or running water. This is called the dry landscape. The dry landscape is created by first constructing the steep edge of a hill or the outline of some wild hillside fields, and then associating stones with it.[53]

The garden without a pond or running water is a further refinement of the widened "garden stream with no pond," and is termed a "dry landscape." It is not an independent style which ignores the pond as a required element, but rather is one in a series of abbreviation techniques that evolved as ways to express the prototype.

As we have seen, the stylization process characteristically involves a degree of abstraction. The dry landscape as an expressive mode was thought to meet the criteria for the prototypical *shinden-zukuri* garden.

Interestingly, the dry landscape–style "garden without water" of the late Heian period, which was attached to a hill or hillside field, shows the makings of Muromachi-period dry landscape–gardens. Abstract gardens did not suddenly appear in the Muromachi period, but were premised on this abbreviation technique of the *shinden-zukuri* garden.

The prototype set forth in *Sakuteiki*'s three overall principles is a grand and very brief treatise on nature. In contrast, interpretations are described in *Sakuteiki* with surprising attention to detail and are offered as techniques for implementing the prototype, premised on natural beauty, in real space.

View Obstruction

The *shinden-zukuri* garden was intended to "provide space for the imperial ceremonies," banquets, and various social functions. For this purpose, the staircase, bridge, island, and artificial hills were to form a single axis originating at the center front of the *shinden.* But since this axis tended to emphasize the shallowness of the site, it was commonly disguised through techniques which provide only partial, or obscured, views. These popular techniques were used in a great variety of interpretations, bringing the further breakdown of symmetry and the rise of a more free-form garden. The main passages in *Sakuteiki* outlining these techniques are as follows:

> [I]n spanning the bridge from the island to the shore of the courtyard, do not bring the centerline of the bridge to fall in the exact center of the staircase of the Main Hall. You should, instead, set the east-side post of the bridge in line with the west-side pillar supporting the roof of the staircase. The bridge itself should be spanned at an oblique angle.[54]

Thirty meters (ninety-eight feet) was much too shallow for a front axial view from the *shinden*. To remedy this, *Sakuteiki* advocates an interpretation which presents the length of the bridge in diagonal profile, creating an illusion of depth.

> The underside of the arched bridge, when it is visible from the direction of the seat of honor, presents a most unsightly view. Because of this, many big stones are placed toward the underside of the bridge to divert such a view.[55]

Creating a sense of vastness in a small site, here by showing an oblique view of the bridge, should not compromise the garden's aesthetics. Scrupulous attention was paid to what would be seen from the *shinden* and specific camouflaging techniques were recommended as necessary.

Some of the other techniques suggested in *Sakuteiki* for achieving this same effect are:

> Do not place the Buddhist trinity stones facing straight toward the Main Hall (*shinden*) of the palace. You should, instead, place them facing a little off the exact front.[56]

> When you make the scene of a hill, do not let the valley point toward the house … In general, the opening of the valley should not face the main front view of the garden, but instead a little away from it.[57]

> In [the hill island] style, the hills on the island should show the outline of overlapped hillocks of varied heights …[58]

> In making the island in [the field island] style, a few streaks of hillside fields (*nosuji*) are built in varied horizontal outlines …[59]

> [W]ater is sometimes made … to fall zigzag to the right and the left by means of placing the water-hitting stones in two or three steps of lowering elevations.[60]

> The Sideways Stone will look attractive especially when placed in a slanting angle to the running direction of the stream, showing its long and heaved middle portion …[61]

> The stones to form the cliff scene should appear as though a folding screen were set up unfurled. Or, it should look as if the door pieces were set in and out against the background hill.[62]

In other words, the view-obscuring techniques described in *Sakuteiki* include averting alignment of the bridge or symbolic stones with the *shinden*'s central axis, rotating the valley opening, offsetting, alternating, overlapping, zigzagging, providing only partial views of objects, and concealing the depth of the site. All have the intended effect of imbuing a restricted space with a sense of limitlessness. The application of these techniques gave rise to some of the most ingenious and effective interpretations of the prototype ever made.

These interpretations combined frontal, unidirectional, static view-obscuring techniques with others that were asymmetrical and more free-form, and became the basis for the post–Heian-period gardens that developed in response to changes in the palace's function and further imposed constraints, and ultimately led to the *miegakure* hide-and-reveal techniques used in the kinetic, multi–vantage-point gardens of the sixteenth and seventeenth centuries.

The Garden As Architecture

Shinden-zukuri buildings were single-room residences in which living space was defined with furnishings. There were no distinct rooms, and the relationship between people and furniture was fluid.

The architectural interior and exterior were partitioned by *shitomido* latticed shutters and *tsumado* paneled doors, both of which swing on hinges. In their open position, these fixtures leave the entire one-bay space between columns unobstructed, and so unite interior and exterior. For this reason the interior and exterior developed in tandem.

Shinden-zukuri living took place in spaces defined simply by movable furnishings, without the designation of specific rooms for specific purposes. By extension, it is safe to say that neither were there fixed positions in the building from which the garden was intended to be viewed.

With *shitomido* in their open position, the structural composition of the *shinden* afforded a panoramic view that encompassed the entire south garden along with the palace interior and exterior. The world that unfolded in this space, including poetry and narrative *yamato-e* painting, was informed by the aesthetic of *miyabi*, or refined beauty, that permeated all of life at the Heian court. Like gardens, painting and poetry of this period also expressed "the natural landscape" and "famous places of scenic beauty."

Yamato-e painting is narrative. Buildings are depicted in the *fukinuki-yatai* compositional technique in which roofs and ceilings are omitted to show interior and exterior scenes from a bird's-eye, panoramic view. Famous places of scenic beauty from the four corners of the capital in the four seasons are expressed on one picture plane connected by mist and clouds in the *kumogasumi* technique. *Waka* poems that extol the seasonal characteristics of these famed places are included calligraphically as part of the painting. With *kasaneirome,* bands of contrasting colors formed by layers of robes worn by Heian empresses and court ladies, providing yet another wash of color, the *shinden-zukuri moya* core building, *hisashi* outer aisles, *sukirō* open corridors, and garden formed a tangible setting for the world of *miyabi.*

As the distance between the *shinden* and *tainoya* opposing annexes on the east-west axis was also condensed, *hajitomi* half shutters, *misu* bamboo blinds, *zeshō* thin summer curtains, and *kabeshiro* heavy drapes were hung, and *kichō* free-standing textile screens placed, to interrupt sight lines. The design approach used for the corresponding *tsuboniwa* courtyard gardens—composed of plants, hillside fields, the garden stream and springs—located between these two buildings shifted from the broad panoramic view used in the south garden to an intimate one-to-one relationship between garden and viewer (see Figure 10.4). This more intimate relationship was to become the mainstream in Muromachi-period garden design (Figures 14.1–14.2).

The aesthetic of *miyabi* arose specifically in the context of the Heian court and fell from favor together with it, whereas the philosophical basis of another aesthetic ideal cultivated during the Heian period, *mono no aware,* retained its appeal and became the basis for the more somber aesthetics of medieval Japan. *Mono no aware*—the capacity to be emotionally moved by "things"—conveys a heightened sensitivity to the ephemeral beauty embodied in nature and human life, and thus contains a hint of sadness.

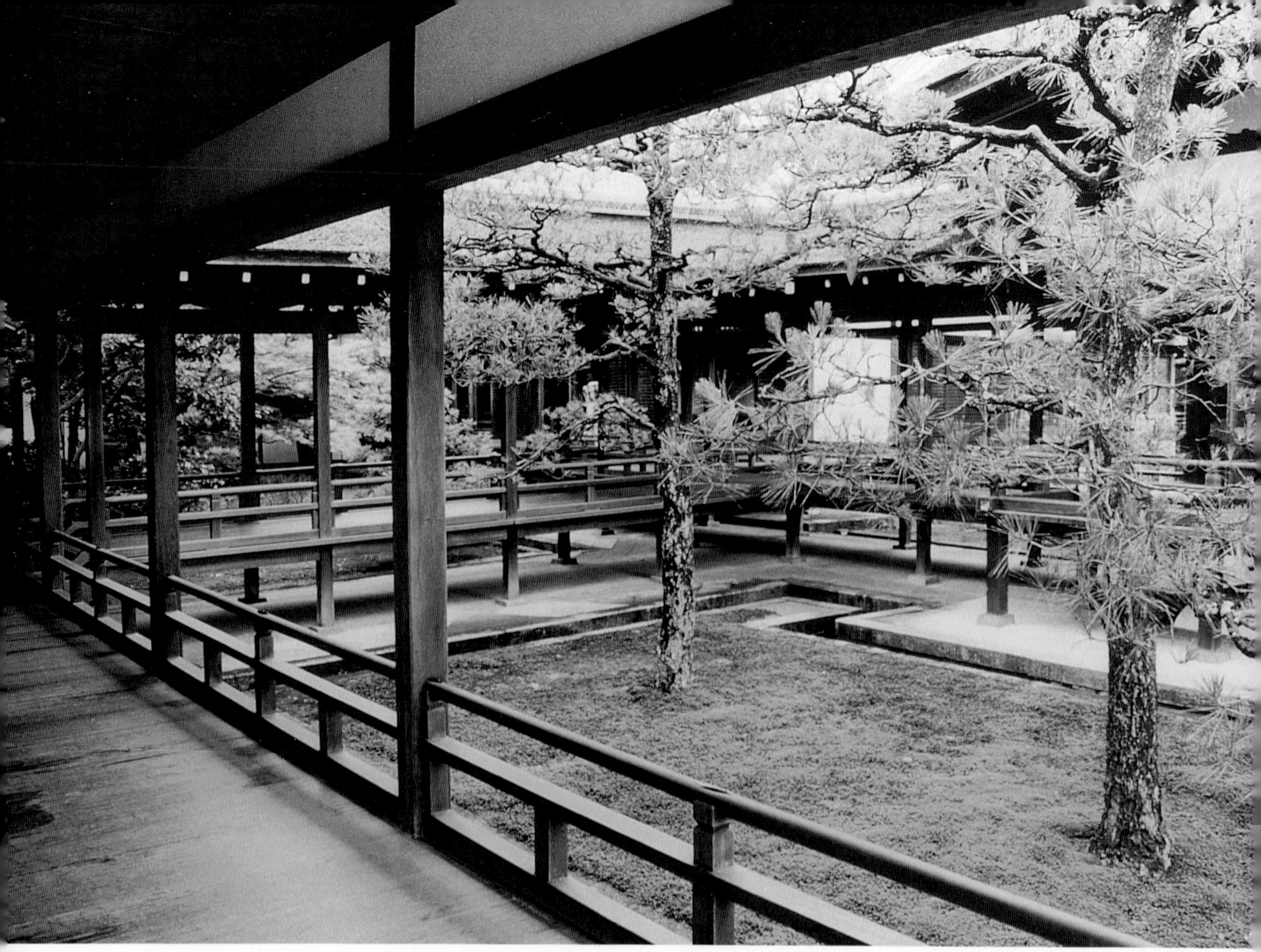

14.1 *Tsuboniwa* bordered by the *shinden, tainoya,* and *sukirō*, Nin'naji, Kyoto.

With the close of the Heian period, the *shinden*—where building interior and exterior were one—was divided into fixed rooms. With the further limitations that arose from the subdivision of the one-*chō* block into one-fourth– and one-eighth–*chō* sites, the relationship between architecture and garden changed radically. An entry appearing in the late-Heian *Nihon kiryaku* (Outline record of Japan) regarding residential zoning restrictions, listed under the year A.D. 1030, states that: "the residences of regional lords shall not exceed one-fourth–*chō*." This was just two years after the birth of *Sakuteiki* author Tachibana no Toshitsuna.

In many respects, *Sakuteiki* reflects the values of the transitional period from the gradual decline of the Heian court life at its zenith to the more austere Japanese middle ages (late Heian, Kamakura and Muromachi periods), and the sweeping structural and aesthetic changes that would be seen in the architecture and gardens to come.

14.2 *Tsuboniwa*, Daitokuji Ryōgen'in, Kyoto. ▶

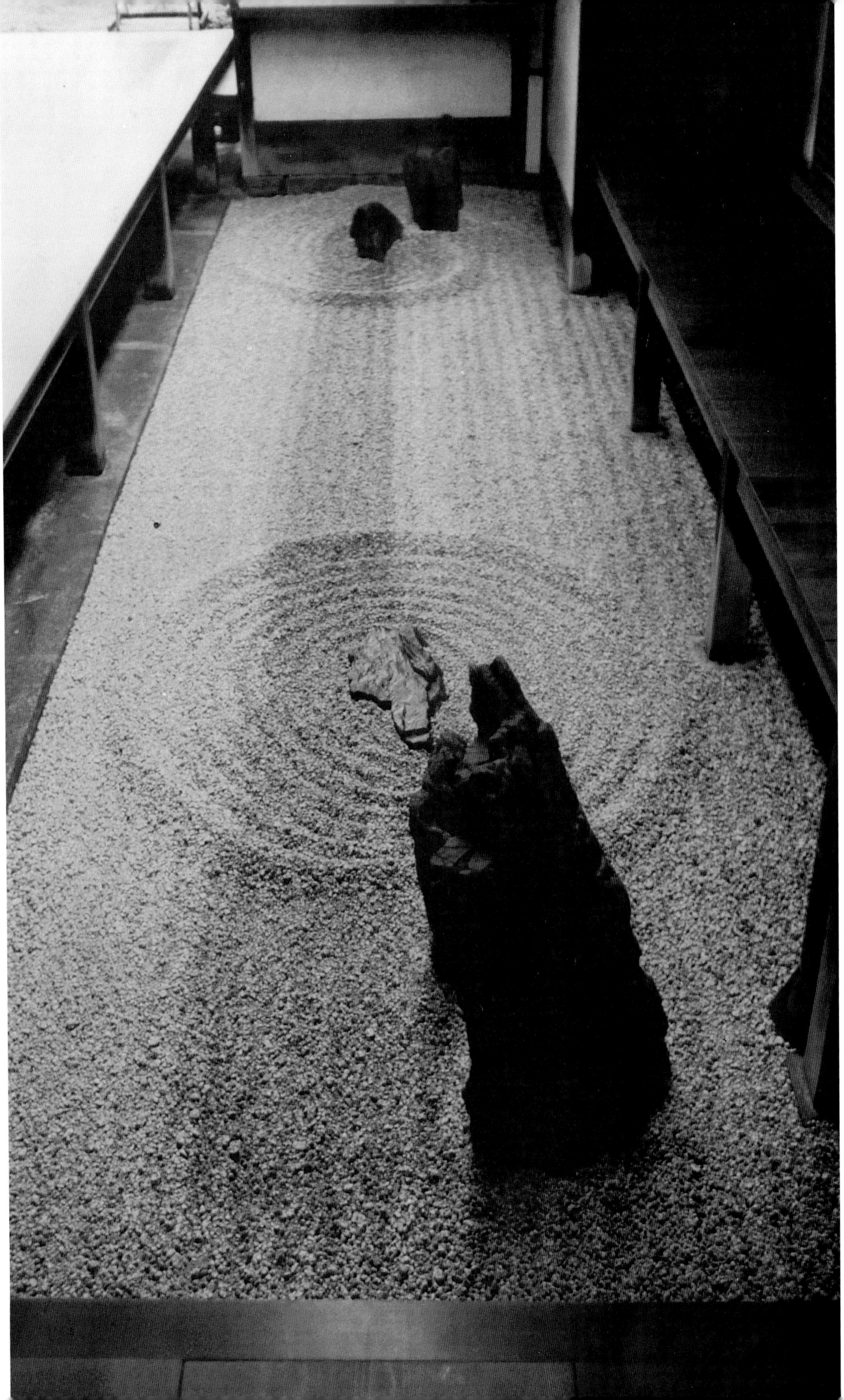

2

Shinden-Zukuri As Prototype, and Two Divergent Interpretations

The next wave of continental cultural influence, following the importation of Tang culture in the Nara and early Heian periods, was that of the Song dynasty (960–1279) during Japan's Muromachi period, when Chinese paintings and wares were imported in astounding quantities. Yoshida Kenkō expresses the tenor of the times in this passage from his classic philosophical miscellany *Tsurezuregusa* (*Essays in Idleness*), written in 1330:

> It is the height of foolishness that Chinese ships should make the dangerous journey over here crammed with cargoes of useless things.[1]

Chinese culture had been transmitted to Japan during the Nara and Heian periods in the form of "images" of the Tang capital and its palaces, whereas the culture imported during the Muromachi period took the form of goods. This bore a direct influence on Japanese residential architecture, where the *oshi-ita* decorative alcove (or *tokonoma* in its later form), *chigaidana* staggered shelves, and *tsukeshoin* built-in desk were constructed for the purpose of displaying Chinese paintings and wares. More indirectly, it led to the subdivision of the formerly open *shinden* main hall into rooms defined by fixed walls and sliding doors, the construction of ceilings and *tatami* mat–covered floors, and a shift from round to square posts. These features define the architectural style which came to be known as *shoin-zukuri.* This second wave of continental influence marked a radical reform in the history of Japanese residential architecture; this reform did not, however, extend to city planning.

By the close of the Heian period, Kyoto's one-*chō* city-block grid had been subdivided into sites measuring one-fourth– and one-eighth–*chō.* This degree of reduction in site size—what might today be called "miniaturization"—would naturally impact the scale and configuration of the architecture and gardens that a site could accommodate, as is evident in the folding screen paintings known as *rakuchū rakugai-zu* (scenes in and around the capital; Figure 15).

Over the course of the Kamakura period, the Tang-based prototype for the palace and garden had faded, although the custom of always basing composition on a model remained. The Heian palaces and gardens of Japan became the new prototype. The transition from *shinden-zukuri* to *shoin-zukuri* began with the north half of the residence. The *shinden-zukuri* style was at first retained in the south half, and the transformation to *shoin-zukuri* was gradual (Figure 16).

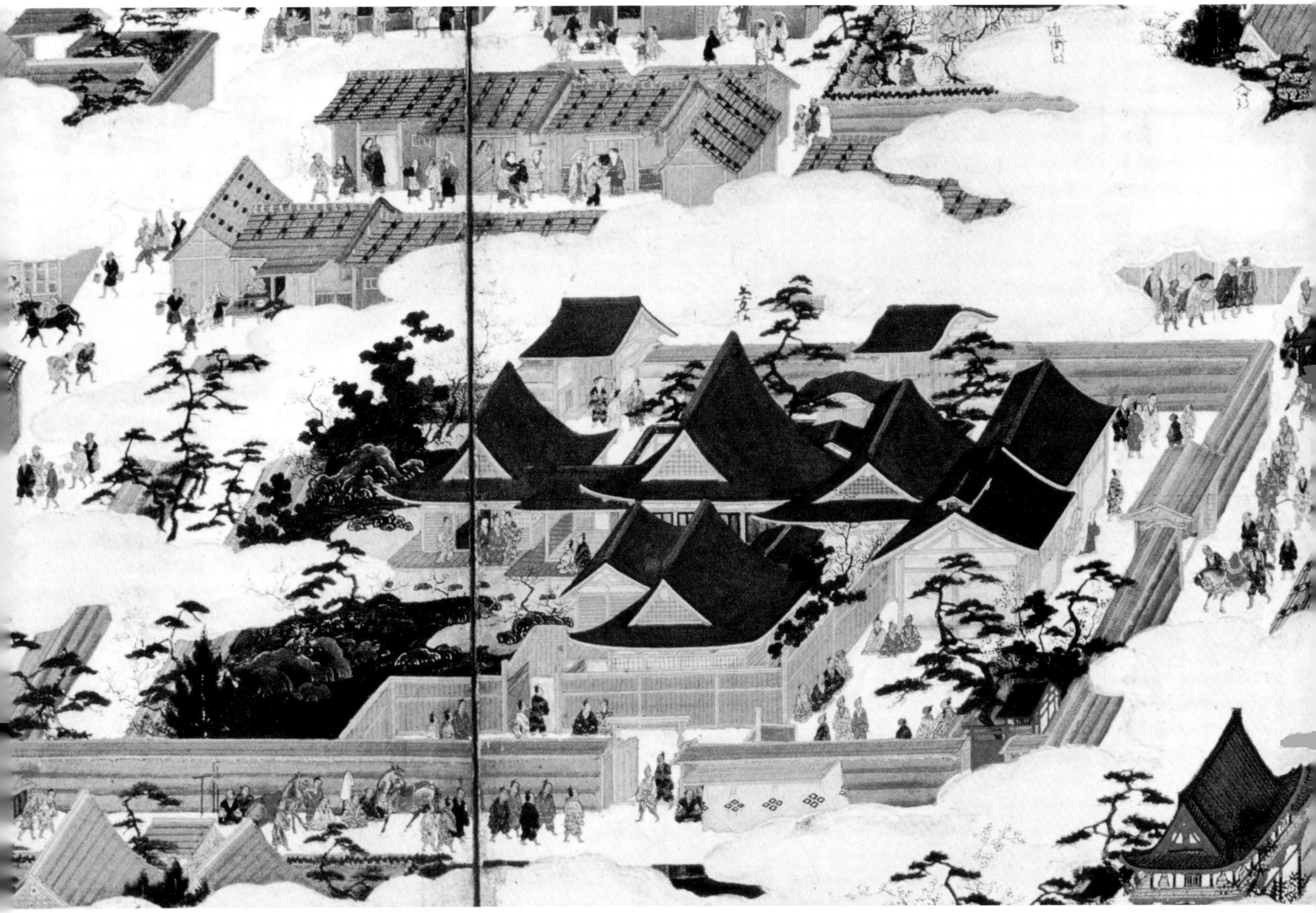

15 Detail from a *rakuchū rakugai-zu* folding-screen painting depicting a shogun estate in late Muromachi-period Kyoto. Property of Yonezawa City, Yamagata Prefecture.

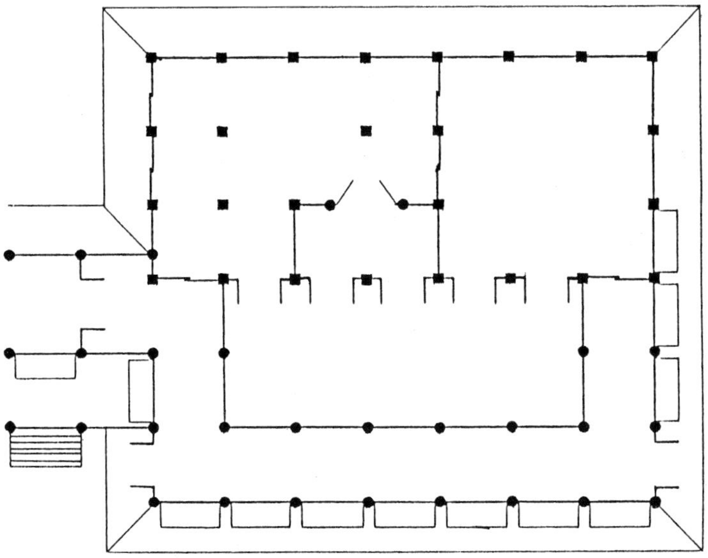

16 Reconstructed plan of the Ashikaga Yoshinori Muromachi villa by Kawakami Mitsugu. Reproduced from *Nihon kenchiku-shi zushū*. (History of Japanese architecture through selected illustrations).

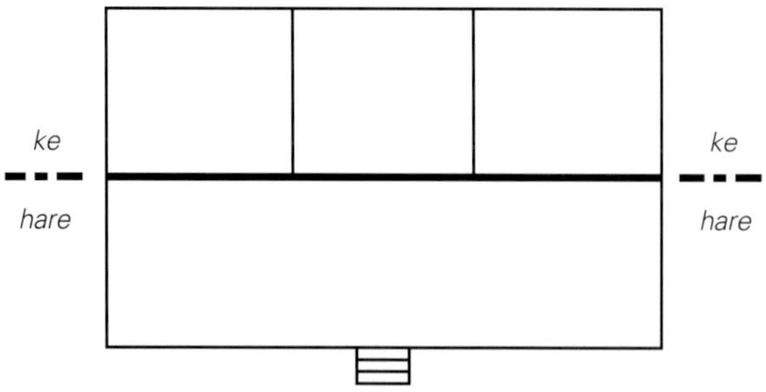

17 Schematic showing the division of the *shinden* into formal (*hare*) and informal (*ke*) halves, and into small rooms along the building's north side.

Sociopolitically, the medieval period saw the formation and development of a feudal society, and the transitional exchange of political power from the aristocracy to the warrior class. Zen Buddhism, also imported from China (where it is known as Chan), stressed self-reliance, discipline, and austerity—attributes that greatly appealed to the military consciousness. The leading aesthetic ideal of the middle ages was known as "*yūgen*" (mystery and depth), and like Zen, it was concerned with the true nature hidden behind the illusory aspects of the world. Yet despite these changing ideals, understanding and expressing the essence of nature remained the keystone of all the arts. In his poetic diary *Oi no kobumi* (*The Records of a Travel-worn Satchel*), written in 1688, Matsuo Bashō looks back in history to masters who exemplified the highest attainments in their disciplines:

> Saigyō in traditional poetry, Sōgi in linked verse, Sesshū in painting, Rikyū in tea ceremony, and indeed all who have achieved real excellence in any art, possess one thing in common, that is, a mind to obey nature, to be one with nature, throughout the four seasons of the year.[2]

The *shinden-zukuri* garden was designed for ceremonial use. During the transitional period, however, this primary function was lost, and the garden became purely ornamental.

From Abbreviation to Abstraction

As was noted earlier, Higashisanjō Palace was based on a bilaterally symmetrical formula but acquired an asymmetrical layout to conform to its two-*chō* site. Small and medium-sized residences, with their greatly restricted sites, were one generation further removed, built with *shinden-zukuri* as their prototype. These were a simplified form of the original, which emphasized the most important features and abbreviated others. The south side of the main hall, having lost most of its official ceremonial functions, was restructured primarily as a venue for the composition of linked verse and other leisure-time pursuits of the powerless nobility.

During the medieval period, in order to adapt to further reductions in site size, the main hall was reduced in scale and the symmetrical pairs of *tainoya* annexes, *tsuridono* fishing pavilions, *chūmon* inner gates, and *sukirō* open corridors were all omitted on one side. Asymmetrical in ground plan, a smaller *shinden* and a single *tainoya* connected by a reduced-scale *sukirō* with *chūmon* became the new standard. This is the compositional form typically seen today in Zen sub-temples, except that the *shinden* is now replaced by a *kyakuden* (guest hall) or *hōjō* (abbot's quarters).

Early examples of *shoin-zukuri* guest halls furnished with *shitomido* shutters and *tsumado* doors—seen for instance on the east facade of Onjōji's Kōjō-in—preserved the *shinden-zukuri* exterior image although this had no functional or stylistic relationship to the *kyakuden* interior (see Figure 33.1).

Ke and the North Garden

In the late Heian period, the most significant change to occur in *shinden-zukuri* architecture was the division of the interior of the *shinden*, directly under the roof ridge, into north and south halves partitioned by sliding doors (*munewakedo*). The south side (*hare*) served as the formal ceremonial space, and the north side (*ke*) was for daily living. The residential area was further divided by fixed walls and *fusuma* sliding doors into small rooms—specifically, the study, the sleeping room and the informal reception room, or *shoin* (Figure 17). This grouping of rooms along

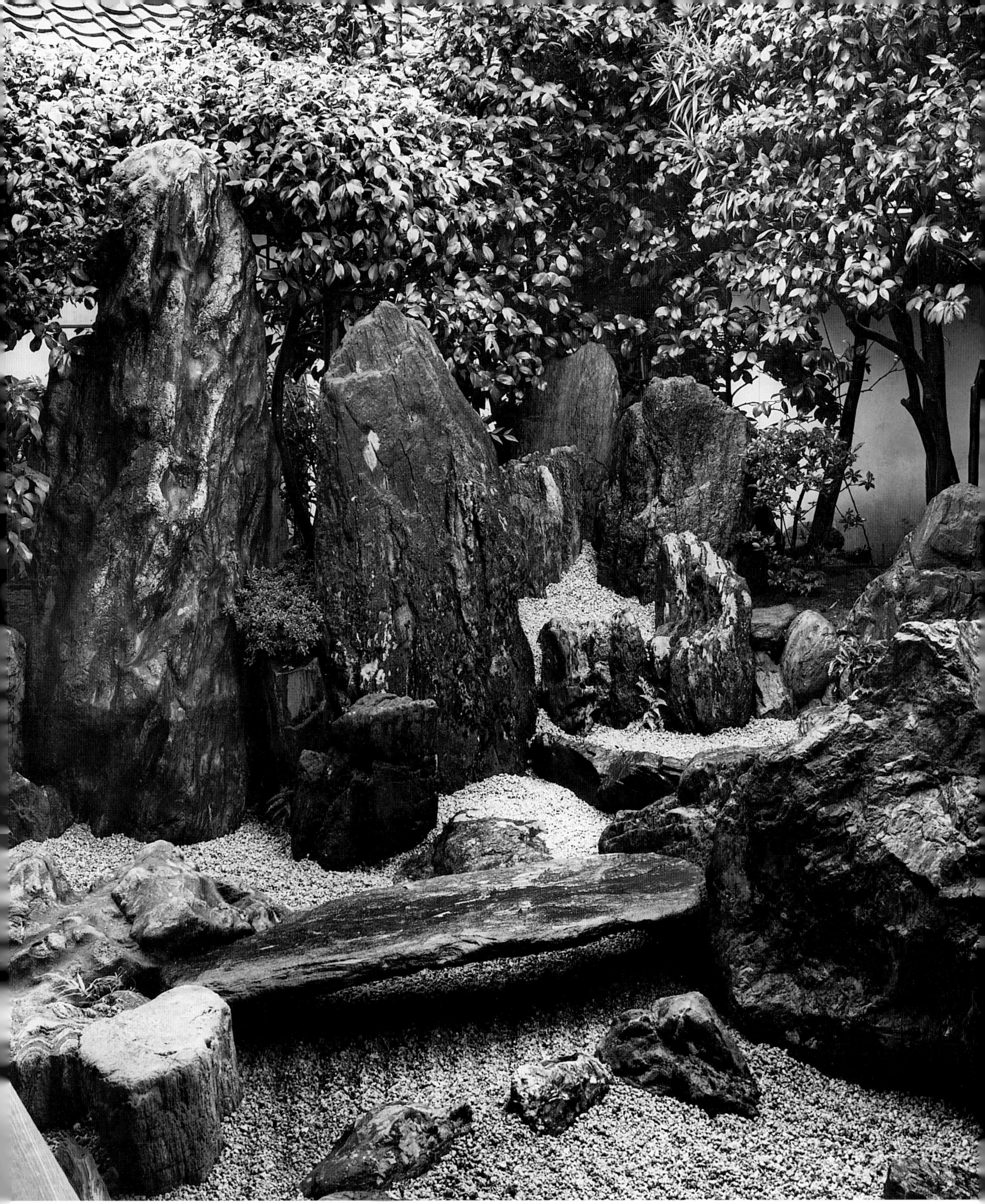

18.1 Dry waterfall and rapids of the north garden at Daitokuji Daisen'in, Kyoto.

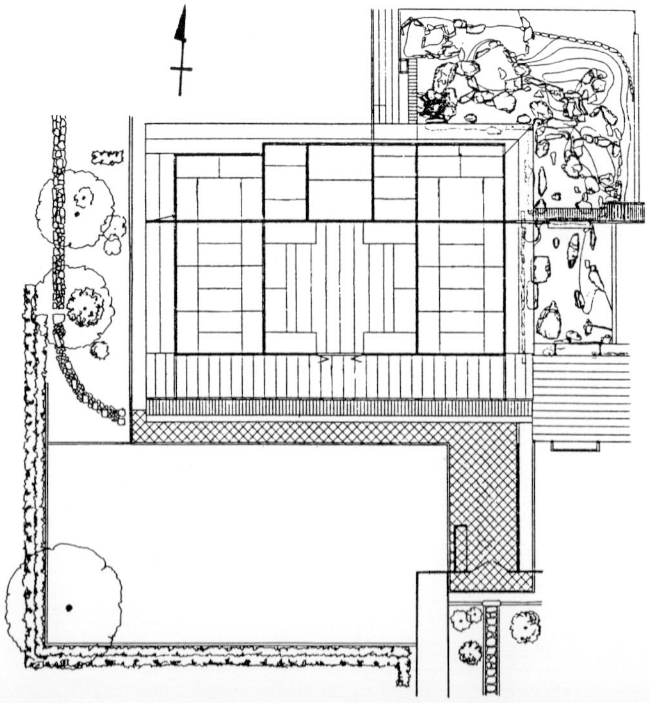

18.2 Plan view drawing of the Daisen'in *hōjō* and the north and south gardens.

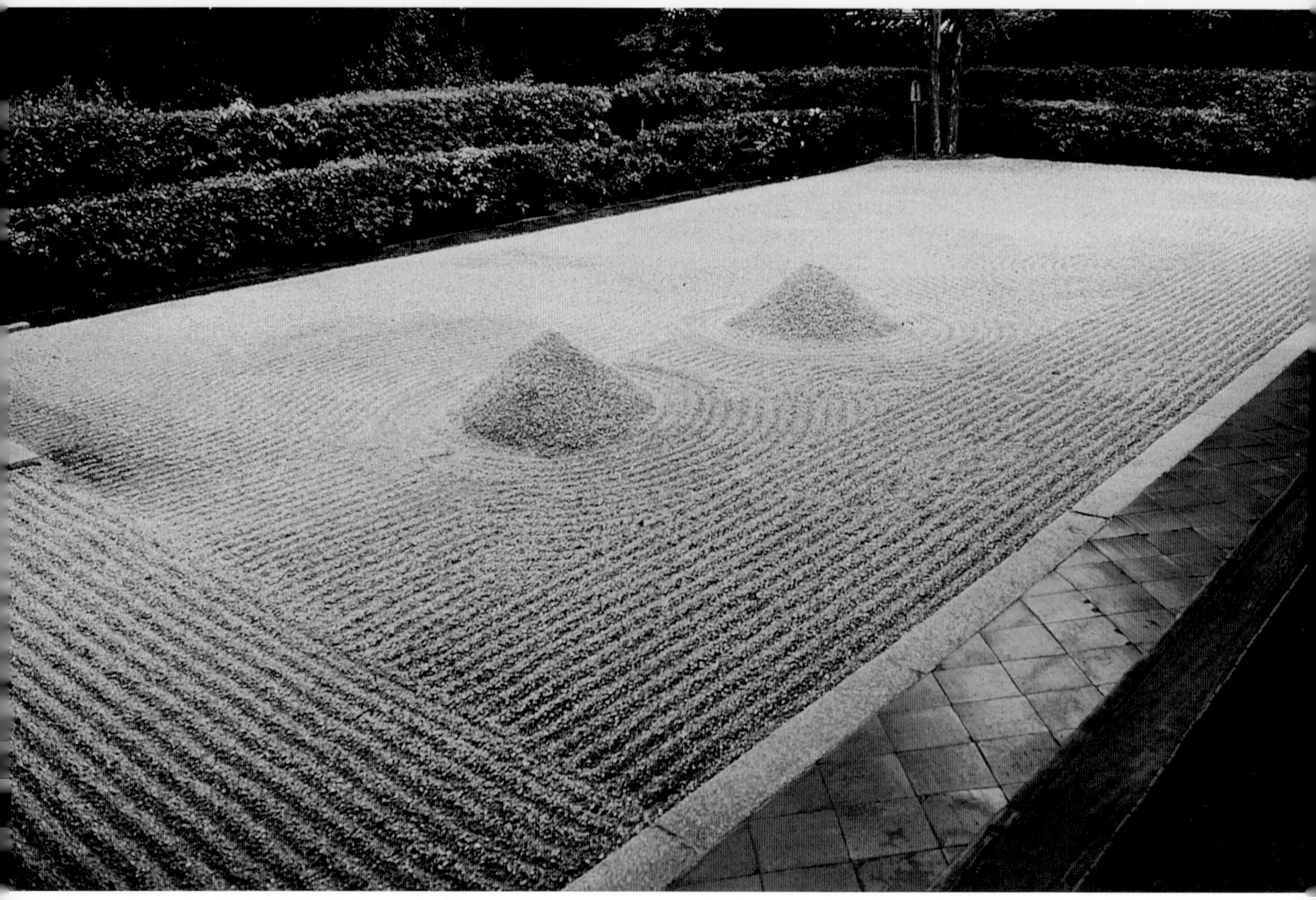

18.3 The Daisen'in *hōjō* south garden.

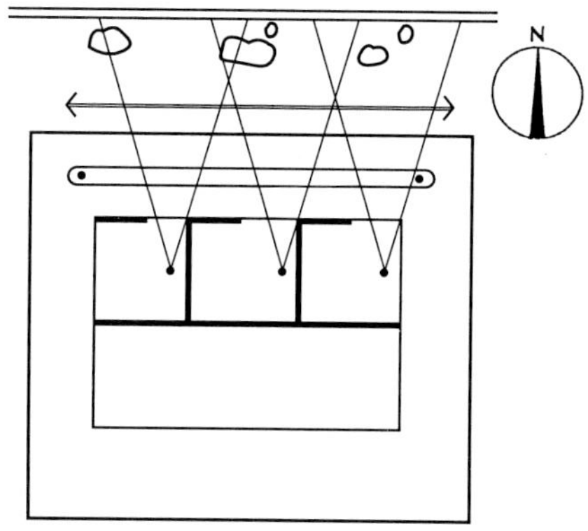

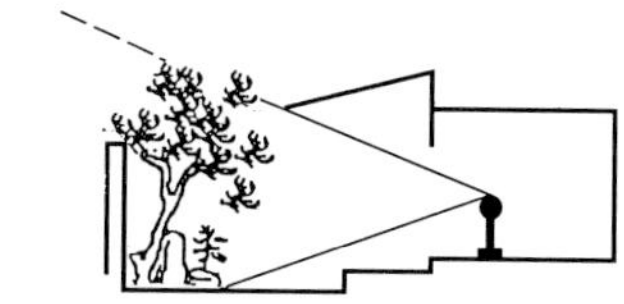

19.1 Plan and section schematics showing views afforded of the north garden through the half-bay openings from the adjacent small rooms along the building's north side and the lateral path of movement on the veranda.

the north side naturally stimulated new approaches to garden design, and is thought to be a factor in the characteristic density of the north garden.

Shinden-zukuri architecture originally had no fixed partitions. When the *shitomido* shutters were raised, the palace and garden were unified, providing a panoramic overview of the entire garden and architectural environment. With the shift to the partitioning of interior space into rooms beginning in the twelfth century, the panoramic field of vision achieved with *shinden-zukuri* architecture was narrowed to a more acute angle. An additional change in exterior fixtures from *shitomido* swinging shutters to *mairado* sliding doors enhanced this tendency.

As opposed to *shitomido*, which swing up on a horizontal pivotal axis, leaving the entire one-bay space between columns open, *mairado* are composed of two wooden doors and one paper screen (*akarishōji*) that slide horizontally in a three-track gutter, so that even in their fully open position a half-bay section always remains closed to the outdoors (see Figures 36.1–36.2). The result is a framed, or cropped, view of a single scene of the garden. The relationship between the garden and the series of rooms with narrowed views gave rise to the unique characteristics of the north garden; the views from inside the rooms demand a garden of considerable density.

Of all the basic compositional elements of the prototypical *shinden-zukuri* garden, the waterfall and rapids of the upper garden stream were best expressed in the high-density north garden. The theme of the gardens of Daitokuji's Daisen'in and Myōshinji's Taizō-in is the "flow" of the garden stream from the water's source—a mountain waterfall with cascading water that flows over, under, and around dams, bridges, and islands, finally exiting under the building, creating an implied continuous flow that pours out into the "open sea" garden on another side of the building (Figures 18.1–18.3). The interpretations for these small narrow strip gardens less than four meters (twelve feet) in depth, replace water with moss and coarse white sand, creating an exquisite, abstract expression of the prototype.

Another compositional characteristic of the north garden was a quality of linear continuity born of the moving vantage point afforded the viewer walking the north veranda. The interactive relationship between the garden and viewer walking on the veranda was an important factor in the changeover during this period to kinetic and bidirectional garden composition techniques.

The garden scenes relating to the views afforded from floor-level seated positions inside the individual adjoining rooms had to be linked so as to create a unified garden that would flow in a linear sequential fashion as the viewer walked along the veranda. The north garden preserved the frontal, single-scene compositions that correspond to fixed vantage points from the room interiors, but at the same time linked one focal point to another, giving the garden a dual composition (Figures 19.1–19.3).

The compositional technique used to bring the spaces between individual garden scenes into play via movement and form a unified garden bears a close resemblance to Sesshū's horizontal handscroll entitled *Sansui chōkan* (Landscape, 1486), in which a series of single scenes are linked into a unified scroll painting through the use of a technique called *zansan jōsui*.

Zansan jōsui is frequently used in ink-wash landscape

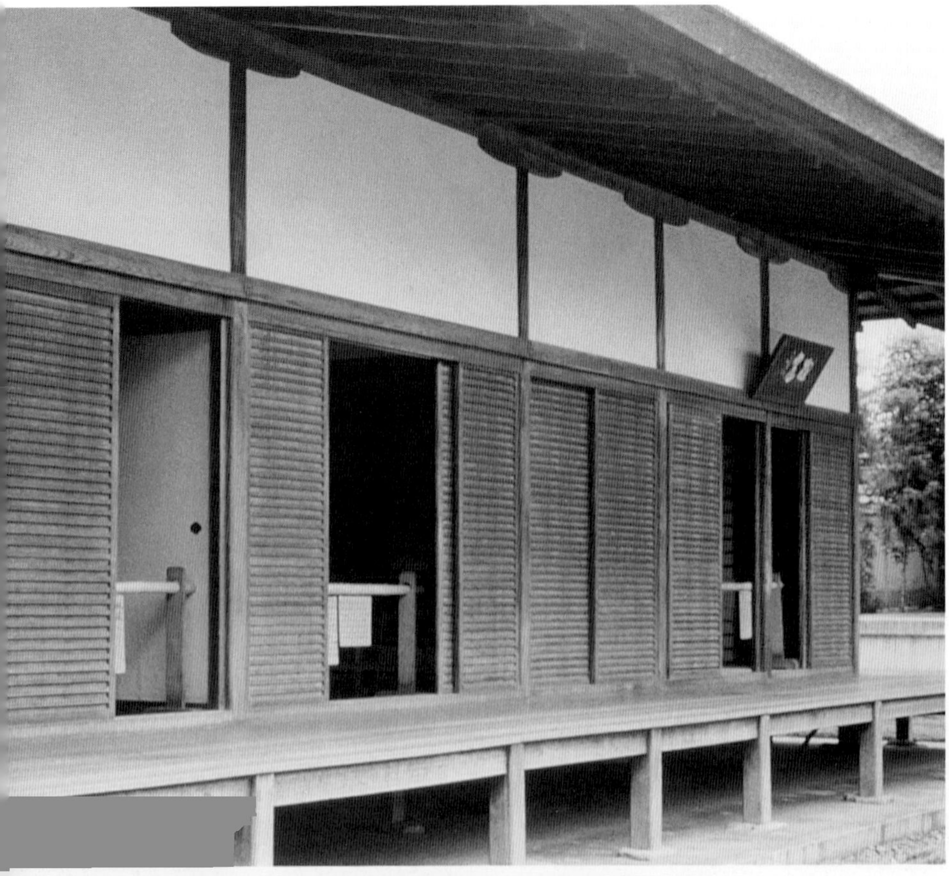

19.2 The Daitokuji Ryōgen-in *hōjō* north facade, Kyoto.

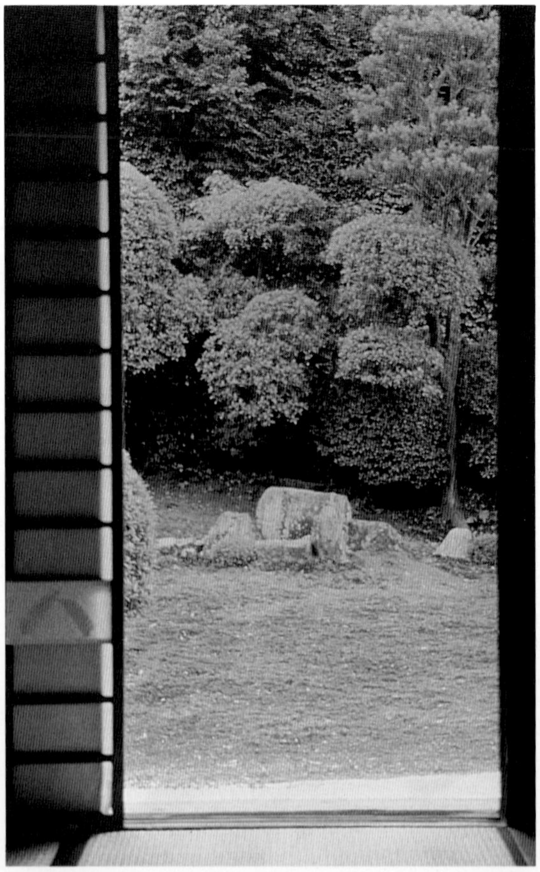

19.3 A view from the room interior of the Tōfukuji Funda-in north garden, Kyoto.

painting to suggest mountains and water slowly receding into the "mist," comprised of segments of white space left open between scenes, linking them into one integrated scroll. This expanse of unarticulated paper is not empty space, but *ma*. The term "*ma*," as used in traditional Japanese performing and visual arts, describes an interval in time or space—a void that by its very absence (whether of sound or of form) asserts its existence, adding to the articulation of the overall space. In Muromachi-period north gardens and ink-wash landscape scrolls, *ma* is an unimposing space that allows for the impression made by the previous scene to fade naturally away (Figures 20.1–20.2).

Just as Heian-period *yamato-e* paintings—in which well-known scenes from the four corners of the capital and the four seasons had been linked by the *kumogasumi* (cloud and mist) technique on a single, all-encompassing picture plane related to the panoramic view of the *shinden-zukuri* garden from the palace, the composition of the Muromachi-period north garden was expressed with techniques similar to those used in the ink-wash landscape paintings popular during the same period.

The *zansan jōsui* technique is adaptable to a garden composed of linked heterogeneous spaces, where each scene is hidden from the next and appears in linear succession, but not to a landscape that can be apprehended in a single sweeping view.

Hare and the South Garden

The simplification of the formal south garden began in the twelfth century with the cessation of imperial ceremonies and the concomitant loss of the *shinden*'s original function. The genesis of the contemplation garden (*kanshō niwa*) began with the abbreviation of the four basic compositional elements specific to the south garden—the white sand area, the pond, islands, and artificial hills. As we have seen in *Sakuteiki's* specification that "where the pond is absent, however, the garden stream should be made especially broad ... in order to make the view of the running stream visible from the palace hall floor," the prototype is not relinquished, but serves as the basis for abbreviated interpretations.

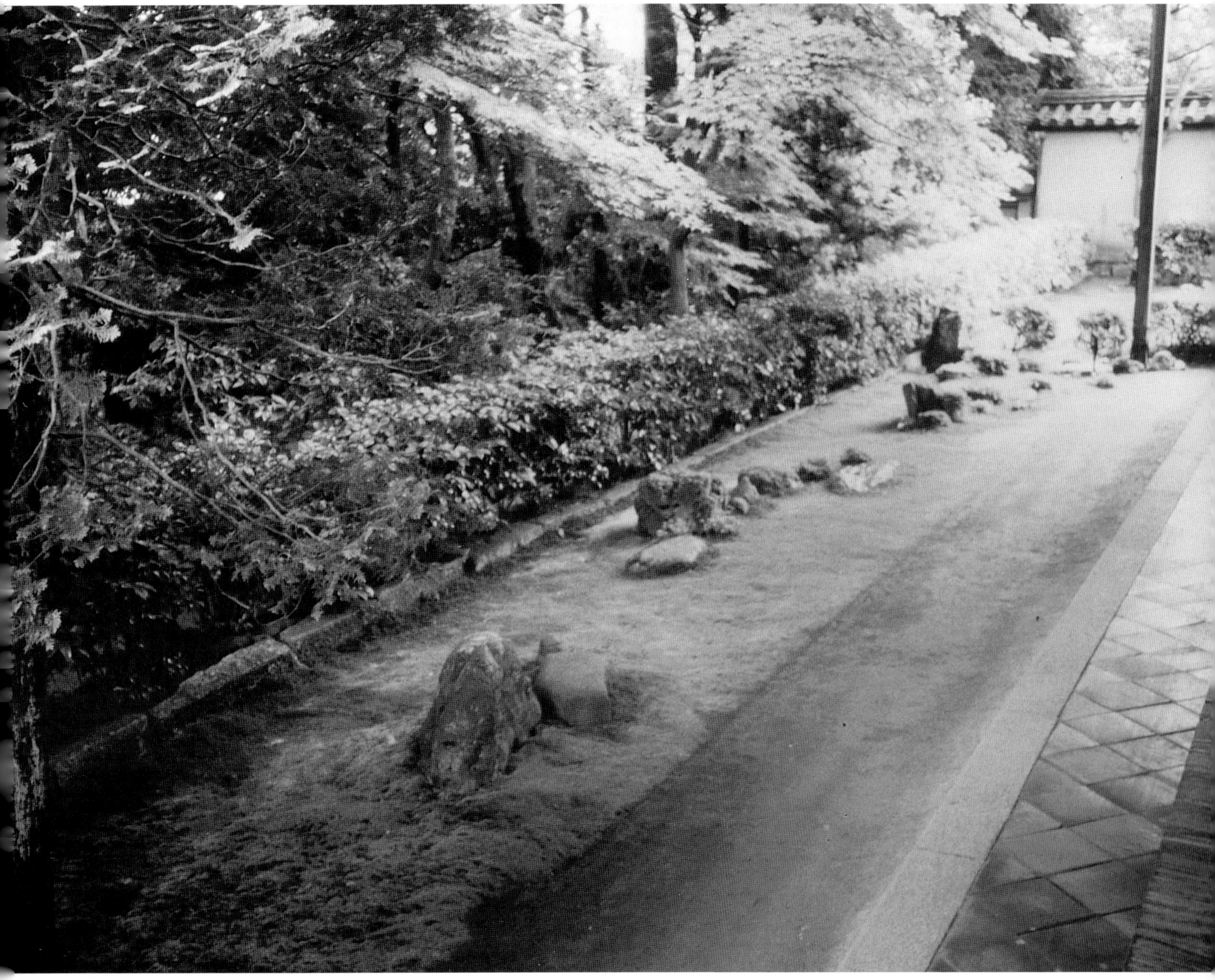

20.1 Daitokuji Shinju-an north garden, Kyoto.

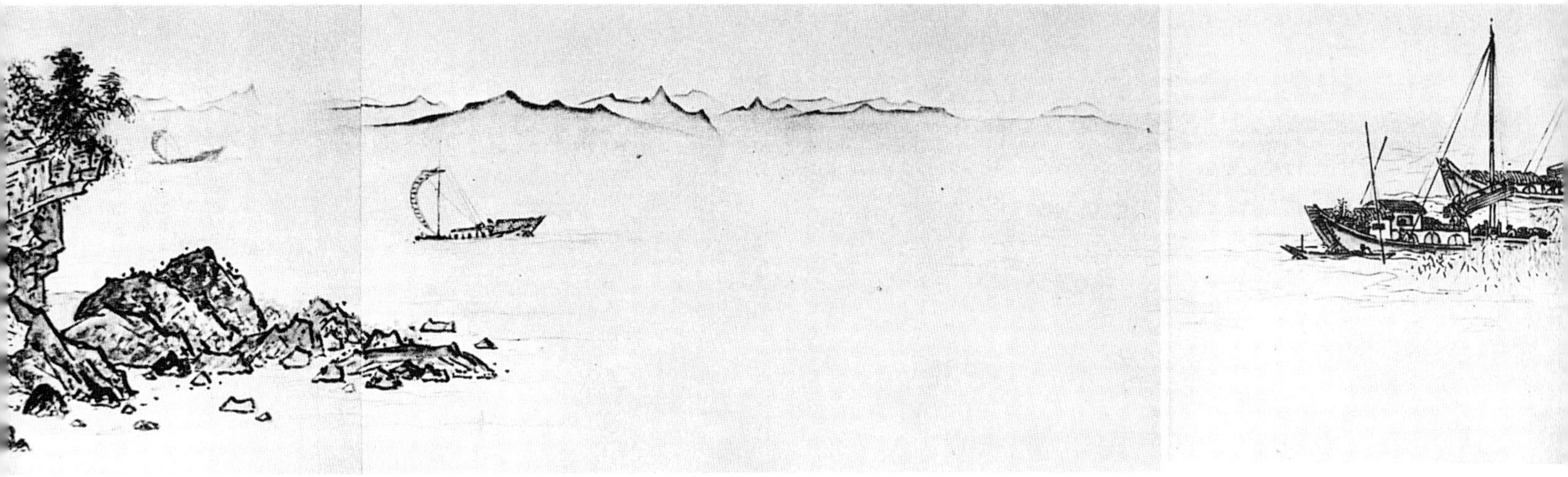

20.2 Detail from *Sansui chōkan* (Landscape) by Sesshū Tōyō, 1486. Mohri Museum.

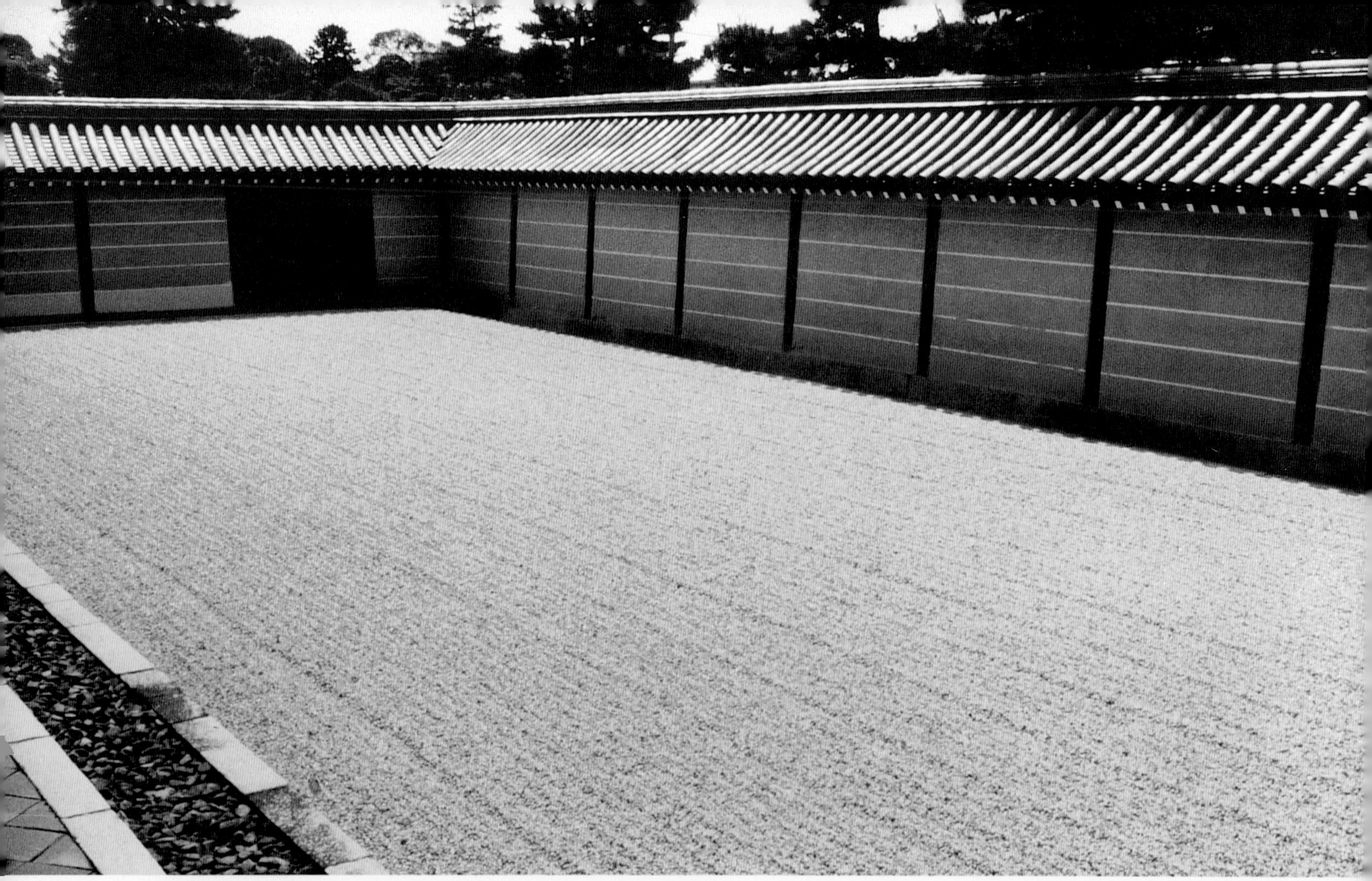

21 Myōshinji Tōkai-an *shiroroji* coarse white sand south garden, Kyoto.

The South Garden in Feudal Zen Temples

The *tsukidai* (moon dais) in front of Manpukuji's central Daiyūhō Hall is a gravel terrace that was used for the Suirikue—a presentation of offerings of food and drink to restless spirits—and other ceremonies. Likewise, the south garden of the Myōshinji Tōkai-an *hōjō* (abbot's quarters) consists of nothing but coarse white sand, although it is not now, and never was, used as a ceremonial area. While patterned after the ceremonial area of the *shinden-zukuri* south garden and the *tsukidai* of Chinese Chan (Zen) temples, the transformation from a functional to a non-functional area is most significant. This is the fundamental reason for the shift from the Heian-period naturalistic expressive style to abstract styles of expression characteristic of the Muromachi period.

Although the south garden of the Myōshinji Tōkai-an *hōjō* was constructed during the Edo period, it represents the most basic form of Zen temple south gardens (Figure 21).

Tōkai-an's south garden (*shiroroji*) omitted most of the main compositional elements of the *shinden-zukuri* south garden, including the artificial hills, pond, and islands, and retained only the white sand area. The highly-polished veranda facing the *shiroroji* served as a *dōjo*, or training ground for seated *zazen* meditation. In response to a question as to how the solid white field came to form the basis of these "gardens for Zen practice," an elderly priest at Tōkai-an offered the following Zen *kōan* (conundrum which frees the mind from conceptualizing):

> Zen monk: Taking the mountains and rivers as my own, I become them.
> Zen master: Taking myself as my own, the mountains and rivers become me.

The coarse white sand can be seen as a canvas on which the image of the "omitted" pond and islands are depicted freely in, for instance, "the ocean style" or "the river style." In his book, *Nihon no niwa* (Japanese gardens), Tachihara Masaaki explains that, "with the development of Zen culture, the dry landscape garden was devised as the Zen monk's ultimate form of recreation."[3]

Muromachi-period Zen gardens also often incorporated distant views of natural features—mountains, water-

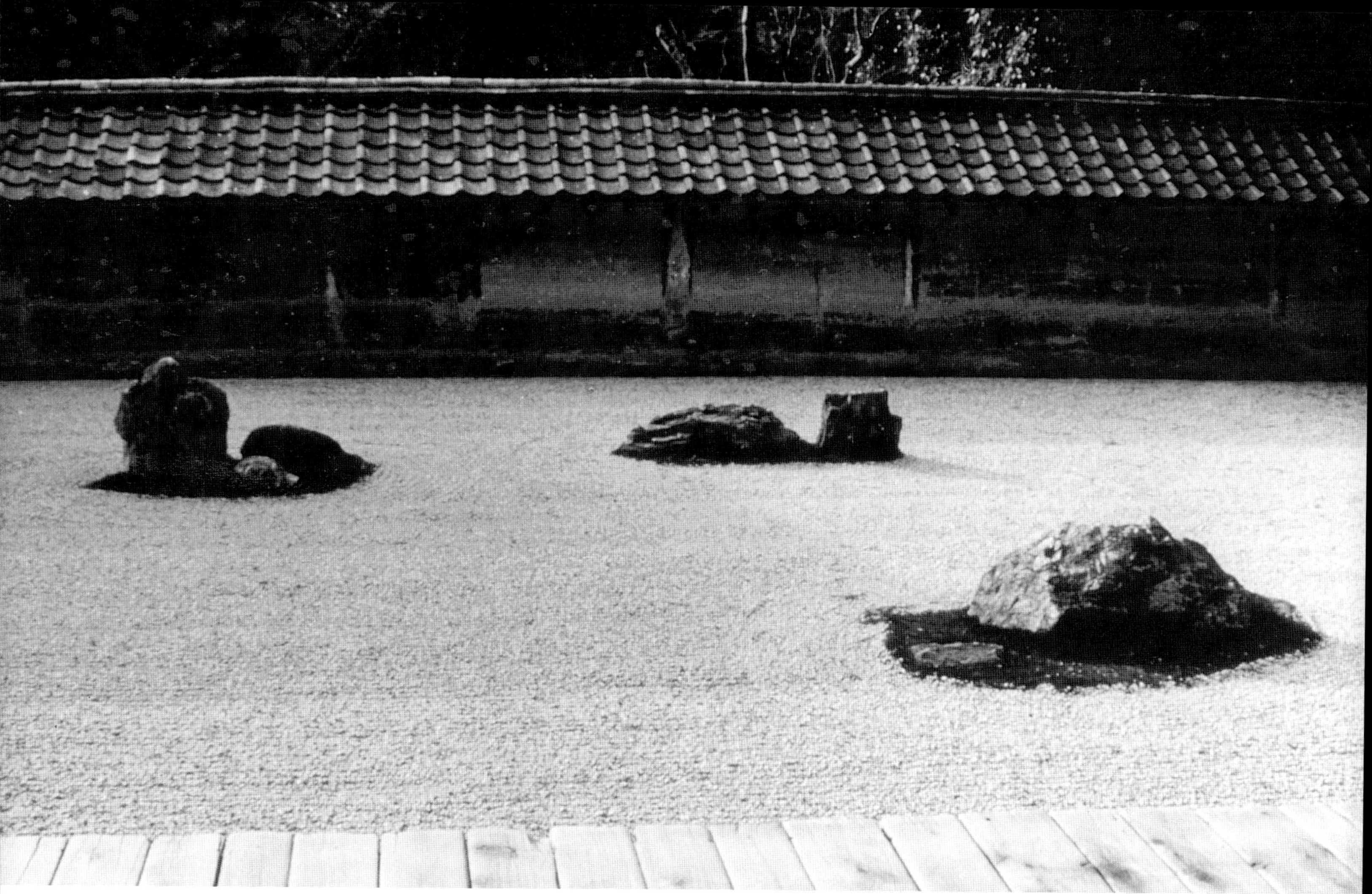

22.1 View from the veranda of Ryōanji's south garden, Kyoto.

falls, even lakes—into the garden's "picture plane" using a compositional technique called *shakkei*, or borrowed scenery. A *shakkei* garden is composed of distinct foreground, middle ground and background planes. The garden site proper comprises the foreground, and the distant feature, the background. The middle ground is composed to frame the "borrowed" feature, which foreshortens the distant view and draws it into the garden, extending the perceived scale of the garden far beyond its own boundaries. Thus the requisite "artificial hills" were added in the form of borrowed scenery (see Figure 22.2).

Fifteen stones of varying size and form placed on a solid field of coarse white sand at the south garden of Ryōanji's *hōjō* turn the space into a "*kōan*" which is also suggestive of *Sakuteiki*'s Hill Island Style, in which "the hills on the island should show the outline of overlapped hillocks of varied heights …"

The south garden of Shōdenji's *hōjō* is composed of large and small clipped bushes used in place of stones. Mount Hiei is incorporated as borrowed scenery cropped by a mud wall and a stand of cedars, making the finite space seem infinite. The south garden of Daitokuji's Kōtō-in is a field of moss upon which undulating waves are suggested by light filtered through quivering leaves of a stand of deciduous trees. Despite their abbreviation of many of the basic compositional elements, all these gardens fulfill the Heian-period garden prototype with remarkable interpretations (Figures 22.1–22.3).

When *Sakuteiki*'s concept of garden design that recreates the magnitude of nature was confronted with space restrictions, the six basic compositional elements for expressing the prototype—the artificial hills, the pond, the islands, the white sand area, the garden stream and the waterfall—were further refined, which led to the abstract and symbolic interpretations in Muromachi Zen temple gardens.

Tracing the course of the development of garden design from Heian aristocratic residences to Zen temples, it becomes clear that naturalistic and abstract expressions of the same prototype are only superficially disparate, and are in essence the same.

Once popularized, however, and executed by designers who were not themselves involved in Zen practice, these

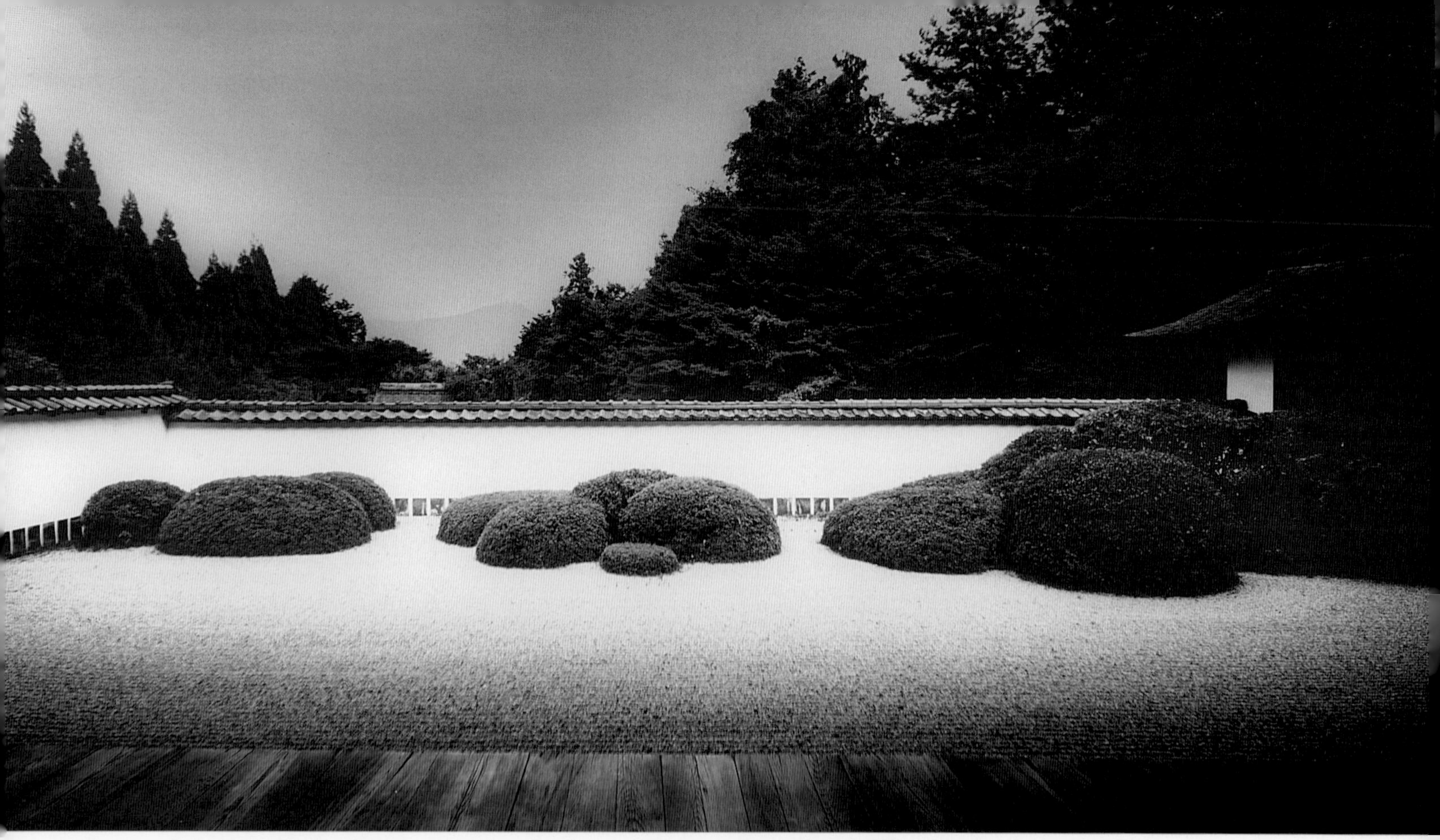

22.2 View, with Mount Hiei in the distance, from the veranda of Shōdenji's south garden, Kyoto.

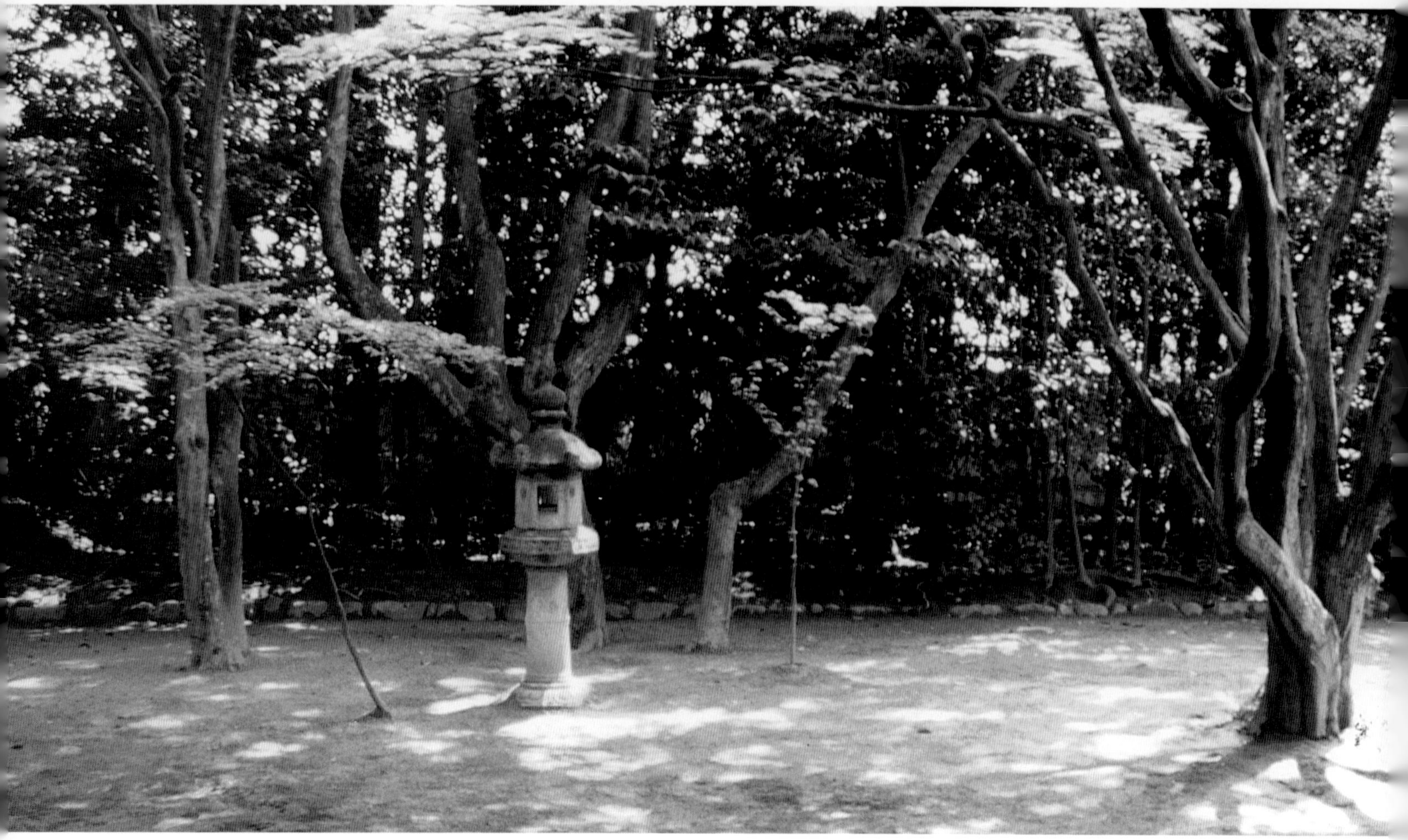

22.3 View from the veranda of Daitokuji Kōtō-in's south garden, Kyoto.

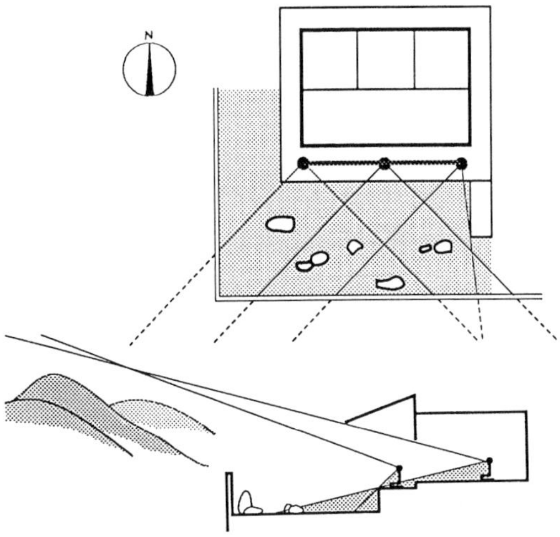

23 Plan and section schematics showing range of view from the room interior and the veranda of the Zen temple south garden.

abstract gardens lost their dynamic quality. "Solid white" as a garden design solution became stereotyped, and stone compositions took on fixed formulas (*kata*) that were passed down as secret teachings.

The Zen temple south garden, as seen at Myōshinji's Tōkai-an and Daitokuji's Daisen'in, retained the original solid white ground form and functioned as a garden for Zen practice. The compositions of these gardens rarely correspond to the views from the three rooms lining the south face of the *hōjō*. For the viewer seated inside the hall, the white sand is obstructed from view by the veranda; only the hedge or mud wall surrounding the garden, and at times, borrowed scenery can be seen from this position (Figure 23). It is only as the viewer stands and walks that the garden gradually comes into view (Figures 24.1–24.3).

The south garden of the *hōjō* of Jōeiji in Yamaguchi Prefecture is another exemplary Muromachi-period garden, in which the *shinden-zukuri* white sand area is replaced by a stretch of lawn upon which numerous large and small stones are set in groupings of three and five, with the entire scene bordered by a pond in the distance. Like a *shinden-zukuri* garden, the composition is frontal and unidirectional, corresponding to a seated view from the building interior (Figures 25.1–25.2).

Conversely, the basic composition of the south garden of Ryōanji's *hōjō* is polarized at the western end and bears no relation to the seated view from the building interior. Its effect is only evident from the veranda. Some hold that the veranda was once connected to a *butsuden* (Buddha hall) to the west; if this is true, this rock garden must be seen as corresponding to a kinetic viewpoint, in addition to the seated view from the south veranda (Figures 26.1–26.2).

In principle, the south garden of the Zen temple *hōjō* was a solid white space cut off from the building interior, composed in relation to the south veranda. At times it represented the final scene of the kinetic north garden, usually conceptually rather than spatially, and as such, also had a multifaceted aspect.

The South Garden of Warrior Residences

The *zashiki* decorative arrangement that came to be known as mature *shoin-zukuri*, in which the main hall was further divided into the *jōdan* (upper level) and the *gedan* (lower level) was not yet fully developed in Muromachi-period warrior residences (*buke*).

A plan-view drawing of Ashikaga Yoshinori's early fifteenth–century Muromachi villa shows that the building interior was divided into *hare* (formal) and *ke* (informal) halves (see Figure 16). The north walls of the small rooms on the informal side were fitted with *mairado* sliding wooden doors, while the formal south-side space basically retained the *shinden-zukuri* style, with *shitomido* shutters on the south wall creating an open, unified garden-to-room environment. The warrior's south garden was thus composed for a frontal, unidirectional view from the seat of honor at the center of the room, where the highest-ranking person present—master or guest—would sit. Despite the shift in the garden's function—from a ceremonial role in the Heian period to a purely ornamental or contemplative one thereafter—the fundamental garden composition techniques applied to *shinden-zukuri* on shallow sites were inherited in these frontally-viewed gardens (Figure 27).

The warrior residence's south garden took a markedly different approach from the abstractly expressed Zen temple south garden, dispensing completely with the white sand area and condensing the pond, island, and artificial hills. This too was a point of transition to the

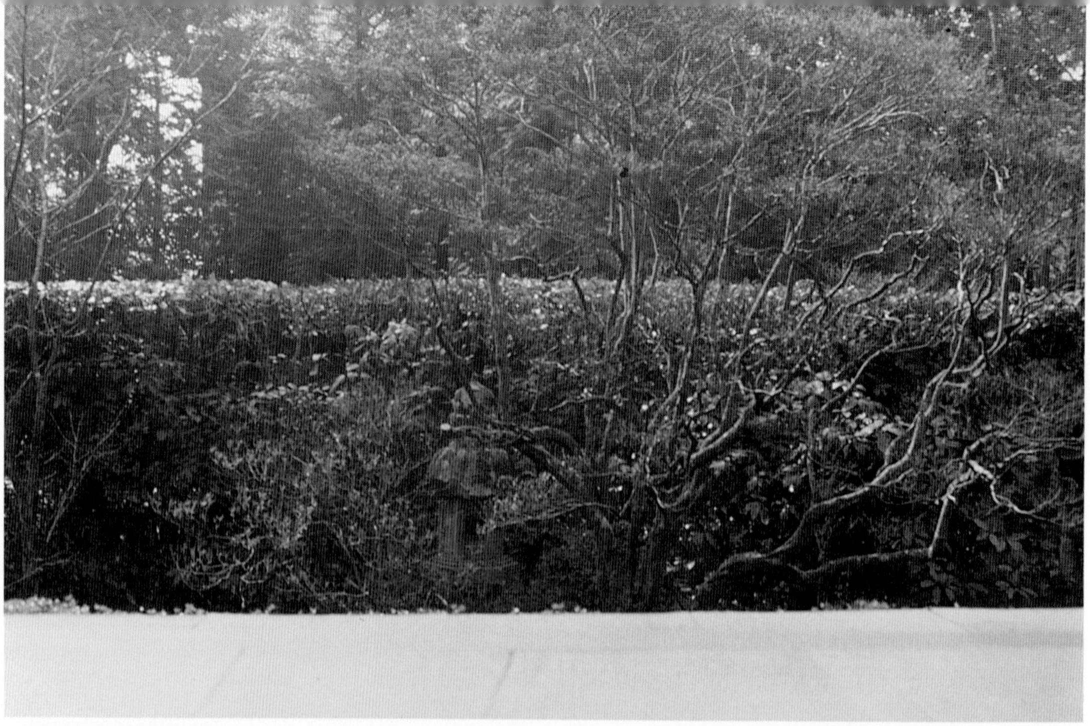

24.1 Seated view from the room interior of Myōshinji Keishun'in's south garden, Kyoto.

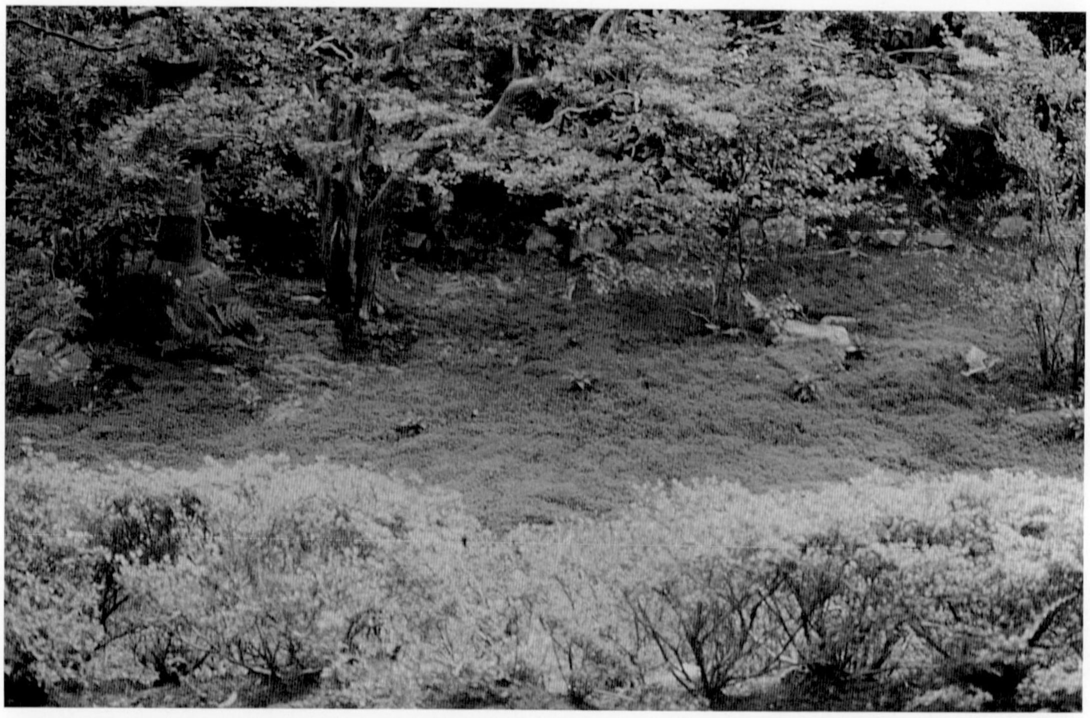

24.2 Standing view.

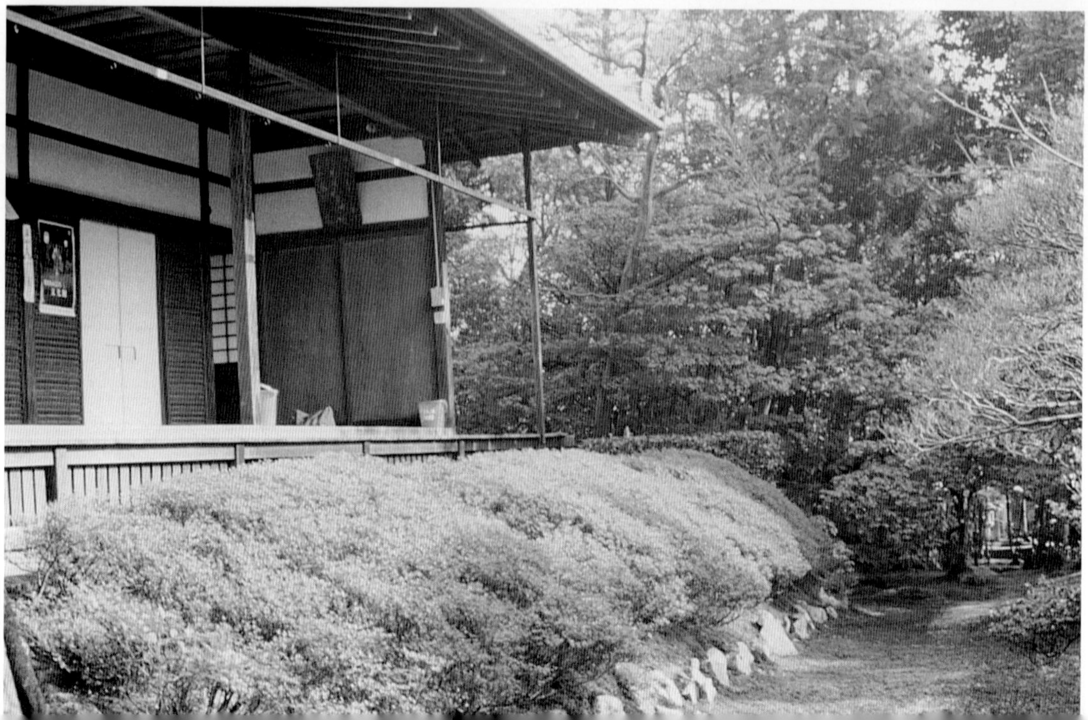

24.3 Lateral view.

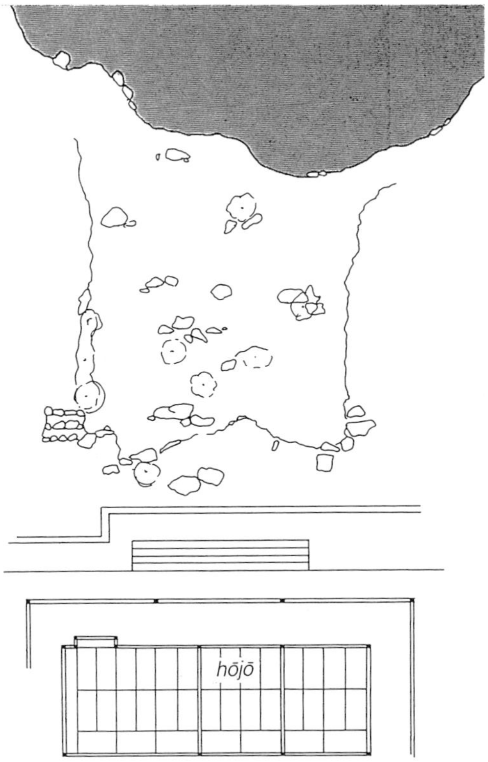

25.1 Plan view drawing of the *hōjō* and south garden of Jōeiji, Yamaguchi Prefecture.

25.2 View from the room interior of the Jōeiji *hōjō*'s south garden.

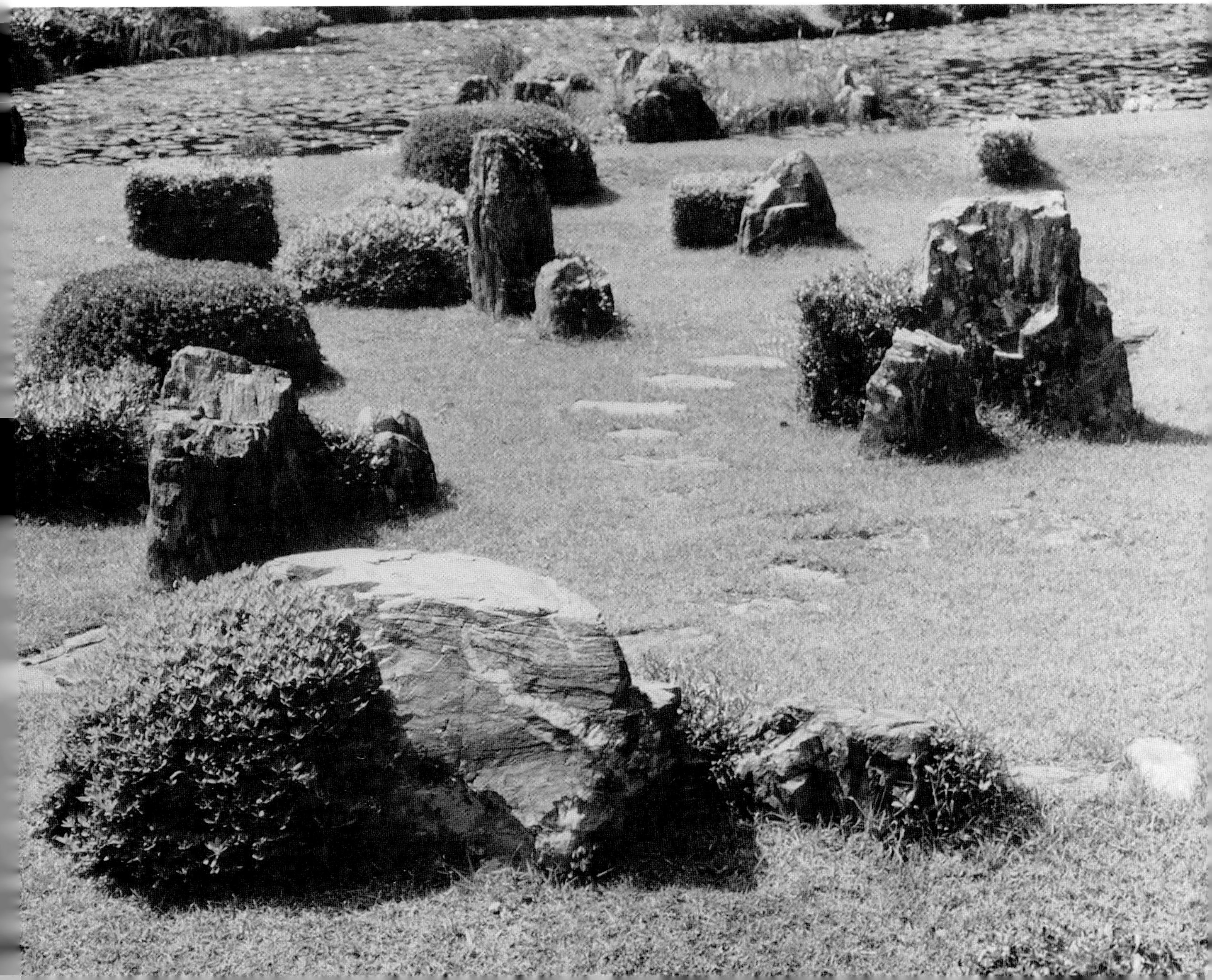

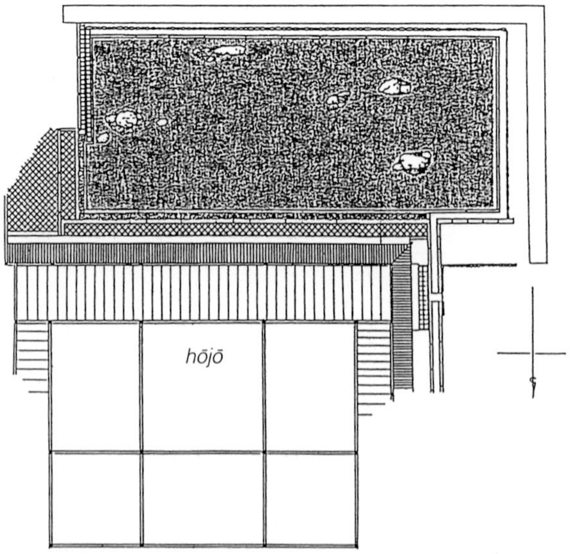

26.1 Plan view drawing showing the relationship between the Ryōanji *hōjō* and the south garden, Kyoto.

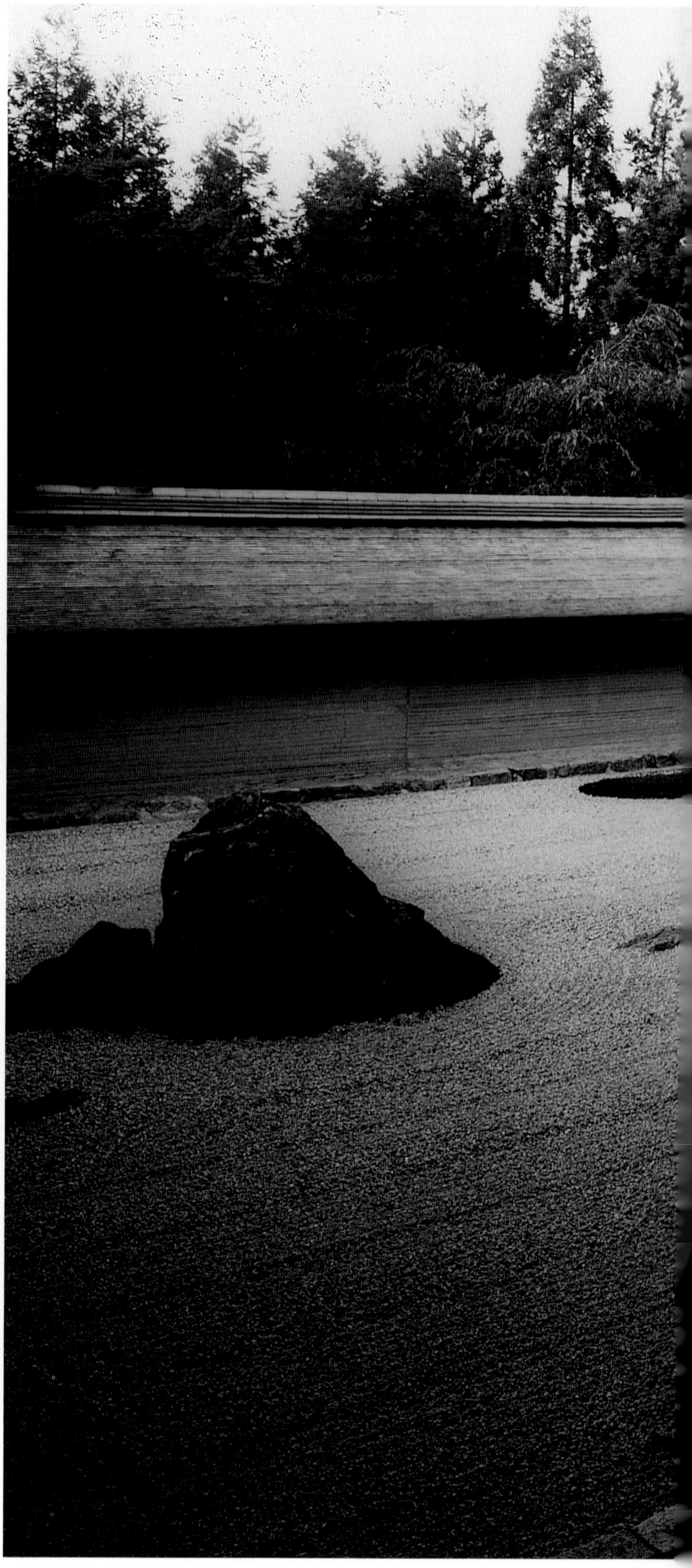

26.2 The Ryōanji *hōjō* south garden.

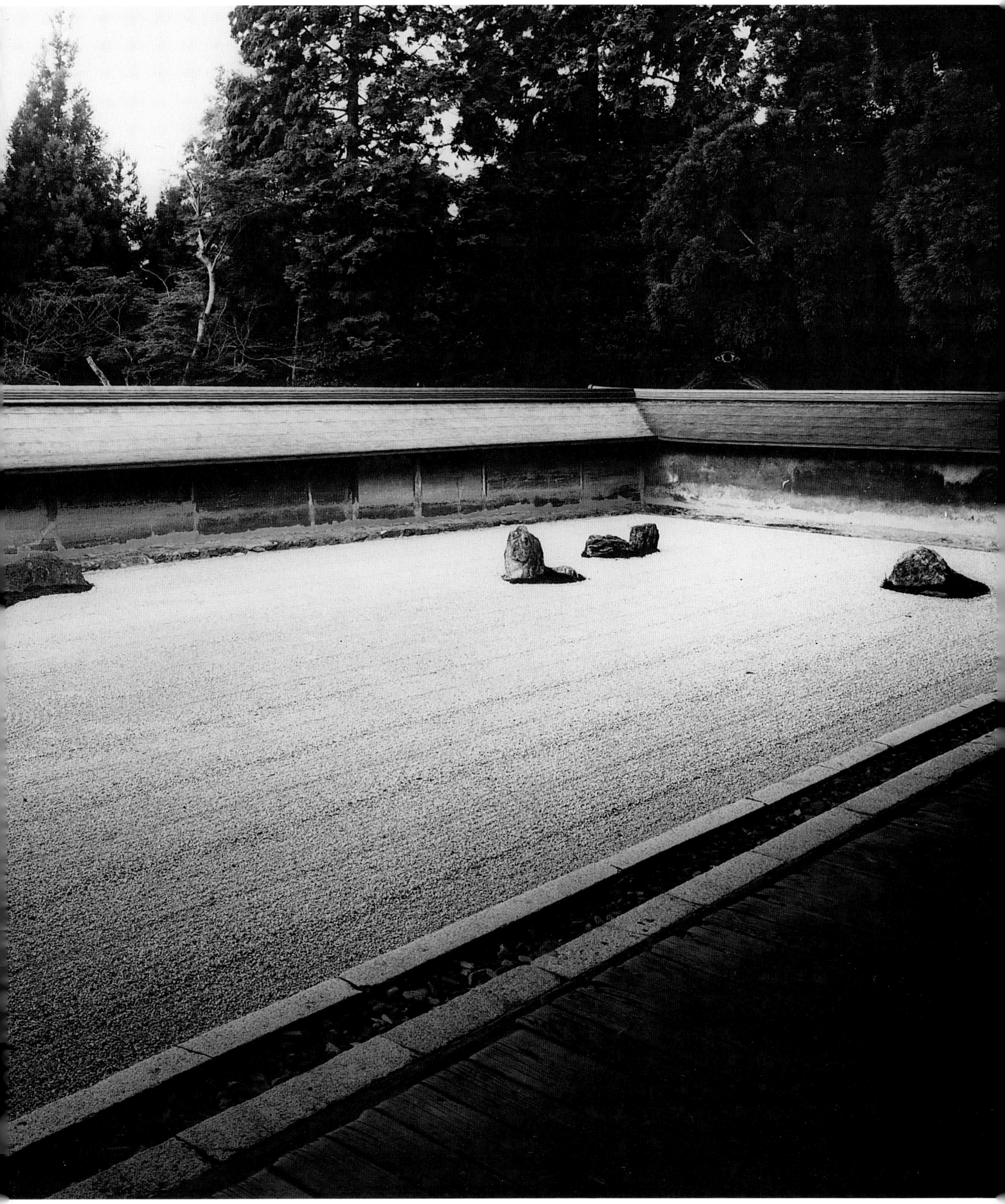

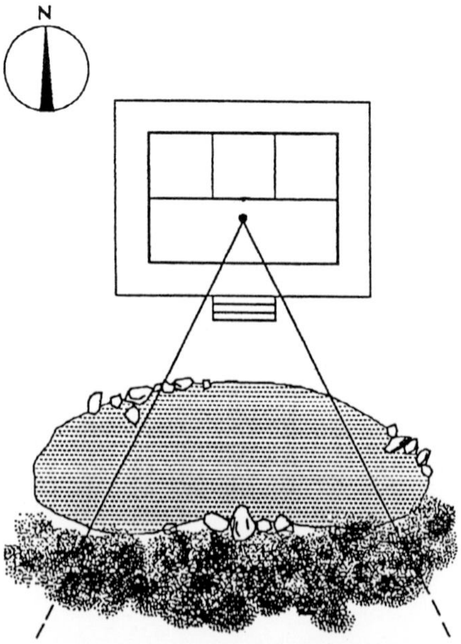

27 South garden of a medieval *buke* warrior's residence, composed for seated, center frontal, unidirectional viewing from the interior of an adjacent room.

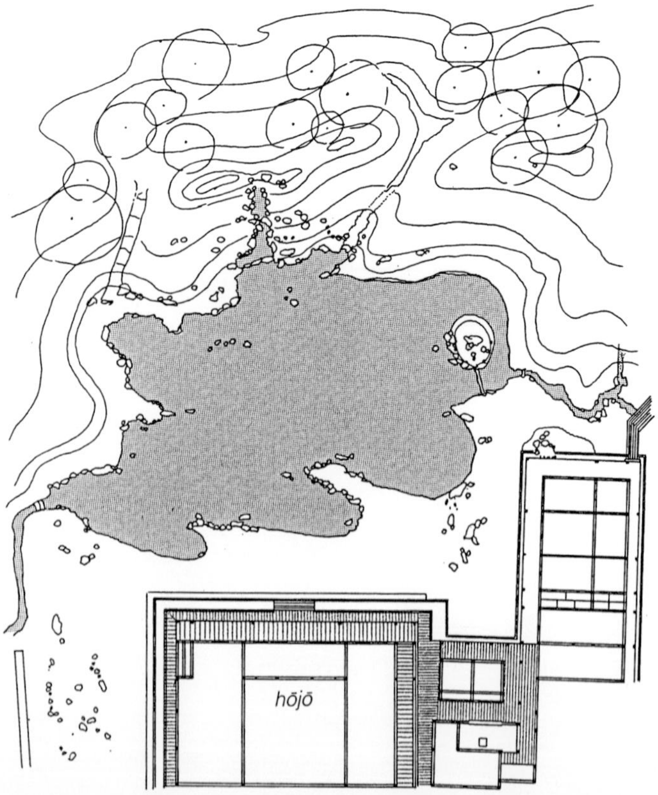

28.1 Plan view drawing of a *buke* south garden, Tenryūji, Kyoto.

28.2 View from the center of the room interior.

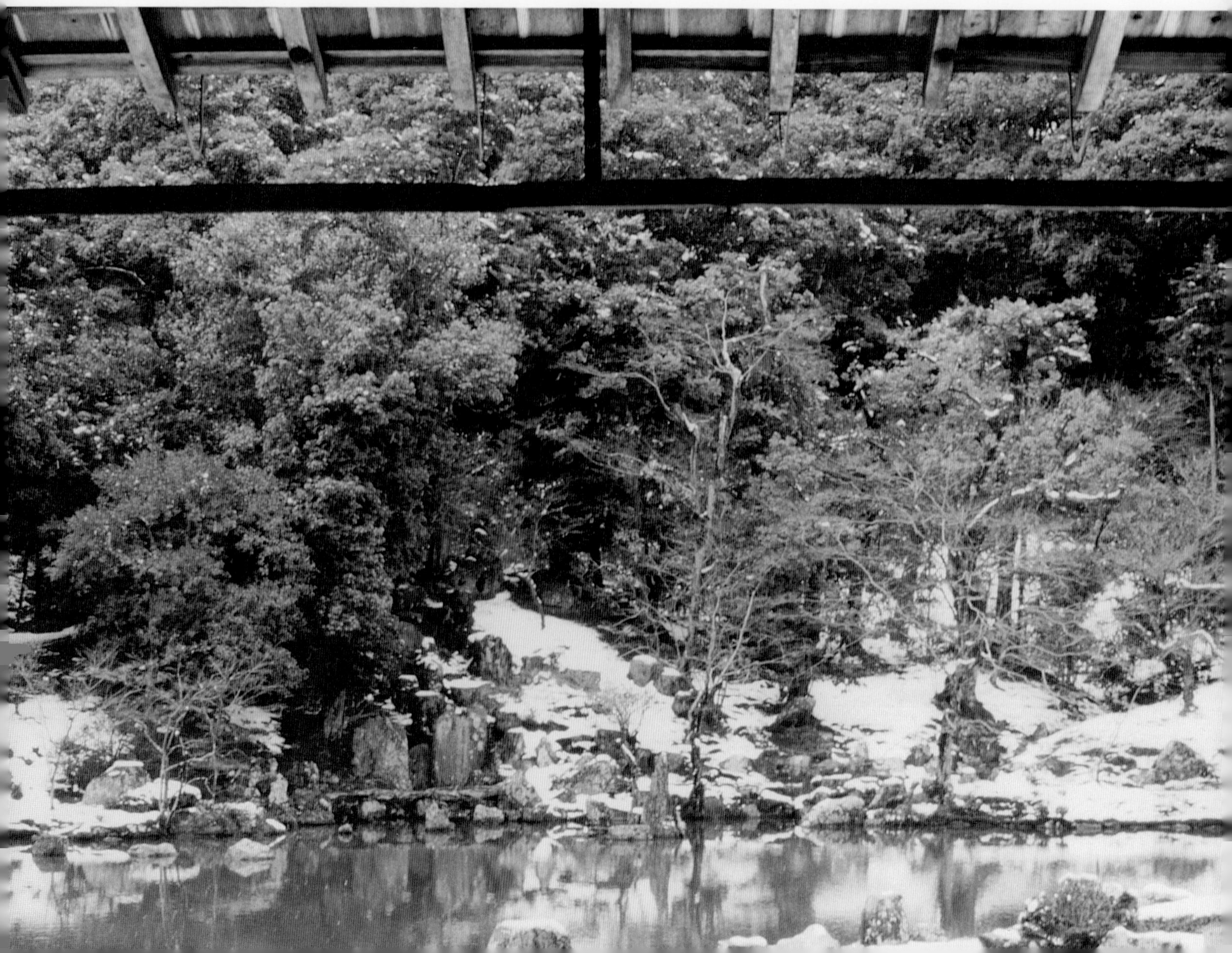

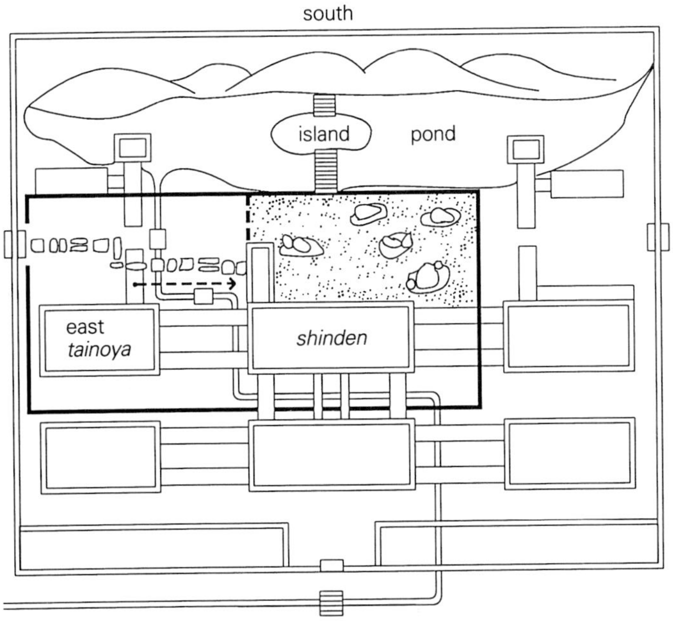

29.1 Aspects of *shinden-zukuri* architecture and gardens retained in medieval Zen temple abstract interpretations.

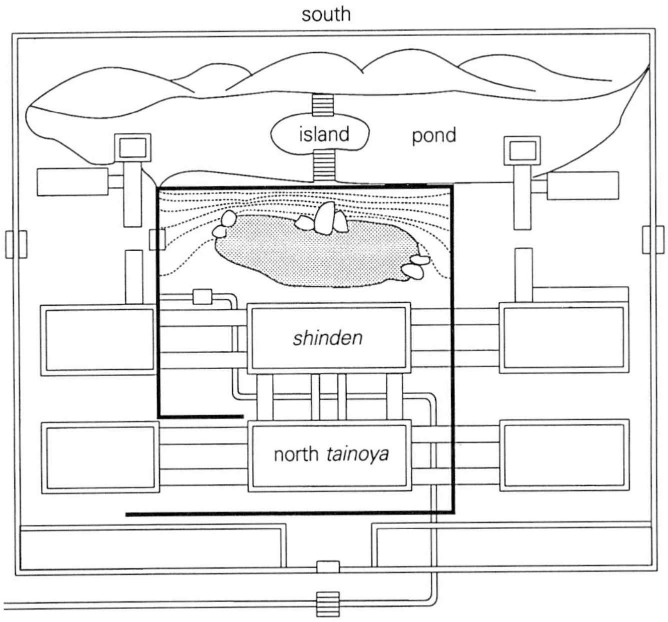

29.2 Aspects of *shinden-zukuri* architecture and gardens retained in medieval *buke* warrior residence condensed interpretations.

mature *shoin-zukuri* garden composition of the period to follow. The Muromachi-period gardens of Tenryūji, Echizen Asakurakan, and the former Kuchigi Shūrinji were all designed for contemplation, and for static, unidirectional viewing from the center of an adjacent room (Figures 28.1–28.2).

Although both date from the same historical period, the methods of expression adopted in the south gardens of the Zen temple and the warrior residence emerged as ostensibly antithetical interpretations of the same prototype. This occurrence was very much a function of the times as well as of the Japanese phenomenon of the garden design's being linked to the functional aspects of the building (Figures 29.1–29.2).

These divergent forms of expression were actually two manifestations, at opposite ends of the spectrum, of the same concept. This is the same process described earlier regarding *yō*, in which the inherently abstract character of stylized forms is implemented differently in accordance with different site conditions and functional requirements, and thus a single stylized form could be expressed in diametrically opposed interpretations.

The influence from imported culture during the medieval period—the direct import of Chinese paintings and wares—was of a different quality than that of Heijō-kyō, where the Tang capital and palaces were transmitted in image. Assessment standards were set and documented by Japanese connoisseurs at the early import stages to handle the large quantities of goods. According to *Kundaikansōchōki*, a late–Muromachi period secret document on the connoisseurship and display of Chinese paintings and wares, the court academic paintings of Southern Song Emperor Hui Cong were assessed at a value comparable to that of the freer ink monochrome paintings of Muqi, and likewise celadon and white high-fired pottery was appraised coequally to oil-spot *tenmoku* (*yūhen*) stoneware—value standards unthinkable to the Chinese. This uniquely Japanese approach to assessment is not unrelated to the ostensibly antithetical abstract and representational expressive forms taking their respective positions in garden making.

Decorative Arrangement of the *Shoin-Zukuri Jōdan Zashiki*

With the rise in importance placed on class rank in feudal warrior society, the main hall, which was used for formal audiences, was subdivided along the east-west axis in the sixteenth century, and developed a formalized order that served as a spatial representation of social hierarchy.

The easternmost position, being closest to the entrance, was the lowest-ranking seat. Seats located closer to the interior of the building indicated progressively higher rank. Rank was also expressed spatially by floor height—the *jōdan* (higher level) was elevated one step above the

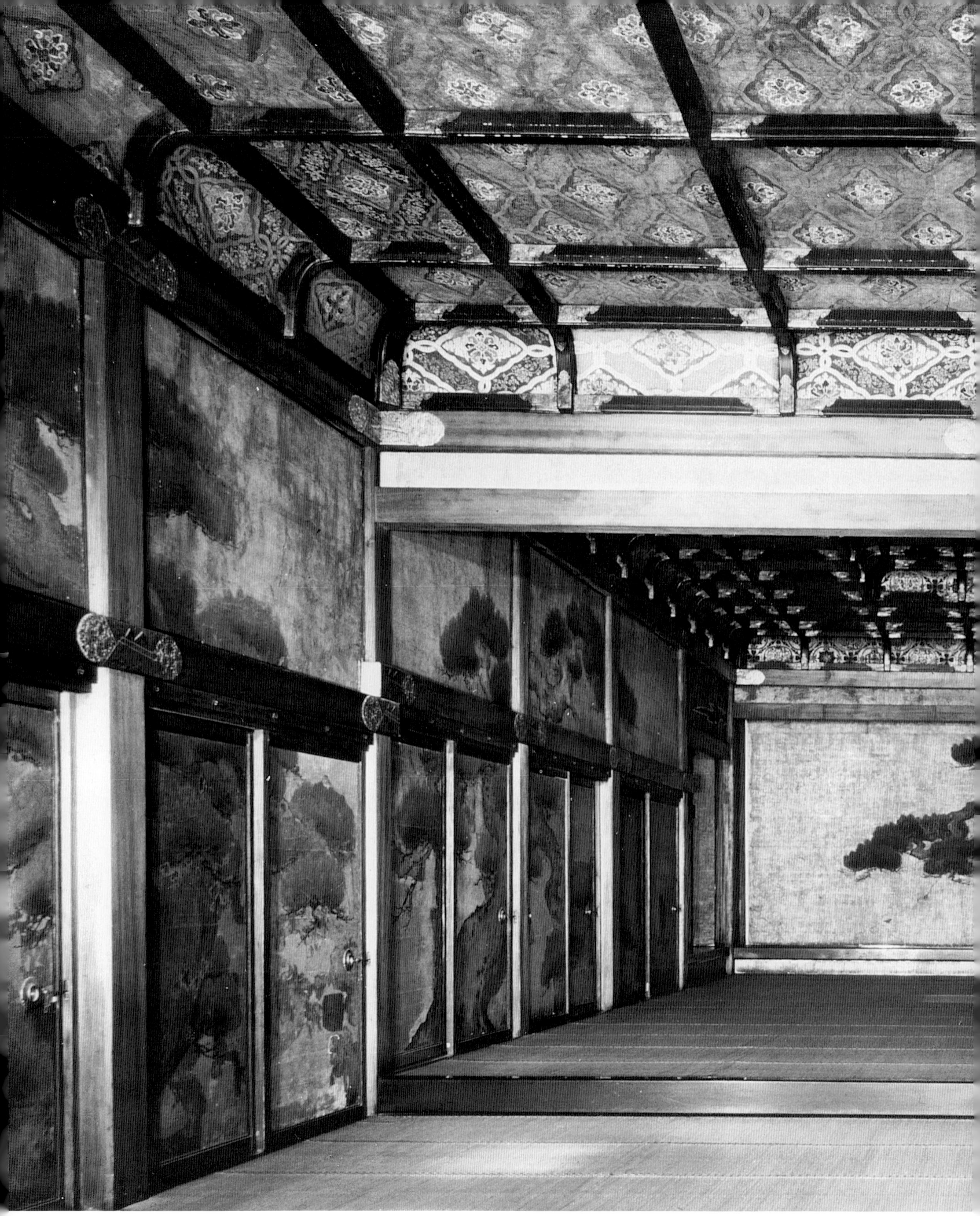

30 The *jōdan zashiki* layout and decoration typical of mature *shoin-zukuri* architecture, Nijōjō, Kyoto. National Treasure.

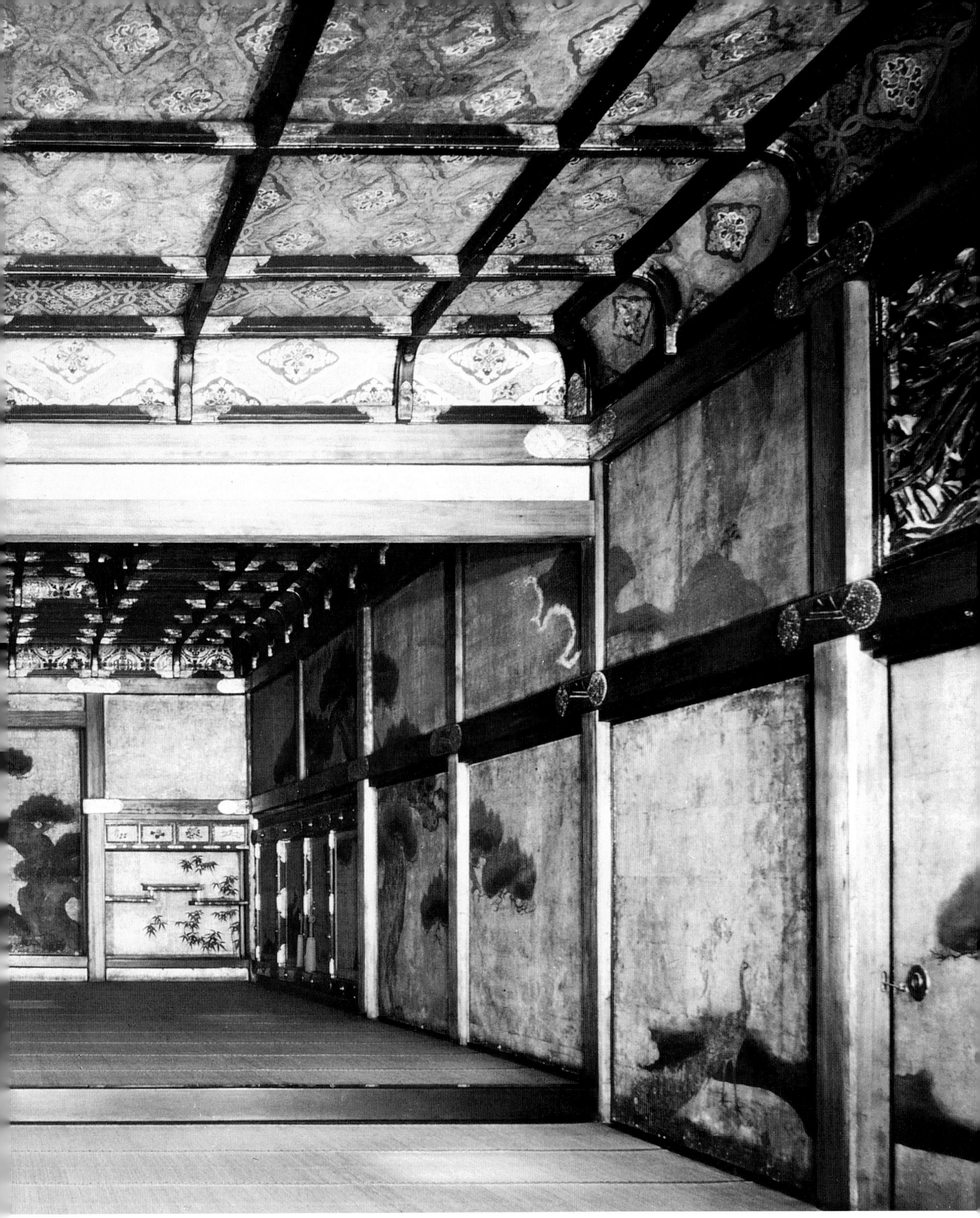

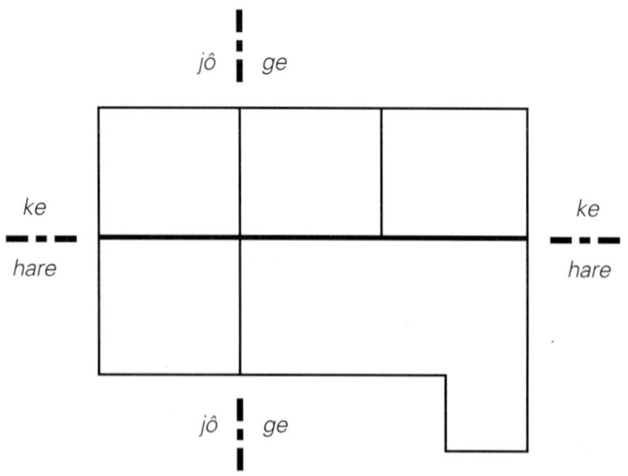

31.1 The further division of the main hall into upper (*jō*) and lower (*ge*) areas in medieval *buke* warrior residences.

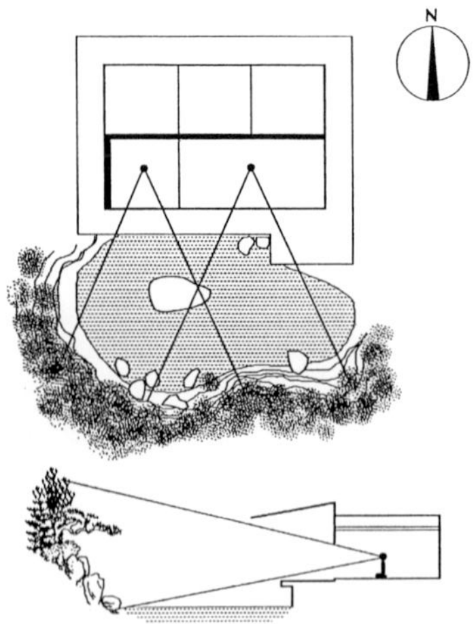

31.2 Plan and section schematics showing range of parallel frontally-composed views corresponding to the *jōdan* and *gedan* in the *buke* south garden.

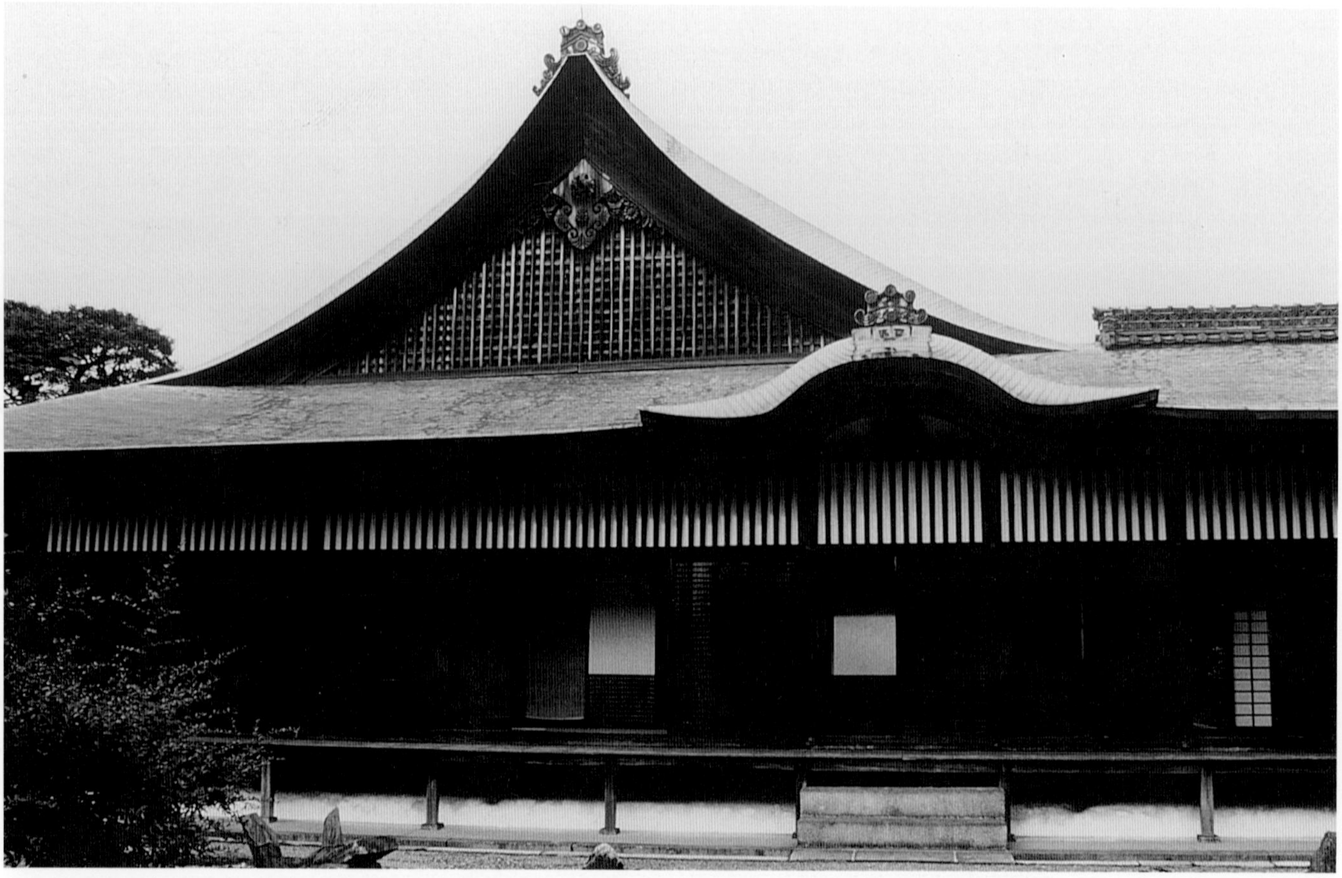

32.1 Tōji Kanchi-in guest hall south exterior facade, Kyoto. National Treasure.

gedan (lower level). Distance was used in the same way: the *jōza* (higher seat) and *geza* (lower seat) were at opposite ends of the room. (The *gedan* and *geza* were later divided into *chūdan* and *chūza*, or middle level and middle seat, respectively.) As a further expression of superior station, the *jōdan zashiki* decorative accoutrements, the *oshi-ita* alcove, *chigaidana* staggered shelves, *tsukeshoin* built-in desk and *chōdaigamae* decorative doors were located around the periphery of the *jōdan*, and the walls and built-in sliding screens were decorated with gold and polychrome paintings by members of the Kanō school. With these developments, the transition from *shinden-zukuri* to *shoin-zukuri*, which spanned the twelfth through the seventeenth centuries, was complete (Figure 30).

In response to such architectural changes to the building interior, the unidirectional, frontally-composed garden designed for viewing from a seated position in the center of the room changed to parallel frontally-composed

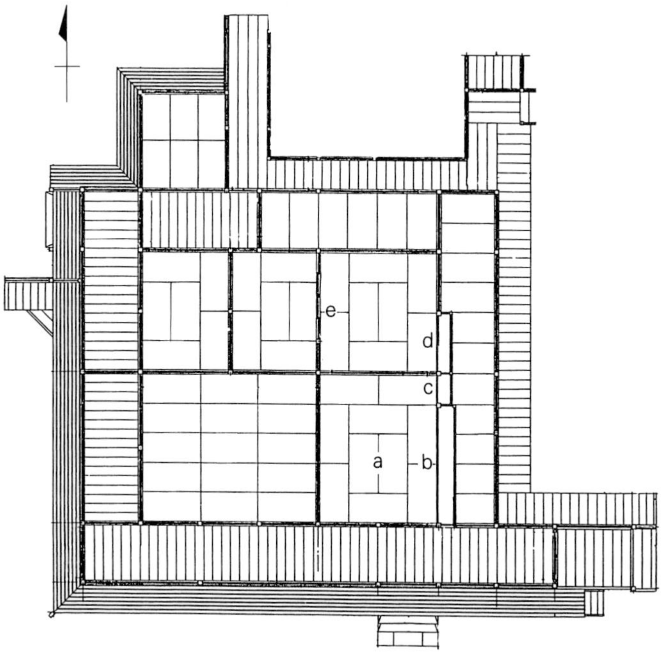

32.2 Tōji Kanchi-in guest hall plan view drawing.
a. *jōdan.* b. *oshi-ita.* c. *chigaidana.* d. *tsukeshoin.* e. *chōdaigamae.*

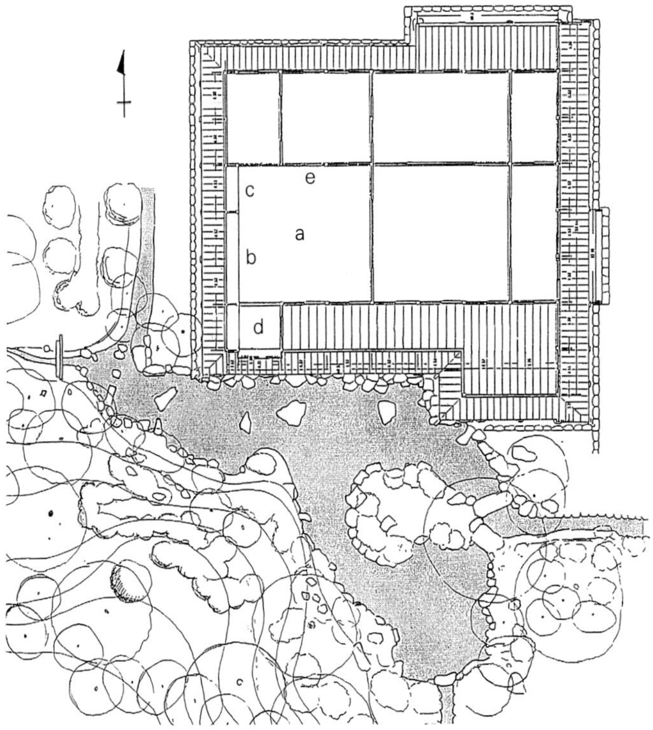

33.2 Onjōji Kōjō-in guest hall and south garden plan view drawing.
a. *jōdan.* b. *oshi-ita.* c. *chigaidana.* d. *tsukeshoin.* e. *chōdaigamae.*

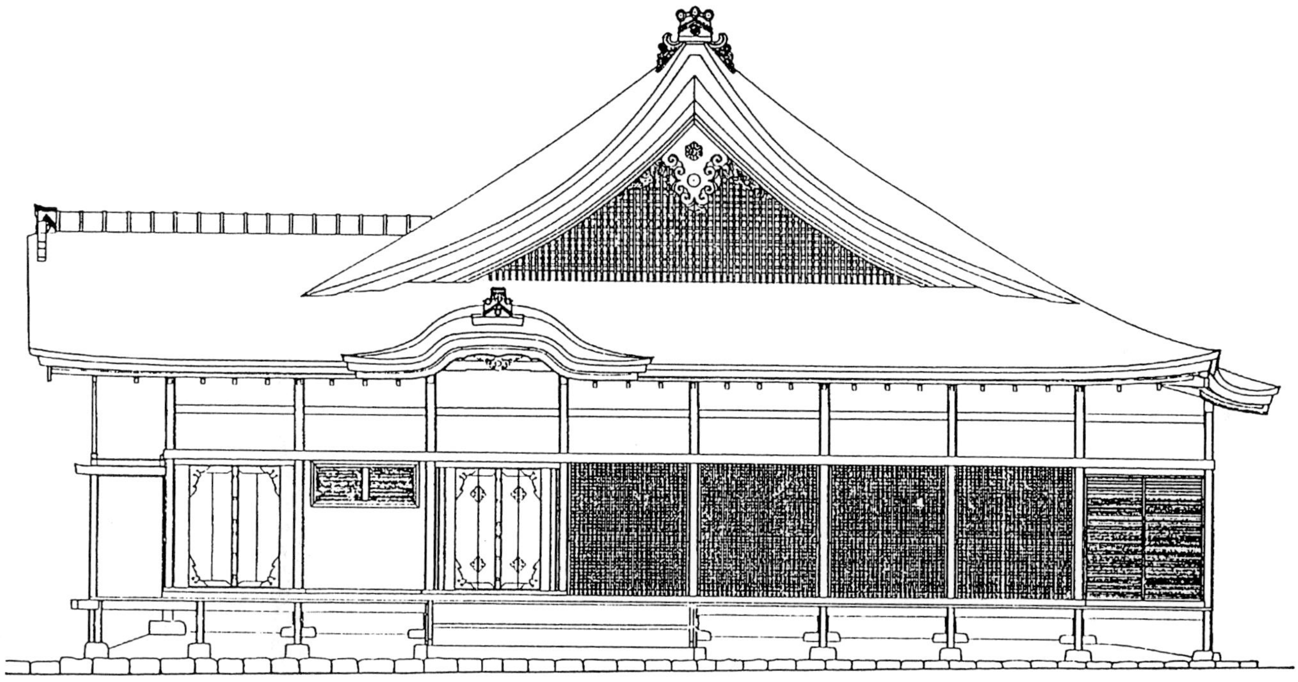

33.1 Onjōji Kōjō-in guest hall east elevation.

views corresponding respectively to the locations of the *jōdan, chūdan* and *gedan* (Figures 31.1–31.2). The related changes in garden and building interior are best examined by comparing the plans of the Azuchi-Momoyama–period Tōji Kanchi-in and Onjōji Kōjō-in.

The Kanchi-in guest hall's formal south side (*hare*) is divided into the Ichi no ma (*jōza*) and the Ni no ma (*geza*). The informal north side (*ke*) is composed of three rooms of eight mats to the east, six mats in the center, and six mats to the west.[4] The Ichi no ma has an *oshi-ita* alcove and staggered shelves; however, the *tsukeshoin* is located in the eight-mat informal study, together with the *chōdaigamae* decorative doors which form the entrance to the center six-mat sleeping room. This arrangement creates a link on the north-south axis between *hare* and *ke,* and another on the east-west axis between *jō* and *ge,* both of which are characteristic of transitional *shoin-zukuri* (Figure 32.2).

The bow-shaped gable (*hafu*) over the entry porch

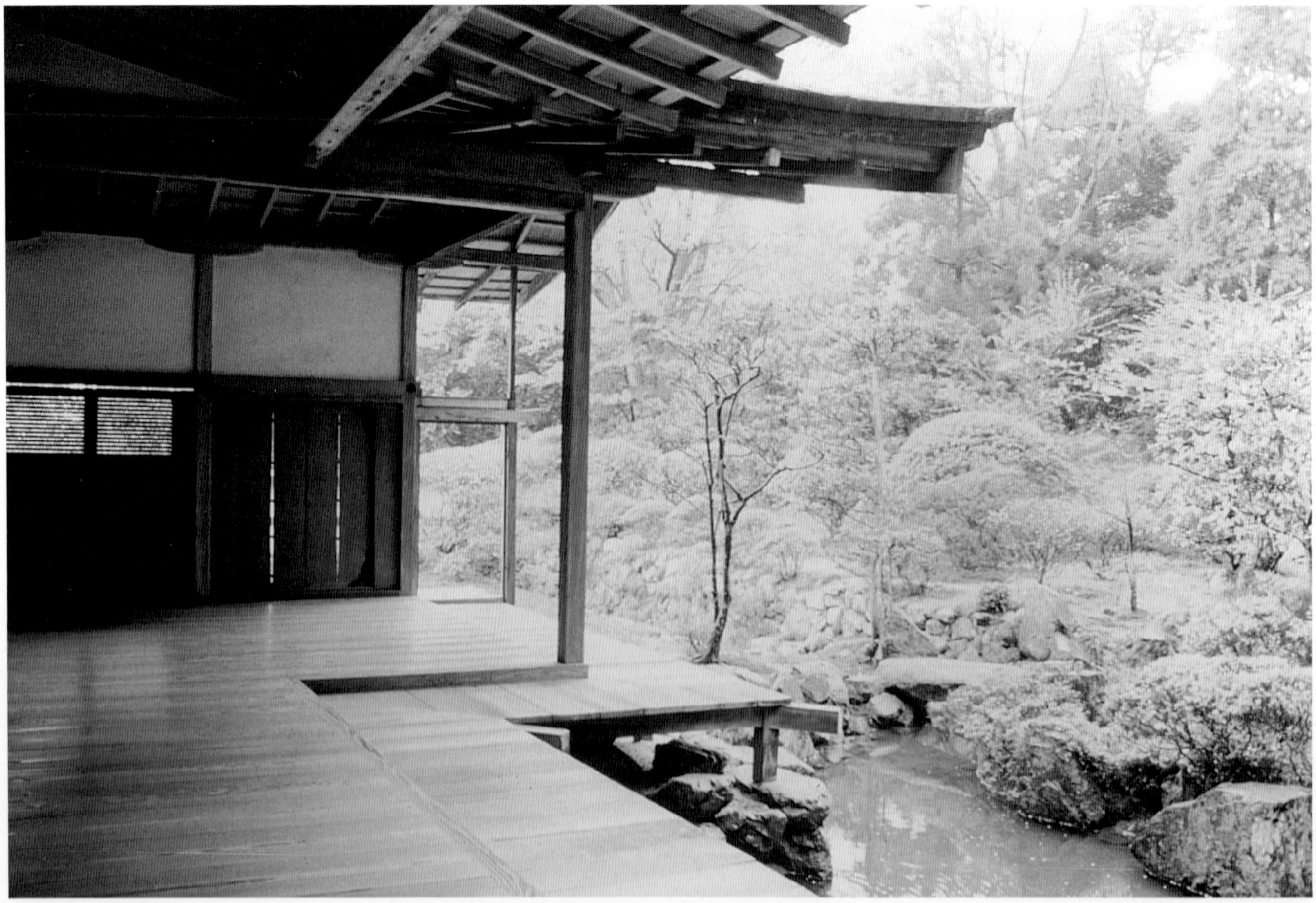

34.1 Onjōji Kōjō-in guest hall east wall interior and south garden, Shiga Prefecture.

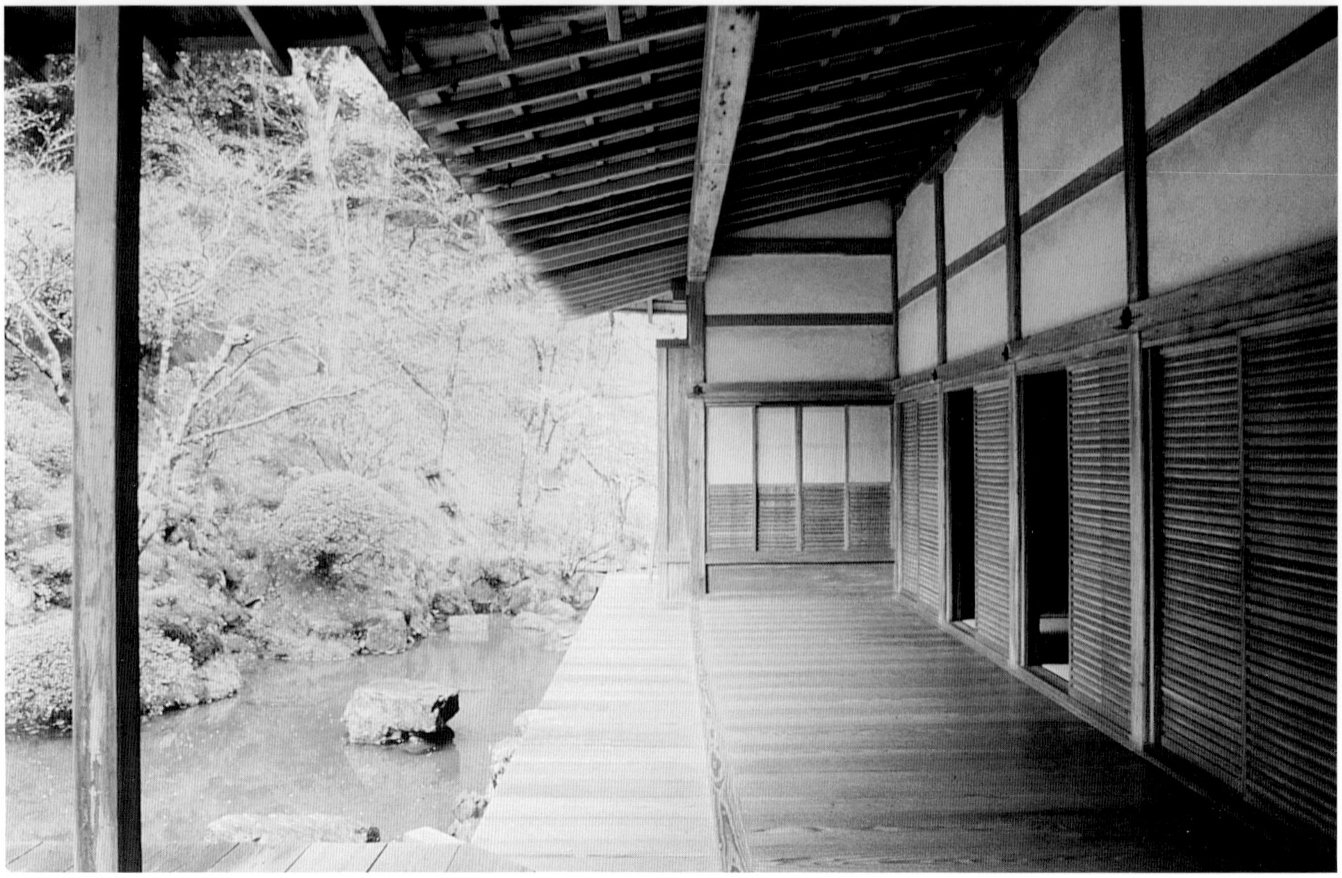

34.2 Onjōji Kōjō-in guest hall south facade and garden.

built into the right side of the south main facade is a vestige of the *shinden-zukuri chūmon* inner gate. The external appearance of the facade that borders the white sand south garden retained the *shinden-zukuri* style, although the garden itself did not (Figure 32.1).

The external appearance of the main facade of the Kōjō-in guest hall closely resembles that of the Kanchi-in guest hall, with the important difference that the former is located, together with the white sand area, on the east side of the building. This same characteristic can be seen in the Daigoji Sanpō-in from the same period.

The east facade displays *shinden-zukuri shitomido* shutters, *tsumado* side doors, latticed windows (*renji mado*) and a transposed *chūmon* entry porch *hafu* gable. None of these elements, however, bears any direct relationship to the interior features (Figure 33.1).

Both north and south facades have sliding *mairado* wooden doors, and the floor plan is in keeping with *shoin-zukuri.*

The *chōdaigamae* and *tsukeshoin* that furnished the east study on the informal (*ke*) side at Kanchi-in were moved to the Jōza no ma on the formal (*hare*) side in an arrangement which, together with the *oshi-ita* alcove and *chigaidana* staggered shelves, forms the standard mature *shoin-zukuri jōdan zashiki* style of decoration (Figure 33.2). The Kanō-school screen and wall paintings decorating these rooms are also characteristic of the early Azuchi-Momoyama period.

The white sand area in front of the east main facade retained the *shinden-zukuri* image, but took on a new function, serving as the approach to the warrior's residence. In the south garden, the white sand area was completely removed, and the pond brought up to the edge of the veranda so that the building appears to float on the water. The pond, islands, and artificial hills were condensed, creating a close-up view from the room interior in which the sky was not visible (Figures 34.1–34.2).

Shoin-Zukuri Gardens and Kanō-School Wall Paintings

Of the garden's six basic compositional elements, the white sand area, which had played a primary role in the Zen temple south garden, was relegated to a secondary role on the east side of the Kōjō-in guest hall, and the pond, islands, and artificial hills, which had been omitted from the Zen temple garden, were here condensed, together with the garden stream and waterfall, into a single, dense landscape scene, and drawn up close to the south side of the building (see Figures 29.1–29.2).

The condensed garden was actually composed of a series of parallel scenes, each corresponding to particular, fixed seated positions in the *jōza, chūza* and *geza* rooms of the guest hall. The early–Azuchi-Momoyama Kōjō-in guest hall and Daigoji Sanpō-in gardens reflect this same design development.

As a further means of representing rank spatially, in addition to the definitive *jōdan zashiki* accoutrements, this room was decorated with coved and coffered ceilings (*oriage-gōtenjō*) and Kanō-school screen and wall paintings (*shōheiga*). The mature *shoin-zukuri* garden became progressively more ornate and representational in expression as a result of influence from these paintings.

The style of Kanō-school screen and wall paintings typically commissioned to decorate *shoin-zukuri* guest halls consisted of rich color against a gold leaf ground. The picture plane was monumental in scale, and the subject—most frequently, trees and plants from the four seasons—depicted at close range with a combination of bold, sweeping strokes and finely detailed brushwork—much like a landscape scene photographed with a long lens. There was no middle-range or distant view, and none of the abstract white space seen in the ink-wash paintings after which Zen gardens were patterned.

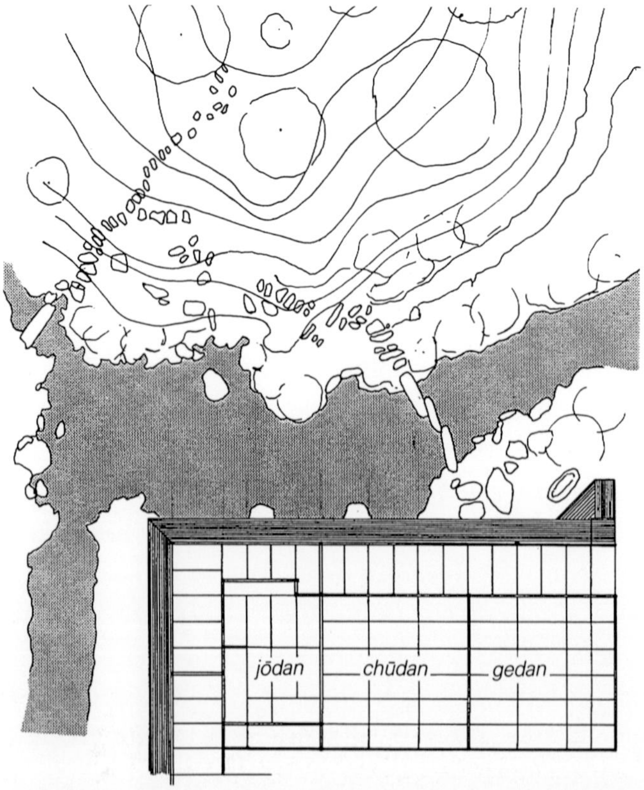

35.1 Plan view drawing of the Chishaku-in *shoin* and south garden, Kyoto.

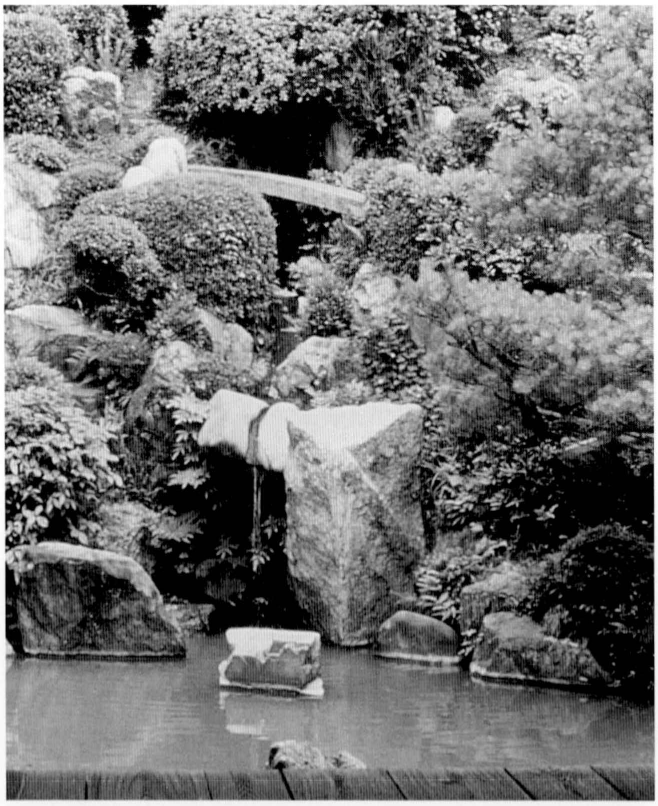

35.2 View from the *jōdan* interior.

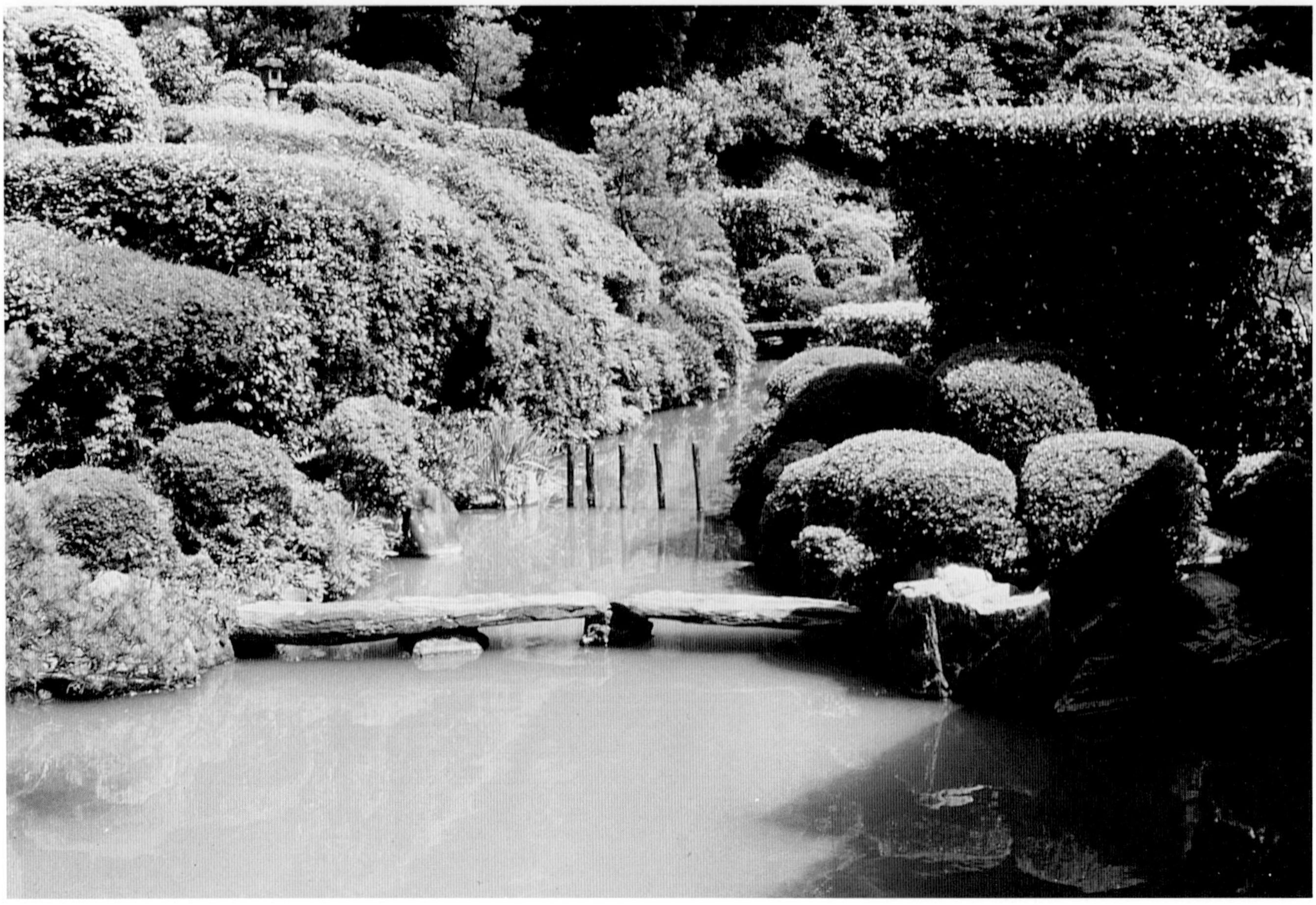

35.3 View from the veranda's southeast corner.

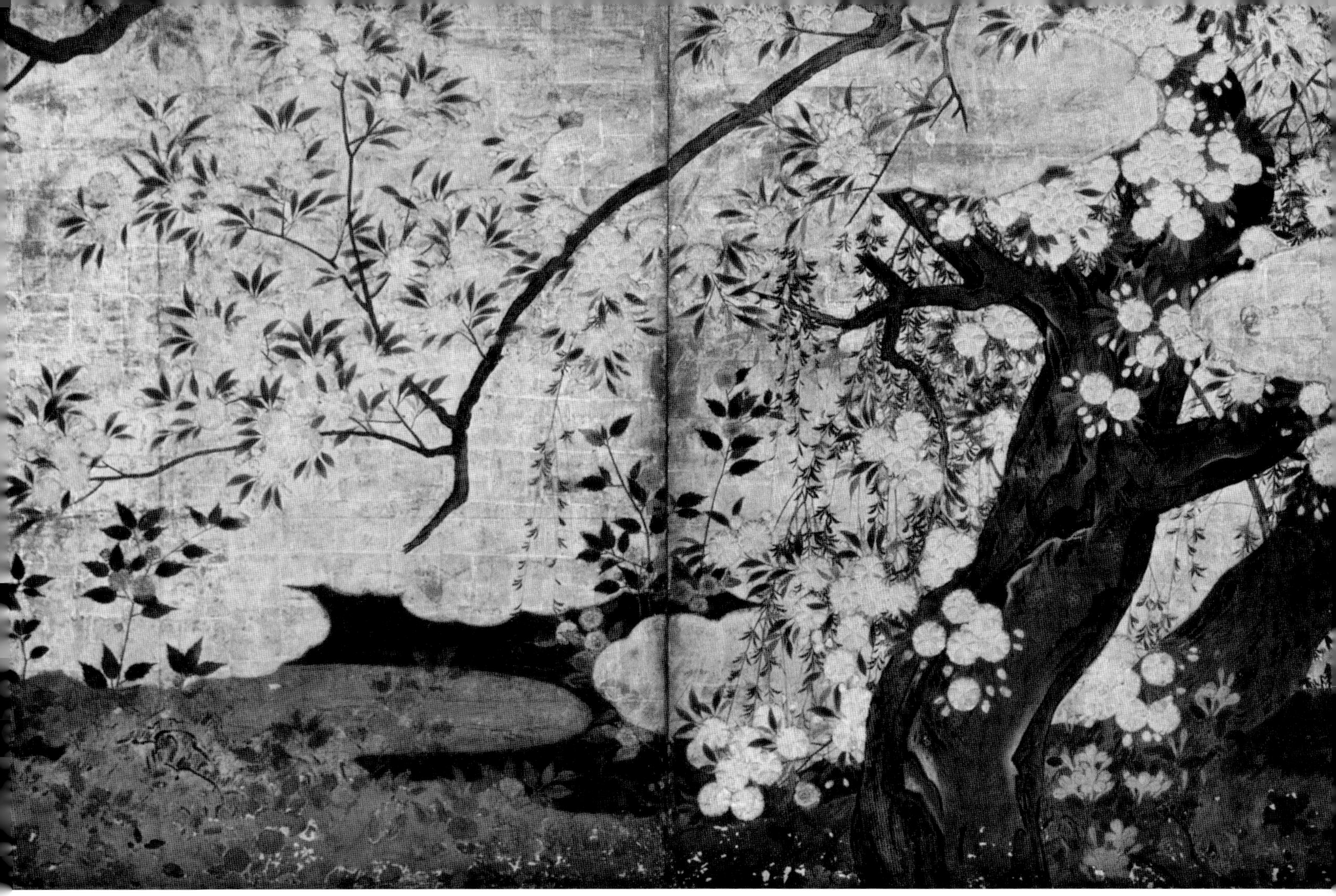

35.4 Chishaku-in *shoin* screen and wall painting, *Sakura* (Blossoming cherry), Hasegawa Kyūzō. National Treasure.

35.5 View from the room interior of the Onjōji Enman'in south garden, Shiga Prefecture.

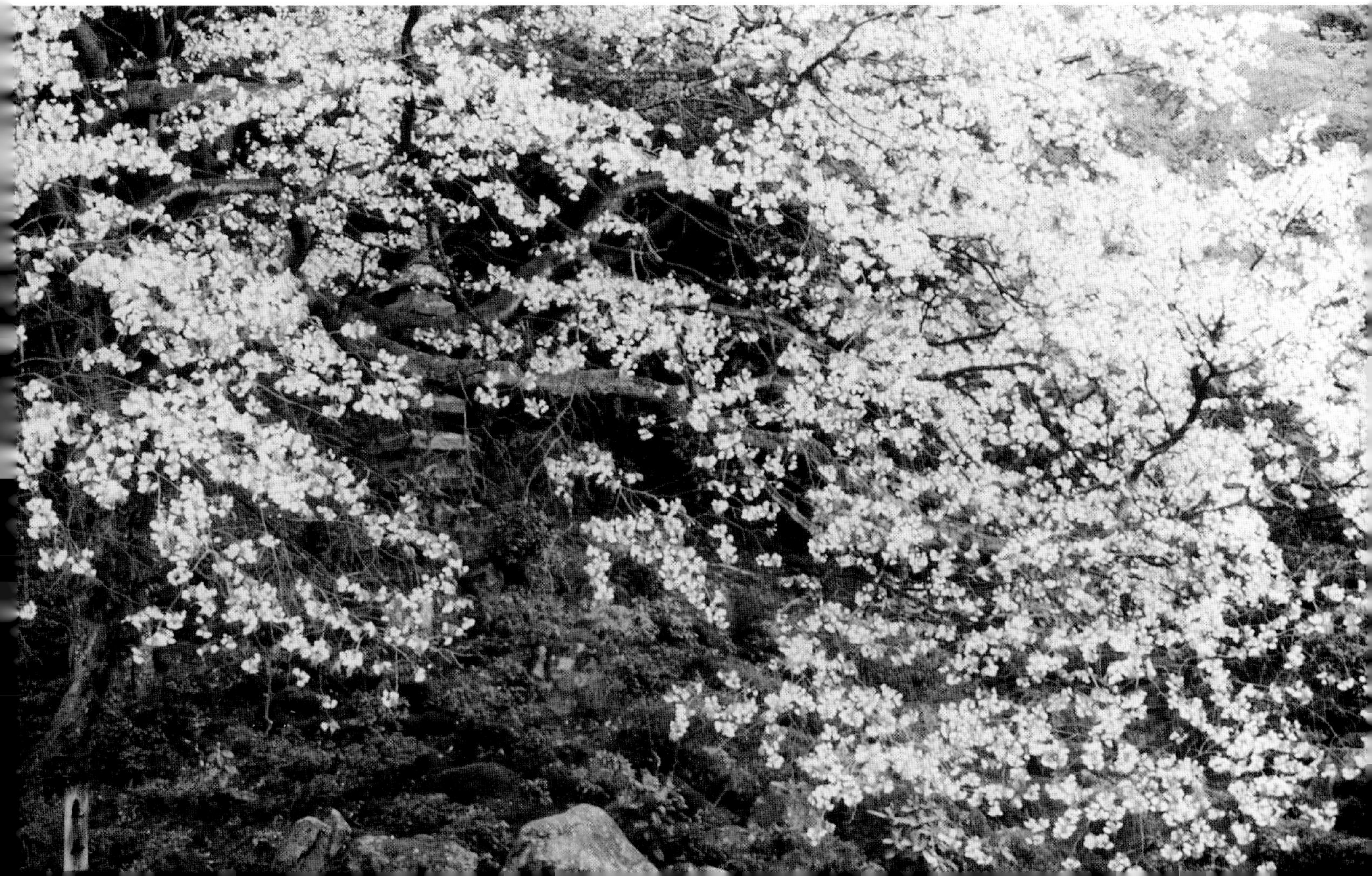

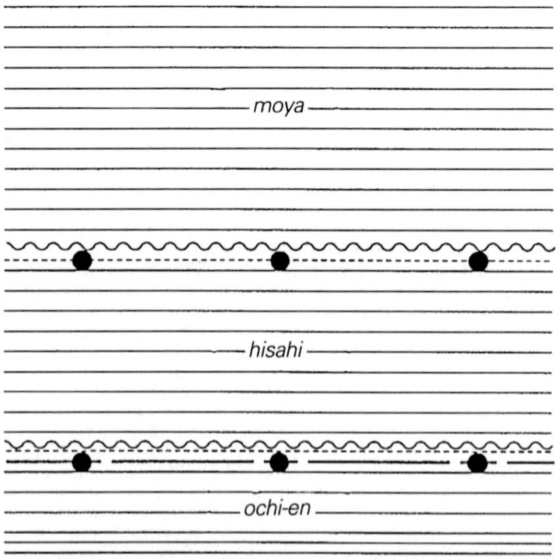

36.1 Schematic showing the interior/exterior threshold with *shitomido* fixtures.

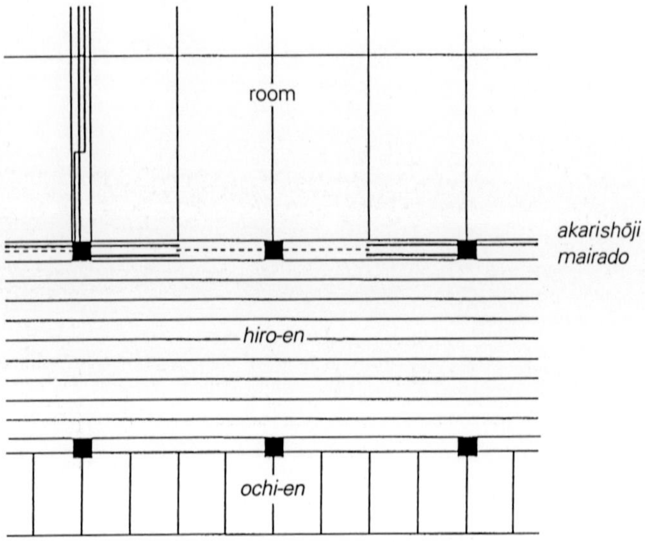

36.2 Schematic showing the interior/exterior threshold with *mairado* fixtures.

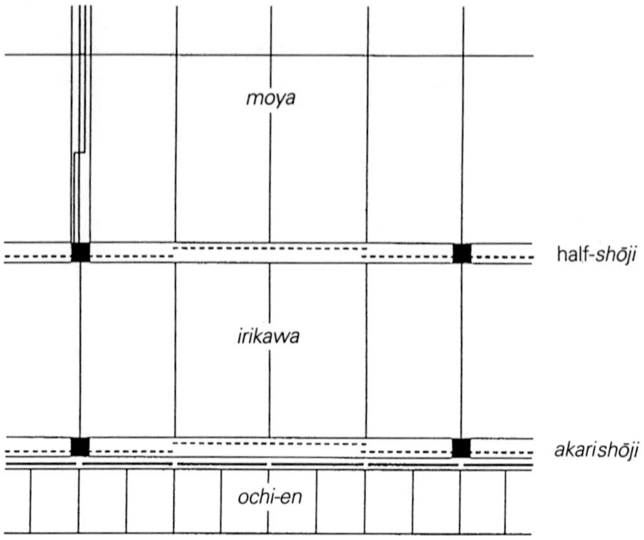

36.3 Schematic showing the interior/exterior threshold with single-track *amado* fixtures.

The interior walls and screens dividing the rooms of the formal *hare* space were covered floor-to-ceiling with these paintings, with the focal point of the overall composition centered on the *jōdan no ma*. The "picture plane" of the garden decorated the fourth, or exterior wall, and like these paintings, it was dense and representational. These qualities were achieved by condensing the hills, pond, islands, garden stream, and waterfall into a single, concentrated scene, and drawing them close to the opening of the building, creating a foreshortened, close-up view. The wall paintings and garden together created a homogeneous, majestic, and ornate "interior/exterior" environment (Figures 35.1–35.5).

The Threshold of the Garden As Architecture

The *shinden-zukuri* main hall was composed of the building core, or *moya*, surrounded by outer aisles, or *hisashi*. The spans between the pillars of the *hisashi* were fitted with *shitomido* shutters, which in their open position left the exterior facade of the *hisashi* totally open, creating a panoramic interior/exterior architectural space. The *hisashi* were used as an extension of the *moya*; an *ochi-en*, which skirted the *hisashi* one step lower in floor height, served as a corridor and was lined with a balustrade on its far edge (Figure 36.1).

With the division of the interior space along the north-south axis into *hare* and *ke* came the further division of the north side of the building into a row of three small rooms which integrated the *hisashi* space and resulted in the breakdown of the *moya/hisashi* structure. This development did not, however, lead to internal corridors, so the basic path of movement still revolved around the periphery of the building. The area between interior and exterior, however, changed from *hisashi* to *hiro-en* (covered

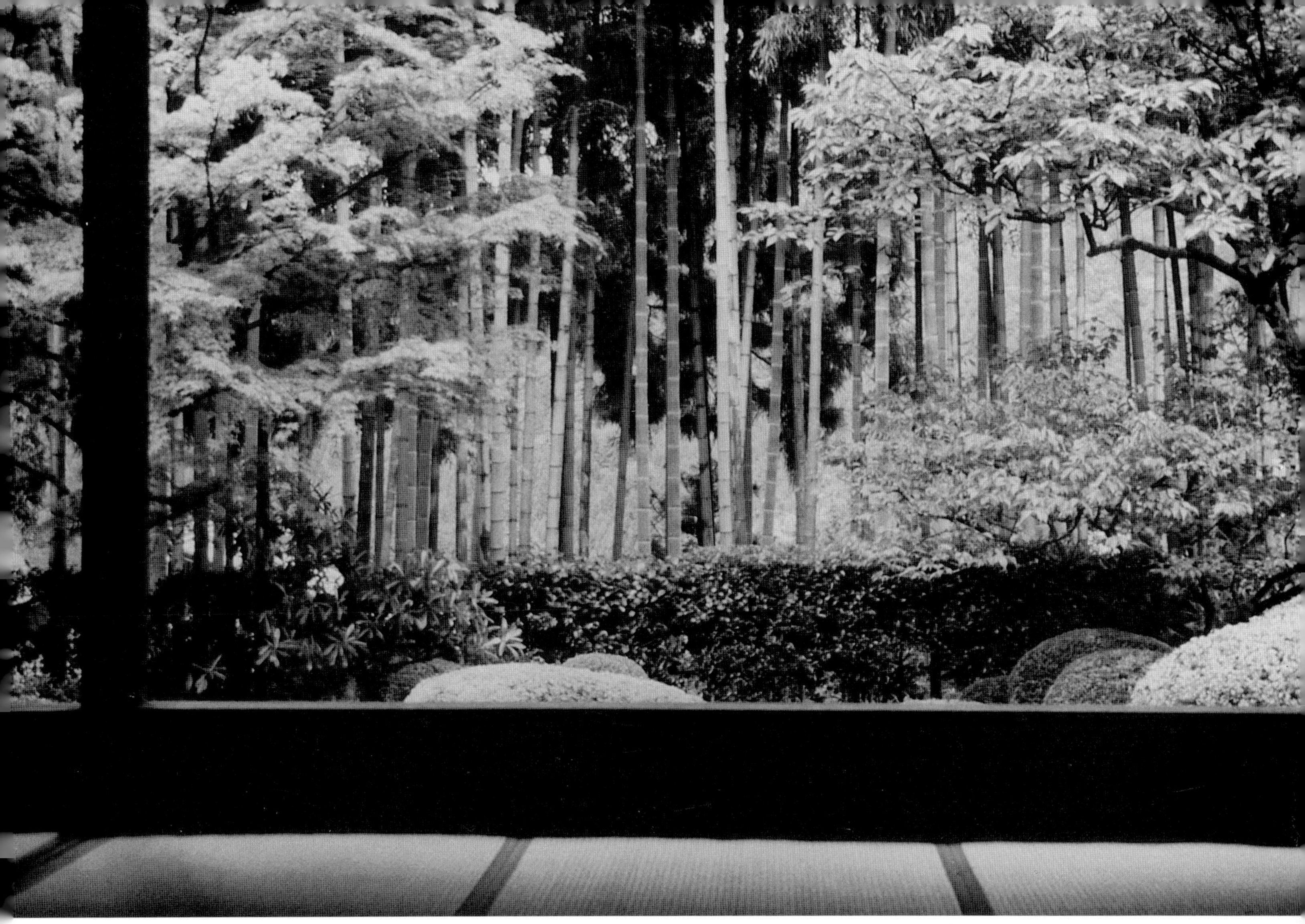

37 Hōsen'in garden viewed from the room interior, Kyoto.

veranda) and *ochi-en* (lower veranda corridor).

The most significant aspect of these changes is that where *shitomido* were installed between the outer row of *hisashi* pillars in *shinden-zukuri*, and so formed a linear demarcation between interior and exterior, *mairado* were installed on the inner row of pillars between the room and *hiro-en*, creating a quasi-interior/exterior space. As noted before, *mairado*—composed of two wooden doors and one *akarishōji* paper screen that slide in a three-track gutter—always leave a half-bay section of wall closed off to the outside, and this cropped view gave rise to the basic characteristics of the north garden. With these architectural developments, the threshold between interior and exterior space became a smaller opening set further back into the building's interior (Figure 36.2).

Early *shoin-zukuri* usually had *hiro-en* not on all four sides of the building, but only on one or two sides; which were closed off on the ends by wooden doors, and there was no balustrade on the far side of the *ochi-en*. While *hisashi* were an extension of the *moya* and formed a single interior space, the *hiro-en* was cut off by *mairado* and had more of an exterior spatial character. Just as the Zen temple south garden was unrelated to the adjacent room, the *hiro-en* and *mairado* structure distanced the room from the garden. Although it is necessary to pass through the *hiro-en* in order to enter the *mairado*-enclosed room, the *ochi-en* skirting the building's four sides corresponds more closely to a corridor.

With the development of single-track *amado* exterior sliding doors in the mid-seventeenth century, the threshold between interior and exterior space moved once again—this time to the outer row of pillars between the *hiro-en* and *ochi-en*, as in *shinden-zukuri*. This also meant that the *hiro-en*, which had previously been delineated from the interior and functioned as something close to exterior space, would again begin to serve as an extension of the interior space. This space, now called the *irikawa*, had *tatami*-mat flooring, further emphasizing its interior character (Figure 36.3). In their open position, single-track *amado* sliding doors allow for a totally open and unified interior/exterior relationship, which is again reminiscent of *shinden-zukuri.*

The view of the garden from the room—arrayed before the viewer like a stage set—is breathtaking. With the appearance of single-track *amado* door fixtures, gardens became increasingly multifaceted, kinetic, and dynamic (Figure 37).

In this way, as door fixtures changed first from *shitomido* to *mairado,* and then to single-track *amado,* resulting changes in the form and location of the threshold between the interior and exterior influenced the relationship between room interior and garden. The room/garden relationship of these purely ornamental, contemplative gardens—which viewers never actually entered—was based on a delicate balance between what was to be shown, and how, and what would be perceived from the principal viewing seat in each of the different architectural styles. The threshold's role in the interior/exterior relationship thus acts as the primary influence on the character of these extremely visual, painting-like Japanese gardens designed to be "viewed from a seated position in the room interior."

3

Kinetic, Multifaceted Gardens and *Miegakure*

Miegakure ("hide-and-reveal") refers to a number of techniques used to configure garden scenes in sequence as visitors walk through a garden. The term was first used in regard to the techniques employed in the small, rustic walkways, known as *roji*, that lead to teahouses. Effects are created that provide a sense of depth and pique the viewer's expectations of the next scene by, for instance, interrupting lines of sight, concealing the depth of the site, and obscuring the overall view.

> In principle, no element of the *roji* is shown in its entirety. Like something intimated in what is left unsaid, the *roji*'s very spirit derives from its suggestiveness, and it is this that gives the garden its profundity. None of the furnishings in the outer *roji* —from the front gate to the *yoritsuki* (changing room), and the *koshikake machiai* (waiting bench), the *setchin* (lavatory) or the other elements—are plainly visible, or shown in their entirety. *Miegakure* plantings half-conceal the forms of buildings, and the partially-hidden, partially-revealed composition is achieved by making the path wind at key places.[1]

This passage from Kitao Harumichi's book *Roji* describes a variety of *miegakure* techniques which were used in making *roji* for tearooms and the effects of which come into play simply by the act of walking. However, this is not the entire extent of this technique's application. *Miegakure* is also a feature of *kaiyūshiki teien* stroll garden design, where it was used to create a continuous series of sequential views. In fact, the concept is still in use today, in both the design of new urban landscapes and the analysis of existing urban environments.

Kinetic, multifaceted compositional techniques created in accord with human motion first emerged with this kind of "walking," or "pathed," garden, which is not to say that the highly sophisticated "hide-and-reveal" mode of expression sprang into being in the late sixteenth century. It had its precursors in the view-obscuring techniques employed in the static, unidirectionally-oriented *shinden-zukuri* gardens described in *Sakuteiki.*

The Zen temple north garden was designed principally for static observation from a seated position, and the added factor of the viewer's walking along the veranda overlooking this garden set up an interactive relationship requiring continuity between separate scenes. The view-obscuring techniques used there contained the seeds of the development of multifaceted, multidirectional garden composition. Nevertheless, they did not go beyond the

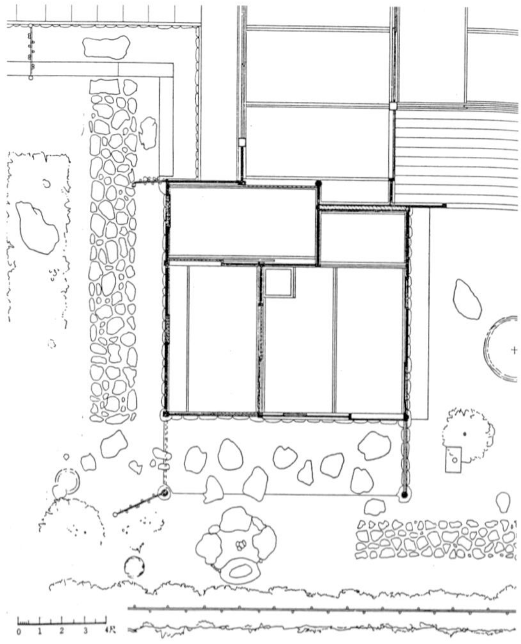

38.1 Plan view drawing of the Myōki-an Tai-an teahouse and its *roji.*

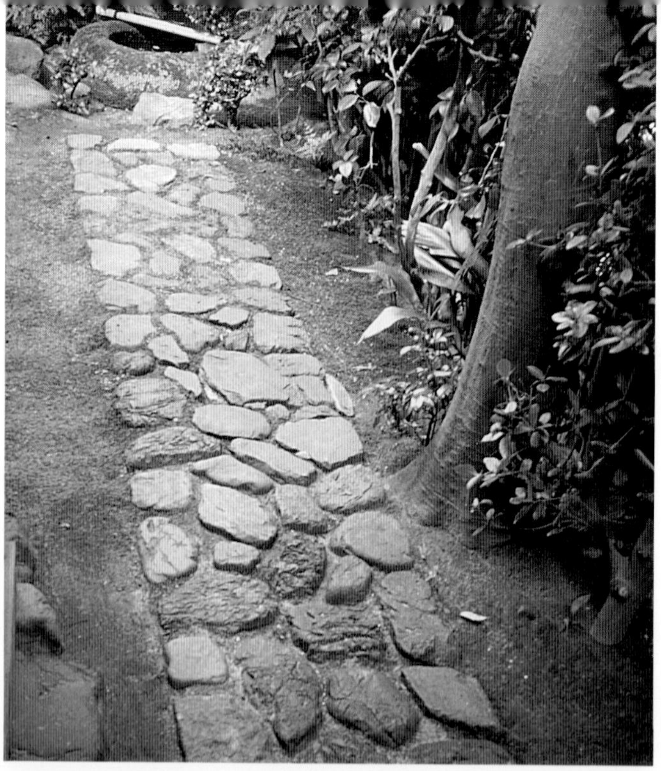

38.2 View of the Tai-an *roji,* Kyoto Prefecture.

domain of parallel motion in spaces that were in essence qualitatively homogeneous.

Walking through a garden has the effect of focusing the viewer's attention. This is especially true of the *roji* and other types of "walking" gardens, which requires the same kind of heightened attentiveness (*kokoro-kubari*) as does the tearoom itself. In the late sixteenth century, as with the *roji,* we find a swift incorporation of this idea of manipulating attention, by controlling movement in garden interpretations.

Miegakure Linking Qualitatively Similar Garden Areas

The act of stepping down from the veranda and walking in the garden begins with the *roji.* The *roji* in its early form consisted merely of a walkway leading to the tearoom, and thus could hardly be called a garden (Figures 38.1–38.2). By definition, the *roji* ("dewy ground") is a path, not a garden, which brings out its essential quality, of being "walked."

As the presence of a ritual washbasin—where guests cleanse their hands, mouth, and, symbolically, their spirit—would suggest, the *roji* played an important role in preparing the minds of those who were about to participate in a tea gathering, or *chanoyu,* and was a point of transition from the mundane world to the realm of tea. The spirit of *chanoyu* was described by sixteenth-century tea master Sen no Rikyū with the phrase "*ichi go ichi e*" ("one life, one meeting"), which suggests that every human encounter is a singular occasion. From the beginning, any elements that might hinder the preparation of the mind were eliminated from the *roji.*

The prototype of the thatched-hut *sōan* teahouse and accompanying *roji* is that of "a mountain locale set within a city." The following verse by twelfth-century ascetic poet-monk Saigyō can be said to describe the atmosphere of the ideal *roji.*

> Leaves of the *kashi* trees,
> Even before they were tinged
> Are all scattered
> Along the path to the mountain monastery
> Lone and desolate.[2]

The solitary, austere quality of the image of a "mountain path" was meant to underscore the fact that the world of *chanoyu* was separate from that of society. It was Rikyū's belief that from a place where there is "nothing," that which is true and genuine manifests itself.

When a *roji* is set within a city, the creation of a mountain path is of course artificial, but still the *roji* is required to express the essence of a mountain locale. This suggests that the *roji* has two fundamental aspects: functionally, it provides a path for walking, while thematically it expresses "the natural landscape" as specified in *Sakuteiki*'s first

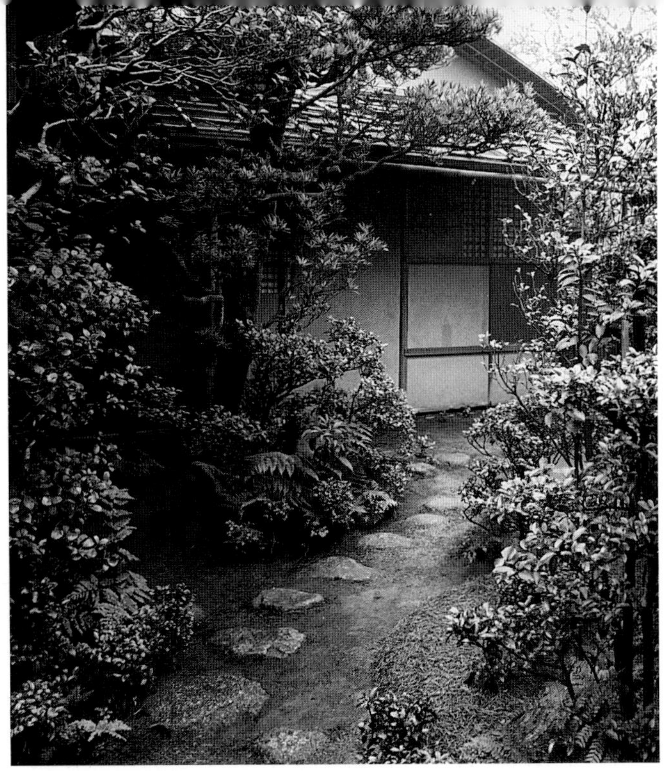

39 View of the Omote Senke *roji*, Kyoto.

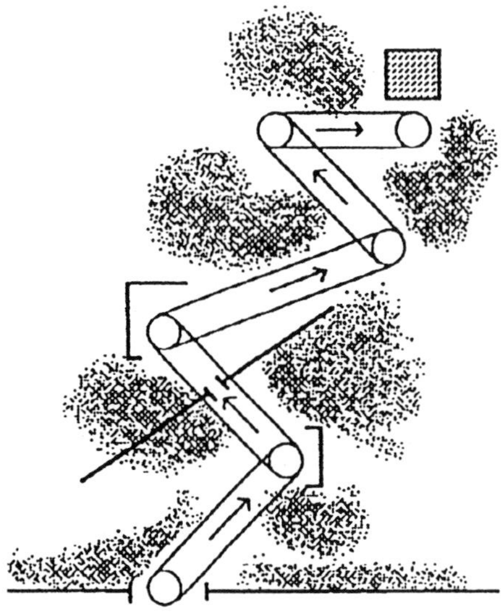

40 Schematic showing *miegakure* as it is used to structure the *roji* path to the teahouse.

principle, of "recalling your memories of how nature presented itself for each feature." It is important to note here that the *roji* possessed both these aspects from the time of its first appearance.

As the art of tea flourished, the *roji* was progressively articulated and developed (Figure 39). It was equipped with various types of facilities for the host to welcome his guests, and likewise for the guests to acknowledge the host's hospitality. It was divided into complex two–and three-section gardens, called double–and triple-*roji*. Indeed, the process of growth did not stop at this point, for the *roji* eventually led to the development of the stroll garden.

Miegakure is a design concept fundamental to *roji* garden making—used for configuring the path that leads from the *roji* entrance and the outer *roji* through the central gate (*nakamon*) to the inner *roji* and up to the *nijiriguchi* (low, sliding-door entrance to the tearoom; Figure 40).

The standard tea garden composition involves a double *roji* with outer and inner sections that are divided by a central gate. Typical features of the outer *roji* start with an entrance gate, which marks the threshold between the *roji* and the outer world, and also include a *yoritsuki* (changing room for removing outer garments), a *koshikake machiai* (covered bench where guests wait to be called to the teahouse), a *setchin* (lavatory), wooden lanterns, and a *chiriana* (small "dust pit" originally used to collect fallen leaves and other debris; now symbolic of leaving behind the cares of this world before entering the tearoom).

The central gate that forms the boundary between the outer and inner *roji* varies from rudimentary *shiorido* gates made of branches to the highly refined *baikenmon* (bamboo lattice doors between stripped cypress pillars supporting a roof of cedar bark). The gate is flanked by short spans of fencing, usually bamboo trellises, on either side. The inner *roji* contains a *koshikake machiai*, a *suna setchin* (lavatory spread with river sand and stones), another *chiriana,* stone lanterns, and a *tsukubai* (a stone basin for ritual rinsing of the hands and mouth). Spans of stone pavements and stepping-stones lead from the garden entrance to the *nijiriguchi* sliding door to the teahouse.

The defining characteristic of *roji* composition is that it does not allow for an open view of the garden in its entirety. Using both tangible and intangible barriers, isolated scenes are alternately displayed and concealed along the path. In this way, space design by *miegakure* focuses the viewer's attention, incrementally revealing the substantial profundity of the entire *roji. Miegakure* here creates settings with intangible barriers to contain the expected, even ritualized, movements of the guests as they visit the facilities arranged within the very confined overall space of the *roji*, while yet establishing continuity with the next movement in the sequence. Thus, the vital integrating factor is precisely the guest's own movement through the garden (Figures 41.1–41.4).

Miegakure as found in the *roji* is an advanced development of the multifaceted, continuous linking of homoge-

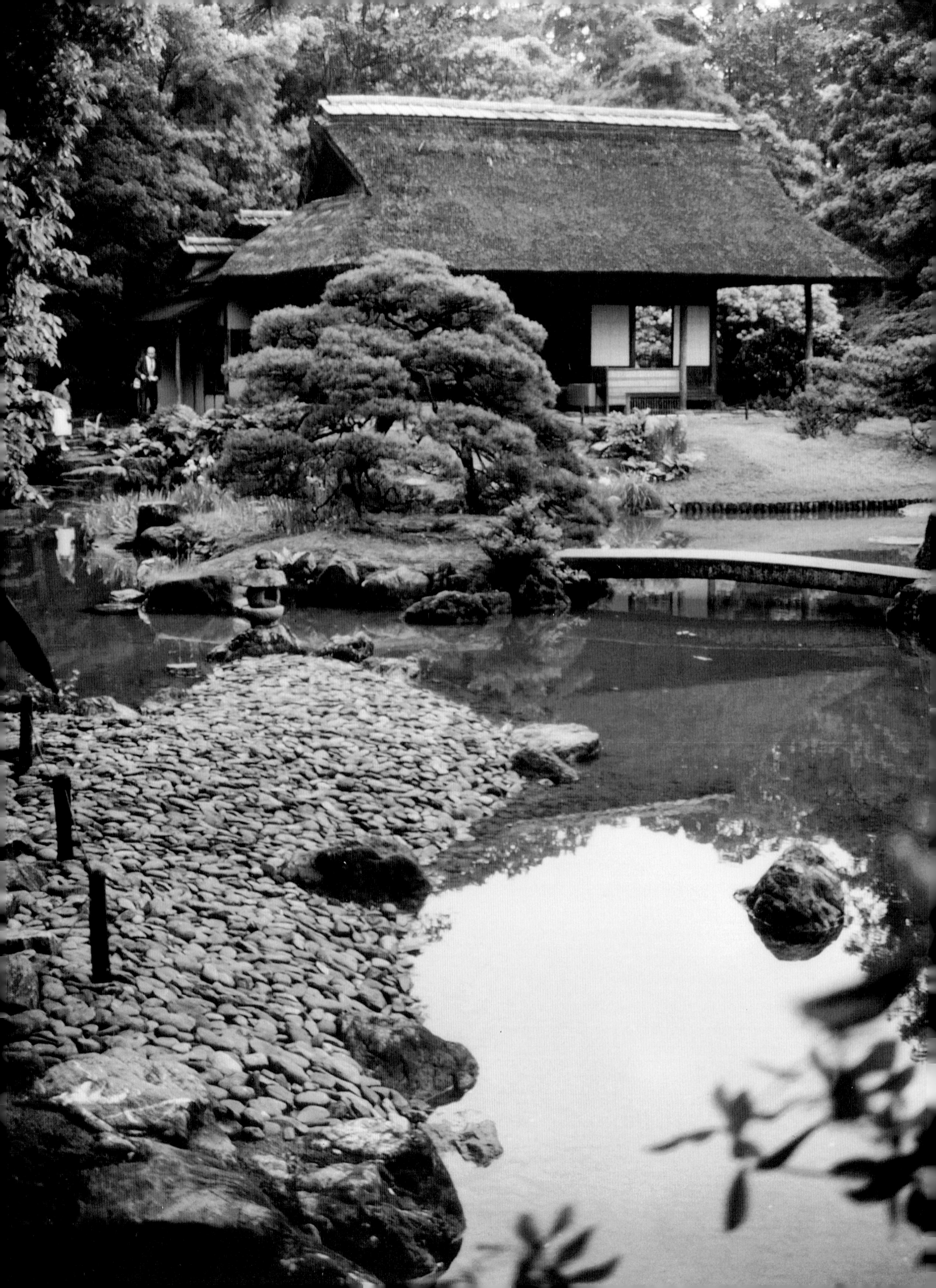

◄ 41.1 *Miegakure* planting screening the Shōkintei teahouse at Katsura Rikyū, Kyoto.

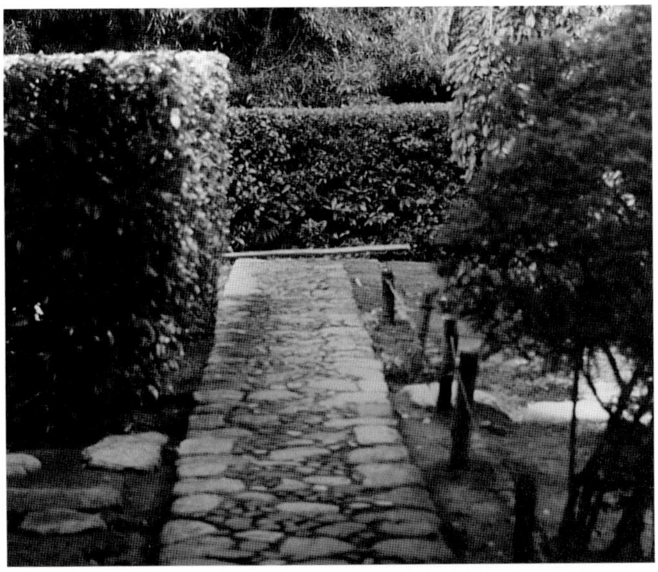

41.2 *Miegakure* structuring the garden path at Katsura Rikyū.

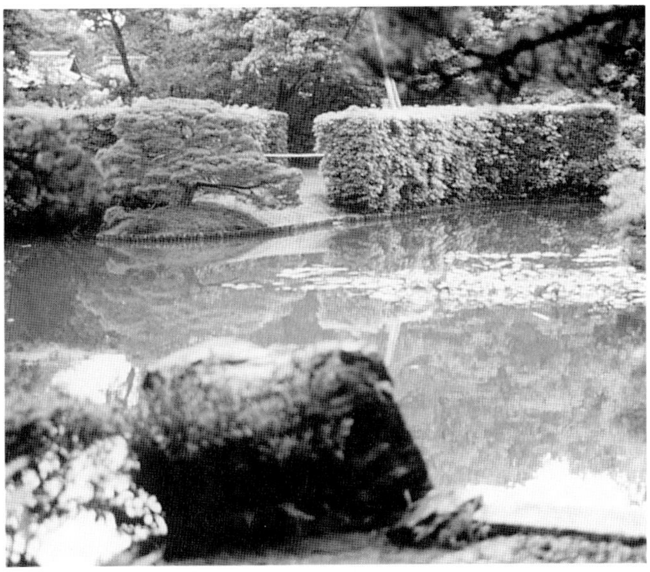

41.3 "Screen pine" as seen from the Shōkintei.

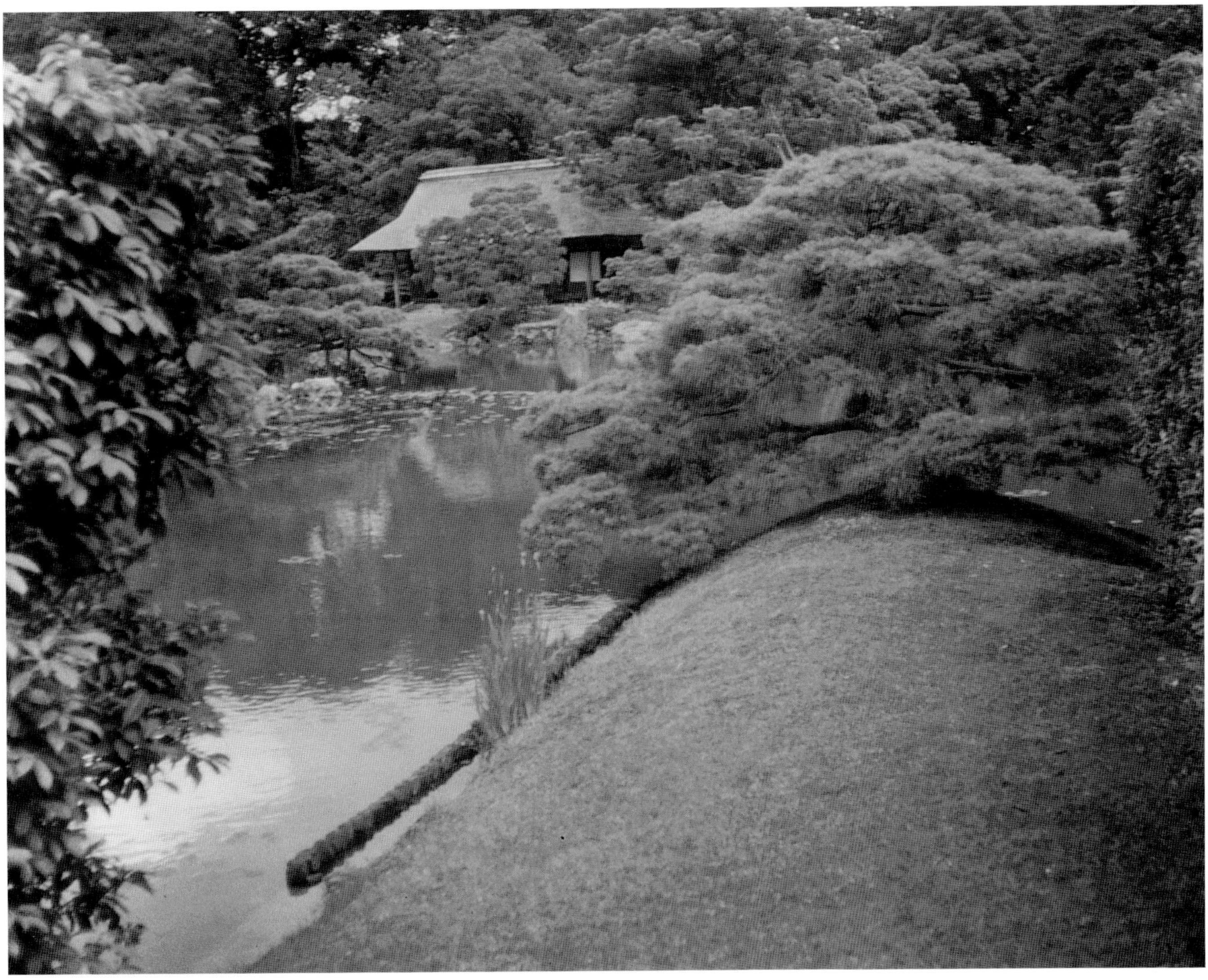

41.4 Shōkintei as seen from behind the "screen pine."

neous points that originated in the Zen temple north garden. It is also part of the developmental process that led to the linking of qualitatively distinct spaces in the stroll garden, which is of course also based on the principle of kinetic, ambulatory viewing.

Rikyū's own *roji* in Sakai was on the coast with a beautiful vista of the sea, but the view was intentionally obscured by trees. Only near the teahouse entrance, in front of the water-basin, did he provide a small opening in the hedge to give a glimpse of the sea. This arrangement corresponds closely to a garden feature described in *Sakuteiki*: " [A]rrange the hills so that the full view of the sea is not seen. Instead, the sea should be made visible only through the small opening of the hills."[3] Here again we can see that *miegakure* evolved from a foundation in the view-obstructing methods used in gardens of Heian-period palace architecture.

As the following didactic poem by Sen no Rikyū suggests, great importance was placed on ensuring that tea ceremony participants' minds were not distracted, but rather focused, by the *roji*.

> Since the Dewy Path
> Is a way that lies outside
> This most impure world
> Shall we not on entering it
> Cleanse our hearts from earthly mire?[4]

The *roji* tea garden was not intended for enjoyment. For Rikyū, it was, like the teahouse itself, a space designed for those who considered the way of tea to be synonymous with Zen practice, and its ultimate goal was to show that "Zen and tea have the same flavor." In this sense the *roji* is distinguished in its spiritual foundations from the later stroll garden, which developed from the more pleasure-oriented branch of tea known as *suki*.

> It is only after many years of practice that you will grasp in its details the fact that everything, from the hundred thousand ways of displaying utensils to the straw-thatched *wabi* tearoom, is governed by the measurements, based on yin and yang, applied in using the *daisu* [utensil stand]. Moreover, since the fundamental intent of *wabi* [beauty amid utter simplicity] lies in manifesting the pure, undefiled Buddha-world, once host and guest have entered the *roji* and the thatched hut, they sweep away the dust and rubbish (of worldly concern) and engage in an encounter with mind open and entire; hence, there is no need to speak insistently of measurements and *sun* and *shaku*, or of formal rules of tea procedure. *Chanoyu* is just a matter of building a fire, boiling water, and drinking tea. There should be nothing else. Here the Buddha-mind emerges to reveal itself.[5]

These words, recorded by a close disciple, show the contradiction inherent in Rikyū's own appreciation of the role of formality, but this is a contradiction that runs right through the way of tea itself.

Originally, drinking tea was a perfectly ordinary, everyday activity; it was a medium for people to meet and chat briefly, and as such included both a social aspect and an aspect of simple enjoyment in its very foundations. Rikyū focused on and rigorously pursued an ideal form of social interaction—direct heart-to-heart reciprocation, through tea. In this pursuit he came to the conclusion that the small tearoom (*koma*) and the *roji* were essential to achieving the necessary attentiveness, and that the *chanoyu* environment should be completed by the proper combination and placement of utensils. However, there were others who focused on tea not as a Zen practice or a pure form of communication, but as a simple form of amusement.

> Sōeki [Rikyū] was the first to construct a tearoom of the virtually minimum size of one-and-a-half mats.

> Although unusual for its time, it was of little use to the ordinary person. It is interesting that Sōeki, being a *meijin* [master], could freely transform mountains into valleys, change west to east, and break the rules of *chanoyu*. But if an ordinary person were to imitate him, there would be no *chanoyu*.[6]

Here Sen no Rikyū's Zen practice is turned into a mere curiosity. Following Rikyū's death, this relatively superficial approach triumphed, and the small *koma* tearoom was dismissed as being too "uncomfortable for the guests." The way of tea came to be viewed as essentially a pleasurable pastime. Not only was the small tearoom rejected, but a *kusari no ma* ("connecting room") was constructed as a place to display utensils, and the concept of "a mountain locale set within a city" was transformed—valued not as a spiritual retreat, but as a pleasant escape from everyday life.

This way of thinking eventually evolved into the spatial formalism known as *sukiya-zukuri*. *Suki*, meaning connoisseurship, initially described a conception of beauty that was unorthodox, but came to refer to the enjoyment of a subtly elegant form of tea ceremony, while *sukiya*, as used in this text, came to refer to the *hiroma* ("large [tea] rooms") in which these ceremonies were performed. The principal factor guiding the design of *sukiya* was the anticipated patterns of people's physical movements and emotional responses within the space.

This architectural approach can perhaps best be expressed as an amalgamation of the spirit of *chanoyu* and the *sukiya* spatial format. The results of adding the element of heightened attention, as cultivated in the walk through the *roji*, to the condensed *shoin* garden were, first, the linking of qualitatively different spaces—the *shōin*, *sukiya*, and *sōan*—and, ultimately, the blossoming of the Edo-period stroll garden, or pleasure garden.

Insight into the social climate that gave rise to the development of *sukiya-zukuri* in the early Edo period is critical to an understanding of the changes in composition of buildings and gardens that occurred with the great transformation of the way of tea after Rikyū's death.

Once the Tokugawa regime had been established, an immensely stable social system divided along rigid class lines, and the peace achieved by a policy of national seclusion gave rise to a varied, vibrant urban society. Lifestyle and aesthetic taste generally fell into one of three discrete cultural realms: the aristocratic culture centered around the court, *buke* warrior culture revolving around the shogunate, and the affluent culture of the urban merchant classes. This is the context in which distinct garden types developed based on the differing lifestyles, emotions, and aesthetics of these three cultural realms.

New aesthetic ideals which arose in this time—including *iki* (an urbane chic with undertones of sensuality), *okashimi* (humor; also, amused recognition that something is ludicrous but inevitable), and *fūryū* (used in reference to both the ostentatious beauty seen in popular arts, and the more tasteful beauty of such elegant pastimes as landscape gardening, flower arrangement, and tea ceremony)—were pregnant with the contradictions of everyday reality. Ironically, the prospering urban merchant class, known as *chōnin*, fostered a vibrant popular culture, despite having been relegated to the bottom of the social scale.

These divergent developments in changing traditions evoked the criticisms of Rikyū mentioned above. Rikyū's way of tea as Zen practice was rejected, and it seemed that the aesthetic ideals that sought beauty in restraint—*wabi* (utter simplicity, or the appreciation of a higher beauty amid apparent lack of beauty), and *sabi* (appreciation of the patina of use and age)—had waned. But they had not disappeared altogether, for in some quarters Rikyū was apotheosized, and the tea ceremony was ritualized and revered as the ultimate aesthetic activity.

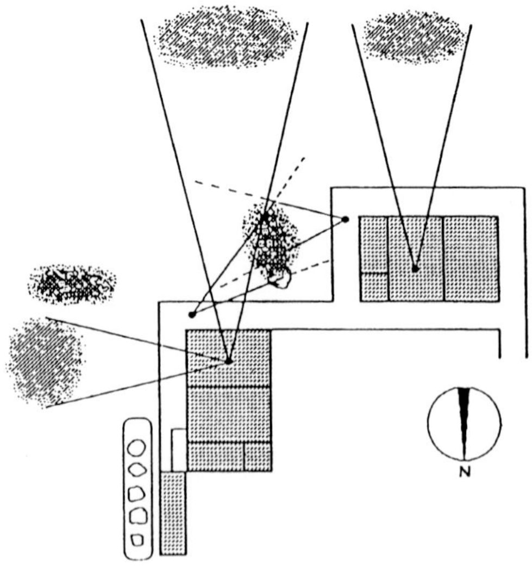

42 Schematic showing *miegakure* as it is used to link qualitatively distinct buildings and gardens.

Combined *Shoin*/*Sukiya*/*Sōan* Structures: *Miegakure* Linking Qualitatively Distinct Buildings and Gardens

After the death of Rikyū in the late sixteenth century, the emergence of the *sukiya-zukuri* architectural style led to a new *shoin* + *sukiya* + *sōan* arrangement, which combined buildings and gardens of these three styles into a single linked structure.

Positioned between the large, magnificent *shoin*, with its formalized decorative accoutrements denoting high status, and the tiny, rustic *sōan* hut which was considered "uncomfortable for guests," was the semi-formal *sukiya*, also known as the *sukiya shoin*. Characteristics of *sukiya-zukuri* include the use of columns with unbeveled corners (*menkawabashira*), earthen walls (*tsuchikabe*), and understated, delicate decoration.

The method used to link these three completely distinct interior spaces and their respective gardens into one continuous building-and-garden form, while barring the view from one to another, was *miegakure*. And the architectural composition used to effect this was the diagonally-stepped "geese-in-flight" formation (*gankōkei*) that had been used earlier in asymmetrical *shinden-zukuri* mansions (Figure 42).

Manshu-in is a *sukiya-zukuri* temple in northeast Kyoto, composed of two *shoin*—one in the formal *shoin* style, and the other in the *sukiya* style—and a *sōan*-style tearoom (Figure 43.1–43.5). The garden, as viewed from the *jōdan* (higher level) of the formal *shoin*, likewise has a formal, highly refined composition centered on a main feature—a single "boat" pine (*funamatsu*).

The recessed *sukiya shoin* is accessed by an external corridor that extends from the veranda of the formal *shoin* in a "zigzagged" form, linking the two buildings. From this veranda, the view of both *shoin* is partially obscured by two trees placed so as to interrupt the lines of sight from one building to another. The main scene in the dry waterfall garden, a Buddhist triad rock (*sanzonseki*) arrangement, corresponds to the view from the *sukiya shoin* (composed of an anteroom called Fuji no ma and a main room named Tasogare no ma).

A dynamic stream of white sand representing the ocean links the two heterogeneous views—that of the representational boat pine garden corresponding to the formal *shoin* and that of the abstract dry landscape waterfall garden relating to the *sukiya*. Tucked into the garden recess formed by these two buildings, a lone island floats in the ocean, hosting the single pine that is the central focus of the overall garden composition and that effects the *miegakure* linking the qualitatively distinct *shoin* and *sukiya*.

A series of stepping-stones extending toward the adjacent mountain then marks the boundary between the qualitatively distinct areas of the *sukiya* and *sōan* and their respective dry waterfall and *roji* gardens.

The side wall of the Tasogare no ma affords a view of the simple *roji* garden, composed of stepping-stones, laid under the eaves, that lead off to the Hassōseki (Eight-window tearoom).

Just as the *shoin*, *sukiya*, and *sōan* structures are combined in the geese-in-flight formation, so are their respective *shin* (formal), *gyō* (semiformal), and *sō* (informal) "sub-"gardens structured by means of *miegakure* into a marvelously integrated, total garden composition.

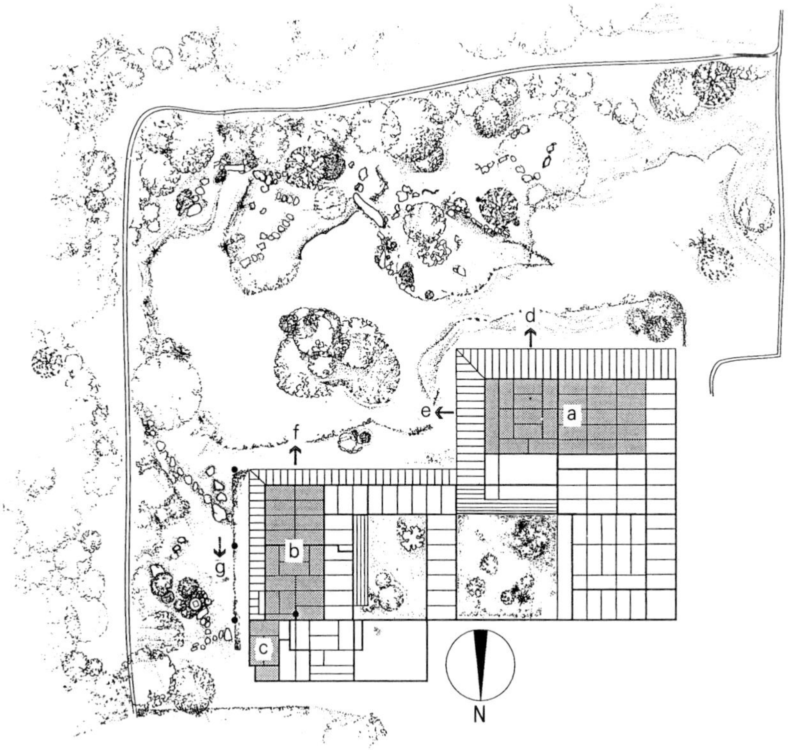

43.1 Plan view drawing of Manshu-in.

a. *shoin*.
b. *sukiya*.
c. *sōan*.
d. formal garden.
e. "linkage."
f. semiformal garden.
g. informal garden.

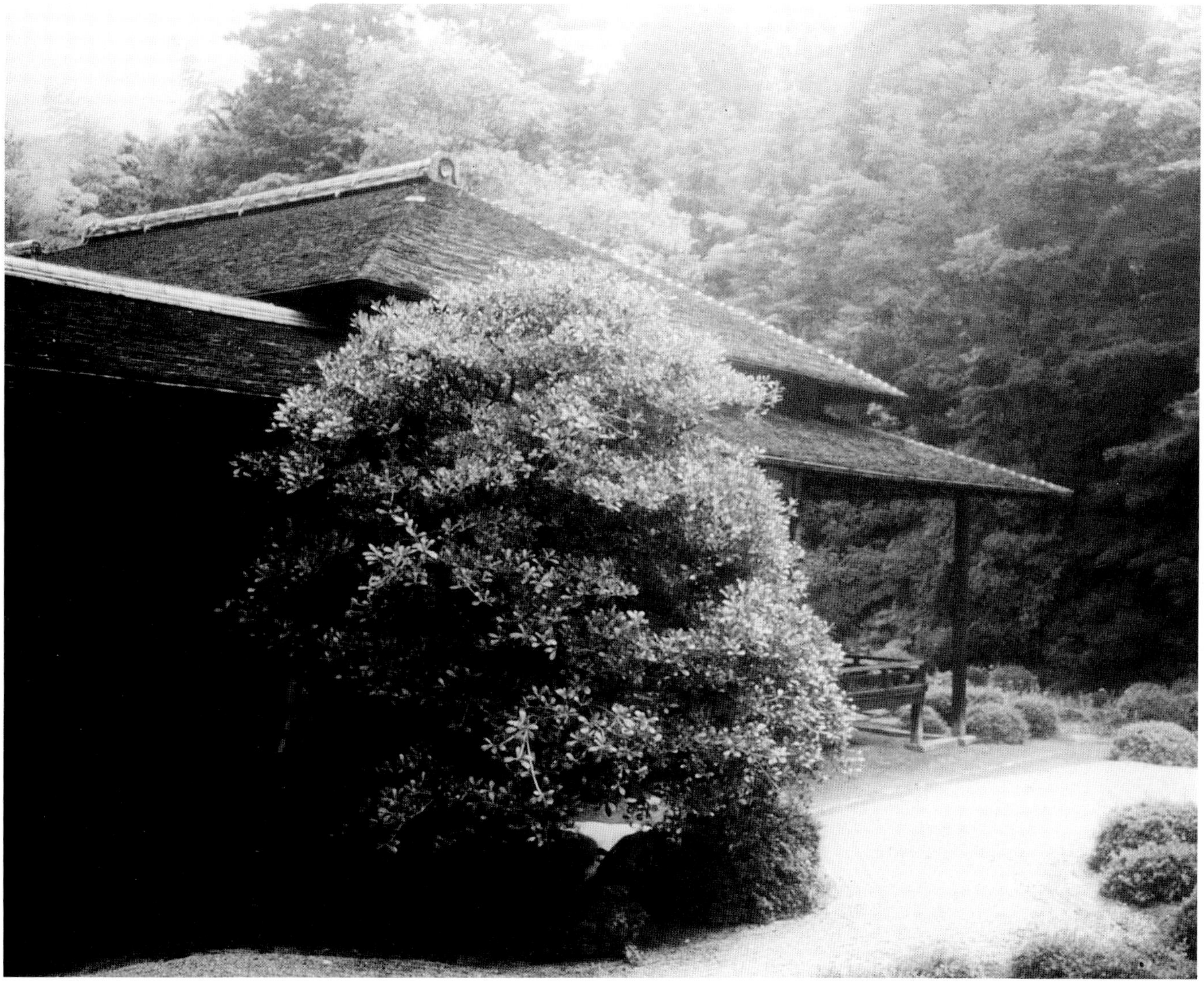

43.2 "Linking/interrupting" tree (b).

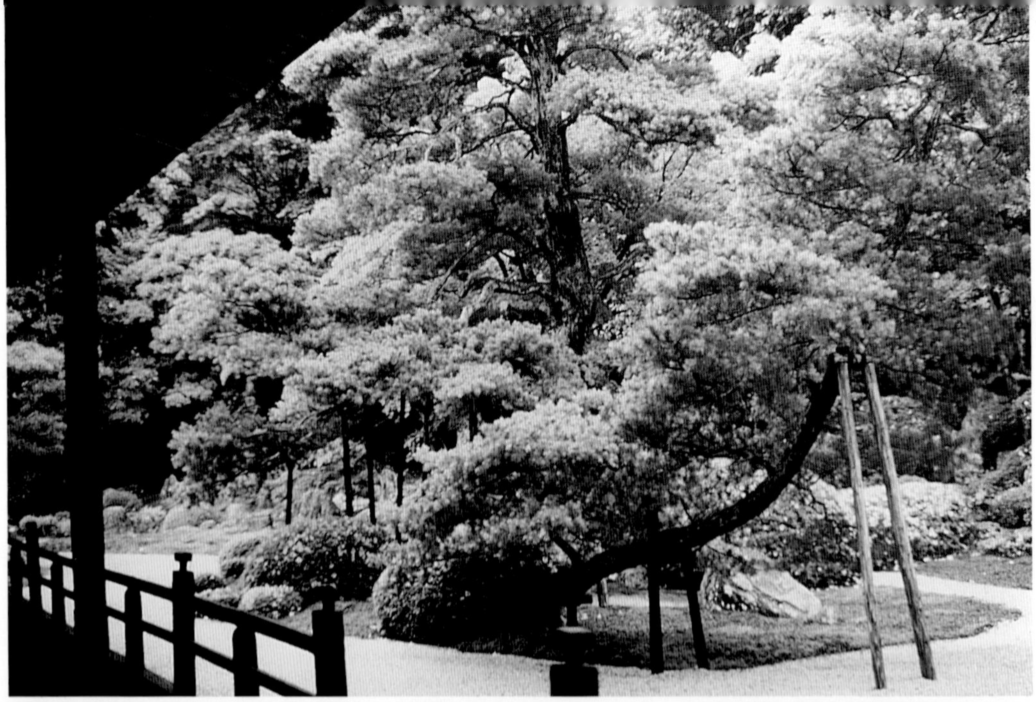

43.3 View from the *shoin* (d).

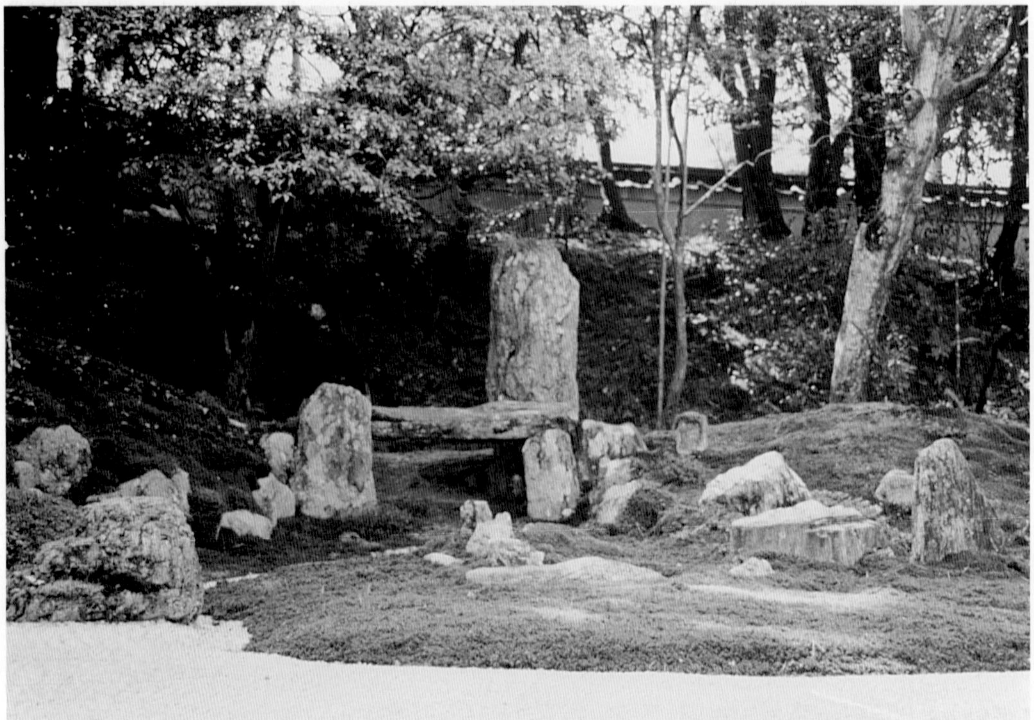

43.4 View from the *sukiya* (f).

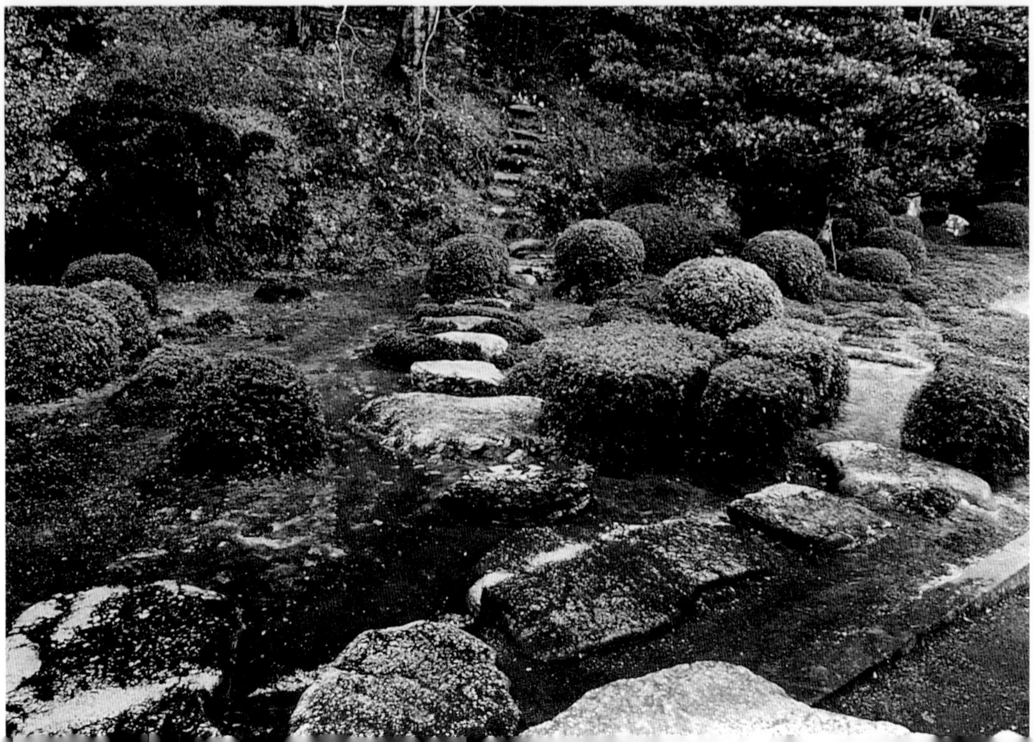

43.5 *Roji* (g).

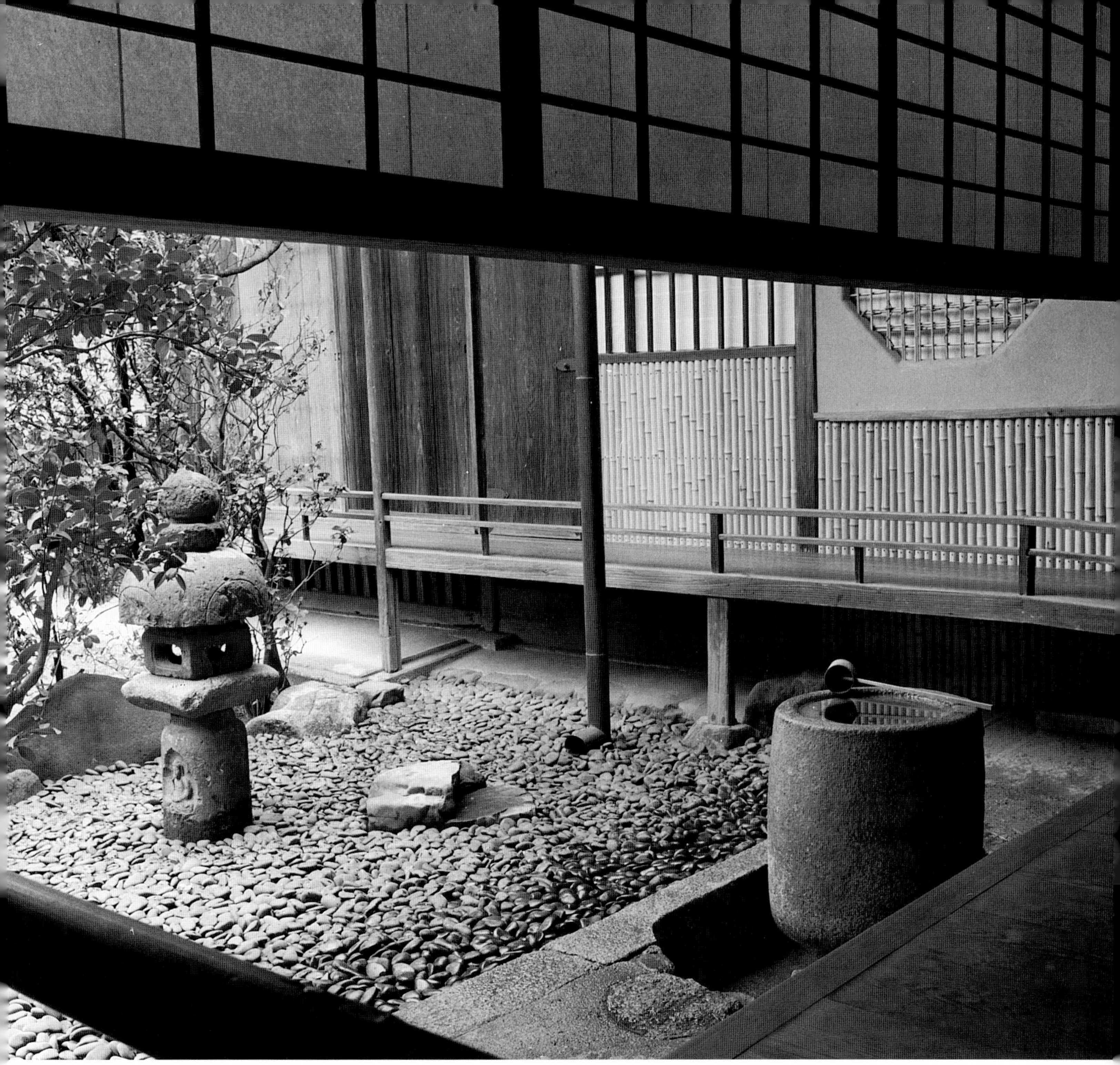

44.1 Daitokuji Kohō-an *roji* to the Bōsen tearoom, Kyoto.

The compositional structure of buildings and gardens of Kohō-an at Daitokuji in Kyoto is similar to that of Manshu-in. The *hōjō*, Bōsen tearoom, *sukiya*, and San'unshō tearoom are linked—with their respective gardens—in the geese-in-flight formation. The garden is a combination of the *hōjō*'s "empty" garden, defined by a double-tiered hedge, and a vast, oceanlike, light-bathed garden called Ōmi hakkei (literally, "eight sights of Ōmi"; Figures 44.1–44.5).

The composition of the Kohō-an garden is marked by the arrangement of some dense and some sparse clusters of trees close to the eaves, designed to conceal and reveal by turns the "oceanic" garden beyond. Thus, a full view of the Ōmi hakkei is not visible except from the veranda of the *sukiya.* The garden's rather vague, "watery" composition may be more easily understood as a backdrop against which the foreground shrubbery is highlighted and silhouetted when viewed from the interior of the Bōsen tearoom; its role is similar to that of gold-leaf grounds in wall paintings of the Kanō school.

As the viewer moves from the *hōjō,* glimpses of the

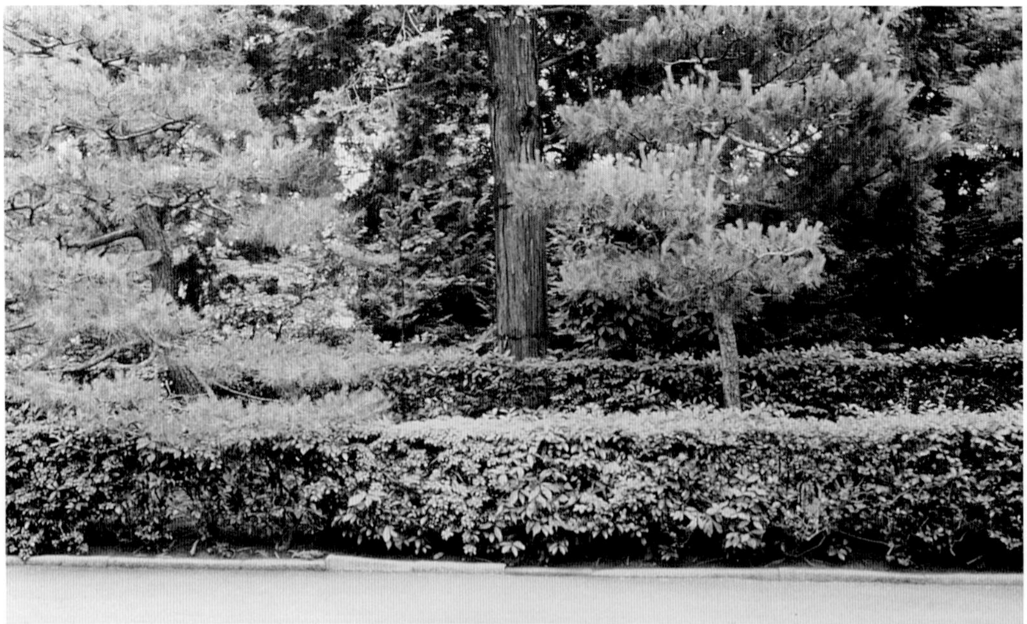

44.2 View from the *hōjō* (d).

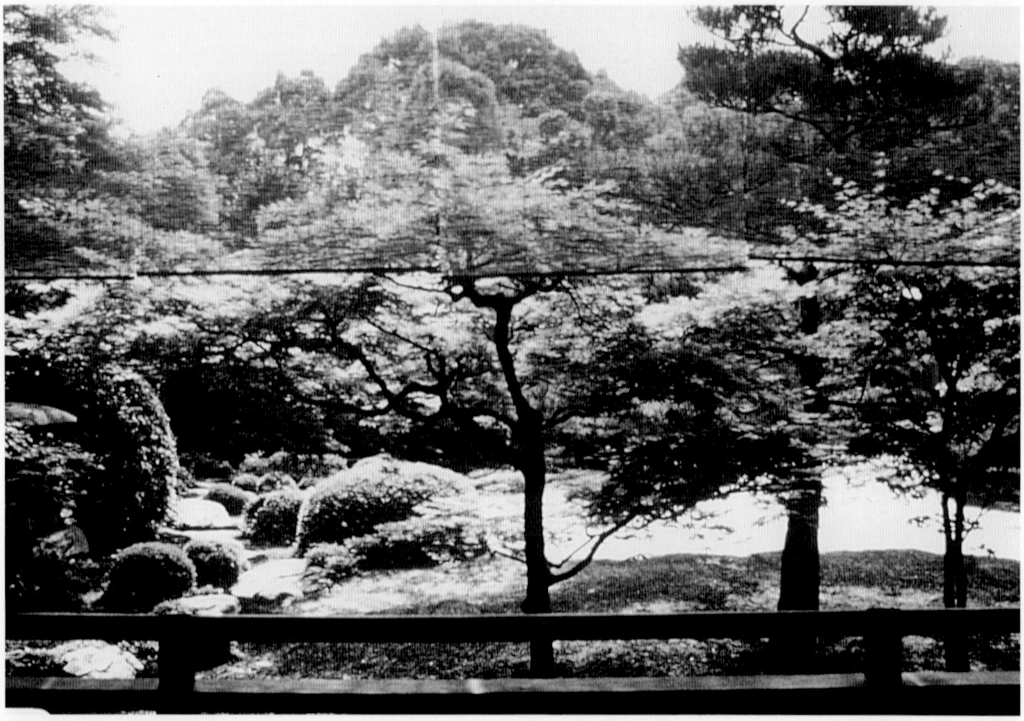

44.3 View of the “linkage” (e).

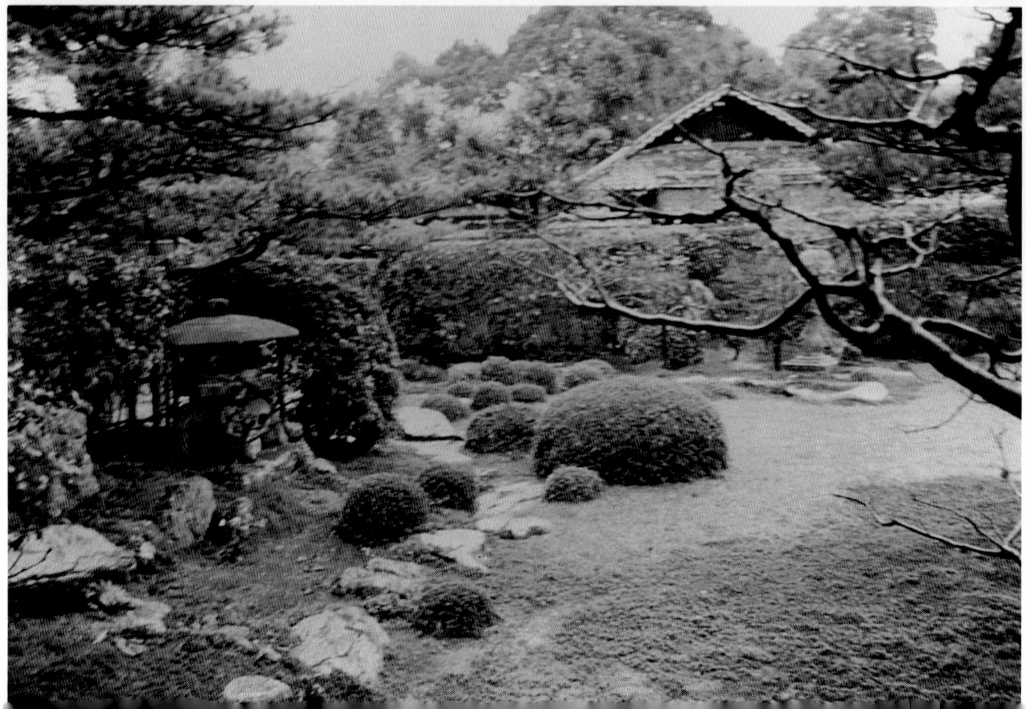

44.4 View of Ōmi hakkei (g).

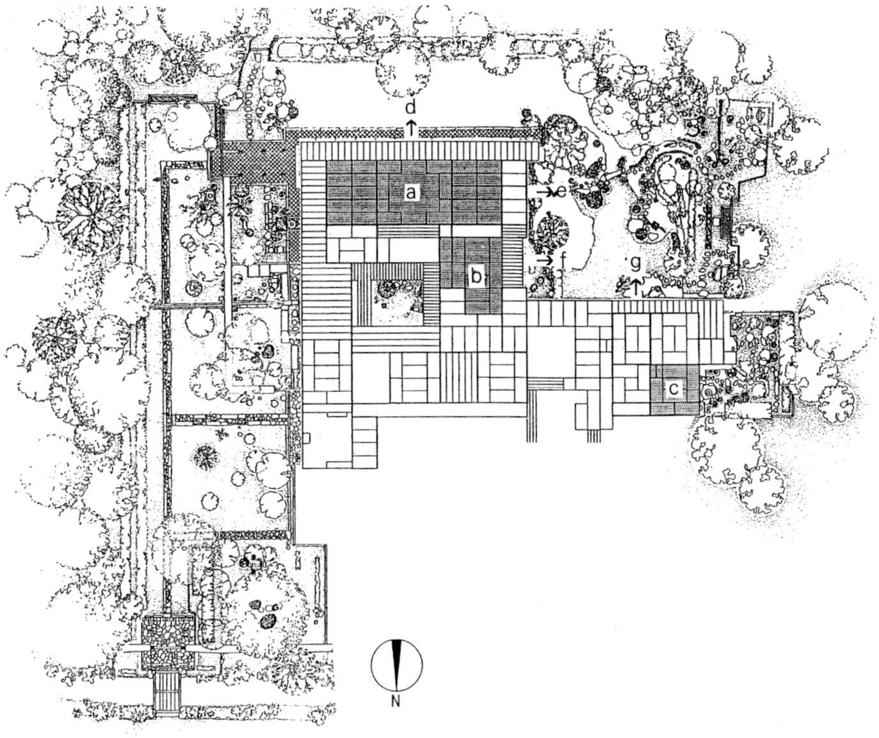

44.5 Plan view drawing of Daitokuji Kohō-an.

a. *hōjō.*
b. Bōsen tearoom.
c. San'unshō tearoom.
d. *hōjō* garden.
e. "linkage."
f. *roji.*
g. Ōmi hakkei.

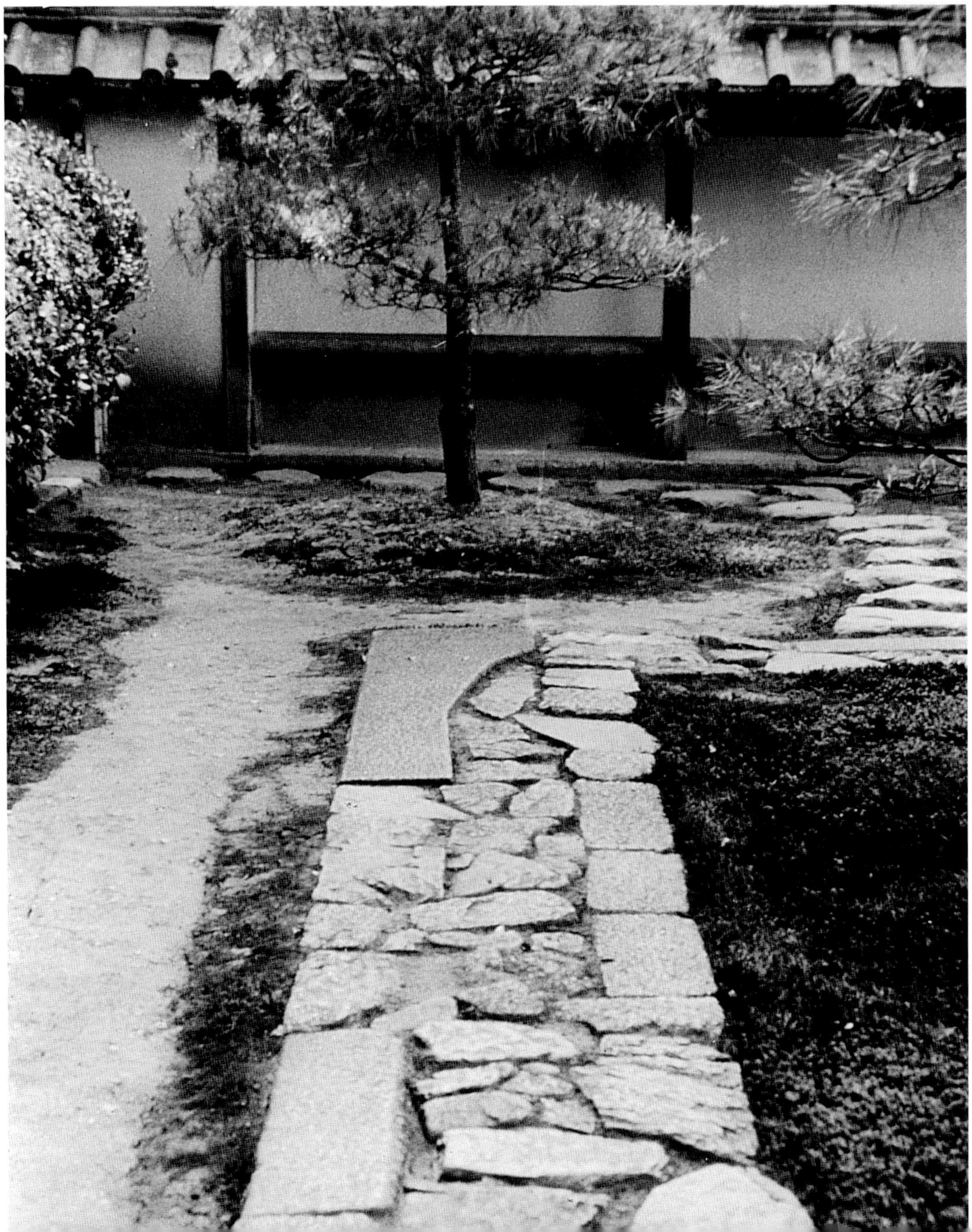

44.6 *Miegakure* as it is used in the approach to Kohō-an.

bright Ōmi hakkei garden are provided through the spaces between the trees, which become incrementally smaller—from one to one-half, and finally to one-fourth—until the row of trees ends at the entrance to the Bōsen. Together with dense shrubbery that obstructs a full view of the garden, a *shōji* screen spanning the upper half of Bōsen's exterior "wall" also blocks the line of sight, while the open lower half allows a suggestion of the Ōmi hakkei to linger and at the same leads the eye into the tearoom. Stepping-stones set in *miwado* cement in the space between the eaves and the row of trees forms the *roji* between the *hōjō* and Bōsen. The open-walled entrance beneath the half-*shōji* is a new and original form of *nijiriguchi* (low entranceway to the tearoom), called the *funa-iri*, or "boat-mooring" style.

While Manshu-in constitutes a basic form of *miegakure* configuration, here we see that same methodology perfected through the superb technical skill and acute sense of modeling of architect, garden designer, and tea master Kobori Enshū. The master's distinctive modeling can also be seen in the composition of the approach to Kohō-an.

First, the stone-lined moat defining the boundary of the subtemple grounds is unique and innovative. The thick, comb-shaped stone bridge spanning this moat is ingenious, as are its central beam, its columns, and the brace stones securing it at both ends. A stretch of stone pavement set in the middle of a bed of cryptomeria moss forms one straight line running between this stone bridge and the outer gate and extending to the waiting bench at the far end of the approach.

On the same axis, just in front of the waiting bench, there is a single "interrupting" tree, around which the stepping-stones arc in a semicircle. The roughhewn stonework in this stretch of pavement is state-of-the-art. A large single stone forms the outer corner of the bend in the path directly in front of the waiting area. Its very form "points" to the right, and so skillfully leads people around the turn to the entrance hall (Figure 44.6). *Miegakure* effected by an interrupting tree that blocks an axial view is a device also utilized throughout the garden of Katsura Rikyū.

The idea of aligning the entrance gate and the waiting area on the same axis, with a single tree interrupting the long sight line, would be unthinkable in *roji* composition; this gives some indication of the originality and freshness of Enshū's insight.

The experience of walking through an environment composed of combined *shion*, *sukiya*, and *sōan* buildings and gardens, such as those of Manshu-in and Kohō-an, is very different from that of walking a *roji*. These combination *shoin/sukiya/sōan* gardens were designed to be viewed primarily while walking within the building confines and represent a development of the technique used to link views of similar quality that was seen earlier in Zen temple north gardens. In *sukiya-zukuri* environments, however, we see the linking of scenes of completely different qualities. When the "walk through the garden" was separated and made independent of the building, the technique of linking heterogeneous garden forms with *miegakure* developed a step further, culminating in the Edo-period stroll garden.

The Stroll Garden: *Miegakure* Linking Qualitatively Different Garden Areas

The stroll garden, or *kaiyūshiki-teien*, emerged amid the stable milieu of the Tokugawa regime and its strict social hierarchy with nobles and feudal lords near the top, and urban merchants near the bottom. The spacious gardens built on the private properties of feudal lords are what is usually referred to as "stroll gardens," but in fact another type of "garden" from this same period can also reasonably be considered a stroll garden—the Pure Land temple garden precincts which became immensely popular as

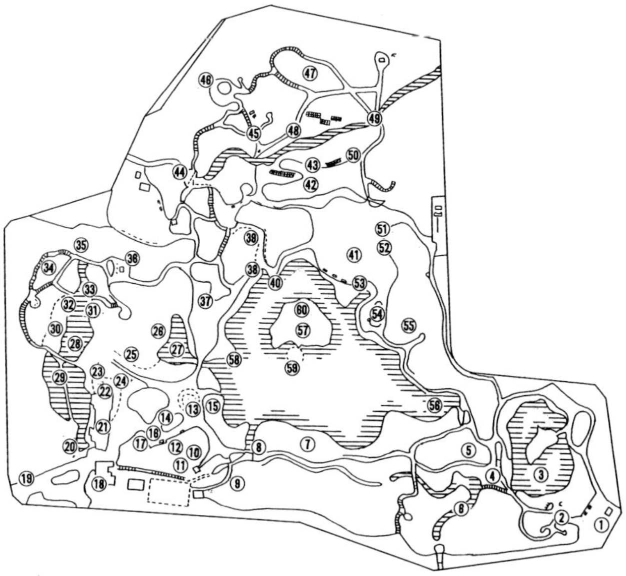

45.1 Plan of Koishikawa Kōrakuen indicating sub-garden themes, Tokyo.

㉑ Little Lushan (China).
㉘ Togetsu-kyō (Kyoto).
㉙ West Lake dike (China).
㉛ Ōi River (Kyoto).
㉟ Tsūten-kyō (Kyoto).
㊱ Chikubu shima (Shiga Prefecture).

recreation grounds with commoners. Thus two fundamentally very similar "garden" styles arose at the same time to serve the needs of two social classes separated by a great social chasm.

Pleasure Gardens of the Daimyō Feudal Lords

The Tokugawa period saw a tremendous rise in popular interest in travel and faraway places, partly because of the general social stability and perhaps also as a result of the government's strict restrictions on travel. In a demonstration of their wealth and station, *daimyō* began to build on their spacious properties huge entertainment-oriented "theme" parks that offered visitors a much sought-after opportunity to "travel." The parklike stroll garden is composed of numerous sub-gardens based on themes of famous locales in Japan and abroad, and well-known settings for classical and contemporary literary works, all arranged around a pond. Just as the distinctly different spaces of the *shoin, sukiya,* and *sōan* were "toured," guests meander along the stroll garden path to tour the qualitatively different garden spaces, and are afforded different views of the pond from strategic points (see Figure 47.2). In most cases, the series of sub-gardens was configured so that people could observe the pond on their right while moving in a clockwise direction around the gardens; this orientation was selected on the basis of simple observation of people's walking habits.

Although the pond is the center of the landscape composition, no view of the pond in its entirety is ever provided. The interpretations expressed in the stroll garden offer a variety of interesting experiences—being drawn deep into the mountains and getting an occasional glimpse of the pond through the trees, descending into a valley, crossing an expanse of lawn that resembles a meadow, and looking out over the pond from a nearby tearoom. As guests proceed along the path, views that are always partially obscured appear and disappear in turn, piquing the viewer's curiosity about the scene to come. The owner's favorite "famous places of scenic beauty" unfold one after another in a kind of narrative with its own continuity, driven by *miegakure* (Figures 45.1–45.5).

The compositional techniques used to create these effects are clearly an extension of *Sakuteiki*'s ideas on "offsetting, alternating, [and] overlapping." The basic difference here, however, is that they are not fixed barriers viewed from a fixed position, but a form of view obstruction based on a moving vantage point that evolves with the walker's progressive movement through the environment. Stroll garden interpretations involve garden-making methods with a new kind of depth. *Miegakure* gained in complexity, amid increased concern for and attention to detail in creating garden paths, and was recognized as an effective method for linking distinct gardens.

The prototype of the stroll garden is unmistakably still the "natural landscape." As mentioned earlier, Edo-period gardens of feudal lords were always based on specific themes—the most popular being well-known scenic locales in Japan and China—which has its basis in *Sakuteiki*'s injunctions to use one's "memories of how nature presented itself for each feature" and to "think over the famous places of scenic beauty throughout the land."

These gardens are pleasure gardens. The stable social

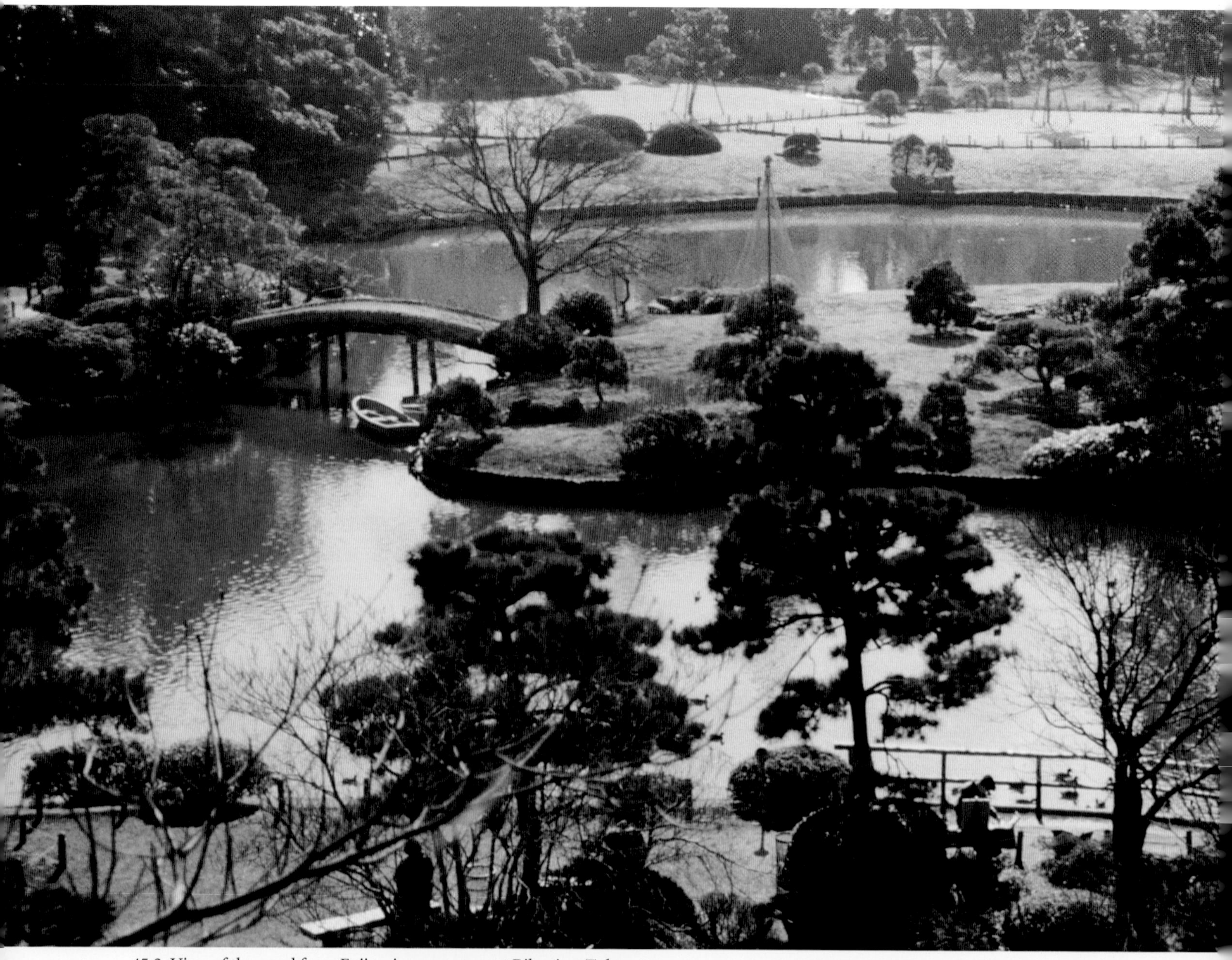

45.2 View of the pond from Fujiyori promontory at Rikugien, Tokyo.

system and peace afforded by a policy of national seclusion provided a sense of liberation from the sublime but severe aesthetics of the medieval period, in which beauty had been confined within extremely strict spatial, formal, and spiritual limits, and allowed an age of the aesthetics of play to blossom.

Pleasure gardens are free of the tension that characterizes Muromachi-period Zen temple gardens, and of the emphasis on status and propriety that was so prominent in *shoin* gardens. Decidedly sensuous, optimistic, and in accord with the injunction to "think over the famous places of scenic beauty throughout the land," they are an animated collection of popular themes. These eminently social gardens were created solely as a form of entertainment.

Pleasure "Gardens" of the Urban Merchant Class

Stroll gardens were made by and for feudal lords and wealthy individuals. Originally, the stepping-stones in these gardens were laid in a single row, which restricted walking to single file and thus formed a path reflective of Japan's hierarchical social order. It has been said that in Japan there has never been a traditional garden style that allowed people to walk two or three abreast, or in larger groups. The exception to this rule, however, can be found in the line of gardens that extend from the Heian-period Pure Land gardens, the temple and shrine precincts that became the grounds for recreation of the urban merchants, or *chōmin*, who had no land holdings of their own. During the rule of the Tokugawa shogunate, the religious pilgrimage—

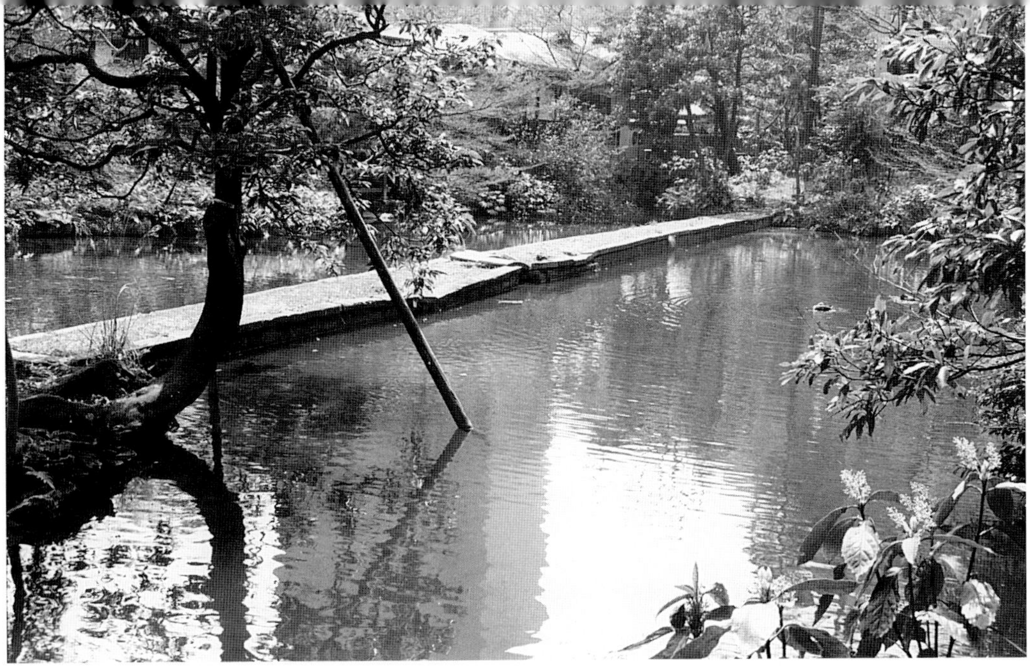

45.3 China's West Lake as a sub-garden theme at Koishikawa Kō-rakuen.

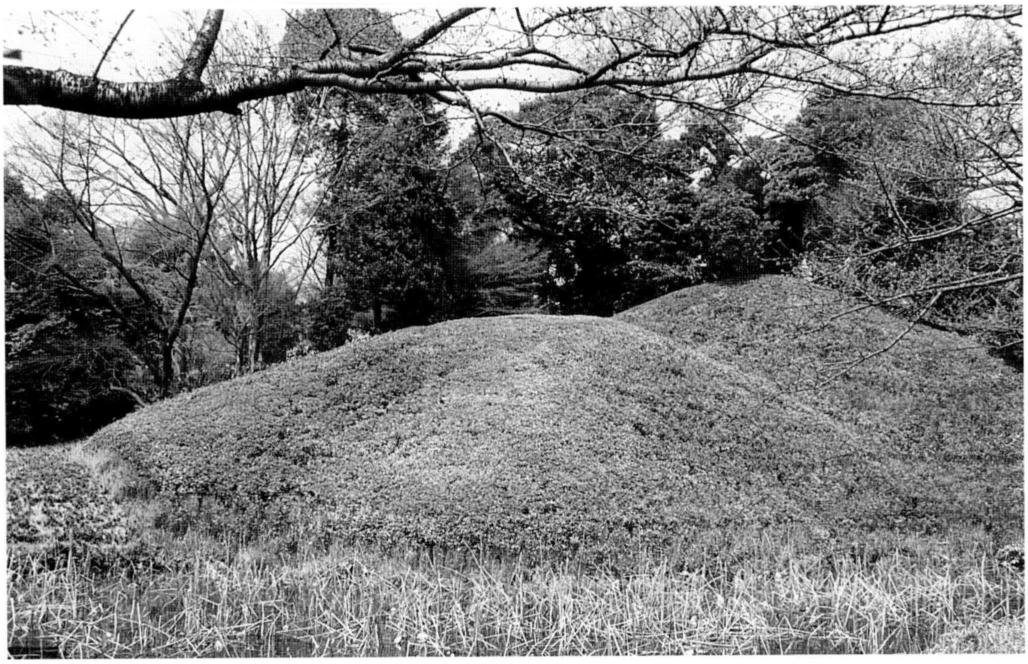

45.4 China's Lushan as a sub-garden theme at Koishikawa Kō-rakuen.

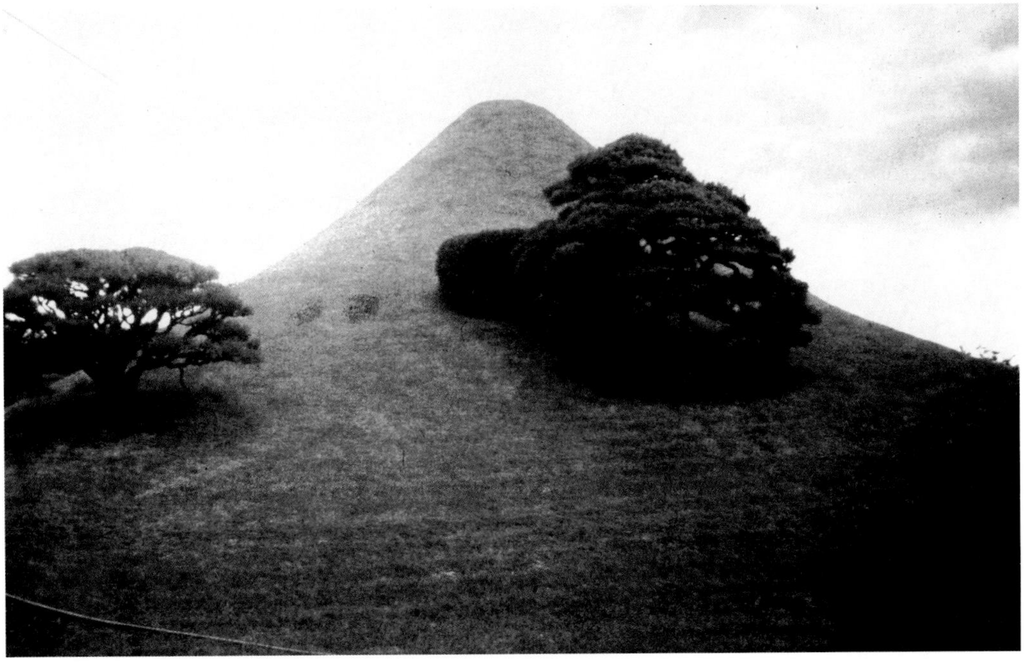

45.5 Mount Fuji as a sub-garden theme at Suizenji Kōen, Kumamoto.

which was exempt from the government's strict prohibitions on travel—gained great popularity. Pilgrimages involved making a circuit, sometimes over significant distances, of temples and other sacred grounds, in a set order.

Hasedera, located in the city of Sakurai in Nara Prefecture, is the eighth stop on the pilgrimage circuit of thirty-three Kannon temples in western Japan, and even today is visited by a constant stream of pilgrims.

There are three points that command a full view of the temple: the main gate, the monk's quarters, and the stage of the main hall. Compositionally these are similar to the views of the pond in the stroll garden. The roofed corridor by which pilgrims gradually ascend to the main hall is flanked by a thick border of peonies which changes—first to azaleas and then to hydrangeas—with each turn of the path. Because of this variety, flowers bloom at the temple year-round. The impressiveness of the view from the front gate gives way to a sense of mystery produced by the inability to make out the full form of the massive eleven-headed Kannon, the primary attendant of the Amida Buddha housed inside the dimly-lit main hall.

Upon turning to leave, the viewer is afforded a magnificent view, from the main hall's raised platform structure, of the Yamato mountain range glistening in the distance—"Western Paradise"—which creates a wonderful contrasting composition.

While Heian-period Pure Land villa-temple gardens were a static, frontal, unidirectionally-composed staging of Western Paradise at the opposite shore of the lotus pond, Hasedera's precincts are composed of a number of qualitatively distinct scenes linked by *miegakure*, which together with the colorful wall of flowers and the incessant chanting of pilgrims produce a highly dramatic and dynamic representation of Western Paradise. Structurally, the "touring" of the temple precincts is the same as the stroll garden's linking of theme-based garden areas. The "ninety-nine–turn" corridor (*kairō*) is quintessential *miegakure* (Figure 46.1).

This kind of *miegakure* landscape composition is seen not only at Hasedera, but also at the Kiyomizudera Kannon in Kyoto (Figure 46.2), the Chiba Kasamori Kannon, the Yanaizu Kokūzō, and other temples. For the most part, temples dedicated to Kannon share this style of composition. Just as the tea of Zen practice became the tea of pleasure, the garden of Zen practice gave way to the pleasure garden. Similarly, just as Heian-period Pure Land villa-temple gardens had expressed faith in salvation by rendering Western Paradise on earth, temple and shrine precincts became the grounds for the recreation of the urban merchant classes—their "gardens" or "parks."

The people of Edo (present-day Tokyo) were known for both their passionate love of flowers and the beautiful ornamental cherry trees which they cultivated. Nationwide, Edo was praised as "the city of flowers"—and it was in this spirit that the "gardens" of urban merchants initially arose from a desire to link faith and seasonal flora. Many temple and shrine precincts famous for their plum, cherry, azalea, or wisteria blossoms have become venues for flower viewing—a favorite seasonal pastime in Edo Japan, as it is today.

At the foundation of the landscaping concept behind the stroll garden lay aesthetic ideals which, like those of the colorful "gardens" of the urban merchants, were radically new. Various movements striving to establish a sense of tradition emerged among the different social classes in the Edo period. Prominent among these within the merchant classes of the cities was a blossoming of the aesthetics of pleasure variously referred to as *iki* (urbane chic), *okashimi* (humor; amusement) and *fūryū* (ostentatious beauty). Both the pleasure gardens of feudal lords and the temple and shrine "gardens" of city merchants show these new aesthetic ideals in full bloom.

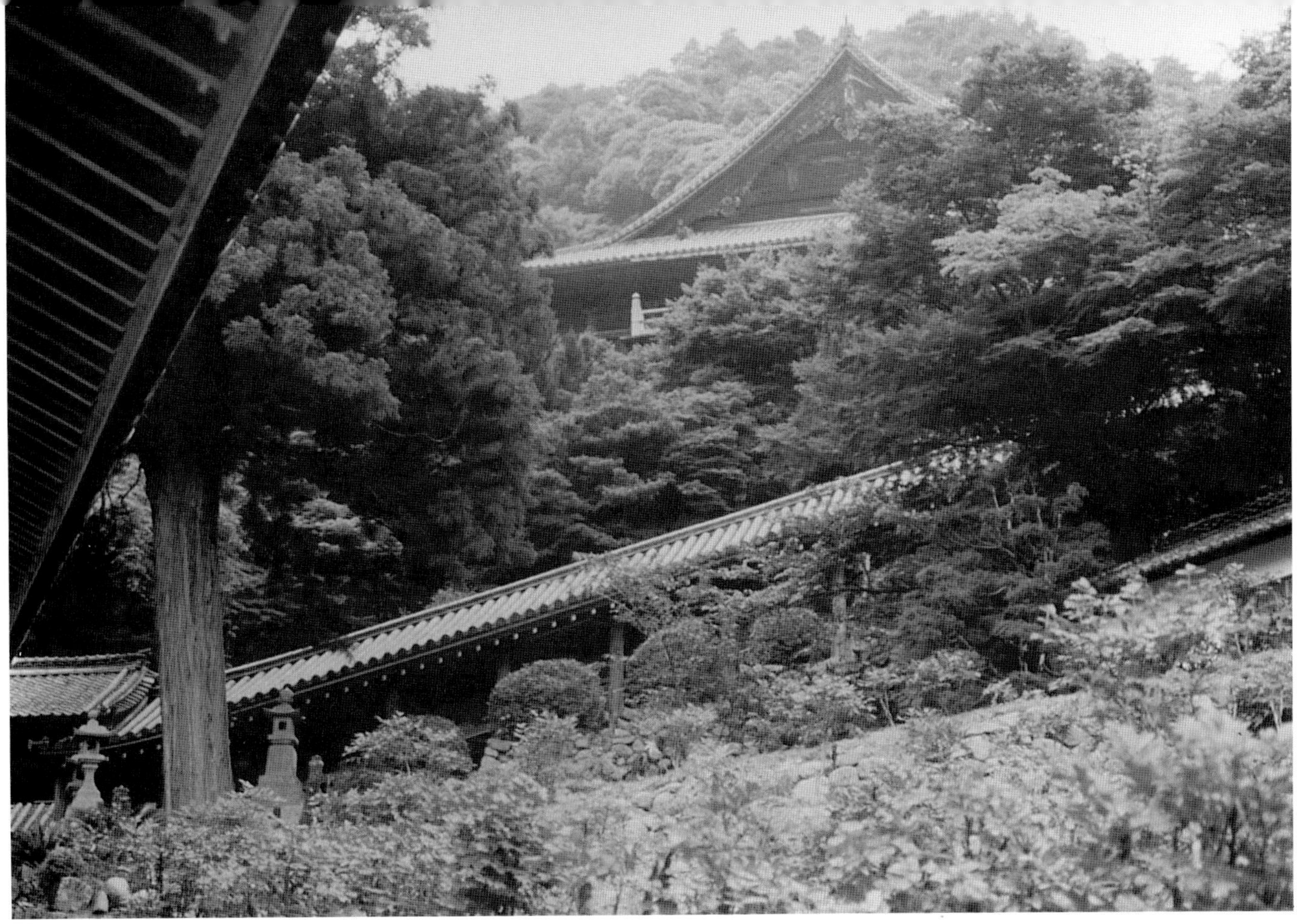

46.1 View from the main gate of the approach and the main hall of Hasedera, Nara Prefecture.

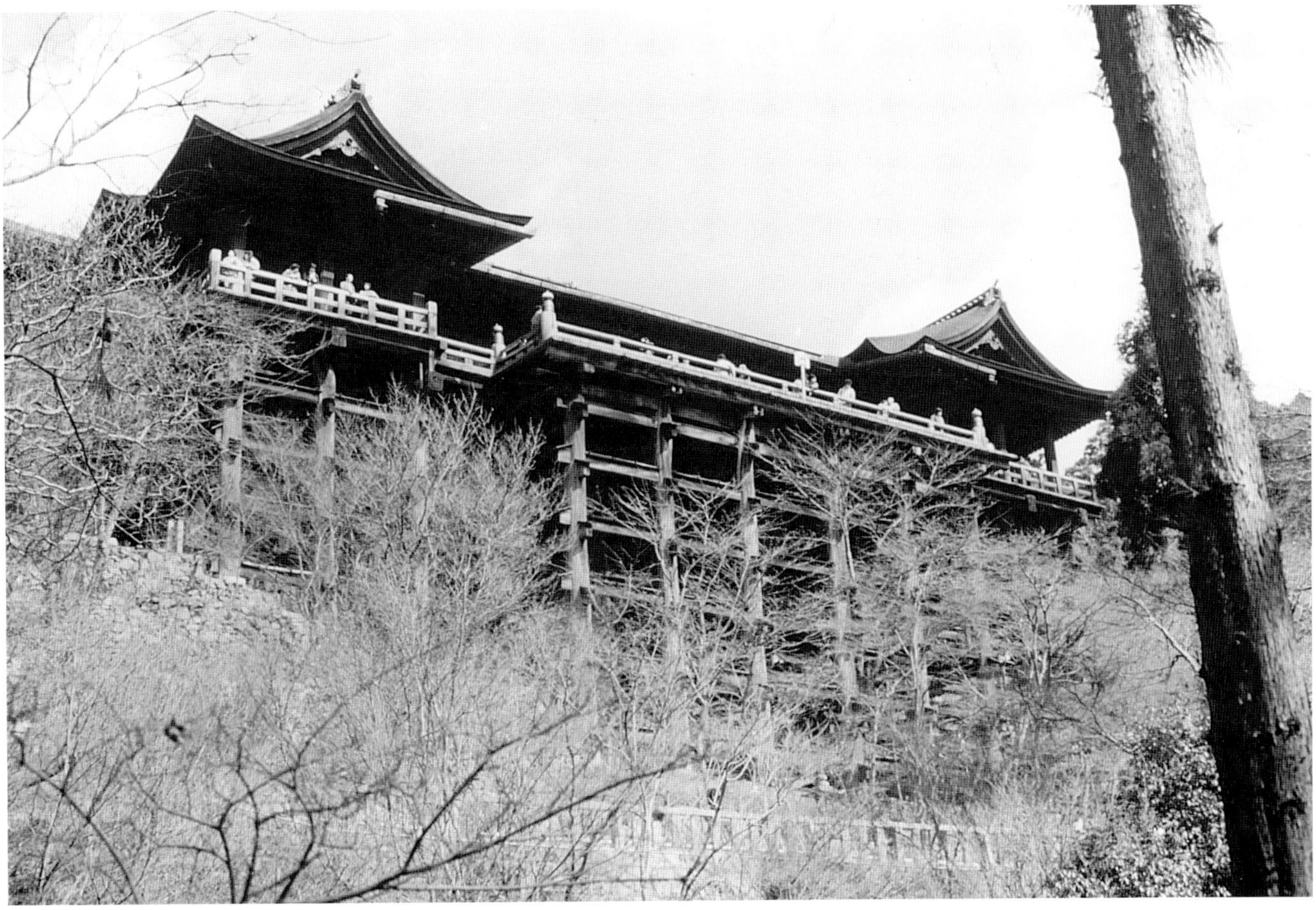

46.2 View of the main hall of Kiyomizudera, Kyoto. National Treasure.

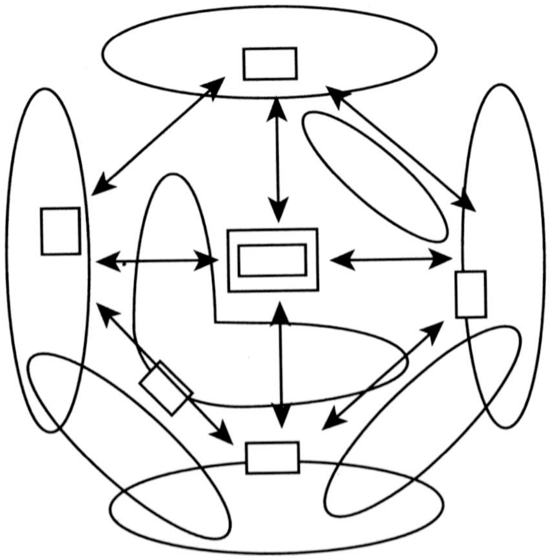

47.1 Schematic showing the correlation between buildings in Chinese *yuanlin* gardens (mutual and intersecting views).

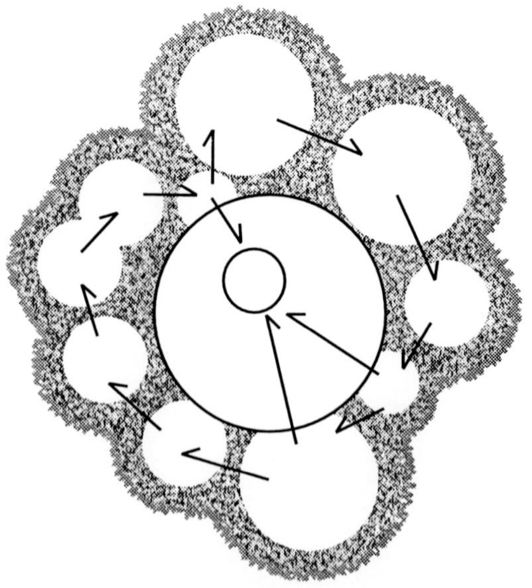

47.2 Schematic showing *miegakure* as it is used in Japanese stroll gardens to link heterogeneous sub-gardens, and views of the pond around which the garden is centered.

The basic composition of the temple and shrine precincts as described above is structured in the same way as are the interpretations seen in stroll gardens—not on a linear axis, but by opening and closing views through *miegakure.* By carefully manipulating the scenes emerging in these intervals, *miegakure* developed as a methodology that was emotionally charged and free of either spatial limitations or set dimensions. Thus, the stroll gardens devised for the pleasure of feudal lords differed from the temple and shrine "gardens" of city merchants in the way they were perceived by their users, but not in their design interpretations.

The stroll garden shares with *sukiya-zukuri* gardens like those of Manshu-in and Kohō-an a basic dynamic of linking heterogeneous components into a continuous sequence. But while Manshu-in and Kohō-an focus on the relationship between buildings and gardens, the emphasis in the stroll garden is on observing scenes—which may include buildings—while meandering through the garden itself. Here the buildings are added as just one of the garden's compositional elements. Prior to the viewer's penetration of the garden space, buildings could not usually be seen from the garden. One exception is gardens in the Pure Land style, a classic example of which is Byōdō-in at Uji, where the Hōōdō hall representing Western Paradise is viewed from the opposite shore of the pond it borders. In "walking" gardens—*roji,* stroll gardens, and the precincts of certain shrines and temples—buildings serve as an element in the landscape. Thus determining appropriate and harmonious forms and locations for them becomes a new requirement in garden composition.

By contrast, the intrinsic importance of buildings to garden scenes is at the very core of European and Chinese garden design. Since Chinese gardens are natural landscape–style gardens, they have many elements in common with the Japanese stroll garden; for instance, both are dotted with pavilions, ponds, and islands. However, the differences between them outweigh the similarities. In the composition of Chinese gardens, the focus is on the arrangement of the buildings. The central element in the Chinese garden is the *huating* open pavilion, which is often open on four sides. Chinese garden makers were required to provide views from and of the *huating* from many different directions and vantage points.

The Japanese stroll garden emphasizes a multifaceted composition of natural scenes with a pond at the center and regards buildings as simply one more venue for the application of *miegakure.* The entire formative process of the Japanese garden is synthesized in the stroll garden.

China

4

Coexisting "Unworldly" and "Mundane" Worlds

Traditional Chinese Dwellings

The Han race, China's racial majority, and the numerous other racial minorities that are scattered across the vast mainland formed distinctive residences in accordance with their respective climatic conditions, economic circumstances, and ethnic customs. For the most part, these diverse vernacular dwellings are closed and introverted in composition.

"*Qing-ming shang-he tu*" (Ascending the river at the Qing-ming season), a painted handscroll by Zhang Zeduan, is a realistic depiction of the main avenue of the Northern-Song (A.D. 960–1126) capital Kaifeng (in present-day Henan Province), from the palace grounds to the outskirts of the city, showing the character of farmhouses, villages and neighborhoods surrounding the palace, and shops within the palace complex (Figure 48). Unlike residences seen in Beijing and Huizhou, which are enclosed by solid walls, the Northern Song–townscape shows similarities to Japanese and Korean residences and villages. The present-day insular Chinese townscape is a post-Yuan (A.D. 1280–1368) characteristic—particularly common during the Ming (A.D. 1368–1644) and Qing (A.D. 1644–1911) dynasties. The examination in this section focuses primarily on Ming-period residences.

The residential styles that will be explored here in an effort to define the fundamental characteristics in the composition of traditional Chinese dwellings are the *siheyuan* residential quadrangles seen in Beijing, and *minju*, or the popular dwellings of Huizhou in central China's Anhui Province. Both have a basic composition comprised of covered interior spaces or halls, and open-roofed exterior spaces or courtyards surrounded by a retaining wall. The exterior spaces within the residential compound are referred to as "*yuanzi*" (courtyard) in Beijing, and "*tianjing*" (literally, "skywell") in Huizhou.

Hall and Courtyard Composition

The Beijing residential quadrangle (*siheyuan*) is composed of a *yuanzi* central courtyard surrounded by four halls: a main hall (*zheng fang*) facing south with wings (*erfang*) appended to either side, an opposing hall (*dao zuo fang*) facing north, and lateral halls (*xiang fang*) facing east and west (Figure 49).

Each hall is a single-story unit of three rooms—a central

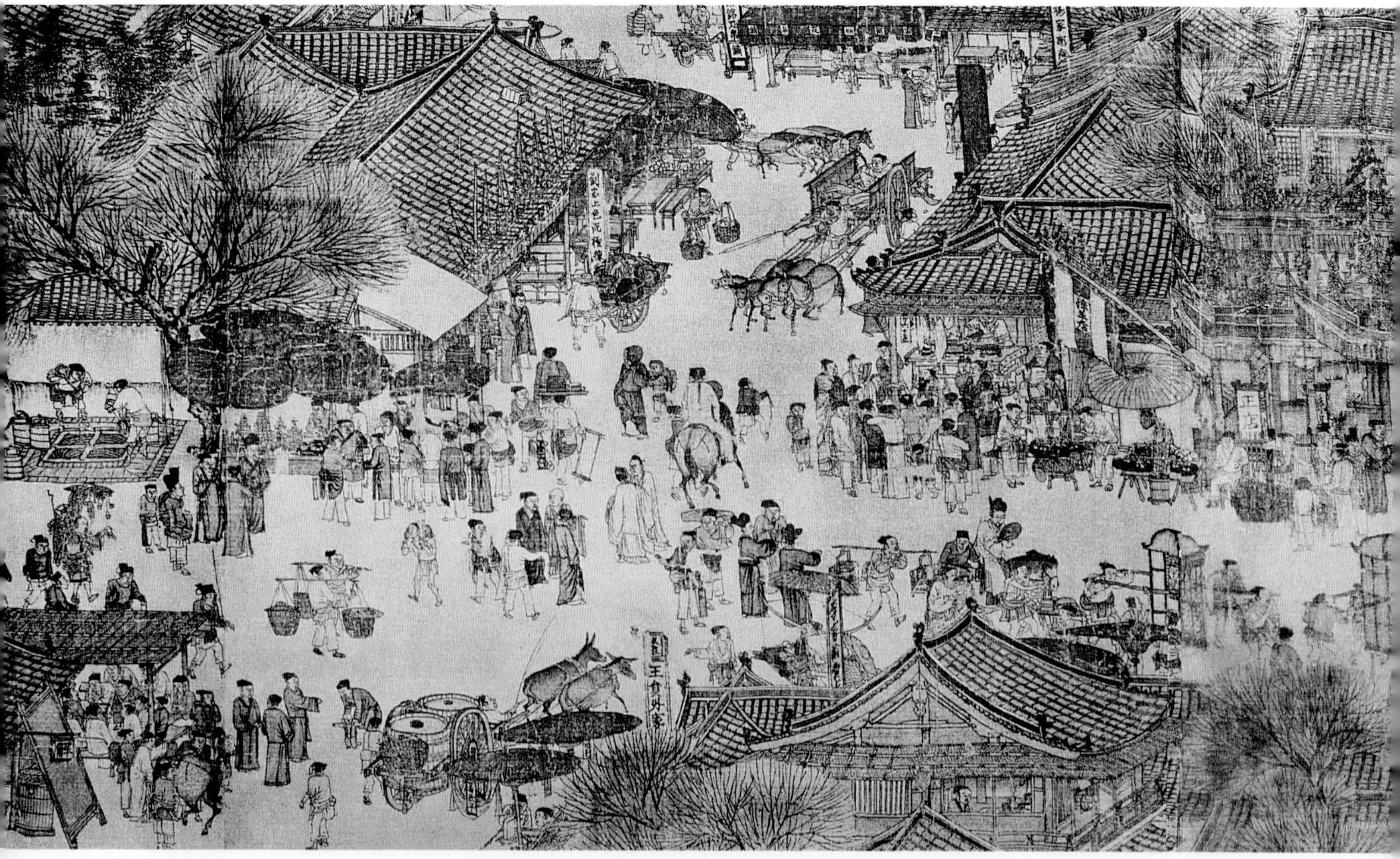

48 A street scene outside the palace gate of the Northern Song–capital Kaifeng from the handscroll *Qing-ming shang-he tu* by Zhang Ze-duan. The Palace Museum.

living room (*tang*) flanked on either side by private/ sleeping quarters (*woshi*). The central room of the main hall, or *zutang* (ancestral room), is where the family ancestors are worshipped, and ceremonial events such as weddings or funerals are held. At other times the *zutang* serves as the living space for the head of the household and his wife, and surpasses all the other halls in its strongly Confucianist, patriarchal coloration. Wings appended to the private quarters of the main hall serve as rooms for female children, or as clothes closets. The east and west auxiliary halls are reserved for the living quarters of the first and second sons and their families, and the hall facing north, nearest the entrance of the compound, is for younger sons or the servants.

From a residential planning perspective, the *tang* of each hall would correspond to what we would call today the living room, or the gathering place for an entire nuclear family. The *tang* is situated at the center of a unit of either three rooms (*woshi-tang-woshi*) or five rooms (*woshi-woshi-tang-woshi-woshi*).

In northern China *woshi* are equipped with a brick sleeping platform heated with internal flues (*kang*) upon which bedding is placed. In central and southern China *woshi* are furnished with beds (Figures 50.1–50.2).

Each hall of the *siheyuan* faces out onto an open-air, nearly square courtyard (*yuanzi*). The *yuanzi* occupies as much as forty percent of the area of the overall residential compound, and is indeed often larger than any of the architectural structures that make up the dwelling.

Huizhou residential complexes are also comprised of three- or five-room halls facing a small courtyard or skywell (*tianjing*). As opposed to Beijing's *siheyuan* quadrangular composition, the halls and courtyards in Huizhou dwellings are aligned on a vertical axis.

These hall/courtyard units (*jin*) are stacked in vertical rows of three or four, referred to as "three *jin*" and "four *jin*." In many cases, second and third rows are added without transfiguring the hall/courtyard unit composition, to form large-scale residential complexes (Figure 51).

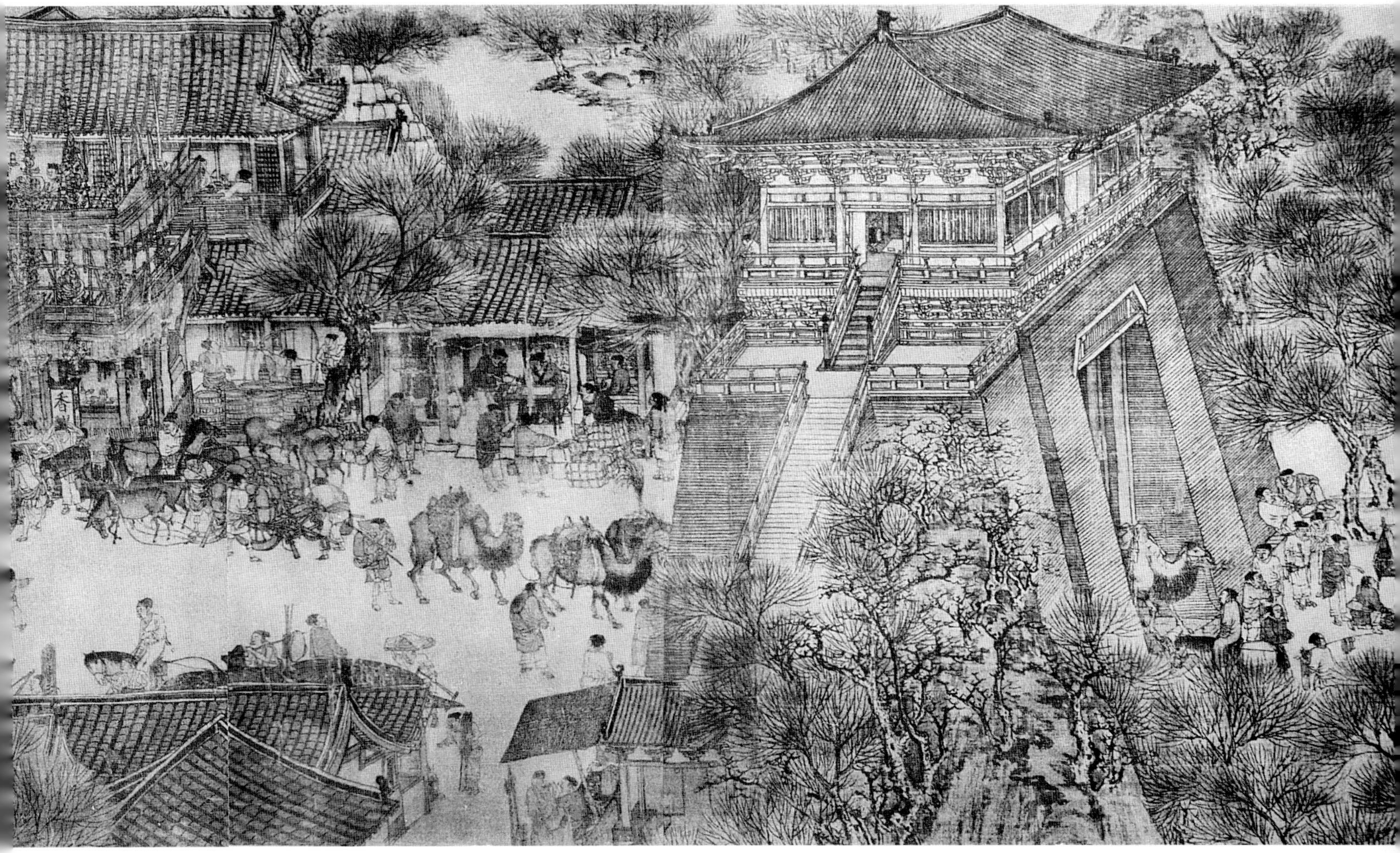

Many of these structures are two, and in some cases three, stories high. The surrounding walls thus become higher, which in comparison to northern China's one-story houses, gives central and southern China villages an overpowering impression.

The square format of the *siheyuan* reflects its adaptation to the constraints of Beijing's grid system of main streets and lanes. Huizhou dwellings are less restricted by city planning regulations, and so are more free-form in plan (Figure 52).

Huizhou residential architecture has a wood-frame structure enclosed by external brick (*zhuan*) walls (Figures 53.1–53.2). Pillars are spaced on an approximately two-by-three or two-by-four–meter (6.5-by-9.8 or 6.5-by-13–foot) grid, far wider than is found in Japanese wood-frame structures. Because wood is scarce in the Huizhou region, beams and purlins are frequently made of composite material, and the peripheral pillars of the frame are bolted to the surrounding retaining wall. Roof tiles are laid directly upon the rafters, without sub-roofing. Glass tiles identical in form to the roof tiles create skylights which are said to have been used since the Qing dynasty. The surrounding wall is made higher where it abuts the gable side of the building, in a decorative, stepped *matou bi* (horse's head wall) or *yun bi* (cloud wall) composition (Figure 54).

Interior wall partitions are all wood-frame panels and fittings, with very little plasterwork. Ceilings are rarely seen in ordinary homes, and when used are usually limited to the *woshi* private/sleeping quarters. When provided in the *tang* central living room they are brilliantly colored and highly decorative. *Woshi* floors are wooden, while all other floors are of stone, brick, or pounded earth.

The main entrance has a small overhang decorated with a carved brick motif and is fitted with heavy metal doors. There are relatively few openings in the high whitewashed walls surrounding the insular, closed residential structure on four sides (Figure 55.1–55.2).

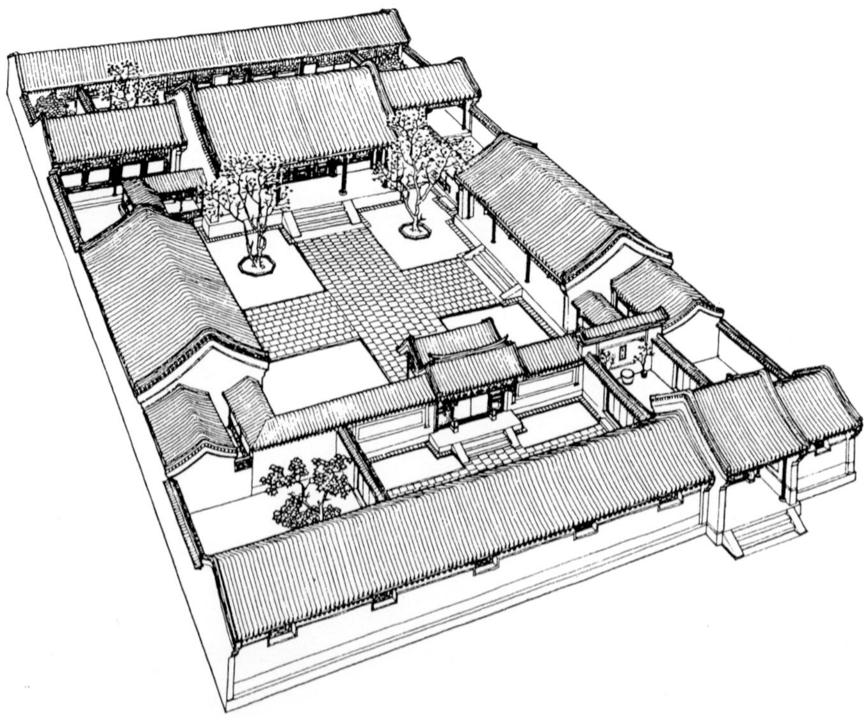

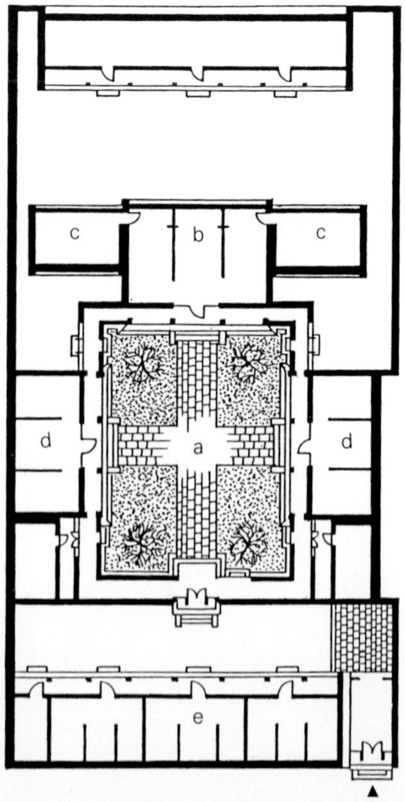

49 Perspective and plan view drawings showing the layout of a typical Beijing *siheyuan* residential quadrangle and a single hall interior.

a. *yuanzi.*	b. *zheng fang.*	c. *erfang.*	d. *xiang fang.*
e. *dao zuo fang.*	g. *woshi.*	f. *tang.*	h. *kang.*

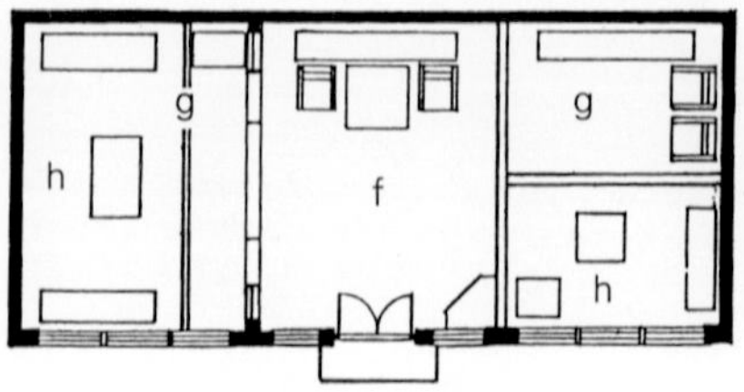

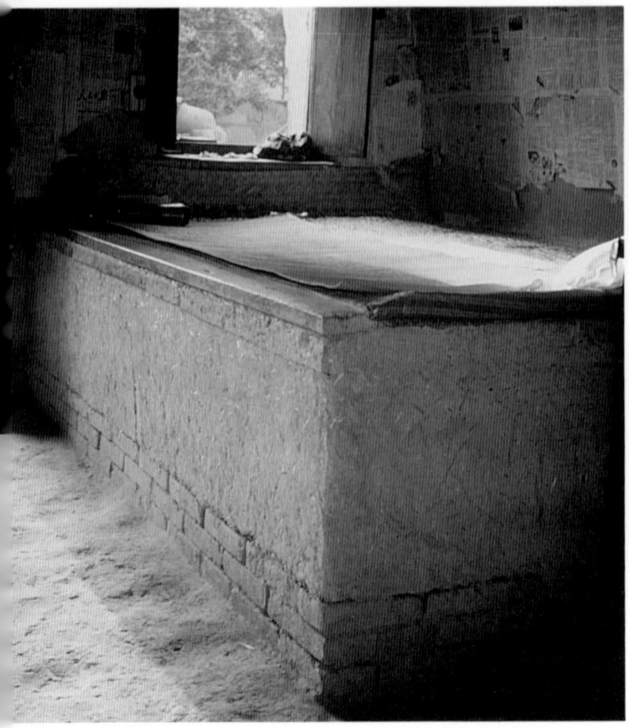

50.1 A *kang* heated sleeping platform in the *woshi* of a Beijing dwelling.

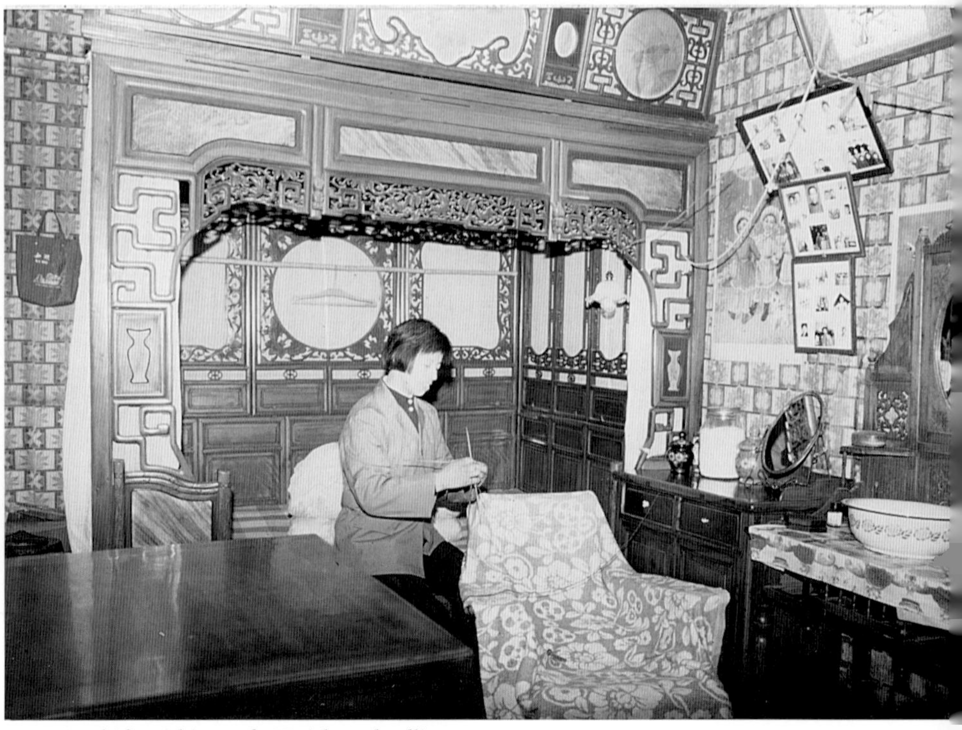

50.2 *Woshi* furnishings of a Huizhou dwelling.

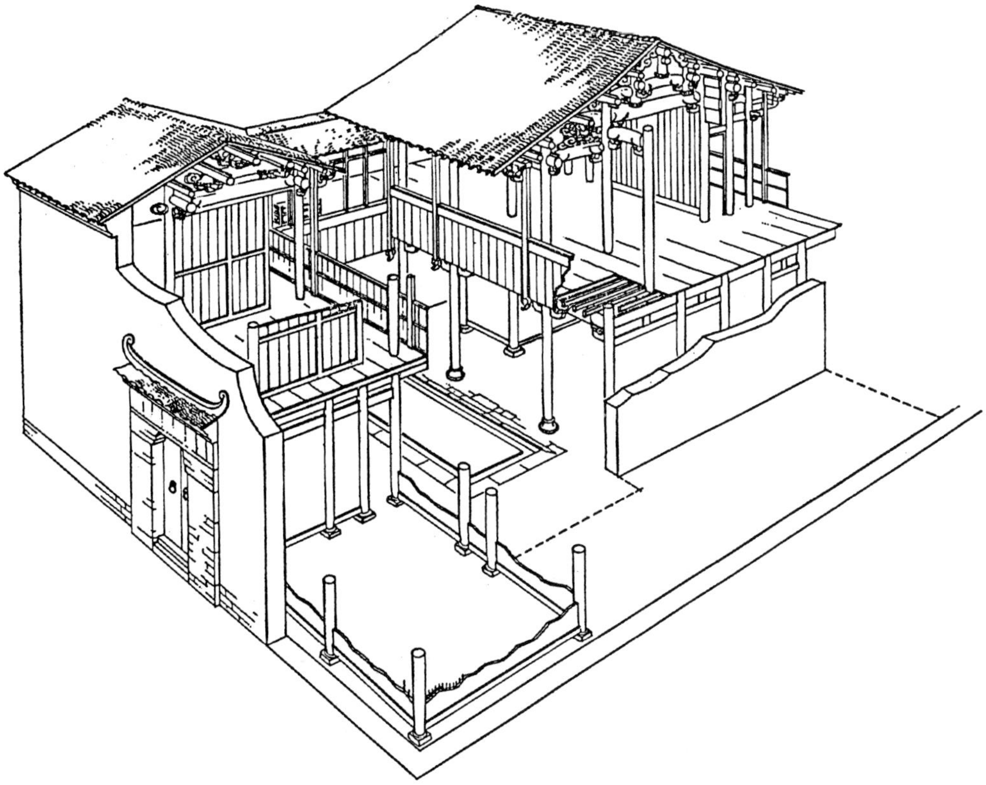

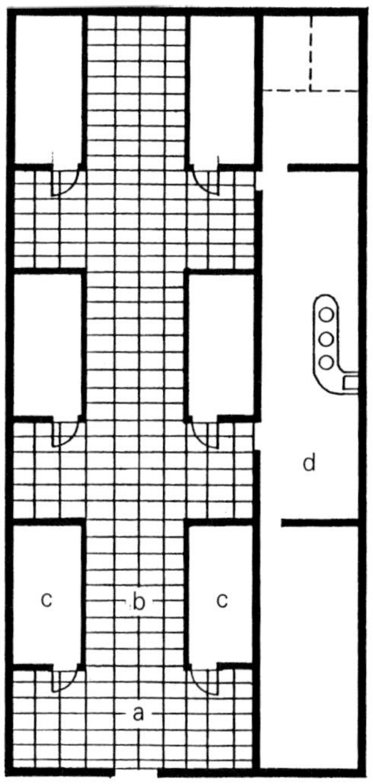

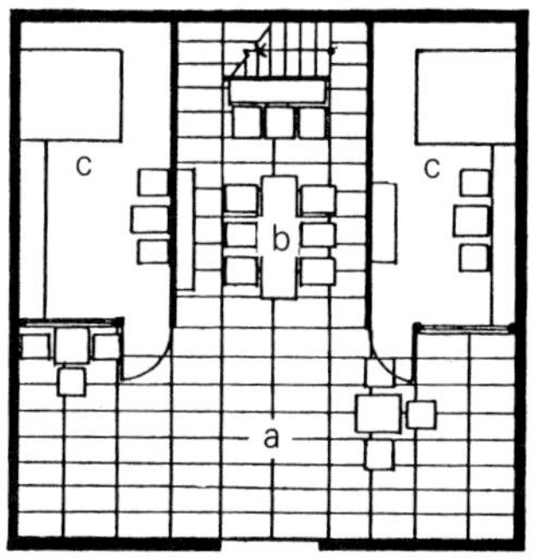

51 Perspective and plan view drawings showing the layout of a typical Huizhou dwelling and a single hall/courtyard unit (*jin*).

a. *tianjing*. b. *tang*. c. *woshi*. d. *chufang*.

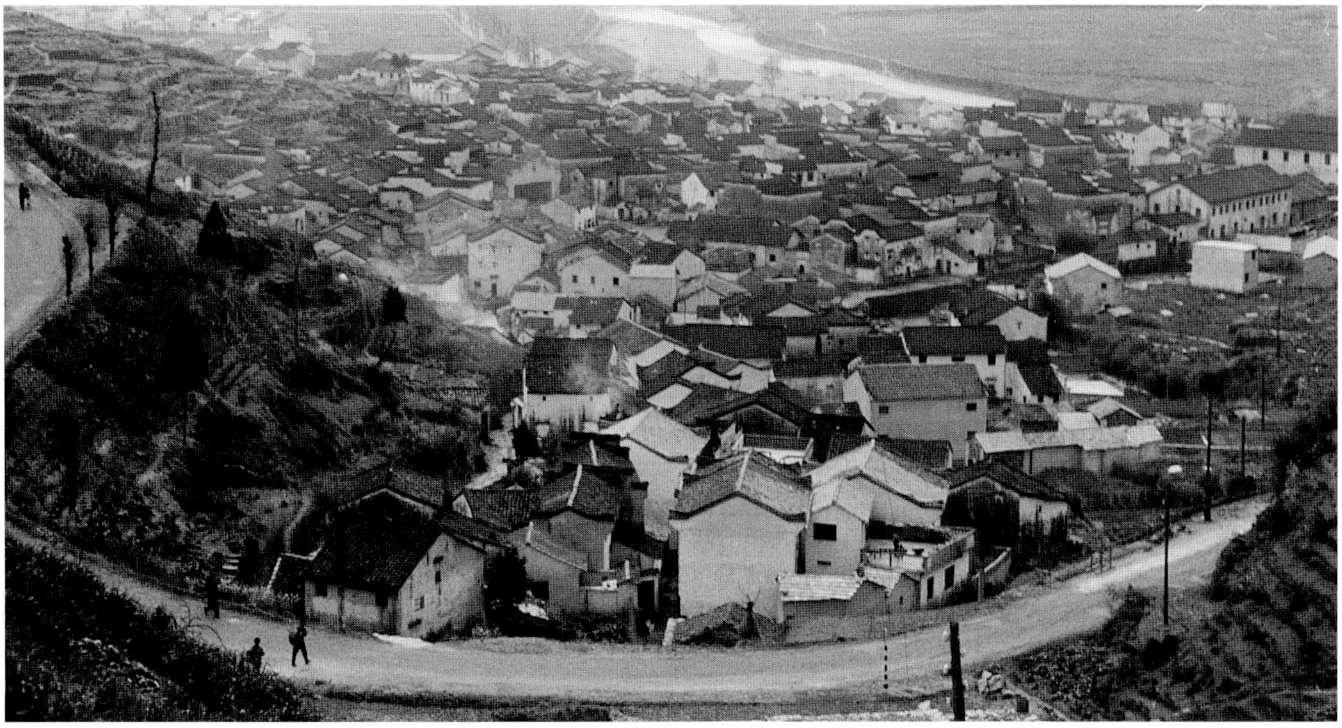

52 View of a Huizhou village.

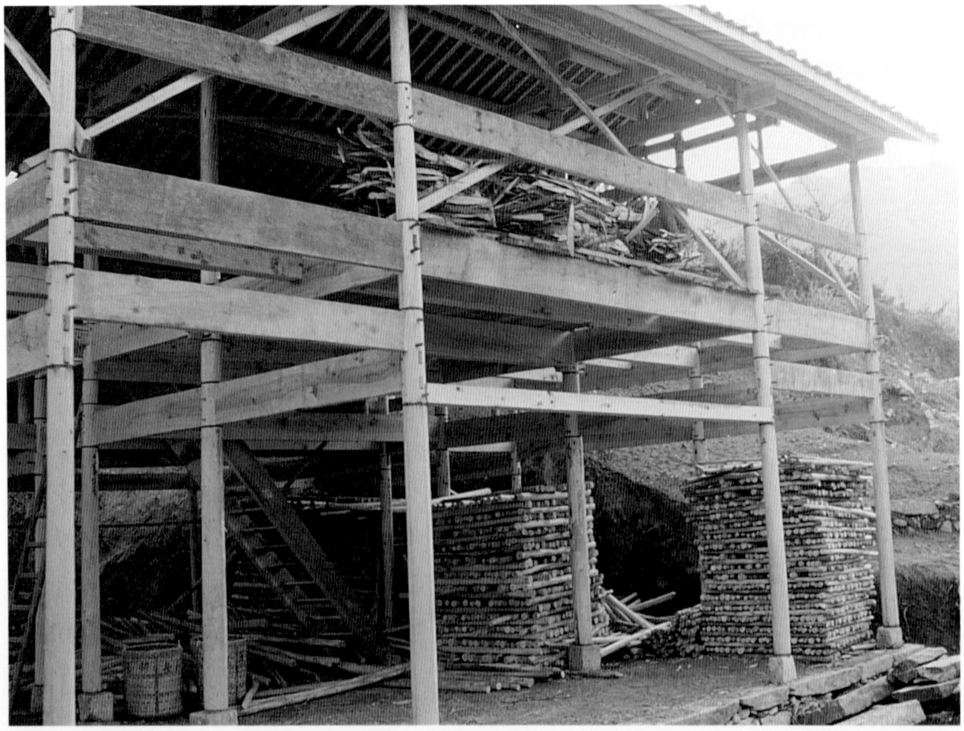

53.1 The wood-frame structure of a Huizhou dwelling.

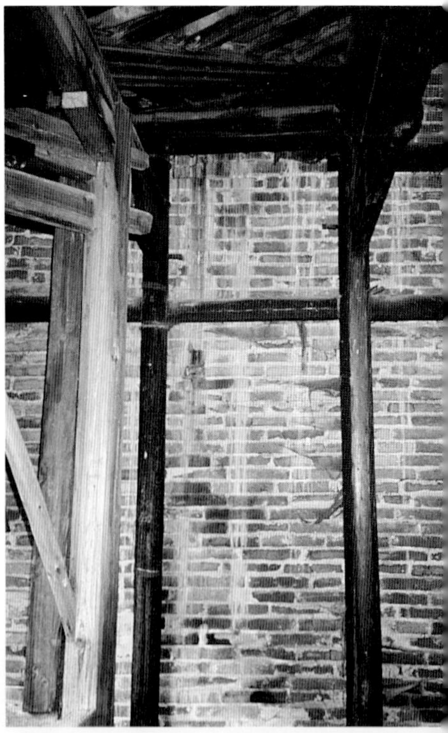

53.2 Wood-frame and external brick wall structure of a Huizhou dwelling.

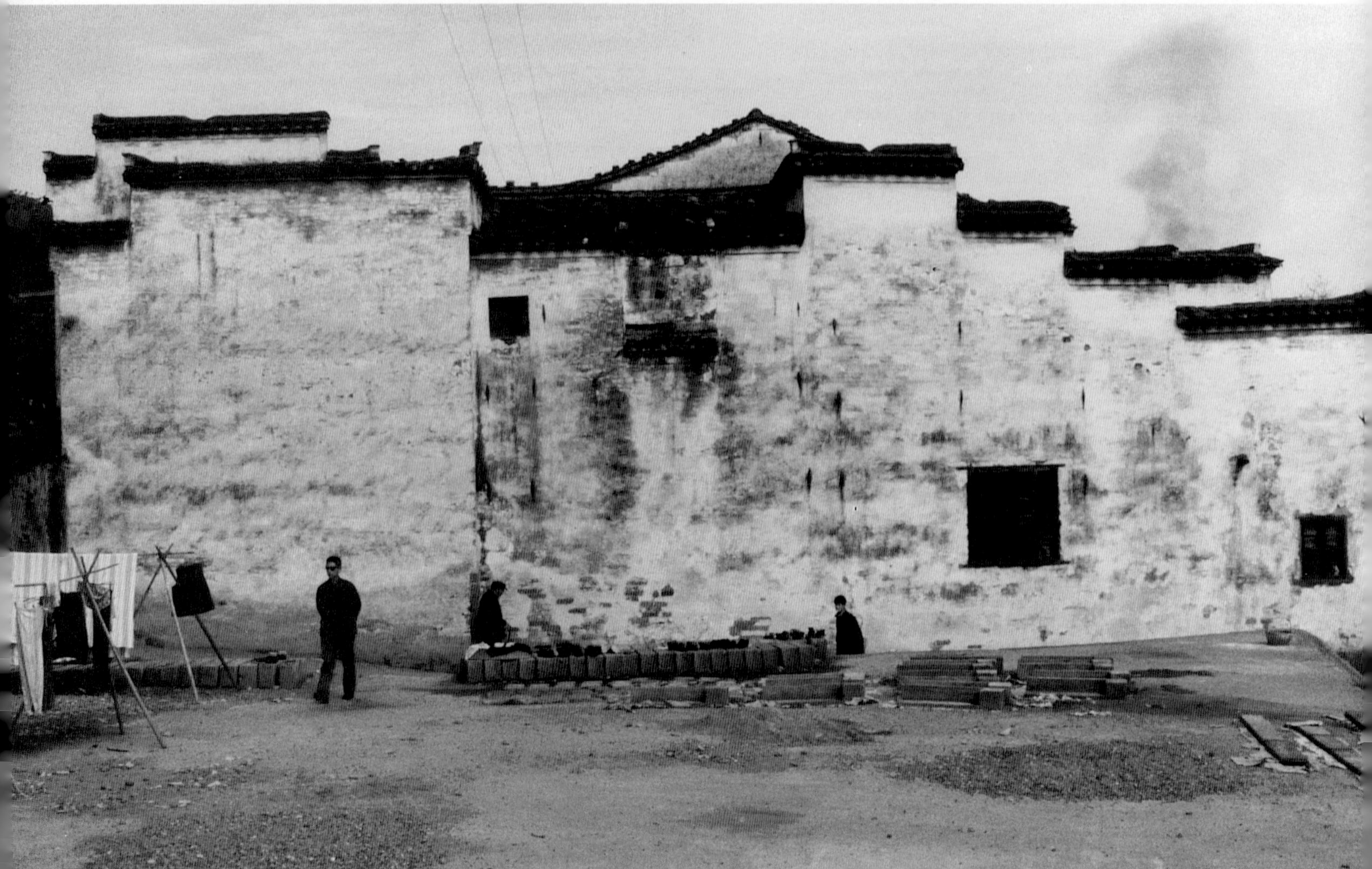

54 A stepped *matou bi* (horse's head wall) on the gable side exterior of a Huizhou dwelling.

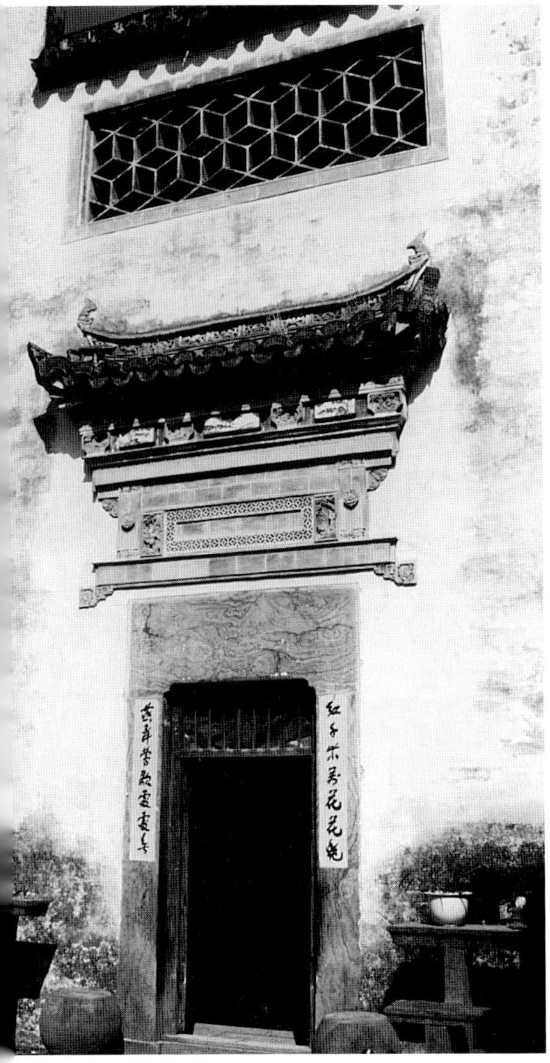

55.1 Decorative detailing of the main entrance of a Huizhou dwelling.

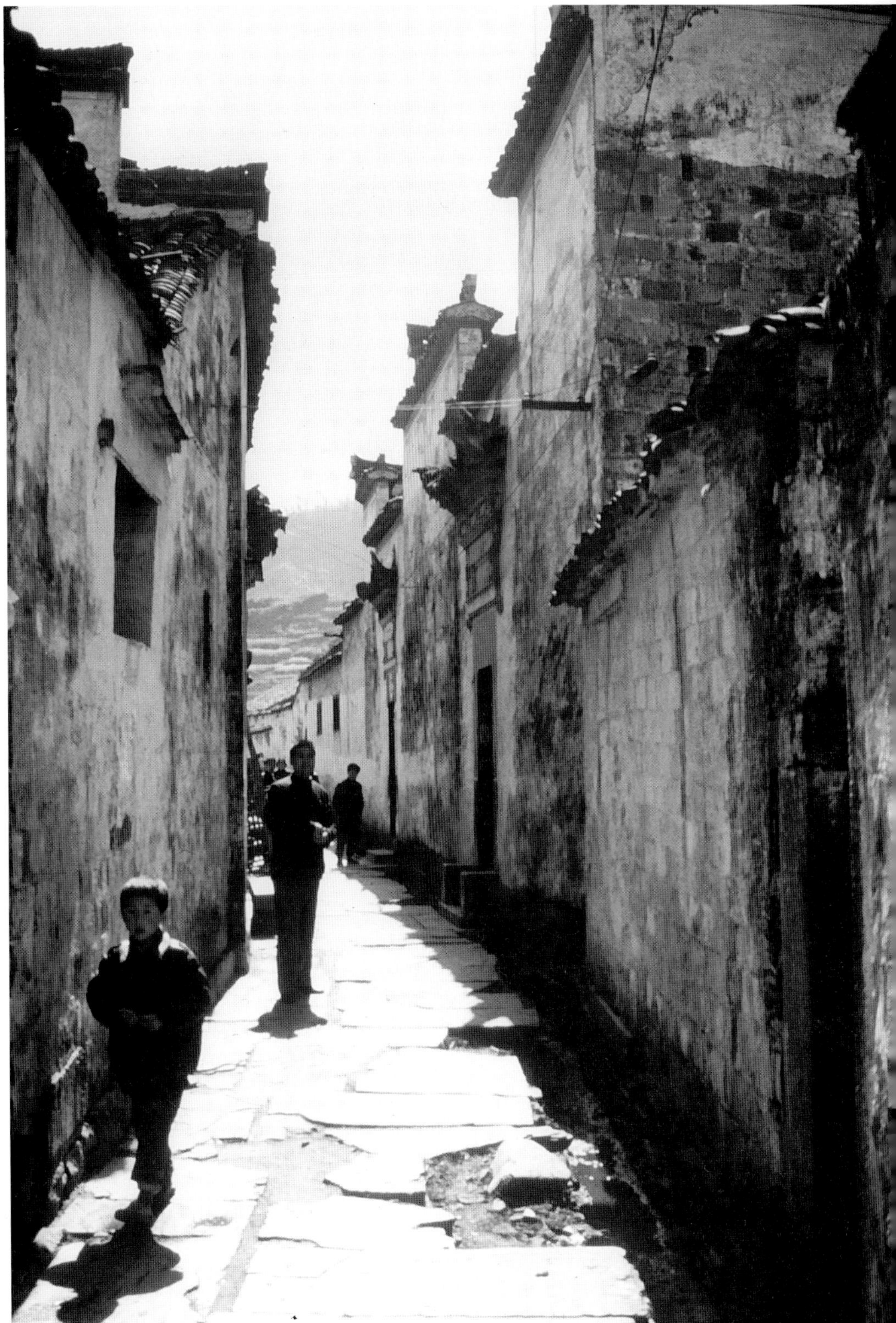

55.2 Streetscape of a Huizhou village.

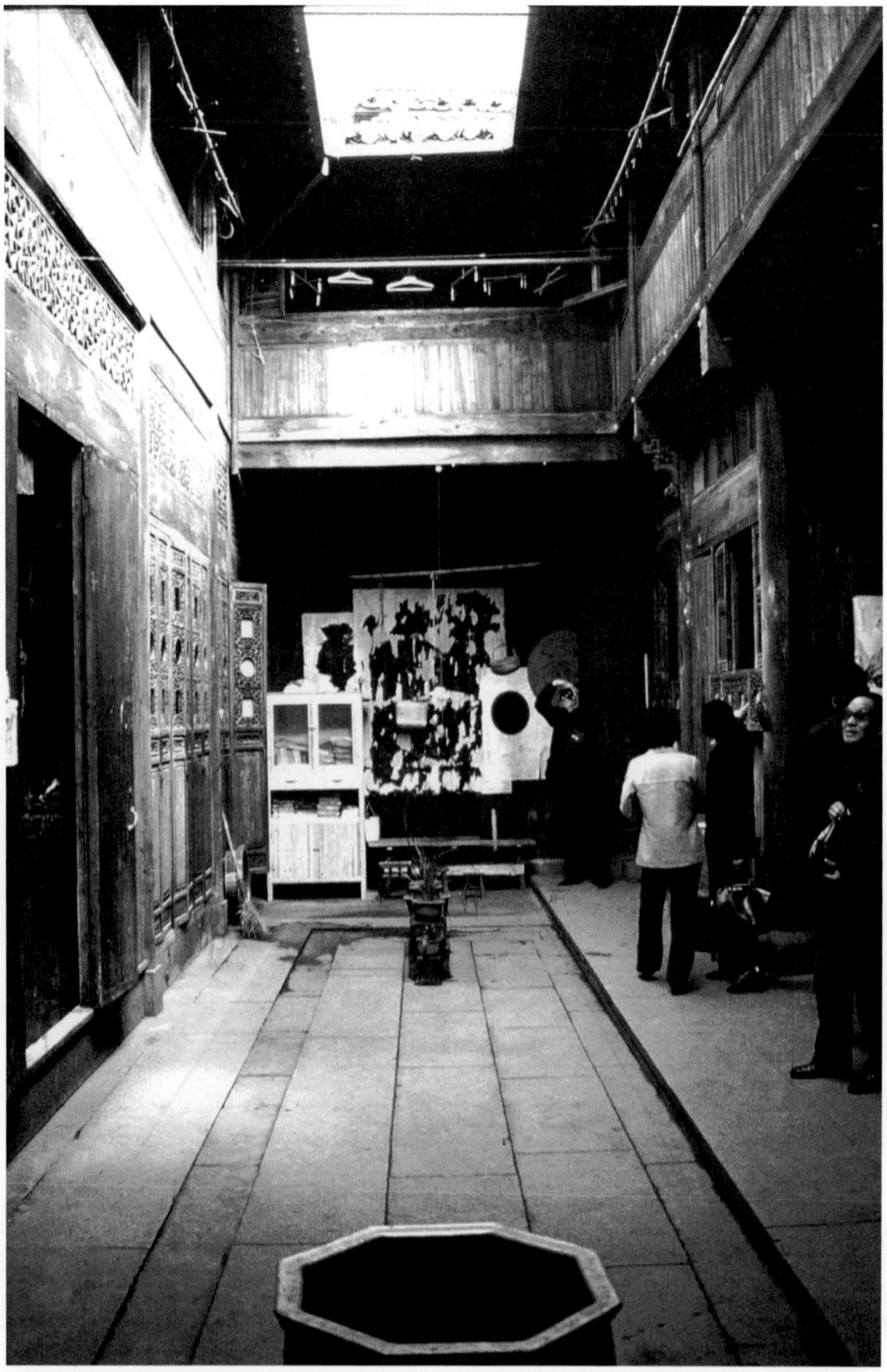

56 The *tianjing* "skywell" provides light and ventilation to the insular Huizhou dwelling.

Climatic Influences

Beijing is located at a latitude of forty degrees north, and Hefei, the capital of Anhui Province, at thirty degrees, which corresponds to the significant difference in Japan between Morioka in temperate northern Honshu, with its severe winters, and Yakushima, a subtropical island south of Kyushu. Hefei has a fairly acute seasonal temperature fluctuation, averaging 29.5° F (–1.3° C) in winter and 82.5° F (28° C) in summer. Its precipitation is similar to that of Japan; its humidity averages seventy percent in the coldest months and eighty percent in the warmest, making it a fairly uncomfortable climate.

High surrounding walls offer protection from winter winds and heat loss. In summer, the walls block high sun rays, which is why inner courtyards were necessarily made deep and narrow. Long, narrow alleyways (*chuan feng lu*; literally, "drift wind lane") between buildings provide ventilation (see Figure 67.2). Huizhou's climate gave rise to both the skywell courtyard contained within the two-story building structure and the high surrounding walls (Figure 56).

In contrast to the Beijing *siheyuan*'s one-story, square composition and spacious *yuanzi* courtyard designed to

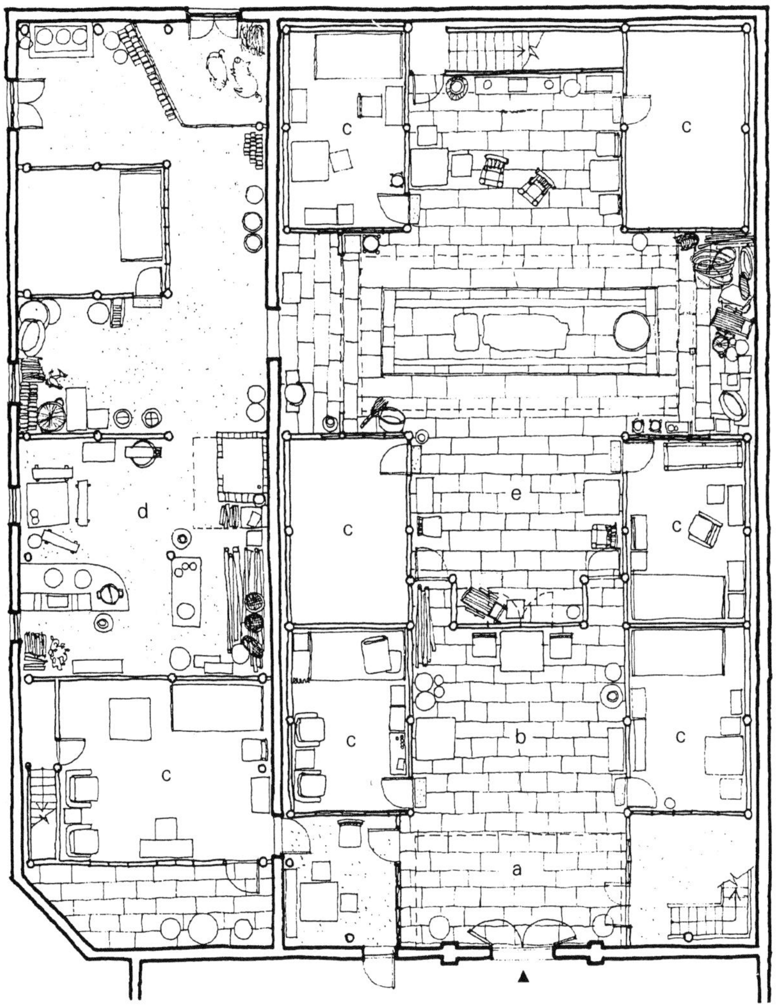

57.1 Plan view drawing of a three-*jin* Huizhou dwelling.

a. *tianjing.* c. *woshi.*
b. *tang.* d. *chufang*.

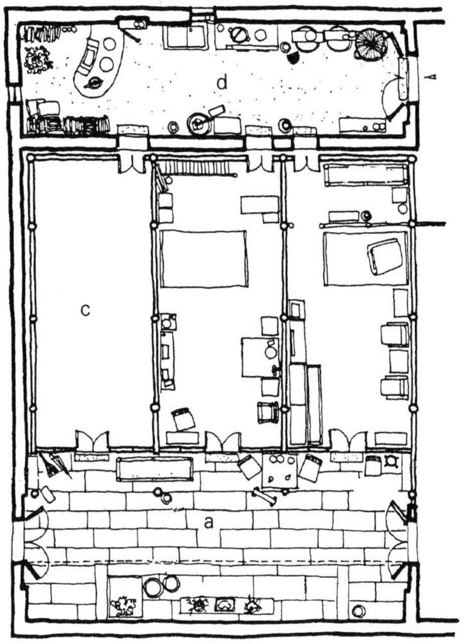

57.2 Plan view drawing drawing of a single-*jin* unit of Huizhou dwelling.

let in the scarce northern China sunlight, Huizhou's well-like, narrow *tianjing* structure is less a transformation of the Beijing *siheyuan* than a matter of the same Han race's preserving the same customs and living habits, in a form of dwelling suitable to the central Chinese climate.

Lifestyle: Hierarchal Private/Communal Composition

According to a Chinese proverb, the cohabitation of "five generations under one roof" brings good fortune. Traditional Chinese collective residential complexes are a hierarchically-arranged series of discrete spaces for each generation, which serve at the same time to link the various generations. The architectural composition clearly and simply positions each nuclear family in a specific ranking within the extended family.

In Huizhou dwellings, *woshi-tang-tianjing* comprise one unit for each generation, containing both private space (*woshi*) and communal space (*tang* and *tianjing*). Communal space is composed with the *tang* of the first generation abutting the *tianjing*, which in turn connects to the *zutang* (ancestor room)—the spiritual center of the entire

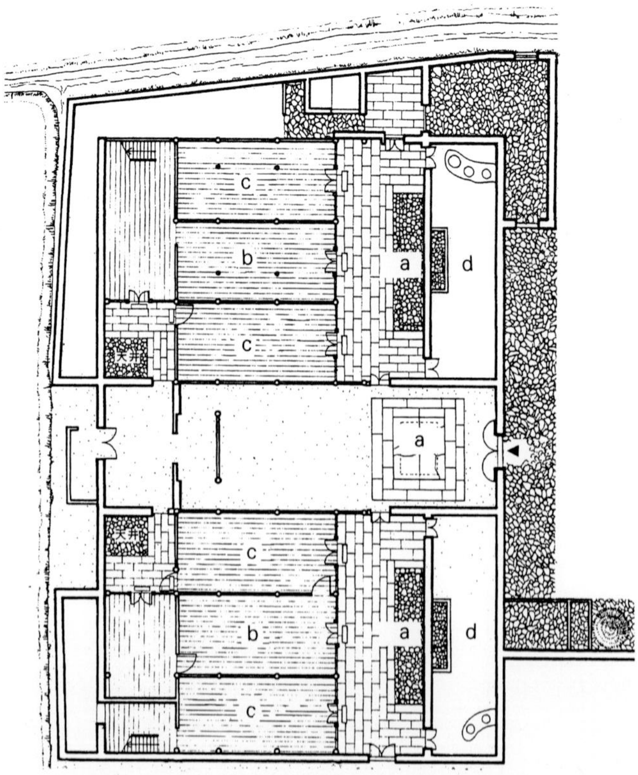

57.3 Plan view drawing of a multiple-family Huizhou dwelling.
a. *tianjing*.
b. *tang*.
c. *woshi*.
d. *chufang*.

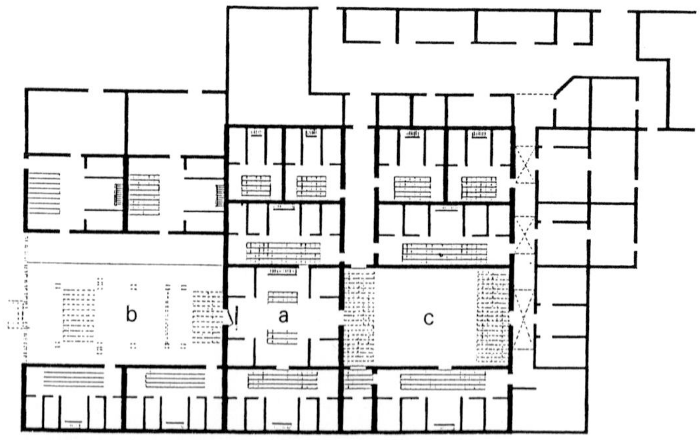

57.4 Plan view drawing of a multiple-family Huizhou residential complex.
a. *zutang*.
b. *Yang* courtyard.
c. *Yin* courtyard.

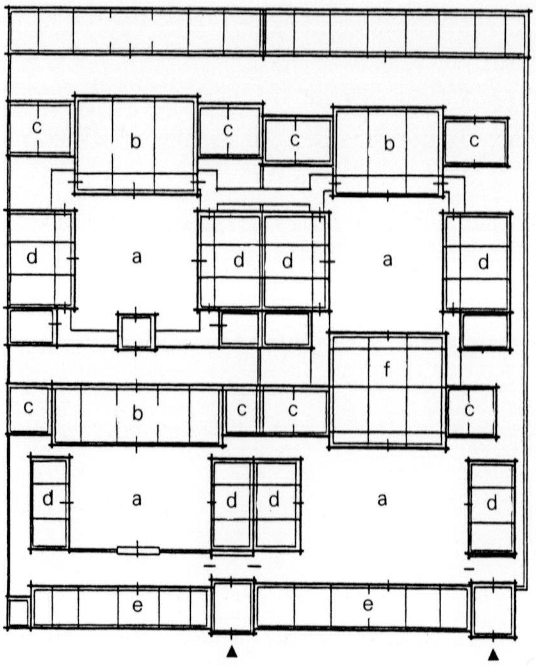

58.1 Plan view drawing of a multiple-family Beijing *siheyuan* complex.
a. *yuanzi*.
b. *zheng fang*.
c. *erfang*.
d. *xiang fang*.
e. *dao zuo fang*.
f. main hall.

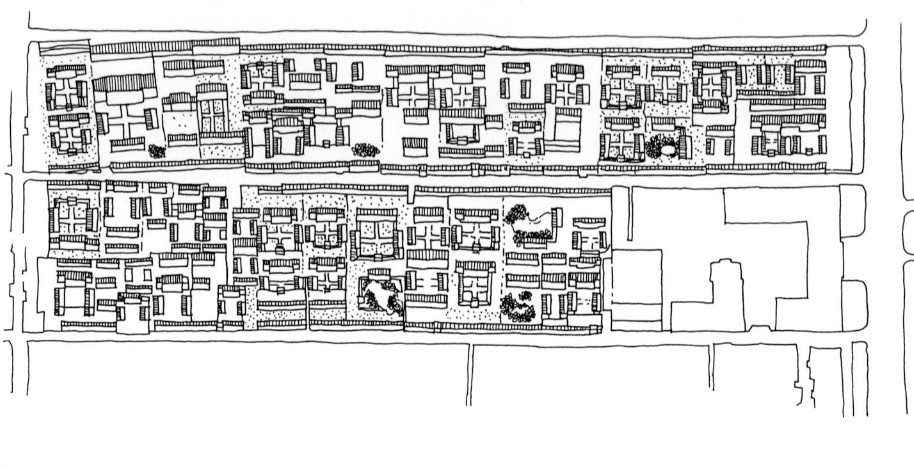

58.2 Ground plan of an extended family collective occupying an entire Beijing city block.

family—located at the physical center of the collective dwelling. All family units link to the *zutang* via interconnecting *tianjing* (Figures 57.1–57.4).

Likewise, in the composition of the Beijing *siheyuan*, private rooms representing the individual are invariably linked to a communal living room to form the unit that houses each nuclear family. Four of these units share a common courtyard space, the *yuanzi*, linking the first generation to his children and their families. Four such quadrangles are frequently combined grouping branches of the extended family, which in turn form sub-units of family collectives that occupy entire city blocks. (Figures 58.1–58.2).

The largest of these collective residential complexes are the three and four-storied *tulou* ("earthen building") built by the Hakka, a Han ethnic subgroup, in southwest Fujian and northeast Guangdong provinces. These structures are generally rectangular or circular in plan, forty to sixty meters (130–195 feet) in diameter, with the ancestor room located at the center of the complex, surrounded by an open communal courtyard from which rooms for receiving guests and utilitarian spaces (i.e., pig and chicken pens, wells, and food preparation and eating areas) are accessed. The small rooms attached to the periphery of the outer wall are used for grain storage on the second floor, and as private sleeping spaces on the upper floors (Figures 59.1–59.6).

The Confucian patriarchal family system—which teaches that morality is rooted in filial piety, or a child's respect for and obedience to its parents (in practice, primarily to the father)—is clearly evident even today in the structure of this hierarchal private/communal spatial composition.

Private Space: Woshi

Facing out on the *tianjing*, *woshi* form insular private spaces. *Woshi* floors are wooden, but shoes are not removed before entering.

Whether the overall residential complex is large or small, all *woshi* are a standard three-by-five to three-by-six meters (9.8-by-16.4 to 9.8-by-19.6 feet) in area, regardless of the resident's generational standing, wealth, or other individual conditions. The three-meter width is said to have been established to provide passage space of one meter around a bed two meters long.

The fact that standardization was scaled to bedroom furniture implies that the room is used strictly as a private bedroom and is not multifunctional. Expansion of the residence does not involve expanding room size, but simply adding on *woshi-tang-tianjing* units.

Communal Space: Tang *and* Tianjing *(Huizhou)/* Yuanzi *(Beijing)*

In contrast to *woshi*, which are self-contained private spaces, communal *tang* adjoin the open-air *tianjing*, which connects to the next *tang*/*tianjing* unit, and so on. Thus the interior of the closed Huizhou residential complex is based on a system which binds "private" to "communal" as one body.

The *zutang*, or ancestral room, has a solemn atmosphere deriving from its many auspicious decorative elements displayed in hopes of bringing good fortune to the extended family. The center wall of the *tang* is decorated with a wide hanging scroll which is flanked by a set of calligraphic couplets and in front of which a flower vase, incense burner, bonsai, and table rocks or table landscapes are set. (Here a relationship is evident to Japanese *shoin-zukuri*, where similar arrangements of imported Chinese scrolls and objects gave rise to construction of the *tokonoma* alcove.) A square table of rosewood, ebony, or another Chinese fine wood is placed at the center of the wall with a chair to either side—the seats for the eldest couple in the extended family. This arrangement characterizes the highly refined central communal space (Figure 60).

A large table placed at the center of the brick- or stone-floored *tang* serves as the dining table for one family and is the place where family members enjoy one another's

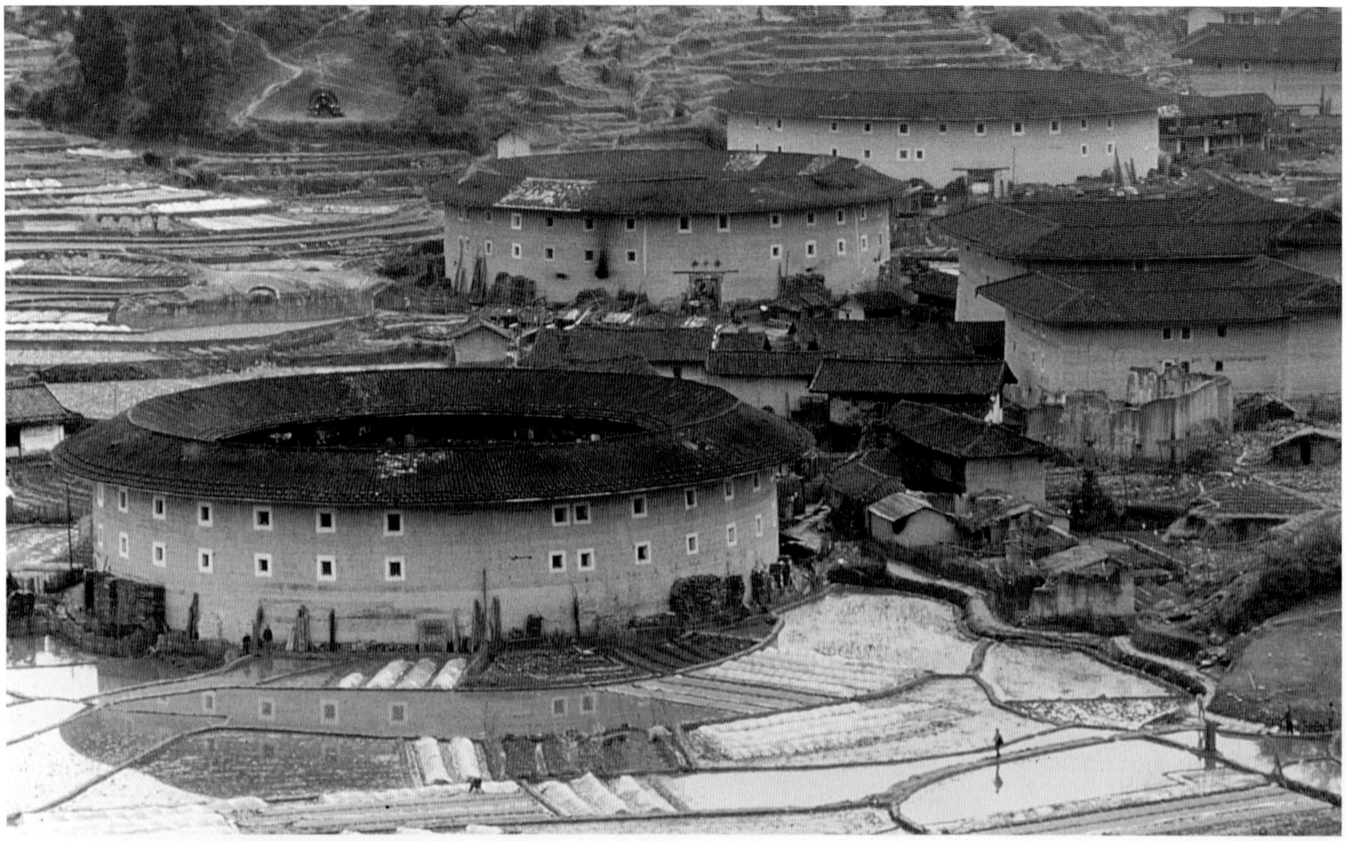

59.1 Circular Hakka residential complexes.

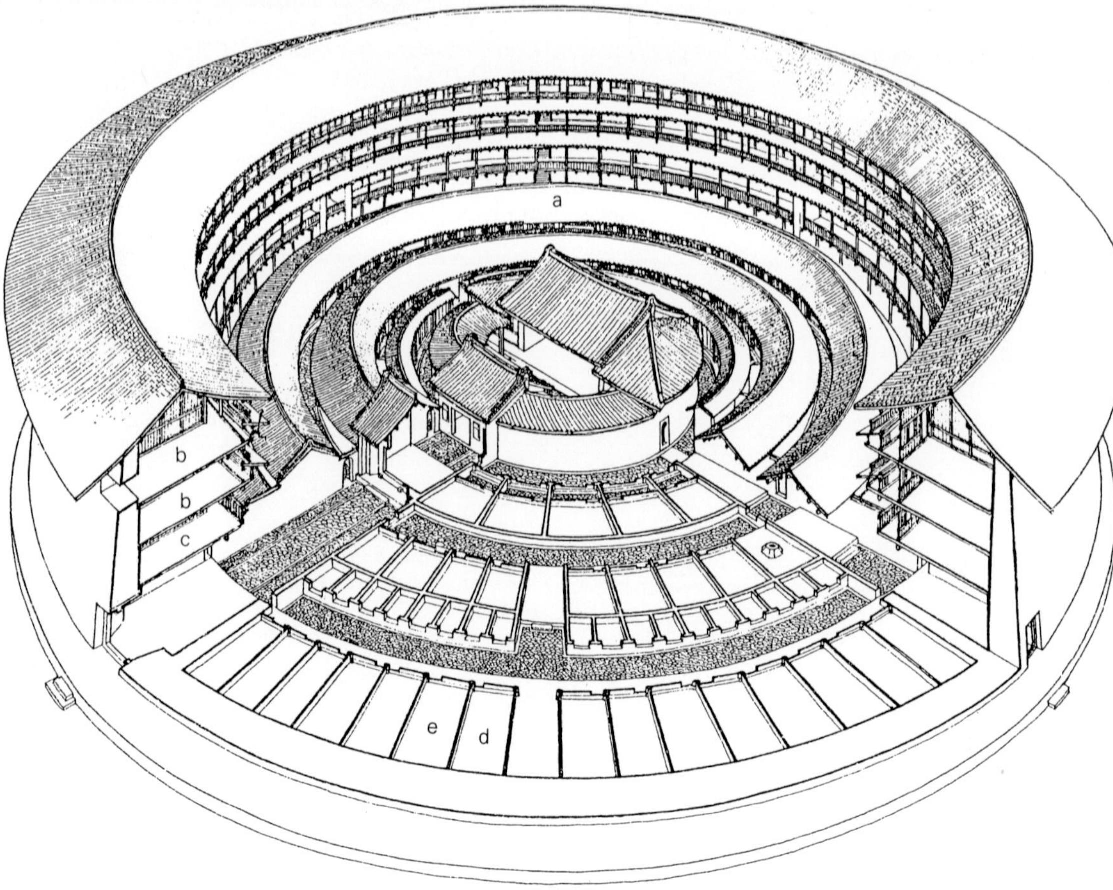

59.2 Axonometric drawing of a Hakka residential complex revealing the structure of the peripheral wall.
a. *zutang.* b. *woshi.* c. storeroom. d. *chufang.* e. dining room.

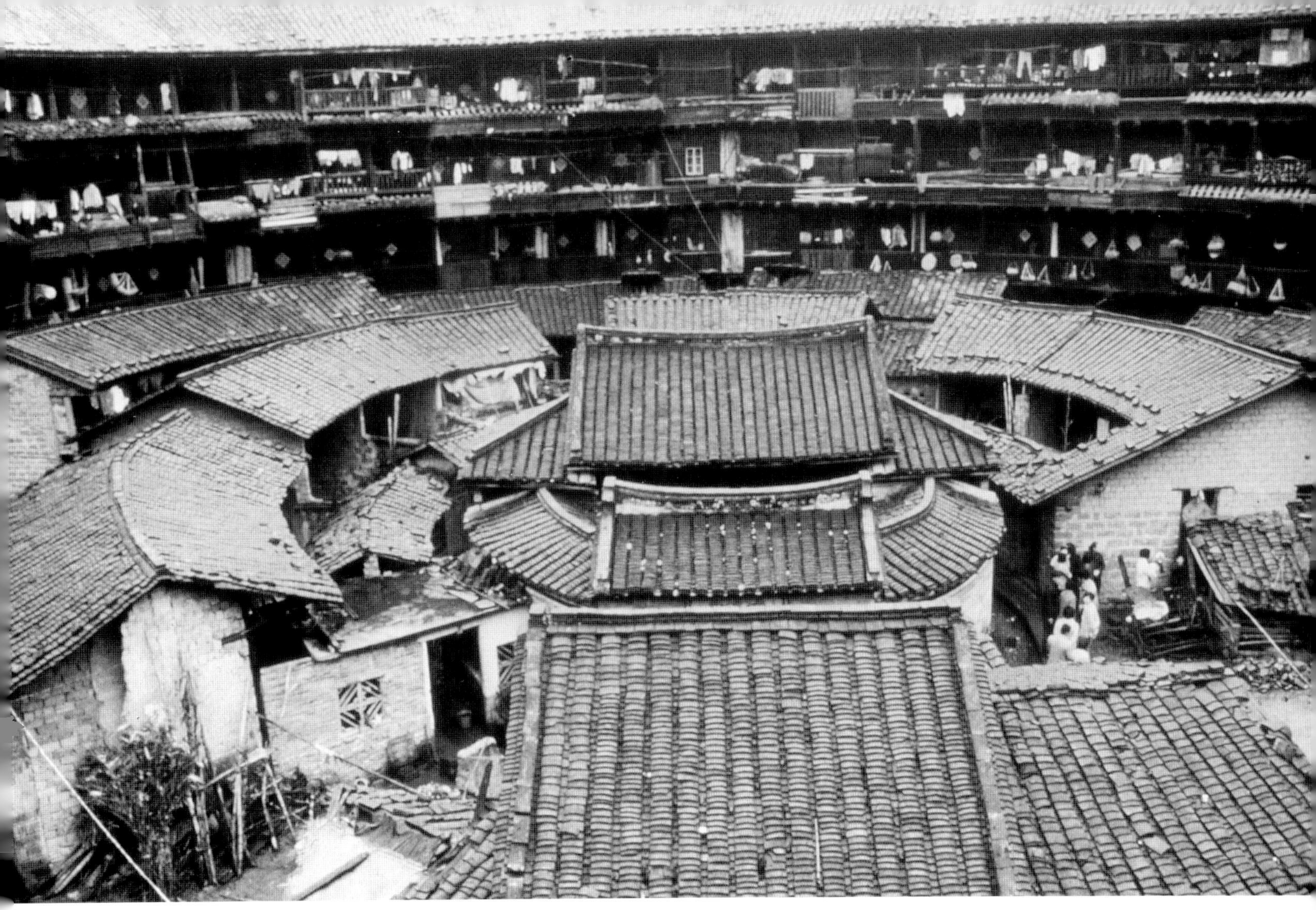

59.3 Interior view of the residential complex.

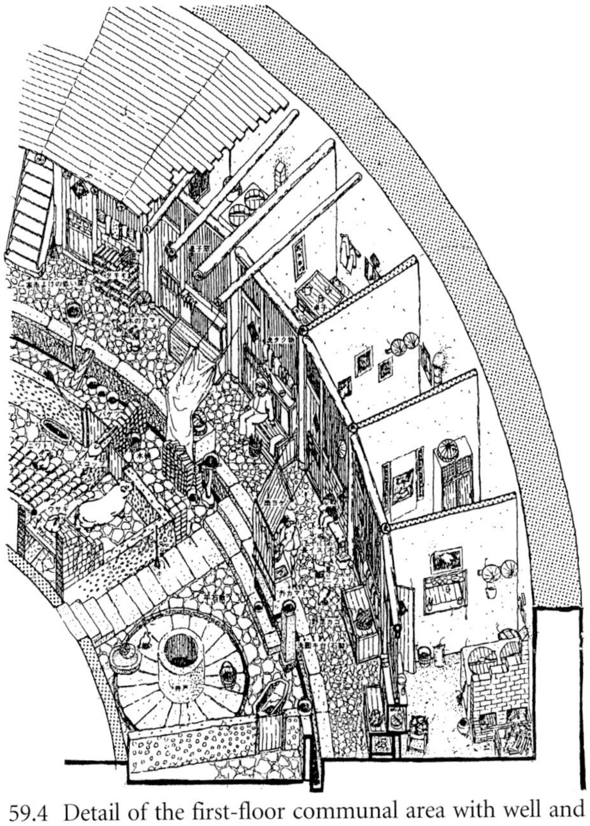

59.4 Detail of the first-floor communal area with well and animal pens in front of the kitchen and dining rooms.

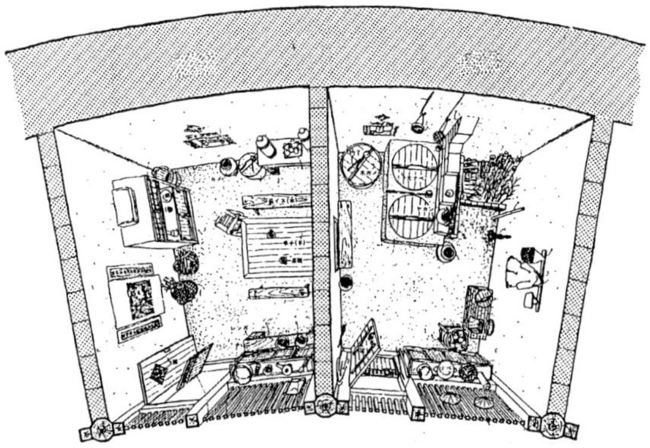

59.5 Detail of the first-floor kitchen and dining rooms.

59.6 Detail of the third- and fourth-floor private *woshi.*

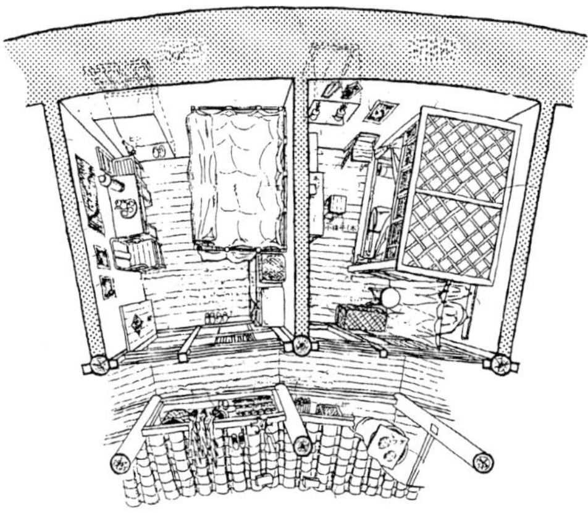

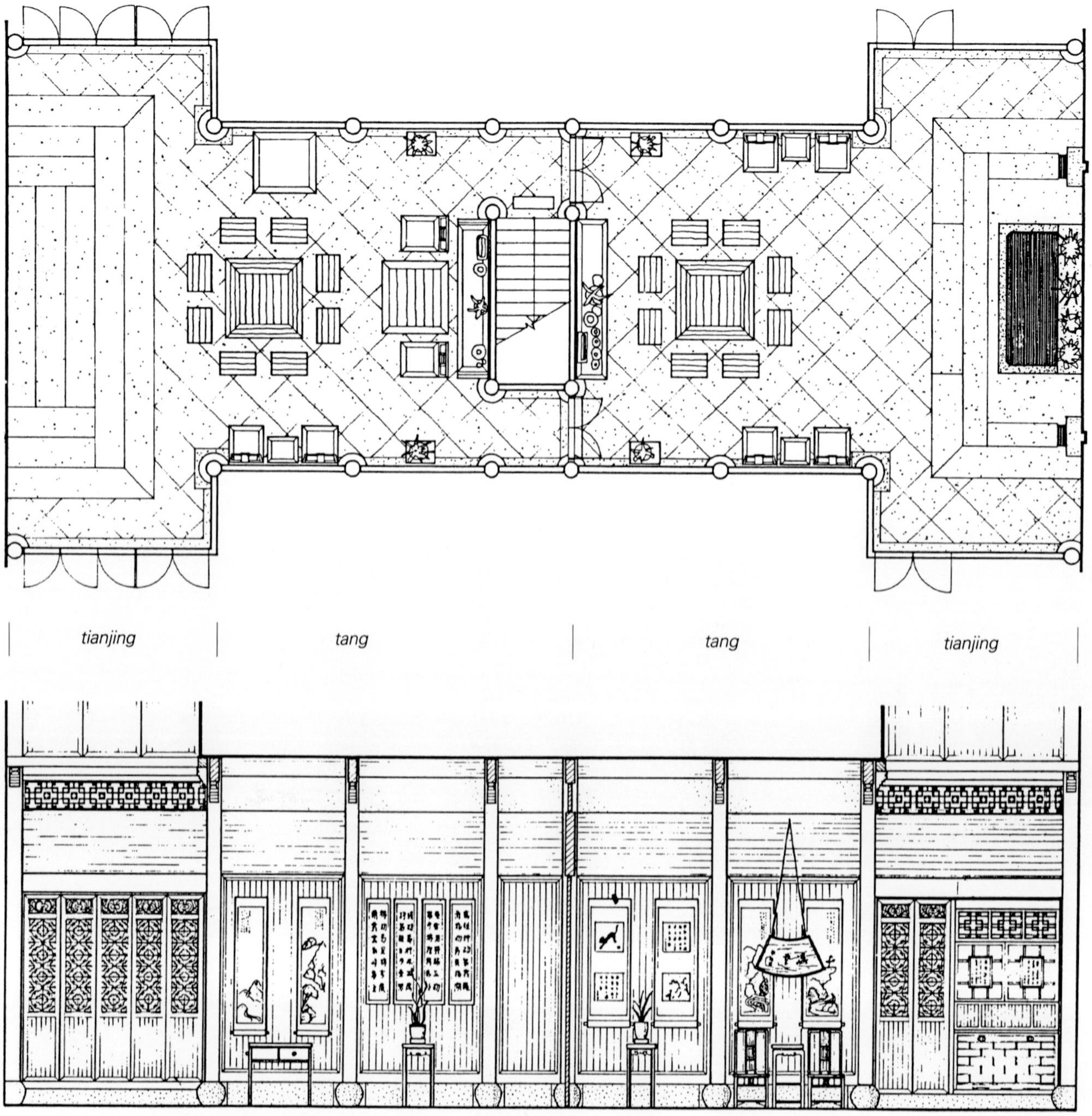

60 Plan view and elevation drawings showing the compositional and decorative arrangements of the communal *tang* and *tianjing* spaces in the Huizhou dwelling.

company. It is also where the elderly pass a large portion of the day sipping tea. An array of chairs, including Chinese fine wood stools, bamboo stools, and folding chairs, collect in this room, at times overflowing into the *tianjing*; at such times the *tang* and *tianjing* become one united environment (Figures 61.1–61.3).

The *tianjing* is not what the Japanese would call a "*niwa*," or "garden." It has the same brick or stone floor surface, and is set at the same floor level, as the *tang*, forming an open-air extension of the *tang*. No plants are planted in this courtyard. As communal space, the *tang* and *tianjing* are essentially the equivalent of a living room—with the simple qualification that the *tang* is closed-roofed and the *tianjing* is open, functionally they are best interpreted as a single space.

With the entire residential complex surrounded by high retaining walls, the communal *tianjing* also serves as a link to the outdoors—a means to enjoy natural light, breezes and rain. To the resident looking up from inside the space, the cropped blue sky is dazzling. The space is isolated from the outer world, and so has a certain solemnity. The same objects displayed in the *tang*—bonsai, and

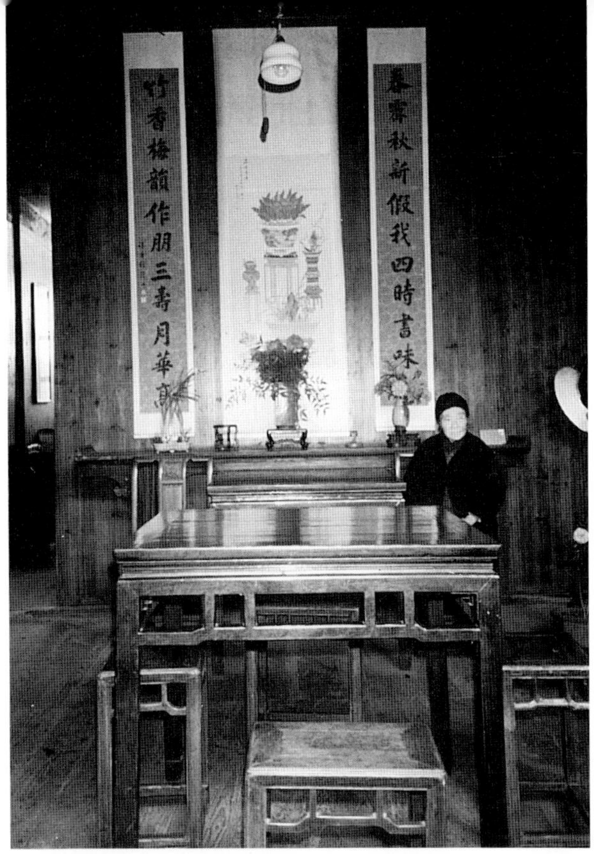
竹香梅韻作朋三壽月華
春霽秋新假我四時書味

61.1 The formal decorative arrangement of the *tang*.

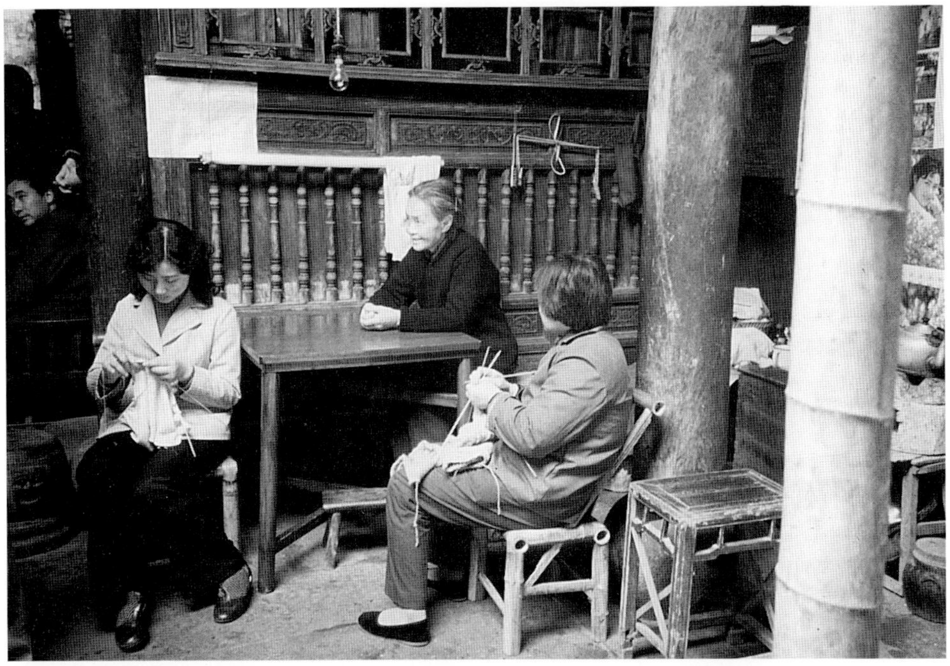

61.2 An afternoon gathering of family members in the *tang*.

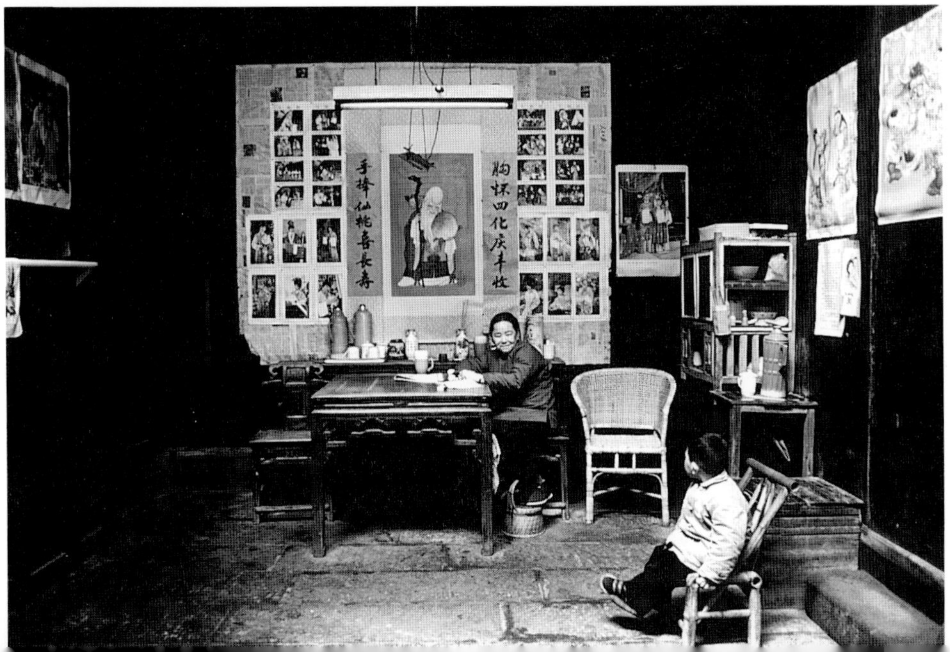
手捧仙桃喜長壽
胸怀四化庆丰收

61.3 A grandmother and child in the *tang*.

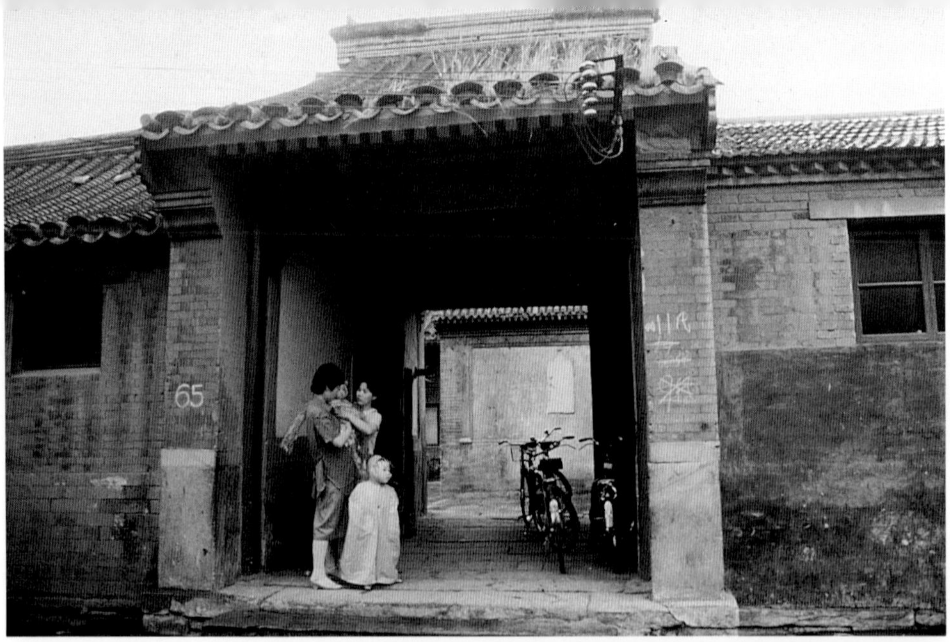

62.1 The main entrance of the Beijing *siheyuan*.

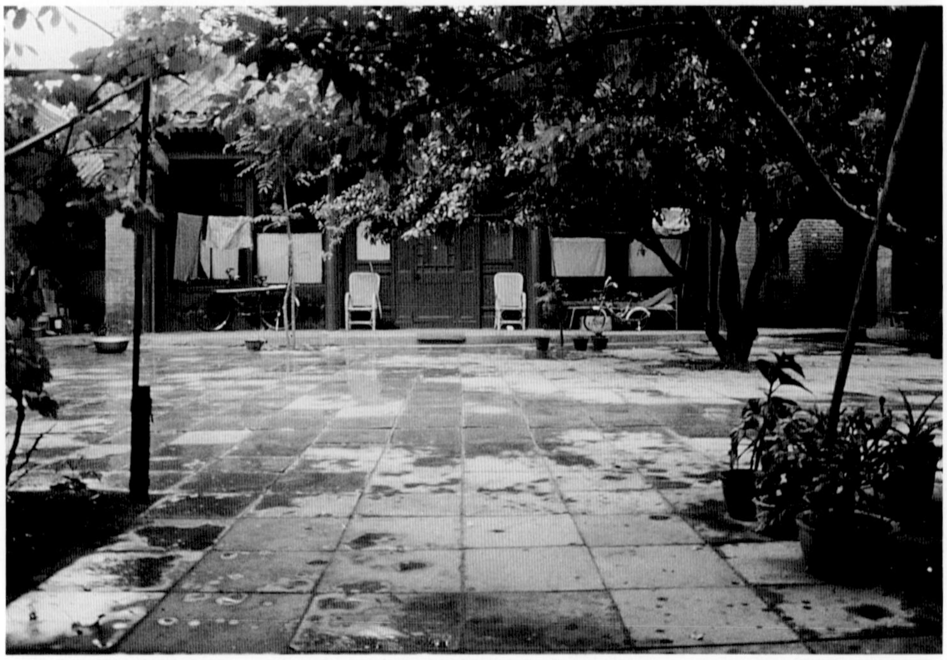

62.2 A Beijing *siheyuan yuanzi* with plantings in its four corners being used here for drying clothes.

table rocks or landscapes—are displayed in the *tianjing*. One specialty of Anhui Province is an almost painfully twisted bonsai; these seem especially well suited to this subdued space.

The Huizhou *tianjing* and Beijing *siheyuan yuanzi* have similar functions as both are forms of communal space. In Huizhou, the floors of the *tang* and *tianjing* are level and have no doors or partitions separating them; there is a greater emphasis on the interconnection between the interior and exterior spaces. In the Beijing *siheyuan*, the *tang* is wood-floored and is raised in height and separated from the *yuanzi* by doors; the sense of integrated space is much weaker than in Huizhou dwellings.

Since the *yuanzi* is nearly square and its surrounding halls all just one story high, it lets in far more sunlight and is considerably larger than the *tianjing*. The *tianjing*'s functional emphasis gives priority to climate control, which restricts its use; the spacious *yuanzi* is designed to serve partly as a work area.

The *yuanzi* is further distinguished from the *tianjing* in that trees and ground cover are frequently planted in its four corners; the composition, however, is very formal, and there is no intent whatsoever to express natural scenery (Figure 62.1–62.2).

Support Space: Chufang *and* Shaichang

A lean-to, sloping roof projects from the exterior of the high outer retaining wall that surrounds the living area of

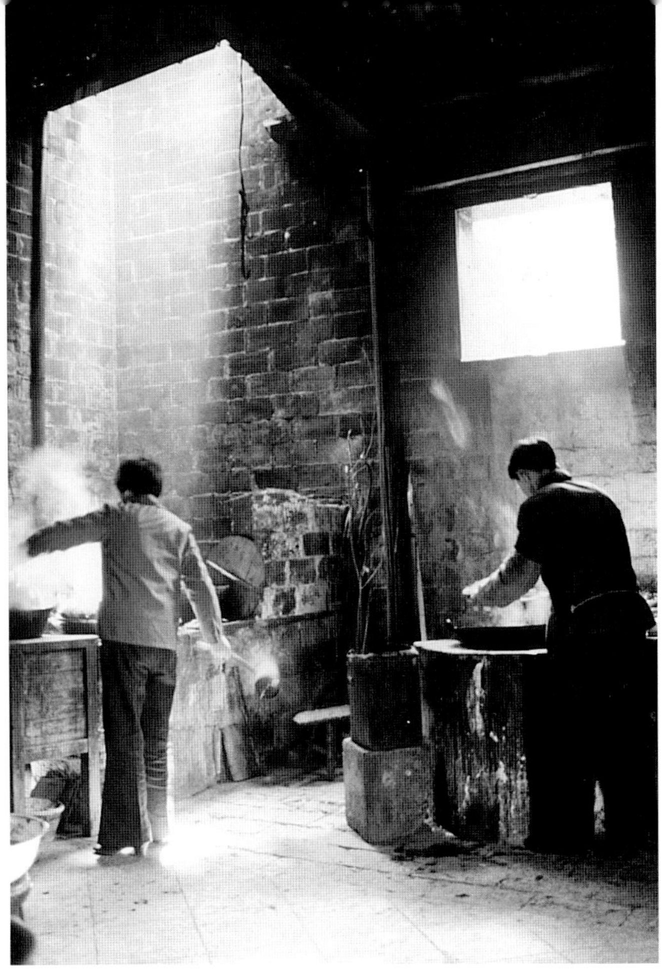

63.1 Skylights and windows used to light the *chufang* in a Huizhou residence.

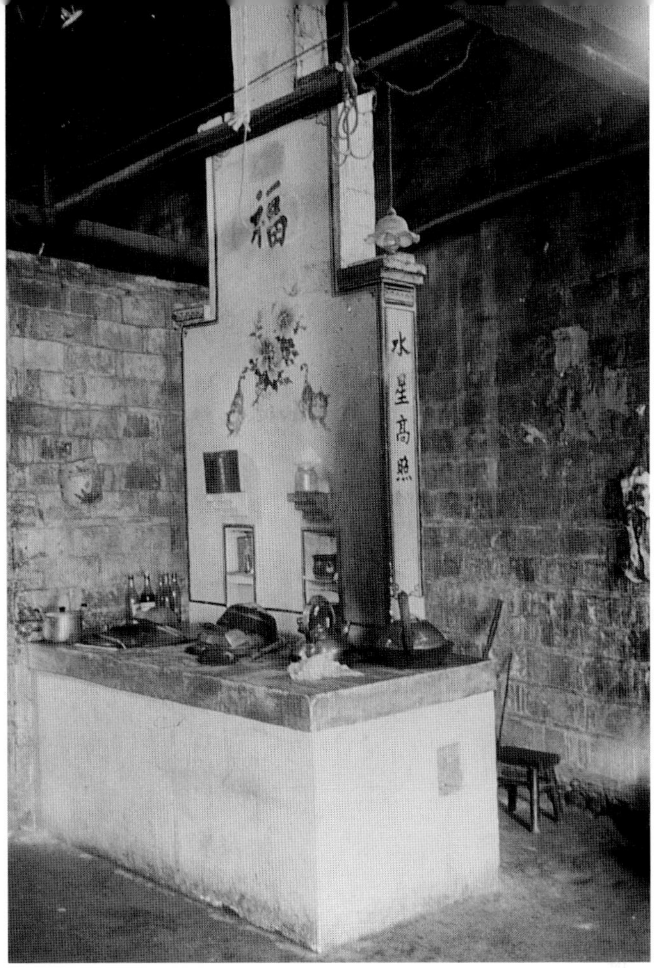

63.2 A stove with decorative motifs.

Huizhou dwellings. Beneath this roof are housed the *chufang* (kitchen), *shaichang* (containing the laundry area, clotheslines, well, etc.), vegetable gardens, livestock pens, and toilet; this entire area is bounded on the other side by another high retaining wall. This roofed, walled area is independent from the living area, giving the living space proper a double-wall construction.

Skylights are the main source of lighting for the *chufang*, with supplementary light provided by small windows cut into the walls at strategic locations. The sunlight that filters in effectively lights the dim, earthen-floored space (Figure 63.1).

The central feature of the *chufang* is the stove, which is constructed of mud. The mortar-covered flues are inscribed with decorative motifs and with prayers for the family's welfare (Figure 63.2). Coke is the primary source of fuel, supplemented by wood and brush. An additional charcoal brazier is often set beside the stove. Cupboards are small and tableware is simple and minimal, strikingly different from the tremendous variety of tableware used in Japanese dining.

There is no designated bathing room in the Huizhou dwelling. Washbasins are used for daily washing and public bathhouses are widely available throughout the cities.

Furnishings

Cabinetry and furniture is extremely simple. Chests are used mainly to store clothing, and these are gradually being replaced by Western-style wardrobes. Chests of drawers are rarely seen.

Sideboards are made of bamboo or wood with screening on the upper portion and slatting on the lower portion. This style is unchanged in old and more recent pieces.

Overall, there is a very large drop in quality between traditional Chinese fine wood furniture in the Ming and Qing styles and everyday furniture. No such drop in quality, however, is seen in Chinese handicraft utensils, for which such materials as wood, bamboo, ceramics, and bronze are used.

There is no built-in heating equipment. Portable, basket-like charcoal-burning foot warmers made of bamboo are hung from the arm when carried (Figure 64.1). Baby baskets are also frequently equipped with similar heating devices (Figure 64.2). Such individual heaters and quilted

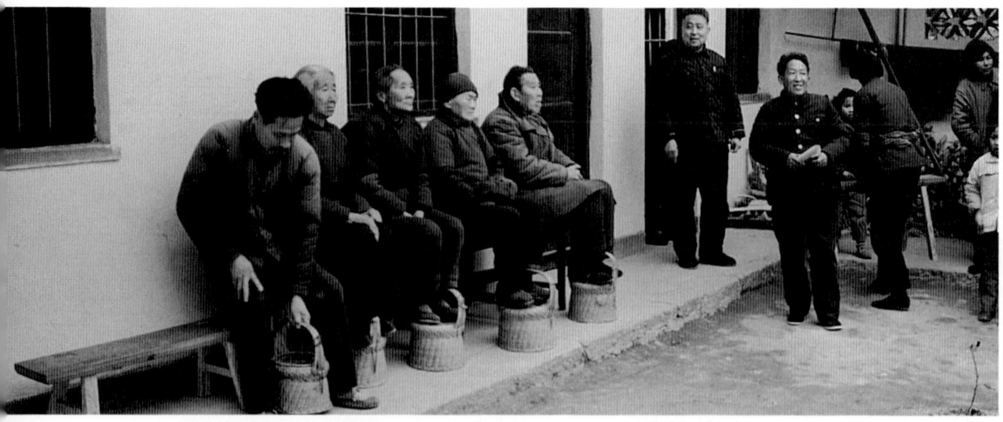

64.1 Portable foot heaters used at a community gathering.

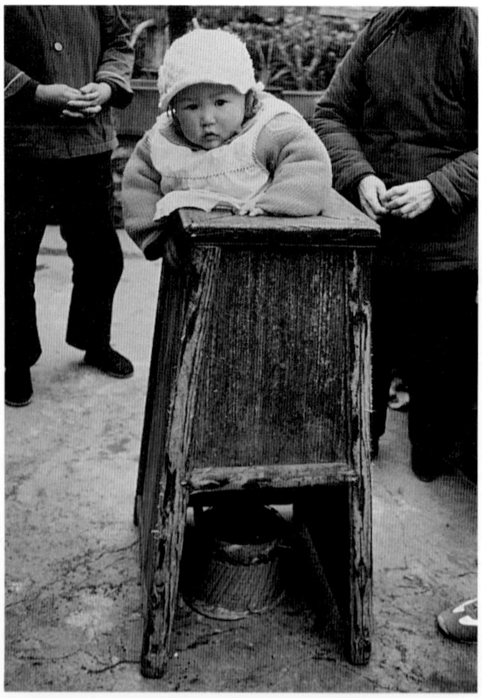

64.2 Baby basket with portable heating device.

clothing are essential to withstand the severe winters of the Anhui region.

Contemporary Housing: Single-Family Style

The majority of recently constructed houses have no *tianjing* courtyard—the *tang* is entered directly from the street. They generally have two stories and are composed of a central *tang* flanked by four *woshi* stacked lengthwise two on each side, with the *chufang* at the rear (Figures 65.1–65.2).

Large window openings are cut into the walls of each room, making the rooms—and the *chufang* in particular—remarkably bright. The standard *woshi-tang-woshi* pattern, however, remains unchanged.

Because contemporary houses are one-family dwellings, they are no longer surrounded by high walls. The *woshi* and *chufang* are fitted with large windows. They are much more open than traditional dwellings. Houses in communities formed of these single-family dwellings face onto a street or plaza that serves as the equivalent of a "communal" courtyard.

As a "communal" space in which much of the heavier, outdoor work around the home is done, the street or plaza also provides an area for chatting and enjoying one another's company—in an expression of increasing freedom from the confines of the Confucianist system, the community has torn down the old walls and is building a new compositional framework around a new courtyard.

Courtyards (*Ting*) Versus Gardens

An overall look at the compositional structure of the Beijing *siheyuan* and Huizhou dwellings, along with documentation from surveys into various Huizhou customs indicates that while the *siheyuan* may be their prototype, Huizhou dwellings formed independently in response to central China's Jiangnan climate.

The *tianjing* is a particularly good example of an adaptive feature that arose independently. "Private" space is condensed into the *woshi*, and "communal" space into the *tang* and *tianjing*—the *tang* is interior and the *tianjing* the exterior extension of that communal space. Though it serves as a very ordinary open-air living room, the *tianjing* is functionally highly sophisticated. It provides necessary ventilation and light that the closed, high surrounding retaining walls would otherwise shut out. This space is clearly not intended to be an object of admiration. It contains no elements of Chinese garden composition as seen in the *ting yuan* (contemplative landscape gardens) which developed into the *yuanlin* (landscape park gardens) that were constructed outside the residential compound. This is not to say that there are no objects for admiration in the

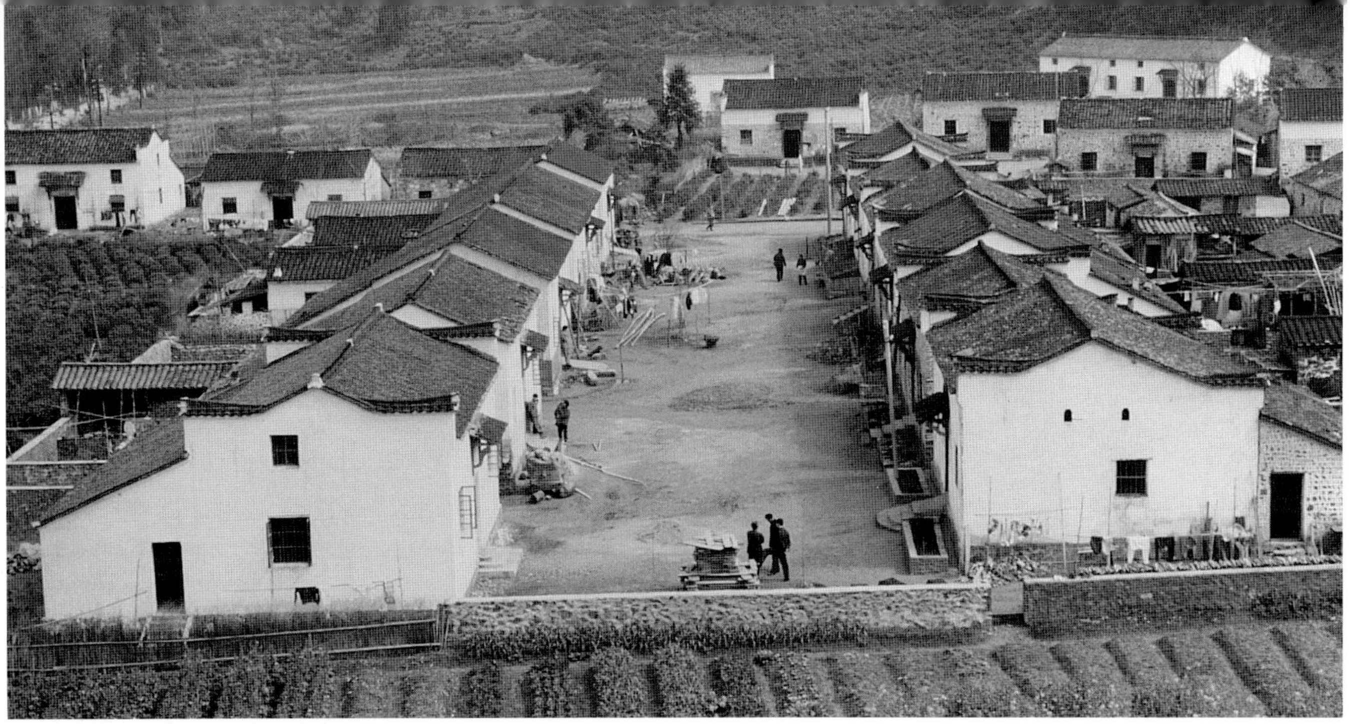

65.1 View and ground plan of a contemporary Chinese community.
a. communal plaza work space. b. communal storehouse. c. water tower.

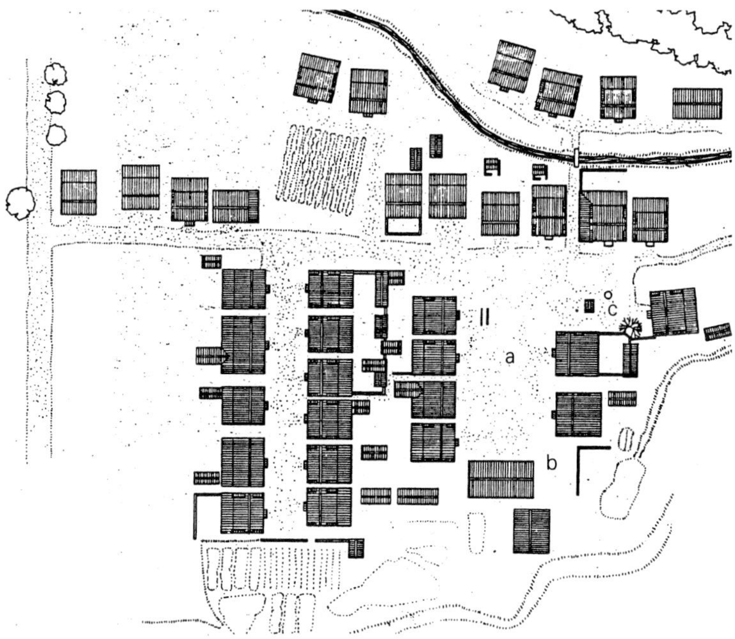

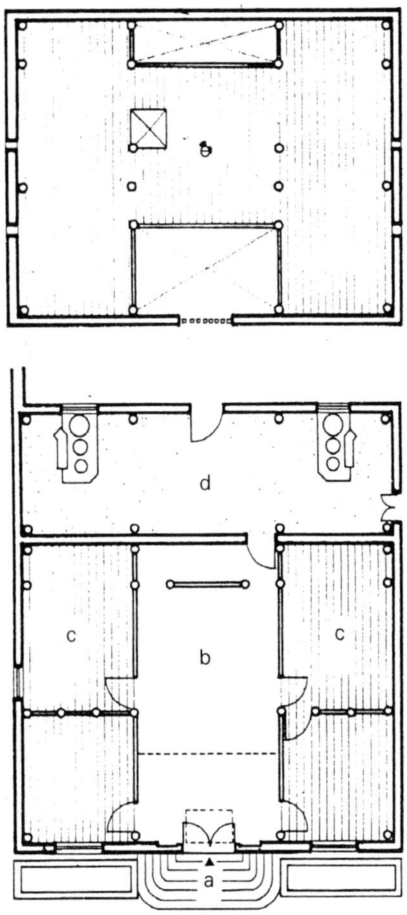

65.2 Plan view, elevation, and section drawings of a contemporary Chinese dwelling.
a. main entry. b. *tang.* c. *woshi.* d. *chufang.* e. storeroom.

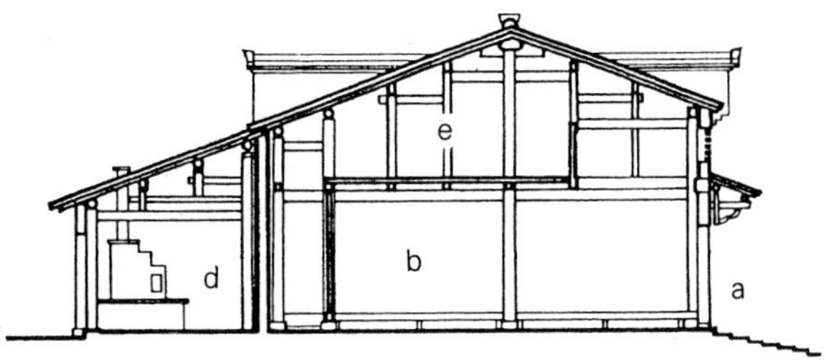

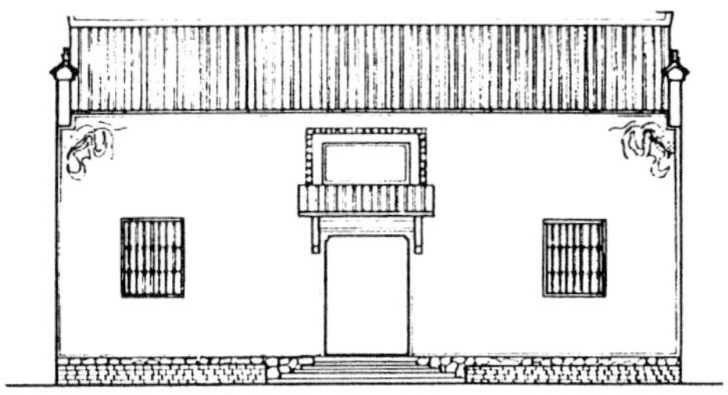

courtyard—bonsai, tray landscapes and rocks are displayed there. They too are an extension of the decorative objects displayed in the interior *tang*.

The word "*ting*" has been used in China since ancient times to refer to a nearly square, vacant space between buildings. According to the Later Han–dynasty (A.D. 25–220) dictionary *Shuo wen* by Xu Shen, "the *ting* lies within the palace confines," and in the Song-dynasty 960–1279) text *Yu hai* by Wang Ying-lin, "the area extending from beneath the *tang* to the gate is called the *ting*."[1] Today this space is called *yuanzi* in the north and *tianjing* in the south. By definition, the *ting* is an open area within the residential complex; it is not a garden, but rather an open-roofed living space.

Clearly, the garden as an object of appreciation and contemplation did not evolve in China from the exterior courtyard space within the residential compound. The formative process of the garden was totally different in China than in Japan, where gardens always developed together with residences as a unified whole.

5

Spatial Composition of the Unworldly

Ting Yuan, Prototype of the *Yuanlin*

The hall and courtyard (*ting*) in Chinese dwellings form one unified, functional, everyday living space. In some homes there is also another important area associated with the residential complex, a *ting yuan* or *yuanlin* landscape garden, which is distinctly partitioned off from the hall/courtyard portion of the dwelling.

The *yuanlin* is a small landscape park, which was enlarged and developed from the *ting yuan*, a contemplative landscape garden.

The *ting yuan* is composed of small buildings—a *shufang* (study), *chafang* (drawing room) or *huating* (banquet hall)—and gardens surrounded by a retaining wall; it abuts with the exterior wall surrounding the residential area, but differs totally in nature from the residential *ting* (courtyard) space (Figure 66).

A total of eight residences with *ting yuan* in Yangzhou, and two in Huizhou, were surveyed, and in all, the residential area—composed of *woshi*, *tang* and *tianjing*—is separated by a surrounding wall from the annexed *shufang* or *chafang* and their corresponding garden scenes composed of plants and arrangements of unusual rocks;

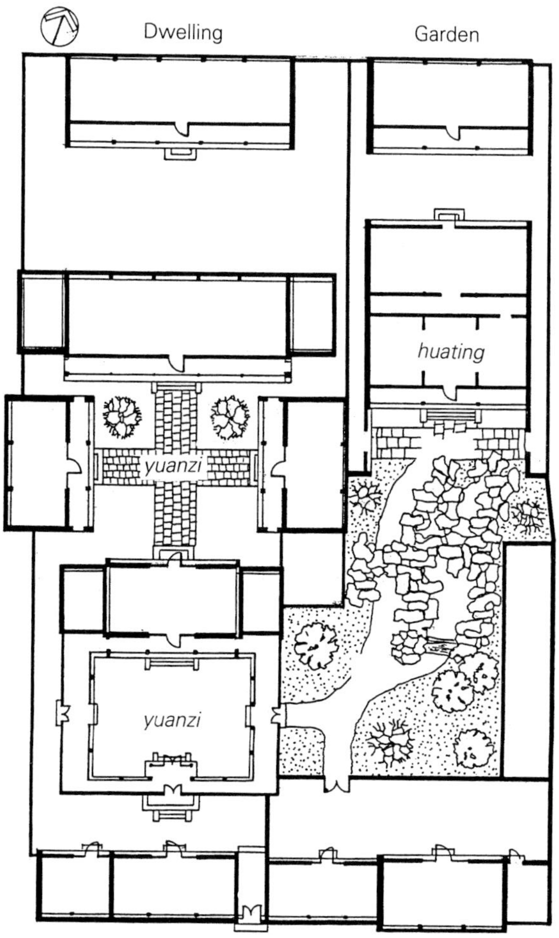

66 Ground plan of a Beijing *siheyuan* residence with a *ting yuan*.

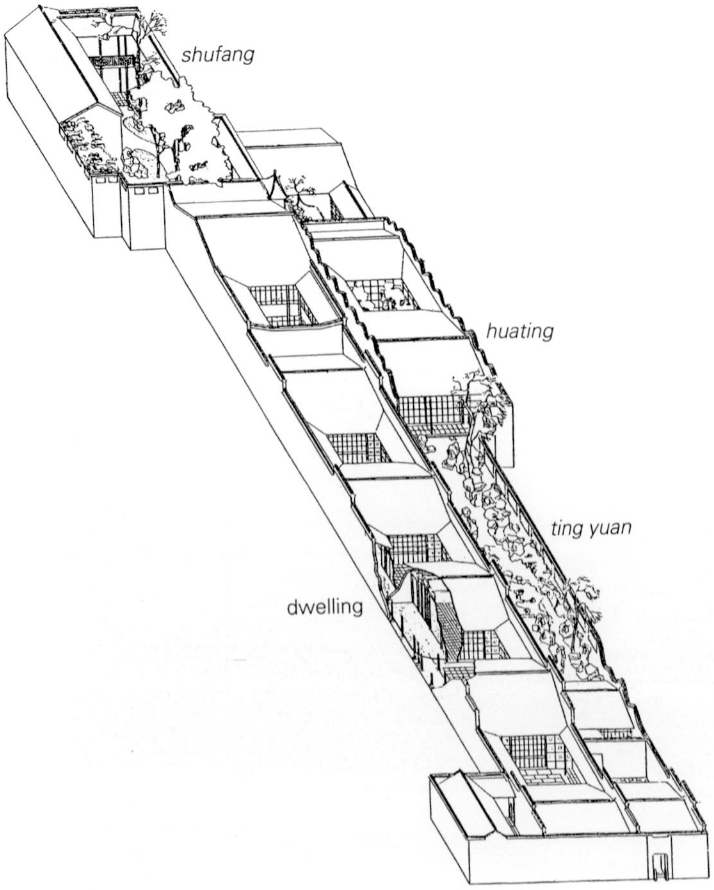

67.1 Axonometric drawing of a residential complex with *ting yuan* gardens.

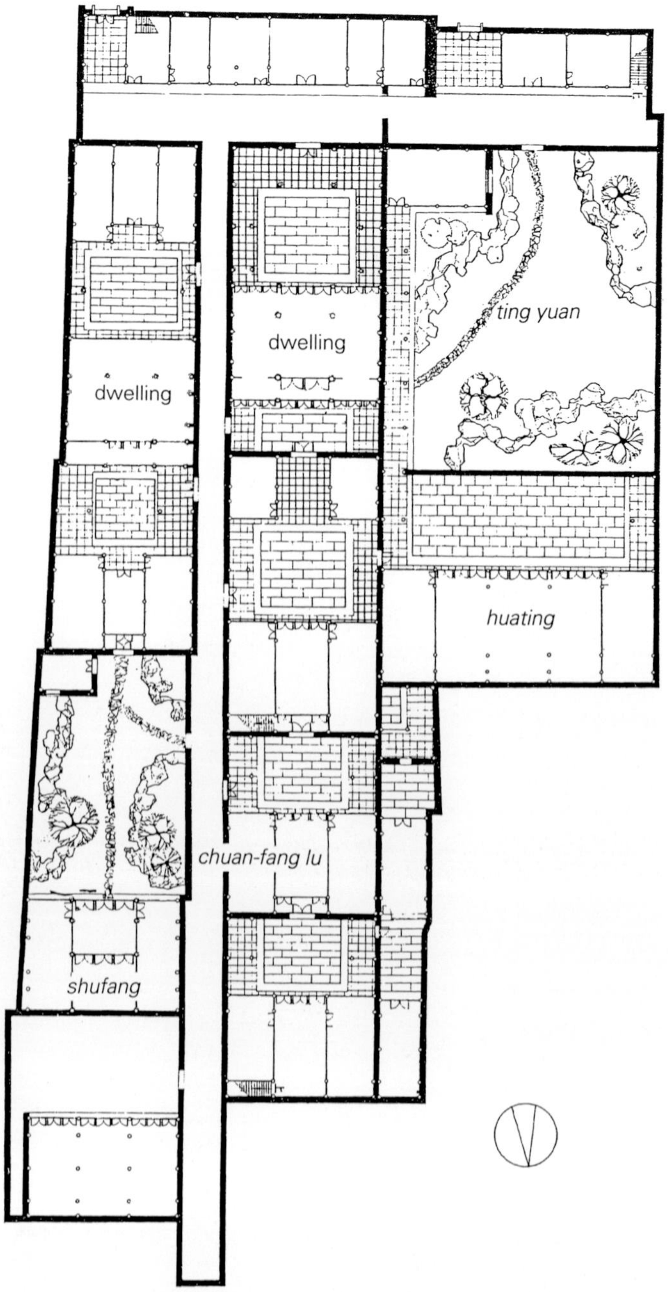

67.2 Ground plan of a residential complex with *ting yuan* gardens.

this annexed area is in turn surrounded by a retaining wall. This structure shows that Chinese gardens did not emerge from a connection to everyday living, but rather in a sphere apart from the functional and mundane. The *chafang* and *huating* (rooms for entertaining guests) and the *shufang* (study) were built outside the living area. The *ting yuan* was always set apart as an object for admiration.

The independent *shufang*, *chafang*, and *huating* were found only in the homes of the literati, warriors, government officials, and the *nouveau riche*, and so were clear indicators of social position. To qualify as an elite space, the *ting yuan* had to be distinctly partitioned off from the mundane spaces of the home. And as an object for contemplation, it set out to give tangible form to a vision of utopia, like the circumstances and spirit portrayed in Chinese landscape painting.

The *ting yuan* is a *hua yuan* (literally, "flower garden"; the term used in reference to ornamental gardens), which differs greatly from the *ting* (which is written with the character used for "*niwa*," or garden, in Japanese.)

In contrast to the *yuanzi* and the *tianjing*, which are functional, outdoor living spaces, the *ting yuan* is purely a pleasure garden, with no everyday functions. Hence it is usually not visible from the residential area; alternatively, it may be partially visible through latticework windows. The residential compound is totally divorced from the

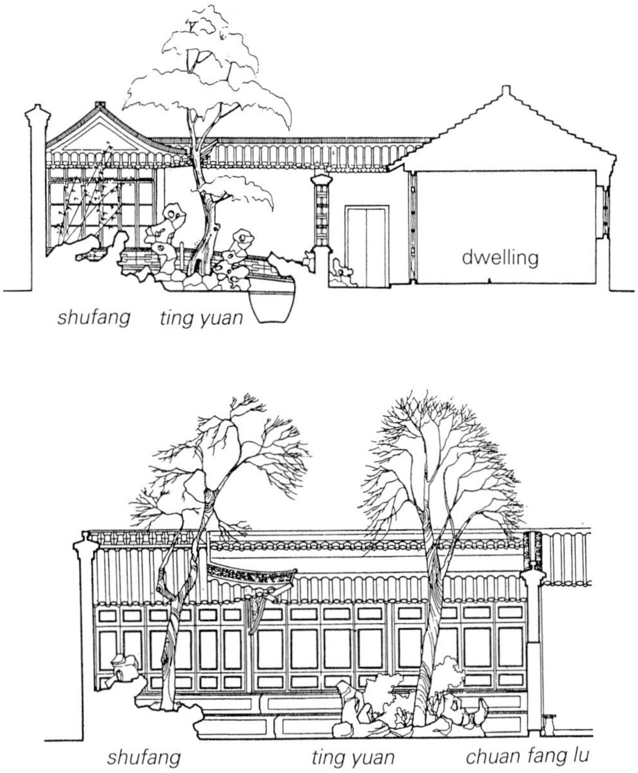

67.3 Section drawings of a Yangzhou *ting yuan.*

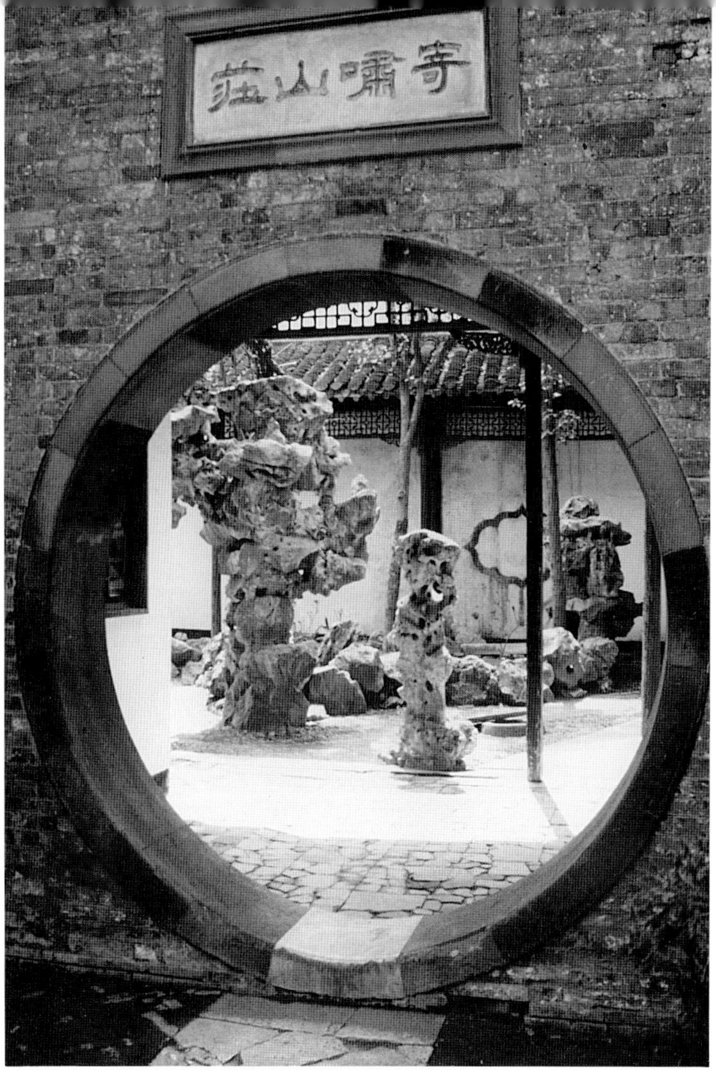

67.4 *Ting yuan* entranceway.

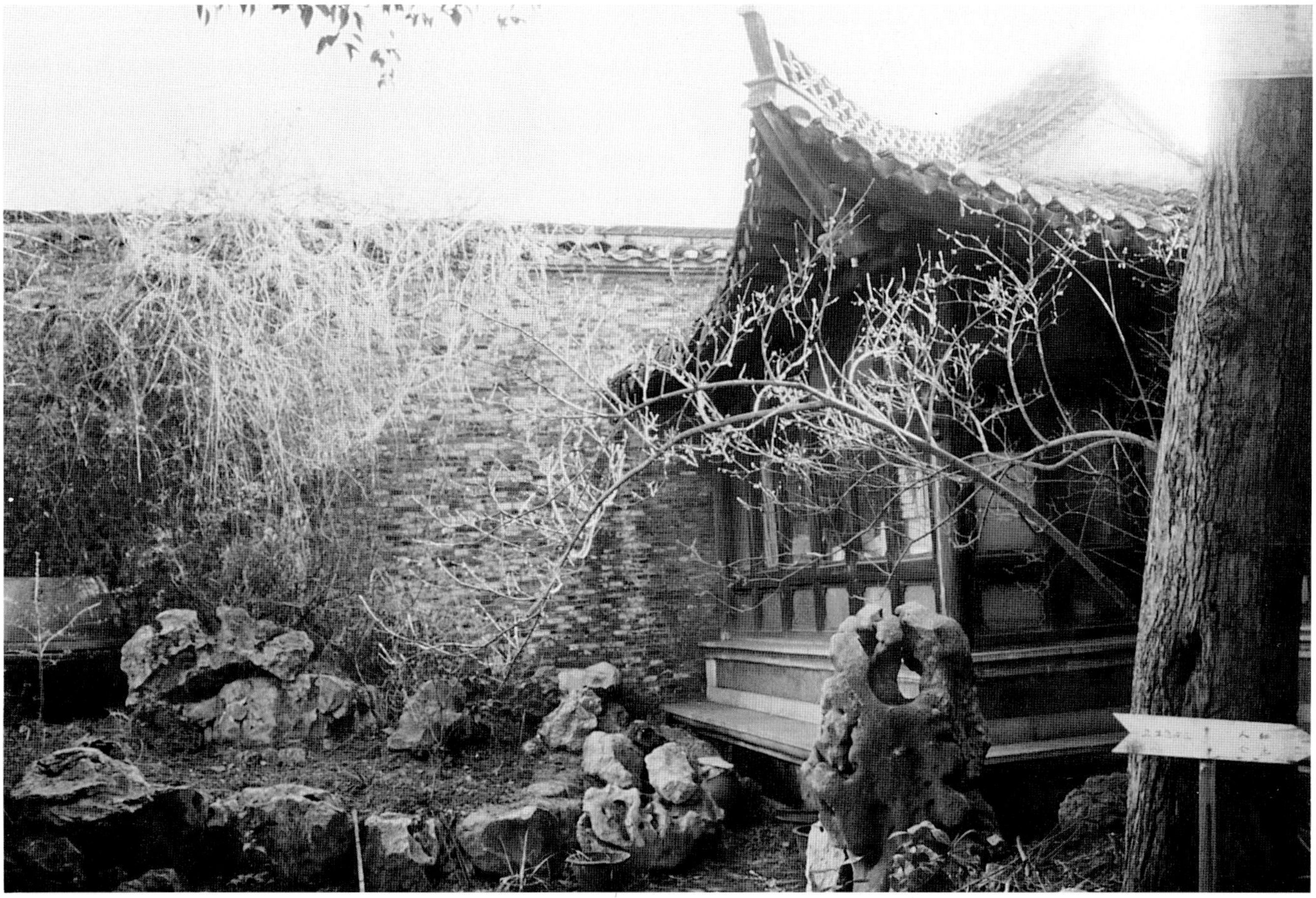

67.5 *Ting yuan.*

ting yuan, separated by retaining walls surrounding both spaces, and a narrow alleyway (*chuan feng lu*) running between them (Figures 67.1–67.5).

Smaller *ting yuan* have a *shufang* or a *chafang* in one corner, together with a garden scene composed of plants, rock arrangements, or a pond corresponding to the viewing position from the main seat inside (Figure 68.1). Larger *ting yuan* contain opposing *huating*, two halls facing one another from opposite sides of the garden with corresponding scenery at the center (Figure 68.2), or a Mandarin Duck *huating* (one central hall separated by an interior wall creating back-to-back halls, each facing out onto different garden scenes; Figure 68.3).

The *shufang*, *chafang*, and *huating* form the core of the *ting yuan*'s meaning as a symbol of elitism, and their corresponding garden scenes contain utopian expressions of the same quality as those seen in Chinese landscape painting. The *ting yuan* stands as the antithesis of the *ting*, in the sense that it is an independent space with no direct relation to daily living.

Garden-Related Terminology

The Chinese terms relating to gardens are defined in the glossary in Sugimura Yūzō's *Chūgoku no niwa* (Chinese gardens) as follows:

Yuan Fruit orchard

Pu Vegetable garden

You Pen in which fowl and livestock are raised, or any fenced-in garden

Yuan (A different character, with the same pronunciation as *yuan* above) This character came into frequent use for garden names during the Han dynasty (206 B.C.–A.D. 9), starting with the Qin-dynasty (221–206 B.C.) Shang-lin yuan. During the Zhou dynasty (1122–770 B.C.), the characters *pu* and *you* were used widely, but from the time of the Han dynasty these were no longer used in association with royal pleasure grounds. In later periods, both characters for *yuan* were used.

Jin yuan (literally, "forbidden garden") Used as a term for Imperial gardens from the time of the start of the Han dynasty.

Hua yuan (literally, "flower garden") The term used for common gardens.[1]

An Outline of the History of Chinese Gardens

Chinese gardens have a long history, which can be roughly divided into two categories: the Imperial forbidden gardens, or Imperial *yuanlin*, and private residential pleasure gardens of scholars, government officials, regional governors and merchants, or private *yuanlin*, which developed from the *ting yuan*.

Most Imperial *yuanlin* were royal pleasure parks linking the Imperial palace to detached palaces. They were sometimes built around natural mountains and rivers with a certain amount of remodeling, and at other times constructed completely from man-made excavations—but in either case they were splendid grounds, built on a vast scale. Private *yuanlin* were built within or on the outskirts of cities, near residences, and were intended exclusively for enjoyment.

The features of the relatively small spaces of private *yuanlin* were minutely detailed; they represented a distillation of the garden-making techniques cultivated in Imperial gardens. The development of the modern urban private *yuanlin* has its roots in the *ting yuan*, an earlier interpretation of the Imperial *yuanlin* prototype.

Imperial Yuanlin

Chinese gardens had already taken form over 2000 years ago, as evidenced in recorded descriptions of the gardens

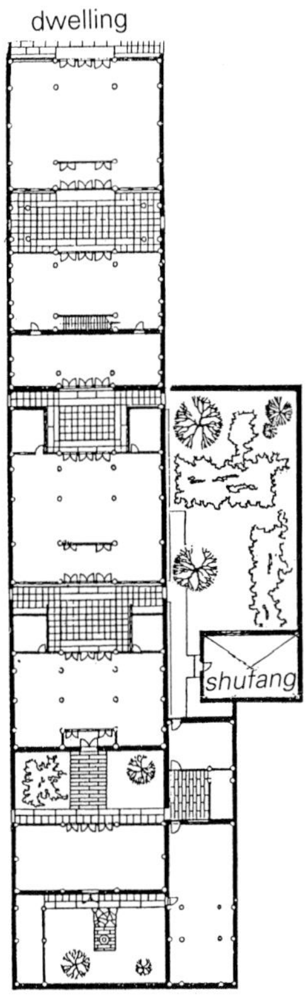

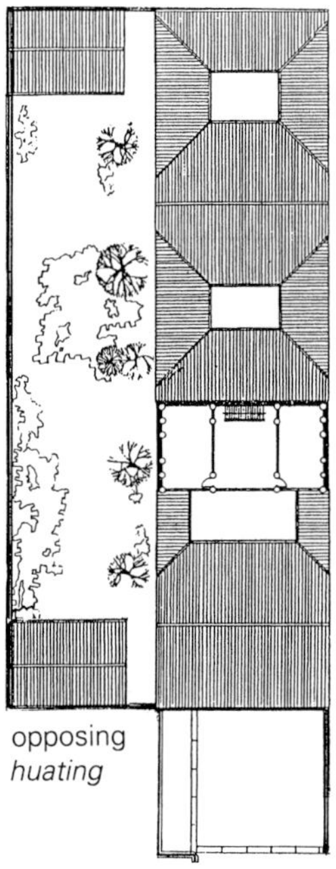

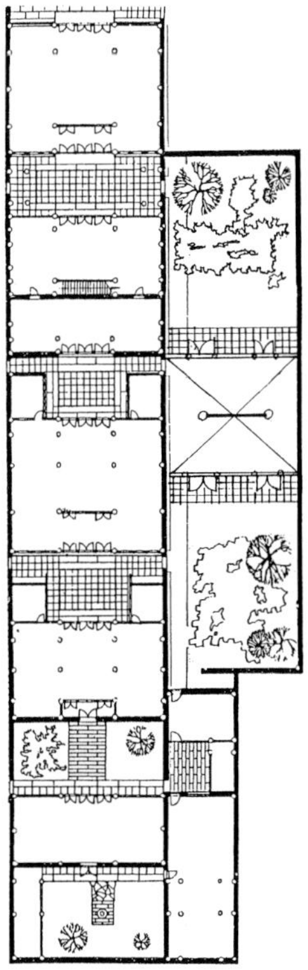

68.1 Ground plan of a residence with a small *ting yuan* composed around a *shufang* at one corner.

68.2 Ground plan of a residence with a large *ting yuan* composed around opposing *huating*.

68.3 Ground plan of a residence with a large *ting yuan* composed around a central Mandarin Duck *huating*.

of E-fang Palace (constructed 213 B.C.) of the first Qin emperor, Shi Huang, and the garden of Han emperor Wu, known as Shang-ling yuan (constructed 138 B.C.).

Shang-ling yuan encompassed more than 300 *li* (a Chinese mile, roughly one-third an English mile, or half a kilometer), had six lakes, over 70 detached palaces, 3,000 varieties of flowering trees, and was stocked with "creatures from all over the world." Hunting parties were held within the Shang-ling yuan grounds. Both it and the gardens of E-fang Palace were ultimately based on spiritual/magical beliefs in the *shen xian*, or Taoist Immortals, whose mist-covered dwelling-places on mountains and islands these gardens were intended to recall.

These Chinese gardens, which borrowed from the natural landscape to express ideological, religious, and literary concepts were profoundly influential as prototypes for later Chinese gardens, as well as for other Oriental—and particularly Japanese—gardens.

Landscape-Style Gardens

Garden ownership reached its height during the Tang and Song dynasties. It was during this same period that scholars and painters appeared in great numbers, leading to the emergence of free-form landscape-style gardens that were supported by literature and landscape painting. The Song dynasty in particular has been called the golden age of the arts, including gardens.

A well-known literary work of the late Northern Song dynasty by Li Ge-fei, *Luo-yang ming-yuan ji* ("The Famous Gardens of Louyang") describes eighteen famous gardens of the time, citing the following as the ideals on which they were designed:

> There are six attributes that do not combine in fine scenery: where magnificence is at work, the subtle and profound is lacking; where artificiality prevails, the patina of age is insufficient; where wooded, watery gardens are featured, panoramas are limited. The only garden combining these six elements is Hu yuan.

As this passage suggests, the successful harmonization of antithetical elements of natural and man-made beauty is an ideal in the design of Chinese landscape-style gardens.

Although none of these gardens survive today, vestiges of their forms are still visible in certain scenes of the gardens attached to the Imperial Palace in Beijing, Bei-hai yuan, Yi-he yuan (known to many as the Summer Palace), and Hangzhou's West Lake.

Private Yuanlin

During the Ming and Qing dynasties, economic development spurred the development of *yuanlin* in the cities, where the aristocracy, government functionaries, landlords, and *nouveau riche* merchants were concentrated,

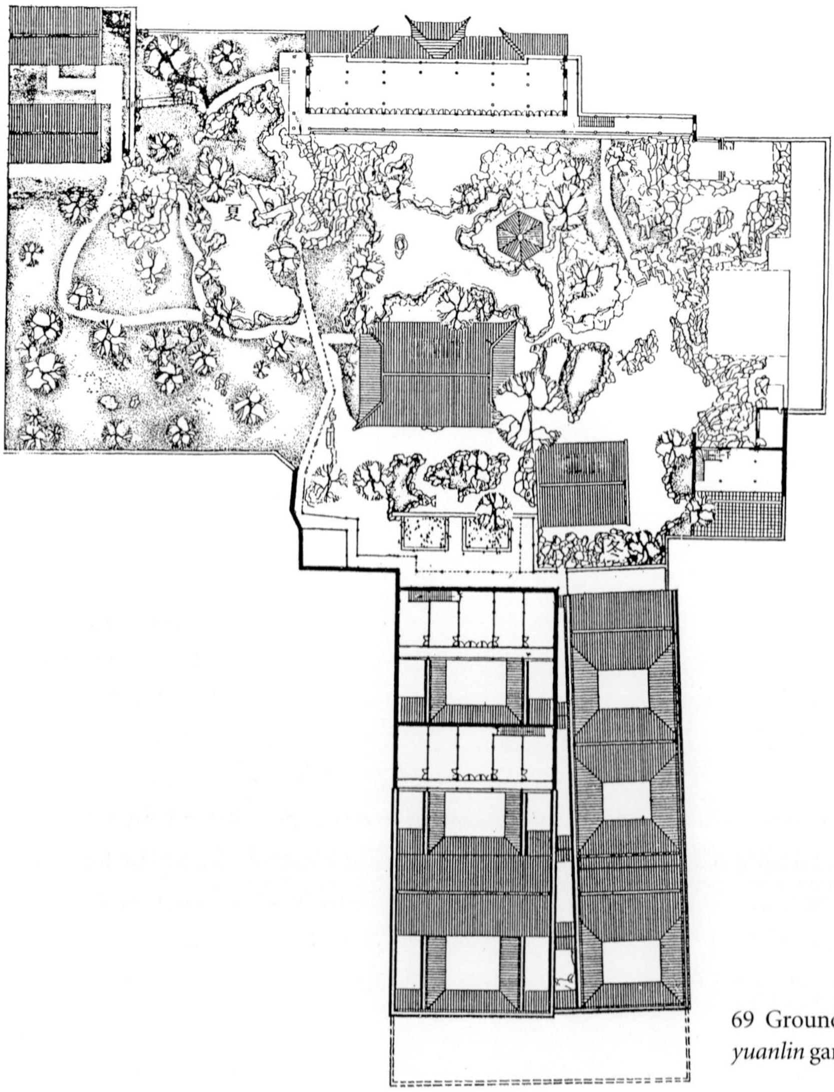

69 Ground plan of Ge yuan, a residence with a private *yuanlin* garden (Yangzhou).

particularly in those cities blessed with a temperate climate and plentiful water supply. Famous gardens of this period still in existence today are concentrated in the Jiangnan region, mainly in Suzhou (including Liu yuan, or "Garden to Linger In"; Wang-shi yuan, "Garden of the Master of the Fishing Nets"; and Zhuo-zheng yuan, "Garden of the Unsuccessful Politician"), and in Yangzhou (for example, Shou xi hu, "Slender West Lake"; He yuan, "He Family Garden"; and Ge yuan, "Isolated Garden"; Figure 69). The main distinguishing feature of private *yuanlin* is that they are urban gardens that are a condensed interpretation of the prototype of the spacious gardens of the Tang and Song dynasties. This process of modeling and adaptation led to the development of distinctively Chinese techniques of garden making. The development of the *yuanlin*'s progress toward the status of a symbol of the elite—completely divorced from the courtyards within the everyday living quarters—may be seen as inevitable in light of the historical circumstances surrounding the formation of Chinese gardens, the influence of social stratification, and the compositional style of traditional Chinese residential architecture.

The Garden Treatise *Yuan Ye*

Garden design theory made great strides during the Ming and Qing periods, and the definitive treatise among the many works produced at this time on landscape gardening in the Chinese tradition—essential to any study of *yuanlin*—is *Yuan ye* (*The Craft of Gardens*), written by Ji Cheng in the late Ming dynasty.

Ji Cheng was a landscape designer from Jiangsu Province, and was renowned throughout that region for his considerable experience in garden planning, and also for his work as a poet and painter. His *Yuan ye* consists of a comprehensive guide in three volumes to garden-making techniques in the Jiangnan region, on the basis of which the reader can deduce the framework and essential points of *yuanlin* garden-making techniques. The following is an outline of the topics which his work covers:

> Volume I. The theory of construction; on gardens: Comments on the overall principles of garden making
> 1. Situation (choice of site): Sites among mountain forests, urban sites, village sites, sites in the uninhabited countryside, sites beside mansions, riverside and lakeside sites. A guide to selection and excavation of each type of site.
> 2. Layout (positioning of buildings and artificial mountains): [Laying the foundations for] the great hall, towers, gate towers, etc. Positioning, scale, and characteristics of buildings within the garden environment.
> 3. Buildings: Gate towers, halls, chapels, living-rooms, chambers, lodgings, towers, terraces, belvederes, covered walkways, etc.—dimensions and characteristics of each. Five-pillared structures, seven-pillared structures, etc.—structural principles.
> 4. Fittings: Description and diagrammatic illustrations of the decorative features of all these types of buildings, including latticework, windows, etc.
> Volume II. Description and diagrammatic illustrations of decorative balustrades
> Volume III. [Structural and scenic features]
> 1. Doorways and windows: Description and diagrammatic illustrations of doorways and windows.
> 2. Walls (exterior walls and hedges): Whitewashed walls, polished brick walls, unworked stone walls, etc.—exterior wall types and their attributes. Description and diagrammatic illustrations of openwork windows.
> 3. Paving (decorative pavements): Garden path ideals, paving materials, and diagrammatic illustrations of paving patterns.
> 4. Raising mountains (artificial mountains): Mountains in private gardens, mountains in courtyards, mountains beside towers, mountains beside studies, mountains beside ponds, mountains in women's apartments, precipitous mountains, mountain rock pools, goldfish tanks, sharp peaks, rounded peaks, overhanging cliffs, caves, mountain torrents, meanderings, and waterfalls. Artificial mountain types—their features and related compositional elements.
> 5. Selection of Rocks: Rocks from Tai hu (the Great Lake), rocks gathered from Kunshan, rocks from Xuanxing, etc.—sixteen varieties of rocks from different regions for use in the *yuanlin* primarily for the purpose of creating the mountain features cited above. Types of rocks and the characteristics of each.
> 6. Borrowed scenery: distant scenery, scenery near at hand, scenery above, scenery below—ways of using these types of borrowed views and the effects they produce.[2]

Note the relative importance the author gives here to buildings and their location in the *yuanlin*, the details of their composition and decoration, and the types of doorways and walls and their decoration. The primary emphasis in garden making is on architectural features, with types and features of artificial mountains (rock mountains) and paved paths playing a secondary role.

The emphasis in *Yuan ye* is on buildings—their position and decoration—and fantastic rocks. One has only to compare the Japanese Heian-period *Sakuteiki*, which concentrates on water and rocks in its description of the definitive features of a garden, to perceive the fundamental difference in the approach taken to garden making in Japan and China. This difference is again confirmed by Edo-period garden manuals that expound at length on rock arrangements, ponds, and running water features, while ignoring buildings altogether. Relevant passages of these Edo-period texts include the section "Complete illustrations of artificial hills, and how to build them" in *Tsukiyama teizōden*, "Constructing mountain and water Landscapes" in *Sagaryūniwa kohōhiden no koto*, and "Methods for the construction of artificial hill mountain and water landscapes" in *Tsukiyama sansuiden.*

Private *Yuanlin*: Compositional Techniques

Private *yuanlin* gardens were associated with, yet positioned outside, and independent from urban dwellings. They were centered around the *huating*, which was used primarily for entertaining, and sought to create a "utopian" atmosphere of separateness from everyday life. From the techniques used to create private *yuanlin* arose a unique method of garden making which was a condensed, intricately detailed version of the most venerable Chinese gardening techniques. *Yuan ye* outlines five principle aspects of *yuanlin* garden making, which are presented here supplemented with original material gathered in the course of this research:

Situation (Xiang-Di)

As expressed in the term *yin-di zhi-xuan* (an exhortation to "follow the natural lay of the land"), the garden is planned around existing topography. Low-lying areas are dug deeper still, and high spots heightened further. The original rocks, water, and plants form the basic garden materials, simply being condensed where they are too scattered, in order to accentuate the naturally formed vistas. This method ensures that even in a relatively flat urban *yuanlin* there will be variations in height, and that the groupings of flowers, trees, and stones will serve as a reminder to the viewer of the beauty of the scenery of that particular region. It is a technique, in short, which utilizes and emphasizes the intrinsic forms and vegetation of the site.

The Ming-dynasty garden Zhuo-zheng yuan in Suzhou was originally a low-lying, swampy area. To maintain the existing features and atmosphere of the garden's site, a large pond was dug in the center, while structures such as halls, belvederes, towers, and pavilions were situated on built-up areas around it to create interrelating views. The emphasis placed on preserving the distinctive characteristics of the Jiangnan region made Zhuo-zheng yuan famous for its water scenes.

Another well-known garden in Suzhou, the Northern Song Cang-lang ting (Pavilion of the Blue Waves) took quite the opposite approach. This site originally comprised paddy fields. Earth and rocks were stacked up in the relatively high central section to create artificial mountains, and the surrounding area was dug to form a pond. It is thus known as a "*chong-fu guang-shui*" *yuanlin*, meaning, literally, "a high mountain aspect and a wide expanse of water."

Layout of Buildings (Li-ji Wu-yu)

The defining characteristic in the design of the Chinese *yuanlin* is that priority is given to the positioning of buildings; the garden is designed around the buildings. *Yuan ye* has the following to say about the layout of *yuanlin*:

> The most important element in the layout of gardens is the sitting of the principal buildings. The primary consideration is the view, and it is all the better if the buildings can also face south. If there are some tall trees around, then keep one or two of them growing in the courtyards. When you build walls you must spread them widely and preserve plenty of open space within them, so that you can arrange and lay out the place exactly as you wish. Once you have picked a site for the main buildings, [*dui-ge* coupled buildings that form counter-opposing views], you can use the

> remaining space for the construction of pavilions and terraces. Their form should follow what is appropriate, and you should cultivate the plants around them carefully. In choosing the direction the buildings face, do not be bound by what the geomancer tells you. But in positioning a gateway, it must be square on to the main hall in its courtyard.[3]

In another Ming-dynasty text, *Chang wu zhi,* author Wen Zhen-xiang writes, "1. Buildings 2. Flowers and trees 3. Water and rocks." He refers here to the order in which a Chinese garden is traditionally planned—first the position of the main hall is decided, then the positions of pavilions, terraces, and towers according to the interrelationship of their mutual views. Plants, mountain rocks, and water features are then added, and the various elements linked by covered walkways.

Nature dominates the Japanese stroll garden, while buildings draw little attention and are of secondary importance. This is evident from the simple fact that in Japan a great many gardens remain famous despite the loss of their original buildings. In the Chinese *yuanlin,* the relationship between buildings is of central importance, and a *yuanlin* without buildings would be unthinkable.

Private *yuanlin*—which developed from the *ting yuan*—were built to satisfy a human need for material and spiritual satisfaction. The focal point of the *yuanlin* is the *huating* hall for gatherings and banquets.

Among *huating* styles are the *simianting* (four-sided hall) and the Mandarin Duck hall, but in larger *yuanlin, simianting* are predominant. This building style comprises an open interior space surrounded by a variety of latticework doors—some large, others long and narrow—without any solid walls. It has open walkways all around, creating an uninhibited space that offers a view on each of the four sides (Figure 70).

The Mandarin Duck hall is divided into two rooms,

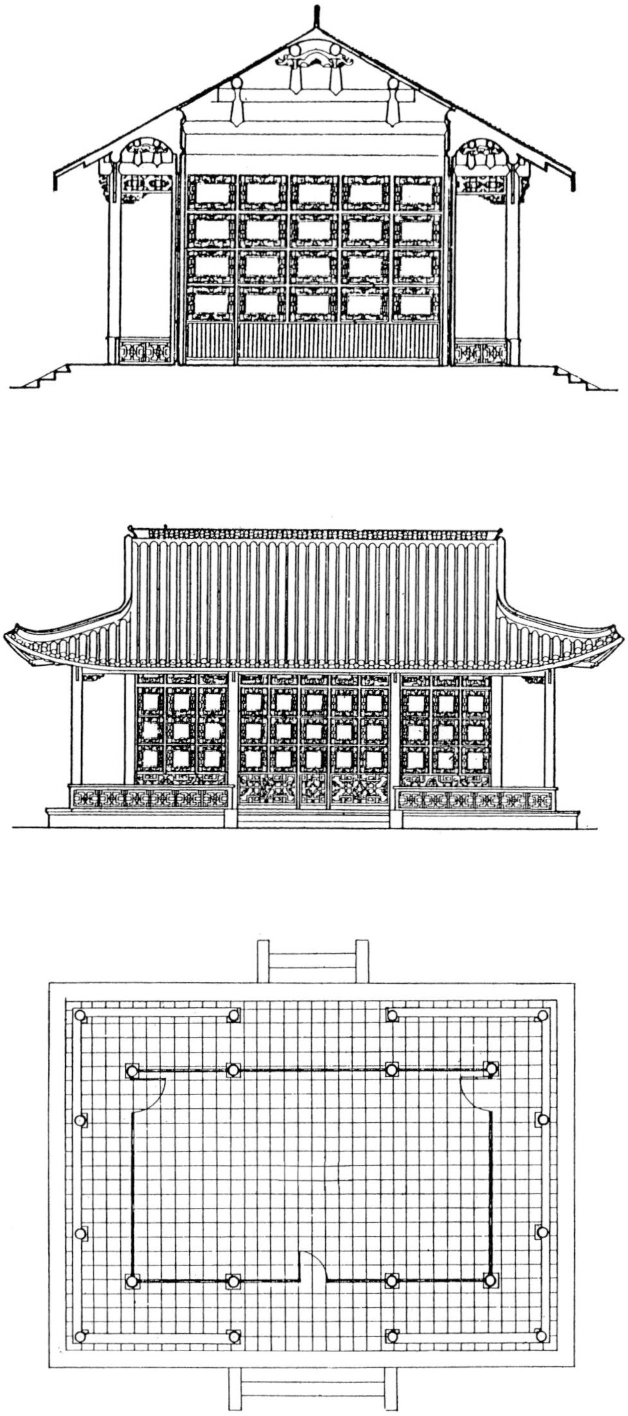

70 Section, elevation, and plan view drawings of a *simianting* (four-sided hall).

front and back, by a sheathed wall with latticework doors. The two rooms are different in ceiling structure and decoration, and are based thematically on different seasons. The room facing south corresponds to winter and spring, and that facing north, to summer and autumn. The gardens facing these rooms are composed accordingly.

A *duiting*, or opposing building, is always constructed as the focal point of each vista. *Duiting* may be halls, chambers, chapels, lodgings, towers, belvederes, pavilions, or other buildings; in many cases these buildings are linked by covered walkways.

The walkway functions not only as a connecting path between buildings, but guides the visitor through the main views of the garden and acts as a device for creating "segmented" scenes.

Qualities of transparency and lightness are intrinsic to the forms of these architectural structures, and the salient characteristic of the technique for composing "segmented" scenes is that these buildings form the pivotal feature.

Huating and *duiting* have a reciprocal relationship, providing borrowed scenery for one another in a series of interdependent views that are both "mutual" and "intersecting." Each building, therefore, becomes an element in landscape composition for others, whether the view be from *huating* to *duiting*, from *duiting* to *huating*, or from *duiting* to *duiting*. For this reason, the central building featured in each view must be both "transparent" and "light" (Figure 71).

The view from inside the building is enjoyed through the latticework surrounding it on four sides, or through open windows. The design of these windows is in keeping with the concept of a utopian realm, since they frame the garden scenery as if it were in a Chinese landscape painting. The famous scenic mountains Lushan and Huangshan are composed of fantastically shaped Tai hu rocks viewed through the frame of this type of window. For such an effect to be successful, the scenery between the *huating* and *duiting*

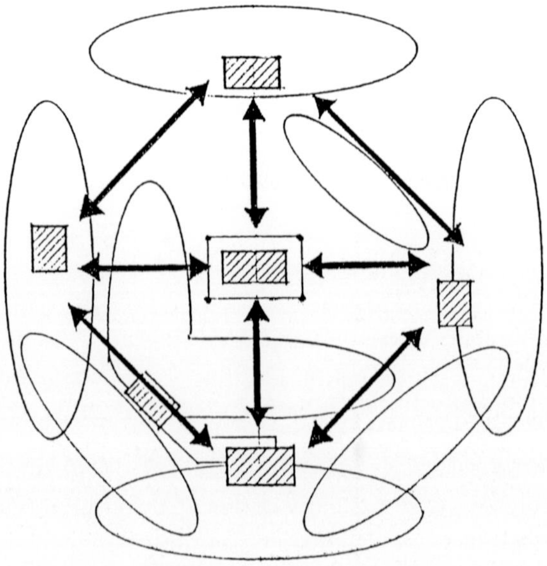

71 Schematic showing the layout of buildings in a *yuanlin* to achieve mutual and intersecting views.

must be highly concentrated, with every inch of space filled (Figures 71.1–71.3).

Screens (Ge) *and Curves* (Qu)

The Japanese stroll garden is a thematically-based series of small garden spaces centered around a pond. It is structured in such a way that as the visitor walks through it, the scenery flows by, with scenes appearing and disappearing sequentially through the use of the compositional technique known in Japanese as *miegakure*.

The Chinese *yuanlin* is also a stroll garden, in which the visitor enjoys different scenes and views while sauntering from the central *huating* to hall, tower, belvedere, and pavilion. Like the Japanese stroll garden, it is composed in the natural landscape–style.

However, as is indicated in the expression *bu-yi jing-yi* ("changing step, changing view"), qualitatively different scenes emerge one by one as the visitor walks, and thus dynamic, contrasting moods and vistas are fundamental means of expression in the Chinese stroll garden.

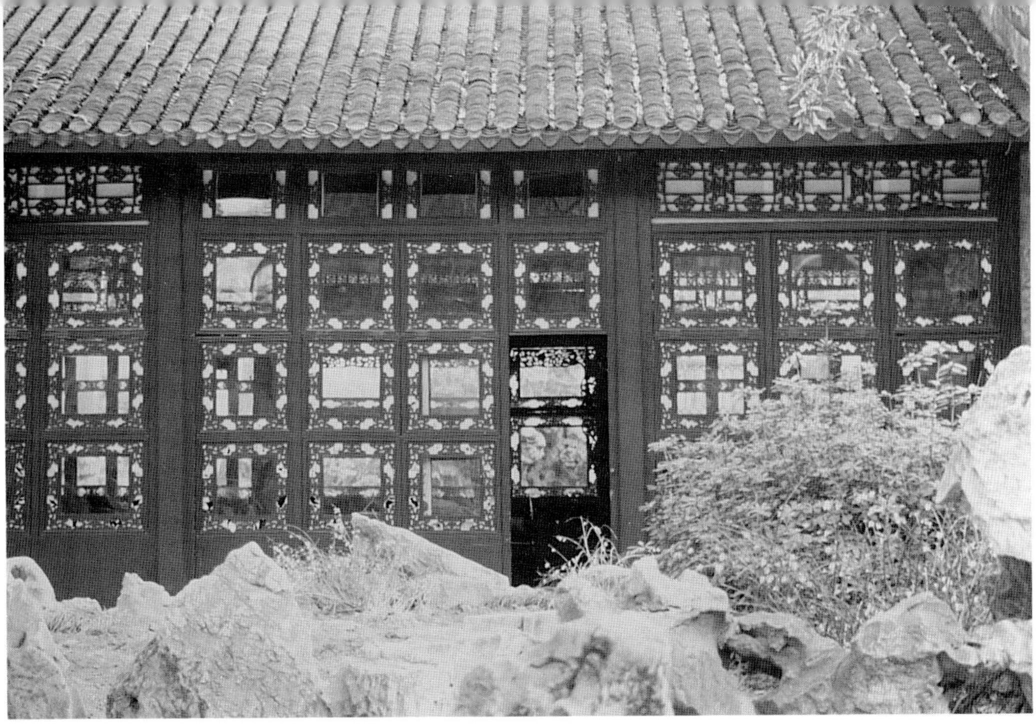

72.1 Latticework doors on the facade of Ge yuan's *simianting* (Yangzhou).

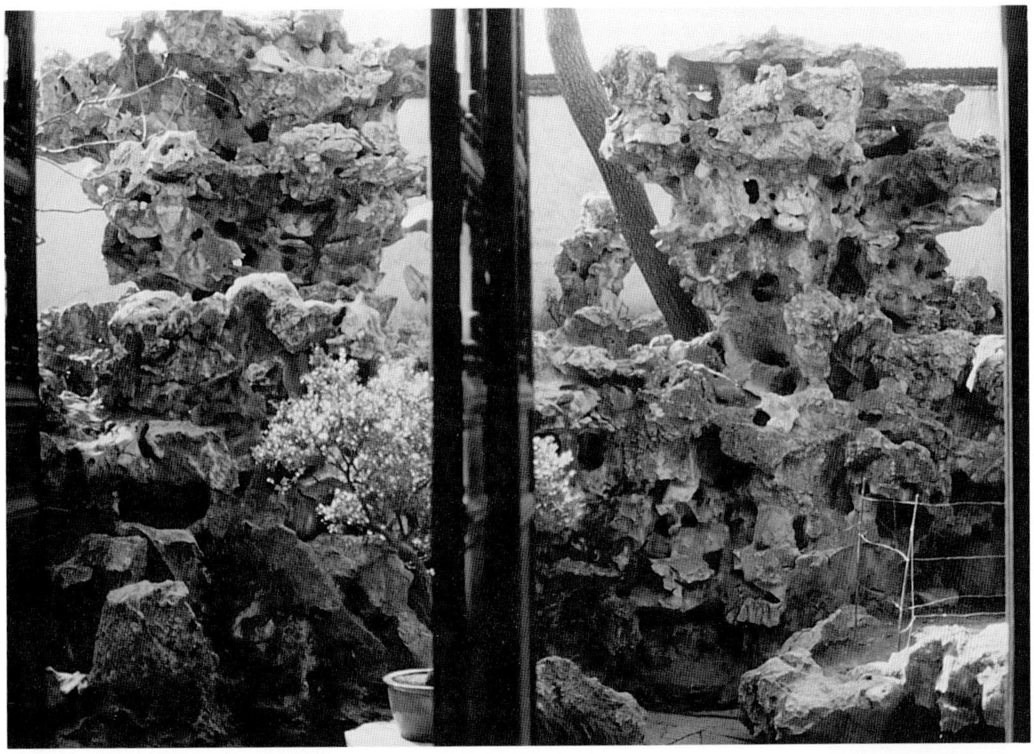

72.2 Fantastically shaped rocks as seen from the Liu yuan *simianting* interior (Suzhou).

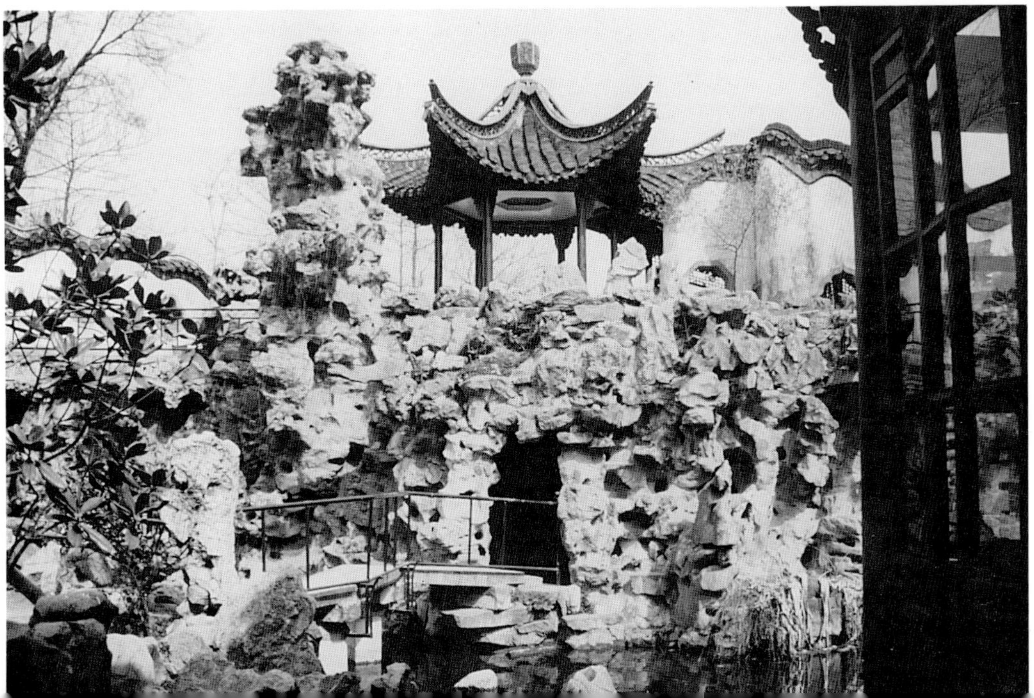

72.3 Mutual views between the *simianting* and a pavilion perched atop a fantastic mountain (Xiao pan qu, Yangzhou).

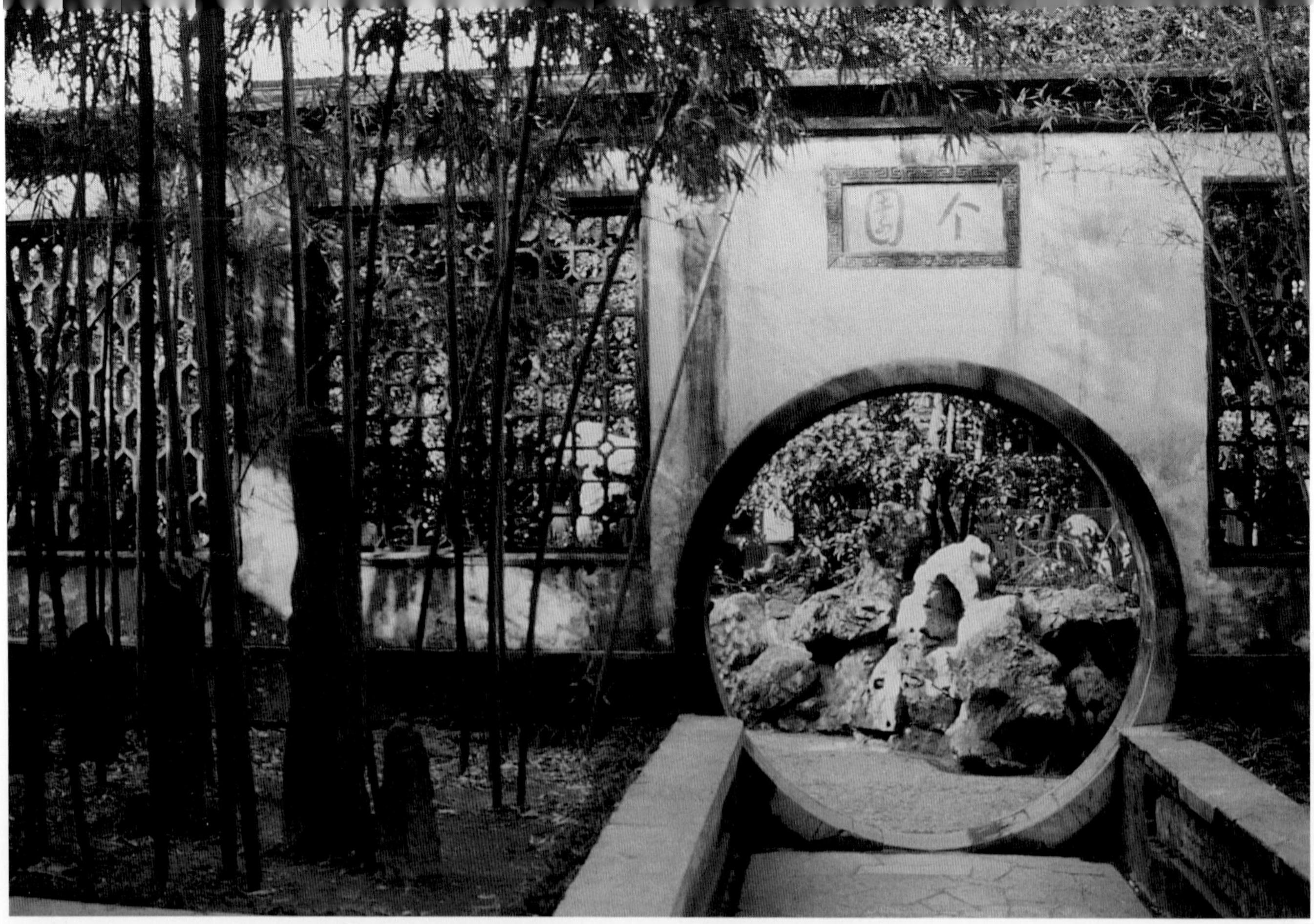

73.1 A gateway used as a screening device to create a distinct garden scene (Ge yuan, Yangzhou).

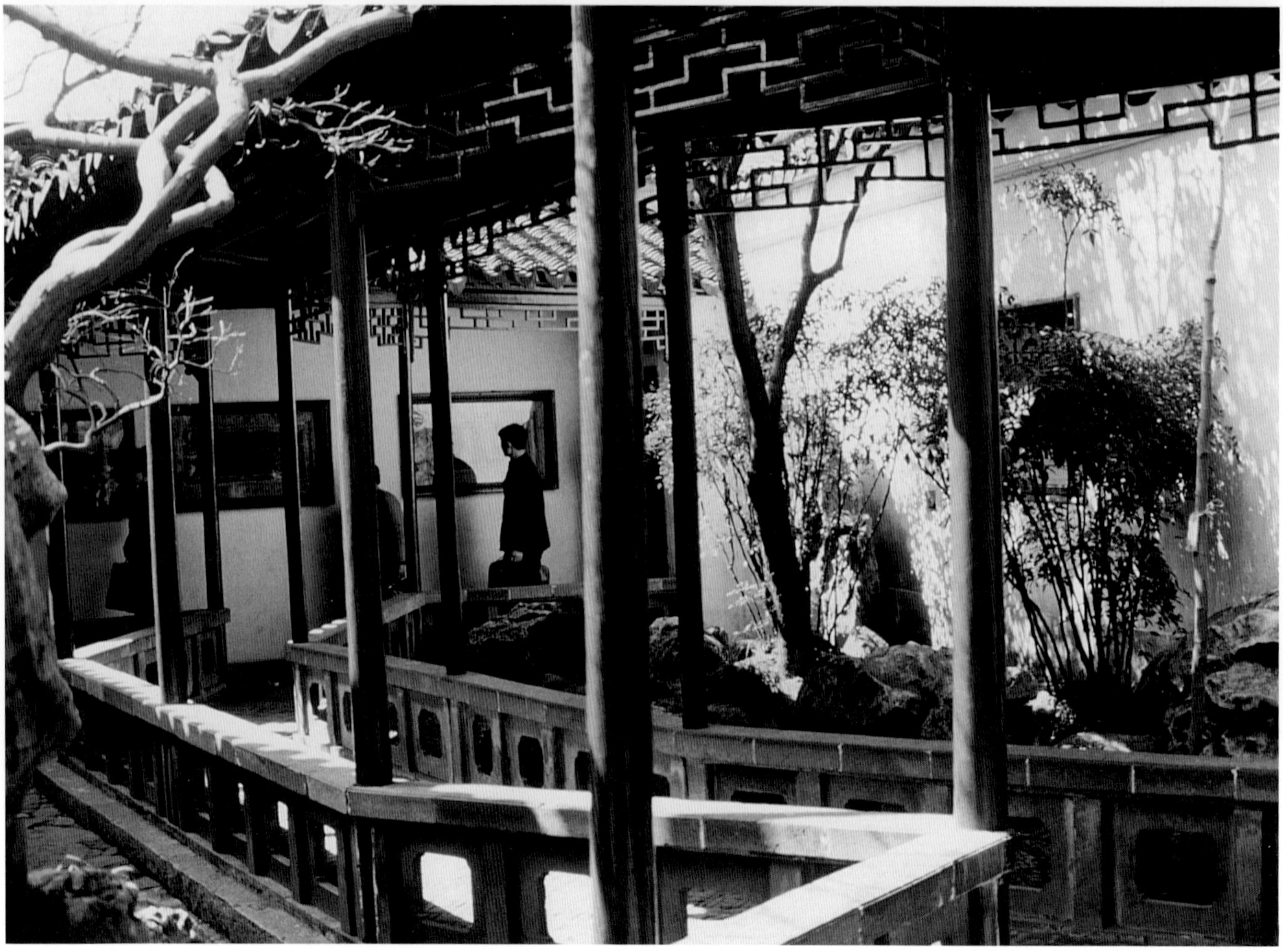

73.2 A covered walkway and wall used as curving and screening devices to create a scenic space cell (Xiao jin shan, Yangzhou).

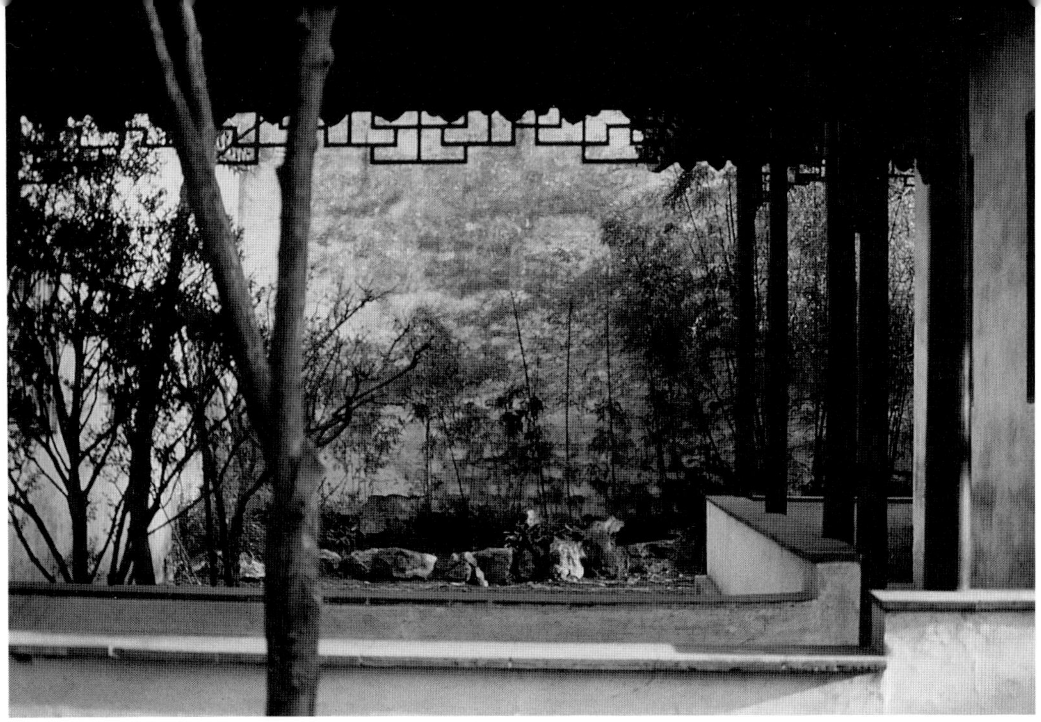

74.1 A "garden within a garden" (Zhuo-zheng yuan, Suzhou).

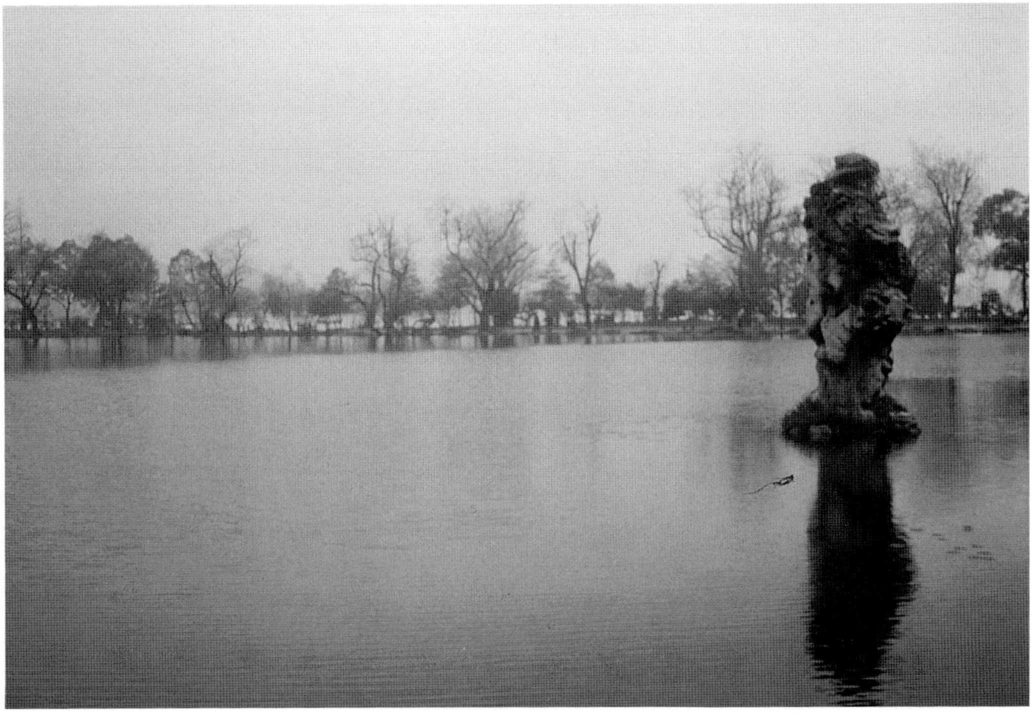

74.2 A "lake within a lake" (West Lake, Hangzhou).

"Screening" and "winding" techniques involving the use of buildings, wall surfaces, fences, caves, gates, and covered walkways divide the entire garden space to create a number of distinct, scenic space cells (Figures 73.1–73.2). Large expanses of water are also converted into a variety of different water features with this method. While these scenes are each different in character, they are also complimentary, and linked into a single environment.

No scene is completely independent of others; each is partitioned and also linked by architectural features—primarily walkways and latticework windows, articulated to prevent oversimplicity or crudeness. This is in direct contrast to the Japanese *miegakure* technique effected mainly with natural elements such as plants. Separate scenes in the Chinese garden are not equal in size; rather the main scenes, forming the core of the garden, cover a larger area and are supported by many smaller scenes providing the necessary opposition. The layout of large and small areas is composed with rhythmical changes juxtaposing expansiveness and concentration. These techniques give rise to expressions such as *yuan zhong you yuan* ("garden within a garden"), and *hu zhong you hu* ("lake within a lake") (Figures 74.1–74.2).

These garden forms, in other words, are an extension

of the idea of *bie you dong tian,* or another world (i.e., the paradise of the Taoist Immortals). Chinese *yuanlin* are composed with ever-changing variety and contrast through the use of garden composition techniques known as *yuan bi ge* ("gardens must have screens") and *shui bi qu* ("water must curve"). The smoother narrative of the Japanese stroll garden can be compared to an "analog" form of expression, in which case the change and opposition marking distinct scenes in the Chinese *yuanlin* would be "digital."

Xie-qu yuan (Garden of Harmonious Interest) in the Yi-he yuan (Garden of Cultured Peace) in Beijing is well known as an example of a "garden within a garden," while the Hua-gang guan-yu (Flower Harbor for Viewing Fish) of Xi hu (West Lake) in Hangzhou is a famous "lake within a lake."

Raising Mountains (Duo Shan) *and Selecting Rocks* (Xuan Shi)

The Chinese *yuanlin* is composed of some views designed to be appreciated from a seated position at chair height inside the buildings, and others designed to be viewed while walking. In the case of Japanese gardens, there was a gradual development from a static, frontal, unidirectional composition in which the garden was viewed from a seated position inside an adjacent building, then first to viewing from two sides, and finally to sequential and even multifaceted compositions as people penetrated and walked through the garden. By way of contrast, the essence of the *yuanlin* centers on interdependent mutual and intersecting views between buildings, so that each element of the garden's composition is multifaceted, multilayered, and kinetic.

The cities in which the greatest concentration of *yuanlin* is seen, particularly in the Jiangnan region, are situated on vast plains, which helped to make the themes of "strange and steep peaks" or "waterfalls dropping from steep cliffs" portrayed in Chinese landscape painting popular elements in garden design. Particularly admired were the fantastic rocks evocative of the "oddly-shaped peaks and strange rocks" of mountainous regions. These rocks of different shapes and sizes had to be "fantastic" in appearance and exude "mystical power," so they were well-suited to the construction of an ideal, otherworldly realm with the *huating* at its center. Garden makers favored vertical compositional techniques such as "layering" (*die*) and "piling up" (*dui*), and pavilions were built on top of piled-up rocks to afford a "high climb, distant view" (*deng gao yuan wang*; Figure 75.1), while caves were cut into layered rocks to provide a space in which to "think meditatively and ponder in silence" (*chen si mo kao*; Figure 75.2).

In Japanese gardens, artificial hills exist as a compositional element used to create scenery, and are not designed to be climbed. Accordingly, they are constructed not to a human scale, but to complement other compositional elements in the scaled-down landscape. In the *yuanlin,* however, mountain features are both part of the scenery and also intended to be climbed, and so they are built to a human scale. In this garden then, the same scale governs both the parts of these natural views and the integrated whole. Rocks are categorized as *tou* (transparent), *shou* (thin), *zhou* (wrinkled, or textured) and *lou* (literally, "leaking"; scattered with small, elongated holes). These criteria for the selection of rocks are a distinctive feature of the materials used in the composition of *yuanlin* (Figure 76).

Borrowed Scenery (Jiejing)

Yuan ye classifies *jiejing,* or borrowed scenery, into four types.

Yuanjie, or "scenery in the distance," includes views of mountain ranges, fields, rivers, and lakes seen from a high vantage point (Figure 77.1). *Linjie,* or "scenery nearby," refers to views of towers, multi-storied buildings, belvederes, and pavilions of adjoining or nearby gardens. *Linjie*

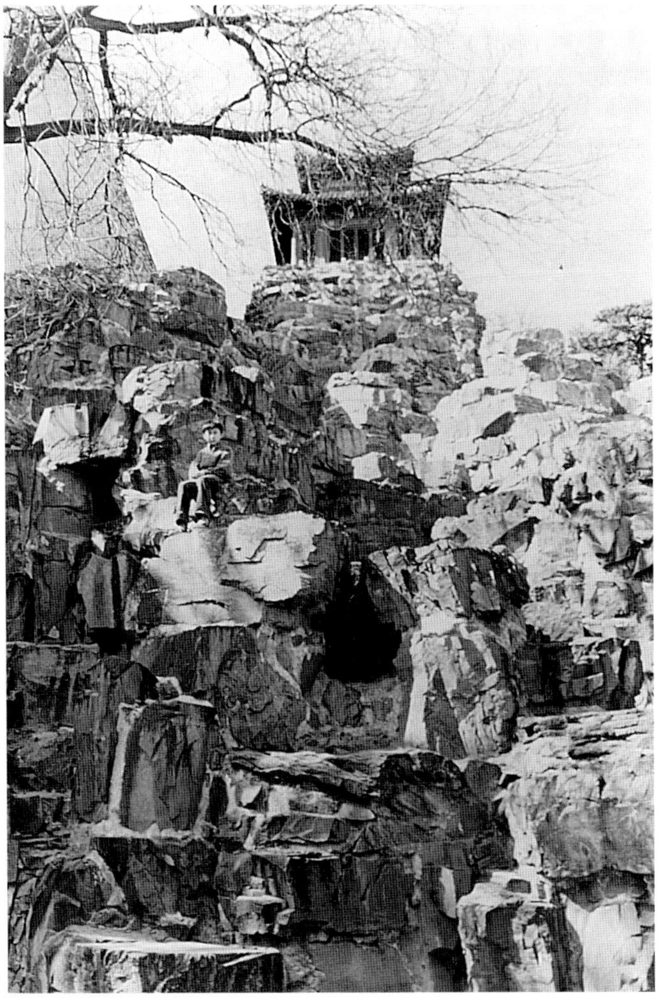

75.1 A pavilion built on top of a piled-rock mountain to afford a "high climb, distant view" (Li yuan, Wuxi).

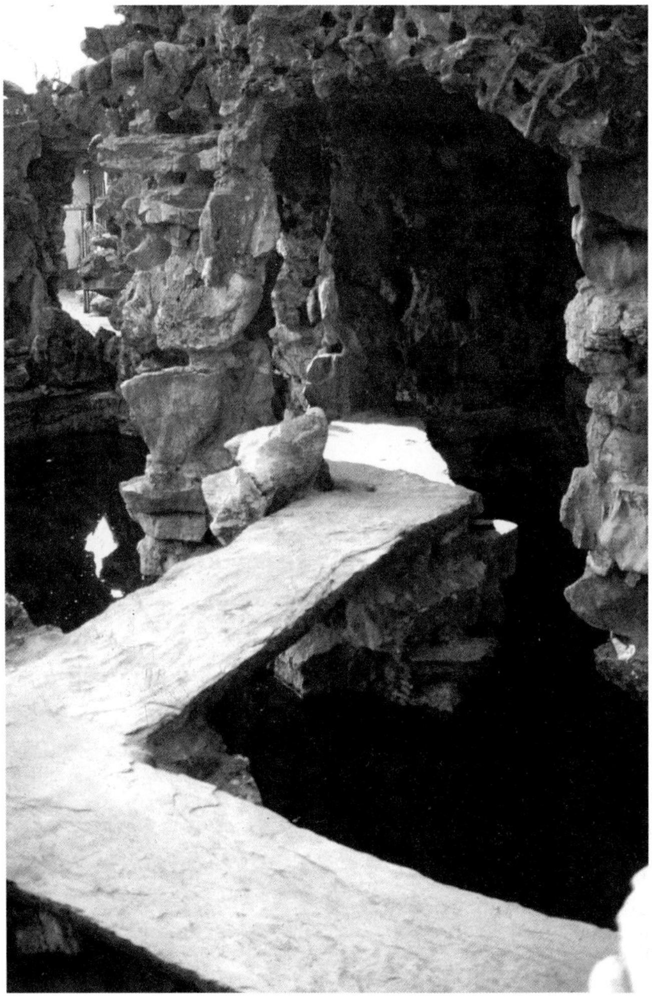

75.2 A cave cut into layered rocks as a space in which to "think meditatively and ponder in silence" (Ge yuan, Yangzhou).

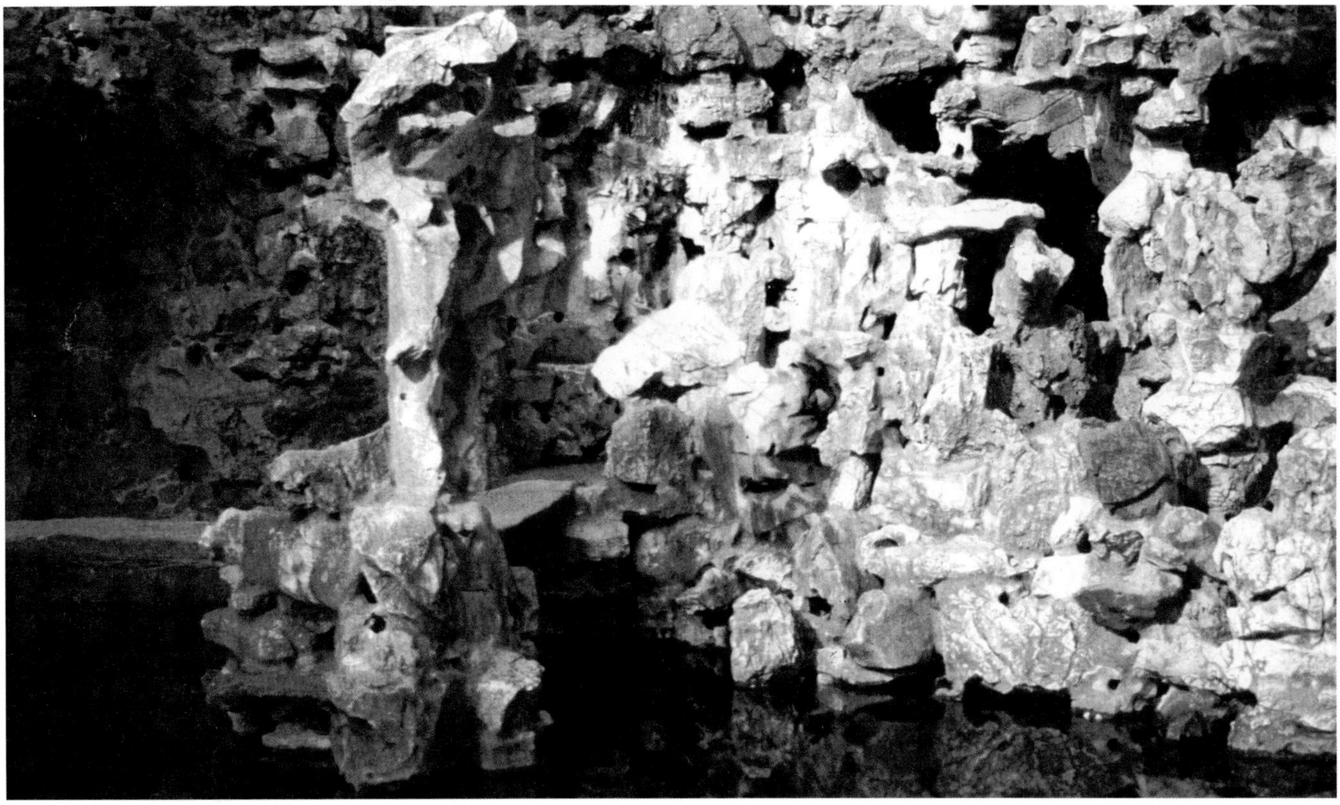

76 A variety of distinctive rocks piled and layered to create mountain features in the *yuanlin*.

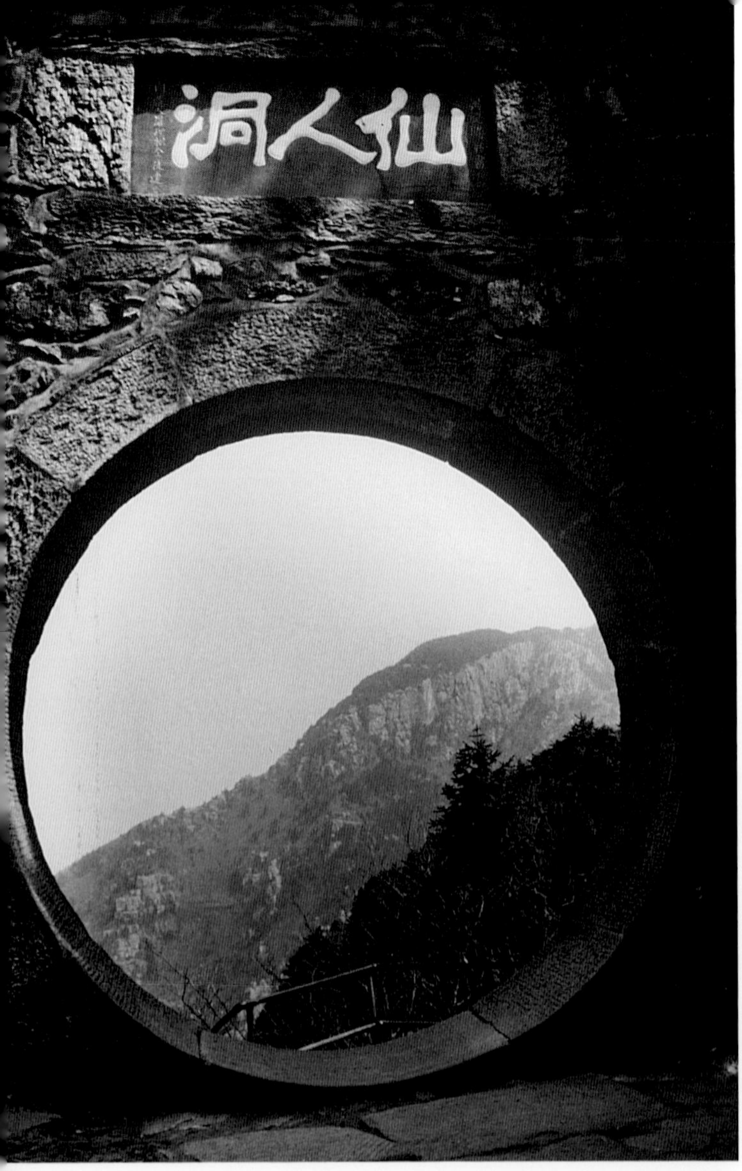

77.1 An open window used to "borrow distant scenery," here the mountain Lushan.

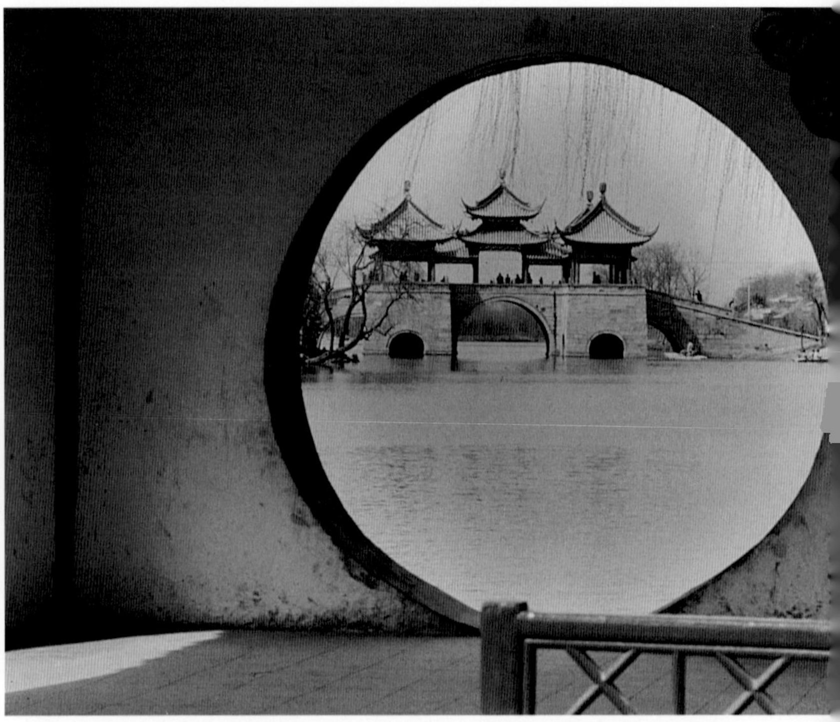

77.2 An open window used to "borrow scenery nearby," in this case the "Five Pavilion Bridge" of an adjoining garden scene (Shou xi hu, Yangzhou).

is mainly the borrowing of buildings as scenery, but the term also refers to views of adjoining garden scenes borrowed through latticework windows (Figure 77.2). *Yangjie*, or "scenery above," describes scenery such as clouds, light, moon, trees, and towers that is viewed by looking up. *Fujie*, or "scenery below," refers to a view of an adjoining garden from above, and is also known as a "stolen view" (*duo jing*).

In the Japanese garden borrowed scenery is distant—for instance, a distant mountain—and is used to impart a sense of the infinite to a comparatively small space, but in the *yuanlin*, the garden within retaining walls is joined to the outside by means of the borrowed view, with the aim being to fuse the garden with the adjoining scenery. In other words, borrowed scenery in the Japanese garden liberates the garden from the confines of its site, while borrowed scenery in the *yuanlin* links one garden scene or "segment" to another.

Private *yuanlin* landscape park gardens developed from the *ting yuan* contemplative landscape garden as an area completely distinct from the everyday living hall and courtyard space. The circumstances under which gardens developed in China suggest that the techniques for constructing *yuanlin* were similar in nature to those used in the garden parks of the nobility. The fundamental purpose of the *yuanlin* was entertainment, which was provided mainly in the *huating*. The *yuanlin* was an expression of the realm of Chinese landscape painting—a real-life version of an ideal world.

6

Ideology and Prototypes

Confucian Thought and Social Structure

The appearance of Confucius toward the end of the Spring and Autumn Period (770–476 B.C.) was the catalyst for the birth of a new culture. A class of Confucian-educated intellectuals became government officials, and with the political life of the nation in their hands a civilian-based feudal order unique to China developed.

During the Han dynasty, Confucianism became the officially recognized state doctrine, and Confucian learning the country's officially recognized form of scholarship, with which the idea of the Confucian state was firmly established. A social and political system based on Confucian ideology was to be the hallmark of the Chinese imperial state for the next two thousand years.

Confucianism and the Emperor

Confucian thought holds that the emperor was given life by the gods who rule the universe, and that he was then charged with responsibility for ruling the earth and governing the people in accordance with the gods' will. It was thought that an immoral or corrupt emperor would be judged by the gods, so the emperor in turn was to act as judge and moral arbiter of people's lives. Since the task of ruling directly over each individual in the state was too much for the emperor to accomplish alone, this responsibility was divided among a number of government officials. Those chosen to be officials were to be the wisest men in the state which, it was hoped, would produce an ideal system of government.

With Confucianism established as the state religion during the Han dynasty, the most able men were gathered from throughout the country and given official appointments after they had passed an oral examination. The Tang inherited this system and established the *keju* system of civil service examinations for candidates from both central and outlying regions.

The Keju *System of Civil Service Examinations*

That someone could enter the civil service with the possibility of advancing to its highest ranks purely on the merits of his Confucian education, rather than through family ties or personal wealth, is indicative of the difficulty of the *keju* examinations, and distinguished anyone who passed the exams as a "learned man." Under these circumstances, having a *shufang* and *huating* became a symbol of an official's learning, and a world separate from that of everyday life was created around these buildings. This was a world accessible only to the educated from which ordinary people were excluded. It is in this social structure that we find the origins of the Chinese *ting yuan* and *yuanlin.*

The *keju* system demonstrated surprising longevity and continued—with modification and changes—to serve as the means of selection of the nation's officials (in lieu of a system of hereditary aristocracy) until 1904. It was over the course of this period that the style of the private *yuanlin* that still exists today first emerged and developed.

What form was the basis, then, for this symbol of the elite? The answer lies in a consideration of the prototype of these exclusive garden spaces.

Prototype of *Ting Yuan* and *Yuanlin*—Chinese Landscape Painting Theory

> ... Though man-made, [gardens] will look like something naturally created ... like a painting ...[1]

> The Chinese garden—from buildings, to mountains and water, plants and trees—is a harmoniously synthesized work of art; it expresses the spirit of poetry and painting. Though man-made, the imitation of mountains and water must become real. Alas, just what is the proper correlation of mountains and water? In short, it should be modeled on nature. Not, however, by merely making scale-reduced scenes from nature, but rather by fully grasping the essential aspects of natural scenery—which is the same principle that applies in painting.
>
> ... [T]rees are not planted to merely provide greenery, but are based on the spirit of painting, that is, they are to express the essence of nature.[2]

These are but short passages from two Chinese garden treatises, but in fact most Chinese theories of garden design start from a concept of the oneness of gardens and landscape painting.

In his book *Zhong guo yuanlin yishu* (The art of the Chinese yuanlin), Chinese garden historian An Huai-qi writes: "The creation of gardens in our country is exactly like literary and pictorial creations, before handling the brush, you have first to fix and determine your spiritual will."[3] Creating a Chinese garden is deemed to be no different than creating a work of literature or a painting, and the creative realm of the garden designer no different than that of the writer or artist. Some works even apply Xie He's "Six Laws" of painting theory to the construction of gardens.

The essence and philosophical context of paintings referred to in Chinese garden treatises relate to the landscape paintings and theories of landscape painting of the Southern Song period, when landscape depiction reached its height of realism and idealism (Figure 78). This vein of painting theory was steeped in Taoist thought and contradicted orthodox painting theories which held that painting was to be valued above all for its use as an "educational tool."

> Now, painting is a thing which perfects civilized teachings and helps social relationships. It penetrates completely the divine permutations of nature and fathoms recondite and subtle things. Its merit is equal to that of the Six Classics, and it moves side by side with the four seasons. It proceeds from nature itself and not from [human] invention or transmission ... Without doubt, [painting] is one of the things which may be enjoyed within the teachings of Confucianism.[4]

The above is excerpted from the introductory chapter, "On the Origins of Painting," from the Tang-dynasty encyclopedic work, *Li-dai ming-hua ji* (Record of famous painters of all the dynasties), compiled in about A.D. 847, which is the main repository of facts about Tang and pre-

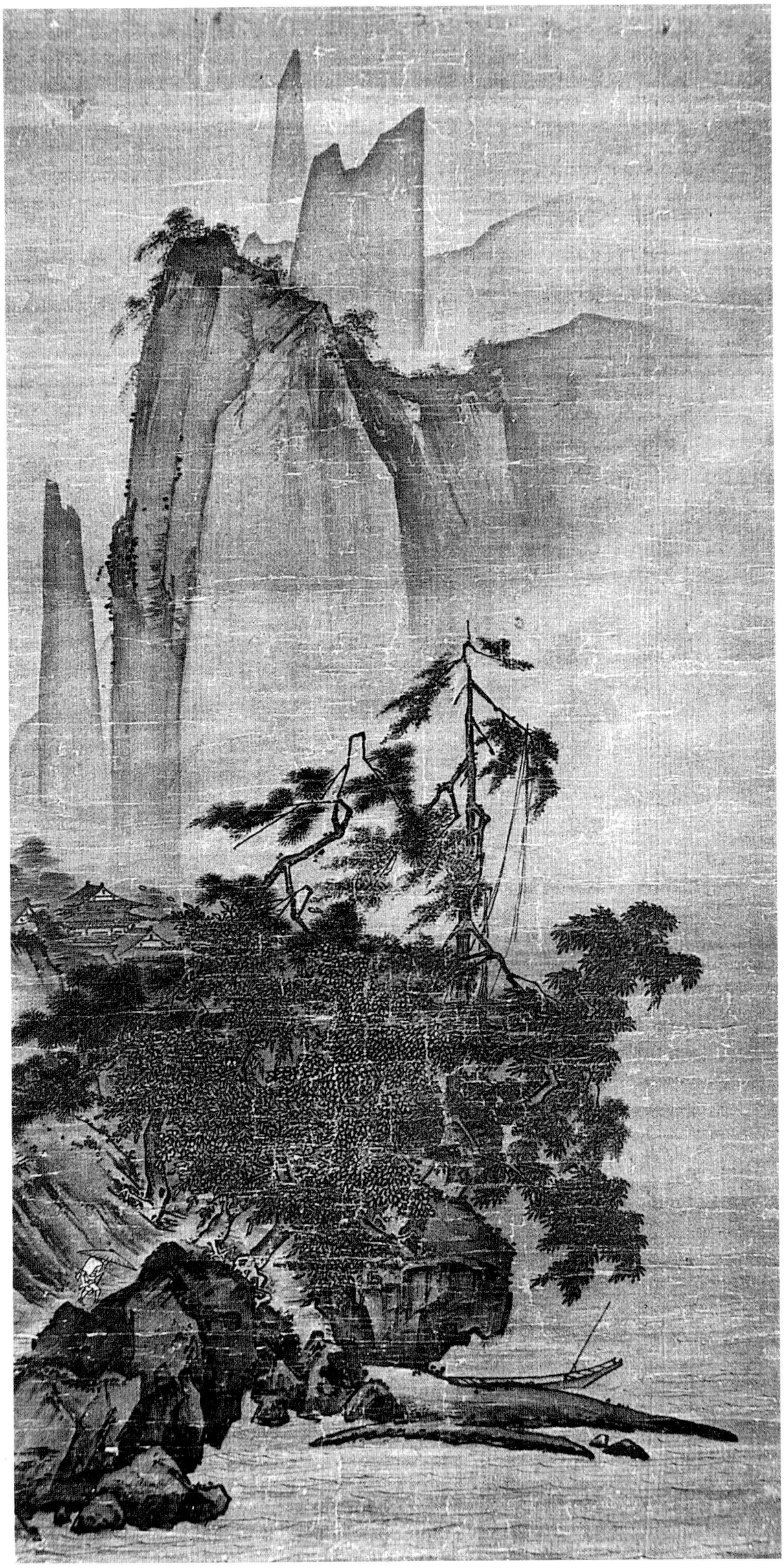

78 A late-Song–dynasty Academy landscape painting by Ma Yuan, *Feng-yu shan-shui tu* (Landscape in wind and rain). The Seikado Bunko Art Museum, Tokyo. National Treasure.

Tang artists. This passage expounds on the idea that the real significance of painting lay in its usefulness as an "educational tool." In the Jin-dynasty (A.D. 265–420) *Lie-nu zhuan fu-juan* (Volume of illustrations for the biographies of heroic women), for example, a subliminal element of didacticism may be detected in genre paintings and paintings of beautiful women.

Li-dai ming-hua ji goes on to comment:

> At that time writing and painting were still alike in form and had not yet been differentiated. Standards for their formation had just been created and were still incomplete. There was nothing by which ideas could be transmitted, hence writing proper came into existence. There was nothing by which shapes could be made visible, hence painting came into being. This was the intent of Heaven, Earth, and the sages.[5]

Statements of this sort suggest that even as the theory of writing and painting as a single entity (that is, painting as a Confucian moral, didactic tool) was developing into one of poetry and painting as a single entity (or painting as an art that transcends formal representation), an undercurrent of utilitarianism and practicality remained fundamental to Chinese painting.

"The concept that helped liberate the appreciation of paintings from their educational role, was that of *woyou* (travel by imagination),"[6] which arose with the advent of landscape painting during the so-called Six Dynasties period (A.D. third through sixth centuries).

> In what does a gentleman's love of landscape consist? The cultivation of his fundamental nature in rural retreats is his frequent occupation. The carefree abandon of mountain streams is his frequent delight. The secluded freedom of fisherman and woodsmen is his frequent enjoyment. The flight of cranes and the calling of apes are his frequent intimacies. The bridles and the fetters of the everyday world are what human nature constantly abhors. Immortals and sages in mists and vapors are what human nature constantly longs for and yet is unable to see.[7]

This idea of *woyou*—of always being close to and enjoying nature—became the pivotal concept underlying landscape painting. It was during this same period that the theory of writing and painting as one (i.e., painting as a didactic tool) developed into a theory of poetry and painting as one (painting as an expressive art), as is suggested in this poem by late–eleventh-century poet and theorist of literati painting (Su) Dong-po (Su Shi):

> When one savors Wang Wei's poems, there are paintings in them;
> When one looks at Wang Wei's paintings, there are poems ...
> [D]u Fu's writings are pictures without forms,
> Han [G]an's paintings, unspoken poems ...[8]

Poems were seen as formless paintings, and paintings as poetry with form. Painting was firmly embedded in the world of literature, and this idea evolved into the primary tenet of Chinese landscape painting.

Landscape painting—its visual and imaginative realms—unfailingly referred to in the introduction of Chinese gardening treatises as the fundamental creative stimulus for garden construction, has its roots in the theory of painting as an expressive art, which in turn is based on the idea of *woyou.* It follows then that the prototype of the private *yuanlin* is found in the circumstances and spirit of Chinese landscape painting (Figure 79). This fact alone, however, does not explain the sharp delineation between the living quarters and the garden, or between the everyday and the unworldly, in the Chinese residence. For this it is necessary to examine the factors linking the origins of *yuanlin* and the concept of *woyou,* by considering the social and

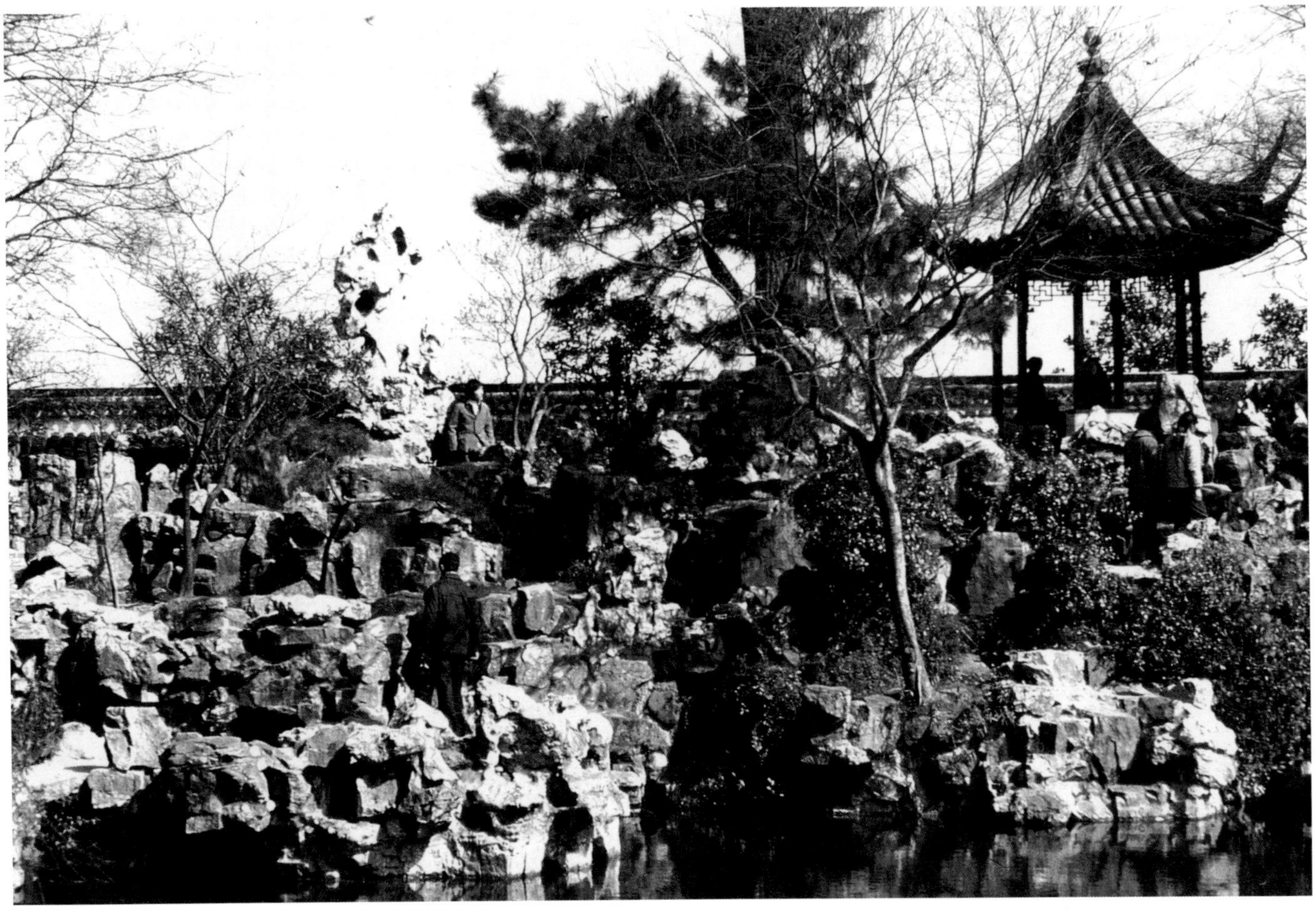

79 A garden scene patterned after the circumstances and spirit of a Song-dynasty landscape painting (Yangzhou).

ideological background of *woyou* and the influence of those factors on the composition of Chinese dwellings.

Landscape Painting Theory and Taoism

The Northern Song–treatise on landscape painting *Lin quan gao zhi xu* (The lofty message of forests and streams), considered the most important of its genre, was written by Guo Xi (after A.D. 1000–ca. 1090), who had studied Taoism in his youth and was the most famous Academy landscapist of his time. In the section of this work titled "*Shan shui xun*" (Advice on landscape painting) Guo discusses the concept of *woyou*:

> It is simply that, in a time of peace and plenty, when the intentions of ruler and parents are high-minded, purifying oneself is of little significance, and office-holding is allied to honor. Can anyone of humanitarian instinct then tread aloof or retire afar in order to practice a retreat from worldly affairs? And, if so, will he necessarily share the fundamental simplicity of [legendary recluses such as [X]u Yu, associated with] Mount [J]i and the River Ying …?
>
> Their songs, such as the "Ode to the White Pony" and the "Hymn to the Purple Fungus" [the latter said to have been composed by the "Four Old Men," who retired from the world in protest against the Qin dynasty, but reemerged to support the Han heir] are of what has passed away and is unattainable. But are the longing for forests and streams, and the companionship of mists and vapors, then to be experienced only in dreams and denied waking senses?
>
> It is now possible for subtle hands to reproduce them in all their rich splendor. Without leaving your room you may sit to your heart's content among streams and valleys. The voices of apes and the calls of birds will fall on your ears faintly. The glow of the mountain and the color of the waters will dazzle your eyes glitteringly. Could this fail to quicken your interest and thoroughly capture your heart? This is the ultimate meaning behind the honor which the world accords to landscape painting. If this aim is not principal, and if the landscape is approached with a trivial attitude, it is no different from desecrating a divine vista and polluting the clear wind.[9]

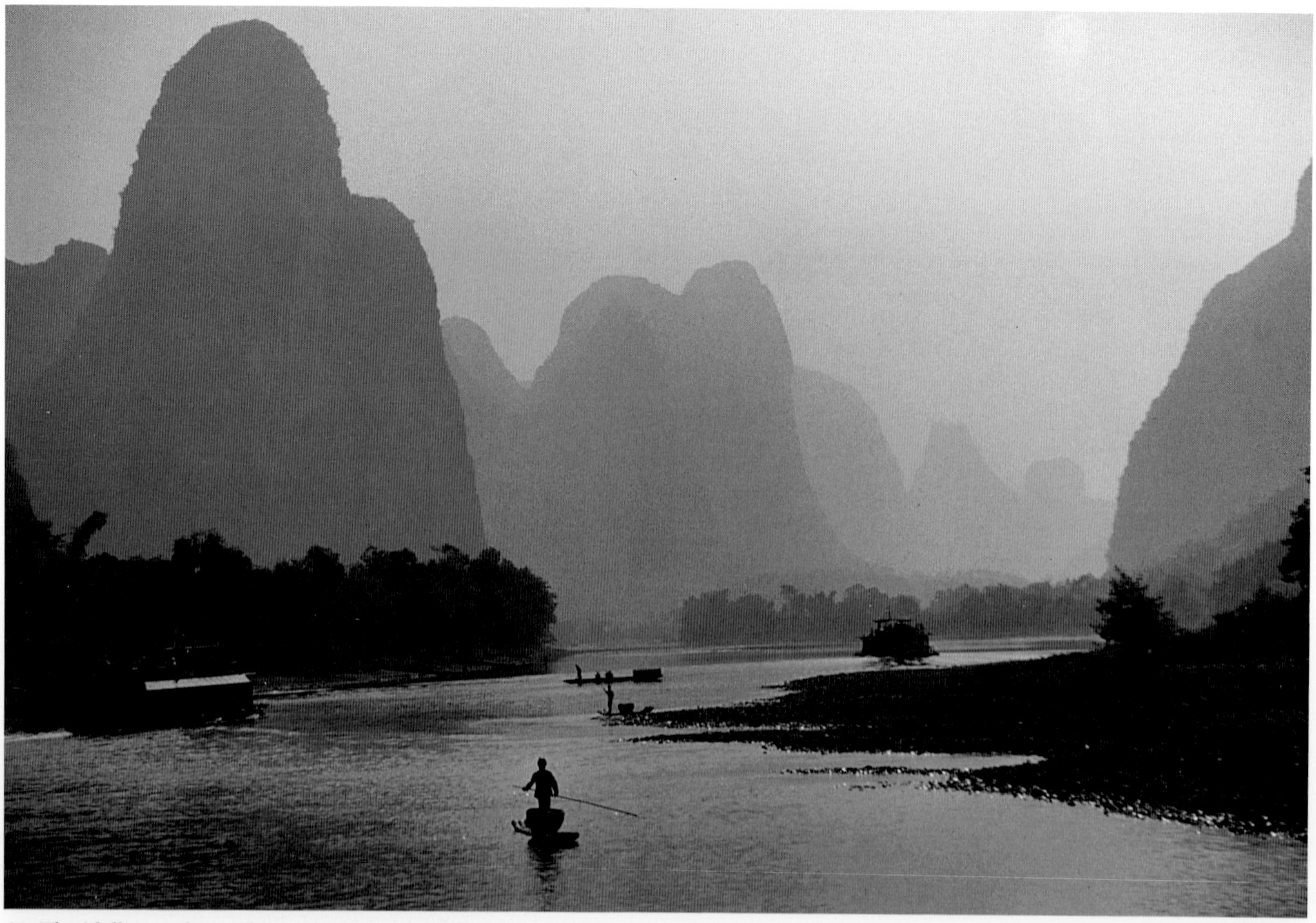

80 The idyllic southern Chinese landscape (Guilin).

The critical aspect of this theory of landscape painting is that the idea of *woyou*—its underlying principle—has seclusion as its ideal state, with Chinese landscape painting as an expression of an ideal world which allows the viewer to "sit to [his] heart's content among streams and valleys." And as expressed in the line "purifying oneself is of little significance, and office-holding is allied to honor," seclusion always stands in opposition to duty and service, with landscape painting playing a part in both realms.

One critic simply states that the theory of Chinese landscape painting "is rooted in Taoist philosophy."[10]

A characteristic of Chinese painting theory is its duality—on the one hand, the objective of painting is to educate or advise in accordance with proper etiquette by Confucian standards, while the Taoist elements of celebrating pleasure and freedom of spirit are also fundamental to the art. This duality has remained the key influence in the development of the theory of Chinese painting. The antithetical philosophies of painting based alternatively on education and *woyou* have both played a part in the formation of Chinese painting theory. The former is the orthodox Chinese thought system based on respect for custom that developed first into a philosophy of morals and later to an emphasis on "education" and "scholarship," and that was established as a social and political creed premised on the teachings of Confucius and Mencius. The latter is related to the idea of *wu-wei*, (non-action, or "no action contrary to nature"), which developed into an opposing philosophy based on the teachings of Lao zi and Zhuang zi.

This idea of seclusion is different from the Japanese concept of a "recluse" in that it bears no relation to the lives of ordinary people, but only to that of the government official. It follows then that the *ting yuan* and *yuanlin*, with their origins in landscape painting theory based on Taoist philosophy, were the domain solely of the educated class (i.e., officials) and for that reason were a symbol of the elite. Obi Kōichi investigates the history of seclusion in his *Chūgoku no inton shisō* (The philosophy of seclusion in China):

> Escape from the duties of service to the state by means of seclusion was a respected lifestyle choice in China from ancient times. A man went into seclu-

sion when he could not carry out his ideas in the way he wanted—in other words when his ideas were at odds with the accepted way of the world. Confucius calls this "the times when our path is not taken." Implicit in this concept of seclusion as escape was reemergence into the world when circumstances improved.

Until the Three Kingdoms period (A.D. 220–265), escape from government service, where the danger of losing one's life was constant, meant quite literally heading for the hills. There was then a shift from this simple flight to a philosophy in which it was considered virtuous to withdraw from the service of the state and go into seclusion when things were not done in accordance with one's beliefs. What had been an issue for the individual became a social custom, the spread of which was encouraged by the ideas of Taoism.

Support for Taoism—The Confucian political principles which were the pillars of the Han empire were a set of rules which reinforced the position of those governing the state. To the person escaping from these rules into seclusion, Confucianism has no meaning—what that person seeks is the freedom of another world. Implicit in this freedom is the need to rid oneself of human artifice and exist within the principles of taking "no action contrary to nature" and being "without self or desire"—the basic philosophy of Taoism. Thus the idea of being "at one with nature" in seclusion came to be much admired.

Shanshui as sanctuary—Gradually the expression for "landscape" (*shanye*; literally, "mountains and fields"), which evoked an image of a wild, inhospitable place, changed to *shanshui*, ("mountains and water"), an expression more evocative of beauty and suggestive of sanctuary.

During the Jin dynasty, the growing popularity of Taoism made people come to think of enjoying oneself in nature as a necessary facet of the educated life of an intellectual. As a result, even for those who did not actually go into seclusion, the act of seclusion in nature was seen as an ideal, and esteemed as a way of finding peace.

The vogue for secluding oneself in natural surroundings gave rise to landscape poetry. Intellectuals actively opposed Confucianism, equating it with the world of the vulgar or "mundane," choosing instead to act in a liberated and uninhibited manner. They set out to challenge the Confucian orthodoxy, with a philosophy exemplified by the "Seven Sages of the Bamboo Grove," who advocated "escape from the constraints of custom." This is clearly a movement for human liberation. The proponents of this philosophy of freedom placed themselves outside of and ignored the accepted conventions, since these conventions represented the world of officialdom rooted in Confucian principles.

The scope of what was counterposed against seclusion expanded from officialdom to include the human world in general. The natural world came to be seen as the one with value, and as this viewpoint gained influence, nature and natural objects (*shanshui*) were termed by the Taoists *ziran* (literally, "that which is so of itself"), and perceived as superior to the "mundane" social world.

Truth and beauty—The rural poet Tao Yuanming declared in the late Jin dynasty that truth could be found in the objects of the natural world. Landscape poet Xie Ling-yun looked at nature with admiration and declared that he could sense its "beauty."

This perception of truth and beauty in nature—a product of Taoist philosophy and the idea of seclu-

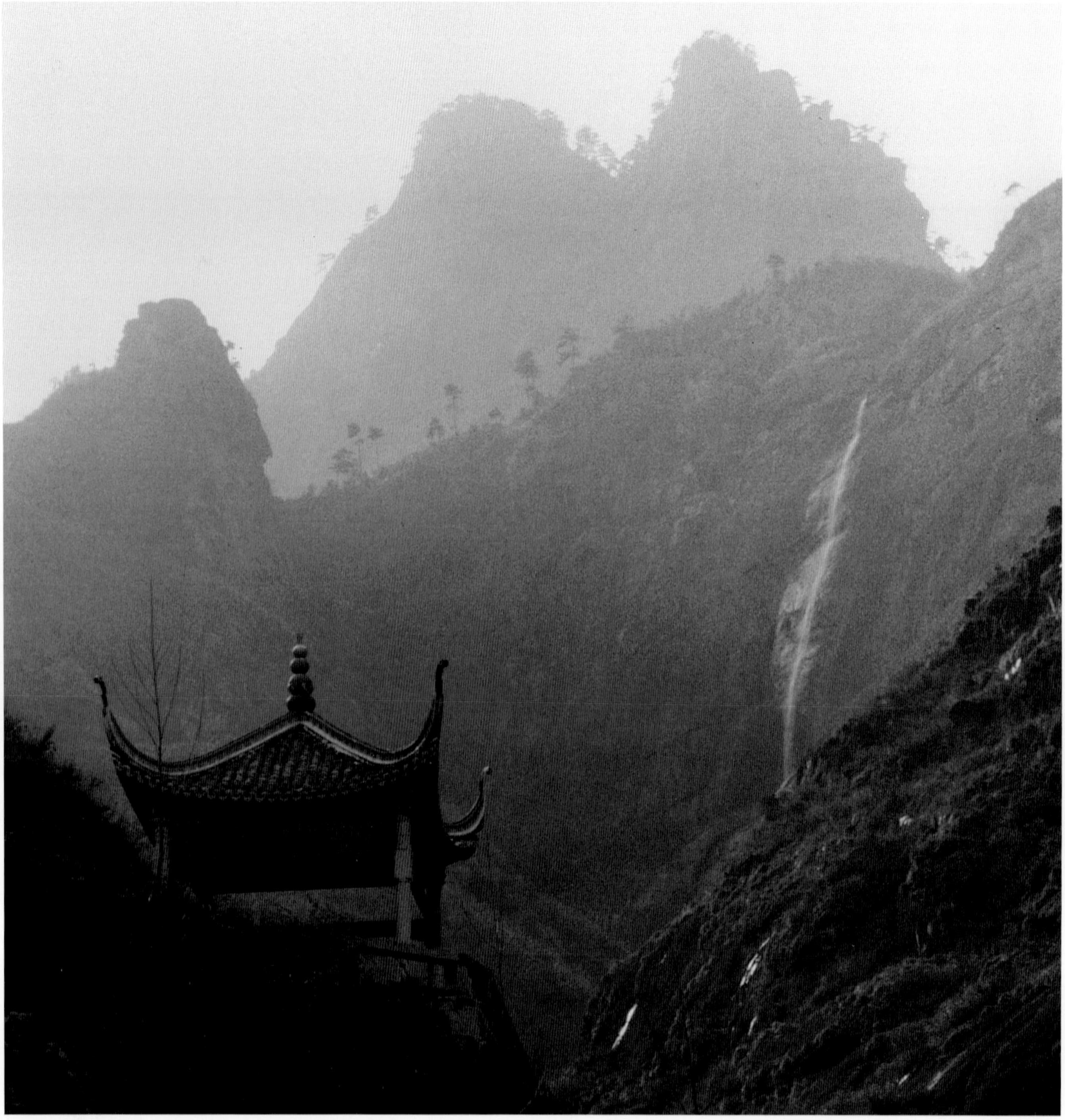

81 A celebrated "waterfall dropping from steep cliffs" scene from nature (Lushan).

sion—spread during the latter half of the fourth and first half of the fifth centuries, taking root thereafter as the traditional Chinese way of looking at nature. By the Tang dynasty, there were people who posed at being in seclusion, with an eye on obtaining a position in the government—pragmatists who used seclusion as a means of entering politics. The development of seclusion into a means of attaining an official position is a surprising turn of events, given the origins of the practice.[11]

This passage charts the development of a view of the natural world whereby escape from official life was an anti-Confucian statement and a form of release from the constraints of the mundane, and seclusion was key to the perception of nature as a worthy object of admiration, the embodiment of truth and beauty. In the realm of the arts, this concept of seclusion was invariably linked to landscape painting as part of the unified entity of poetry and painting.

However, as was noted above, seclusion was also used

by officials to achieve their own more worldly objectives, a fact of major significance for this study, since the extant *yuanlin* constructed during the Ming and Qing dynasties are not direct reflections of *woyou* or of the ideology of the period in which this theory of landscape painting was developed, but products of a "prototype" of landscape gardens formed over a thousand-year period.

The concept of the *yuanlin* as a garden form separate from reality developed from the Taoist idea of *wu-wei*, or "non-action," which arose to challenge the orthodoxy of Confucian social and political thought, giving rise in turn to the concept of *woyou* upon which landscape painting theory and the theory of painting as an expressive art are based.

The idea of seclusion was developed using compositional elements from the natural world to create a style of garden scenery in which views of mountains and valleys "could be enjoyed without leaving one's seat." The prototype for these gardens was found in poems and paintings; however, during the Ming and Qing dynasties, as social conditions reduced the idea of seclusion to a shell of its former self, the interpretation of "seclusion in nature" became one formalized, widely recognized style. Techniques of garden construction such as those outlined in *Yuan ye* are thought to have developed freely in the private *yuanlin* which survive today, within the framework of the prototype of this style.

Hierarchical Dwelling Composition

The traditional composition of Chinese dwellings, whereby a number of units are joined to form a residential complex is a design influenced by a feudal patriarchy rooted in a class system. Confucianism was key to the maintenance of this feudal order. As explained earlier, Confucianism became the orthodox system of thought in Chinese history, developing from a respect for custom to a values system based on filial piety, then to "education" and finally to "scholarship." It was a political system in which everyone, from the emperor down to the lowliest commoner, had their place in the order of things, so it was only natural that a hierarchy of residential units—from the communal, housing an extended family centered around the *citang* (ancestral shrine), to individual units—should, along with the class system, become an element in the composition of villages and residential complexes.

In the Beijing *siheyuan*, the central *zheng fang* was reserved for the head of the household and housed the ancestor room; *erfang* on either side were for female children; *xiang fang* to the left and right were for the first and second sons; and the *dao zuo fang* was for the younger sons or the servants. Of all the buildings in the complex, the inner hall facing south was the highest ranking, followed by those to the left and right and the one in front. In Huizhou residences the innermost row (*jin*) was the most important, and the ancestor room was placed in the center of the middle row.

This "sacred" order based on Confucian principles was—in the context of the Taoist idea of being unconstrained by custom—"mundane."

The "Mundane" and the "Unworldly"

The *keju* examination system for entering government service was part of the mundane world. During the early Qing dynasty, there existed also a system known as *zhike*, which worked in parallel with the *keju* system. The *zhike* was a system which relied not on examinations, but on promoting people who were in seclusion. This was known as "the course of seclusion in the mountains and forests."[12]

Even in light of the prevailing orthodoxy, the government intellectuals who had passed through the *keju* system and themselves functioned within a mundane world saw no contradiction in the parallel existence of a "way of seclusion." During the thousand-year period that followed the establishment of the *keju* system, philosophical developments led to the acceptance of these seemingly contradictory methods of recruitment.

Areas for everyday living took on standardized forms as the "mundane" corresponding to the Confucian order, while areas removed from everyday life—the *ting yuan* and *yuanlin*—became stylized, "unworldly" realms in accordance with the elements of landscape painting. Everyday living space was then a tangible manifestation of the Confucian-based patriarchal system with custom as its prototype, while the unworldly realm of the *yuanlin* was a stylization of the visual and philosophical realms of landscape painting which had the Taoist concept of *woyou* as its prototype. Neither of these contrasting areas overpowered or absorbed the other: instead, from them arose a style of building composition in which they coexisted as representations of their respective prototypes.

Korea

7

Traditional Korean Residences and Their Gardens

Traditional Korean gardens are said to always have an "untouched" or "natural" appearance.

> People taking a strictly Japanese view might say that there is no such thing as a formal garden in the Korean tradition. They would also say that there is really no artificial ornamentation in traditional Korean architecture. All a Korean garden consists of, they would claim, is enclosing the necessary area with lengths of carved granite or walling off an area of sloping ground. The far side of the garden might feature a lone tree and one or two strangely shaped rocks. However, the true character of the Korean garden can be seen in the rear garden of the Ch'ilgung Palace at the foot of Mount Pukak in Seoul. This is not a garden in the usual sense, but merely a part of the hillside around which a wall has been built to bring it into the orbit of the palace buildings.[1]

> ... This was not the work of architecture scholars or landscape architects who had traveled to foreign lands to study [the art of landscape architecture]. It displays a purely natural and native skill and requires no explanation to be understood.
>
> ... Unfortunately, these gardens have been defiled by people who ... have abandoned the traditions of their ancestors. When we look at these and other famous gardens today, they have inevitably lost all sense of being untouched due to the indiscriminate introduction of Japanese gardening techniques developed for the representation of nature in miniature.[2]

The above quotations are taken from *Han'guk mi ŭi t'amgu* (A study of Korean beauty) by Kim Wŏn-yong, and *Han'guk ŭi p'ung'a* (The elegance of Korea) by Ch'oe Sunu respectively. As they both demonstrate, the overt forms, the expressive techniques, and the *raison d'etre* of Korean gardens are completely distinct from those of Japanese, or Chinese, gardens.

Most traditional Japanese garden forms—the Zen temple, *shoin*, and *sukiya*—were invariably designed with the primary aims of unifying the building interior and exterior and providing a view for a person sitting inside an adjacent room to gaze out onto. The stroll garden first created in the Edo period was intended to be "walked," and therefore developed from a predominantly outdoor perspective. In both cases, regardless of the garden's size, the environment achieves an overall unity of space based on the relationship between inside and outside; this approach has been adopted widely in the composition of homes and gardens of the common people.

The manifest form of the traditional Chinese residental garden—designed to be admired from inside a room—bears no relation to the basic hall and courtyard composition that forms the infrastructure for daily living. In China, gardens are completely removed from the business of ordinary life, which is reflected in their being built independently from the living spaces. These gardens were strolling gardens—the *ting yuan* (contemplative landscape garden) and the larger *yuanlin* (landscape park garden)—centered around a *shufang* study and *huating* banquet hall, and were symbols of high social status exclusive to aristocratic families as well as literati, governing officials, landowners and the *nouveau riche.*

Whereas the garden in Japan was somehow linked to people's daily activities, Chinese culture created the *yuanlin* as an exclusive place quite apart from everyday living spaces.

If we define a garden in one or the other of these traditions, the Japanese or the Chinese, then it would have to be said that gardens did not exist in the traditional Korean residential setting.

A number of uniquely Korean "conditions"—not present in either Japanese or Chinese settings—underpin the layout of traditional Korean homes and gardens. Since the formation of the Korean building/garden environment as a whole is based on these very conditions, they produce a number of fundamental factors that affect the composition of Korean dwellings.

Influences on the Composition of Traditional Korean Residences

The practices and customs that have developed in the historical circumstances and social environment of the Korean peninsula have influenced not only the way Koreans live their lives but the way that they have composed their dwellings. There are five basic factors that influence the form of the residential environment. These are: location (factors based on the geomantic principles of *p'ungsu*), social status (factors based on the traditional hierarchical class system), social mores (factors based on Confucian principles), function (factors based on the *ondol* system of heating), locality (factors related to the dwelling's locale [urban versus rural]).

The composition of all traditional Korean dwellings is based on a combination of these five factors, which are discussed in greater detail below. The focus of this research is on extant dwellings and gardens, so the investigation of these factors here is limited to the six hundred–year Chosŏn period (A.D. 1392–1910).

Location: Factors Based on the Geomantic Principles of *P'ungsu*

One of the strongest impressions that visitors to China remark on is the enormous number of bicycles in Beijing, Shanghai, and the other major cities. Visitors to Korea, on the other hand, are often surprised at how few people they see riding bicycles in Seoul, Pusan, or Kyŏngju. This contrast reflects the fundamental difference between the two countries in terms of the topography of the cities, towns, and villages.

The Korean Peninsula is a region of undulating but relatively low mountains and hills scattered with numerous small basins of flatland. Approximately seventy-five percent of the terrain is mountainous, but there are not many fast-running streams or rivers. Similarly, about seventy-five percent of the settled land in Korea stands at the foot, or on gentle southern slopes, of mountains or hills. Indeed, the rustic charm of farming villages nestled on

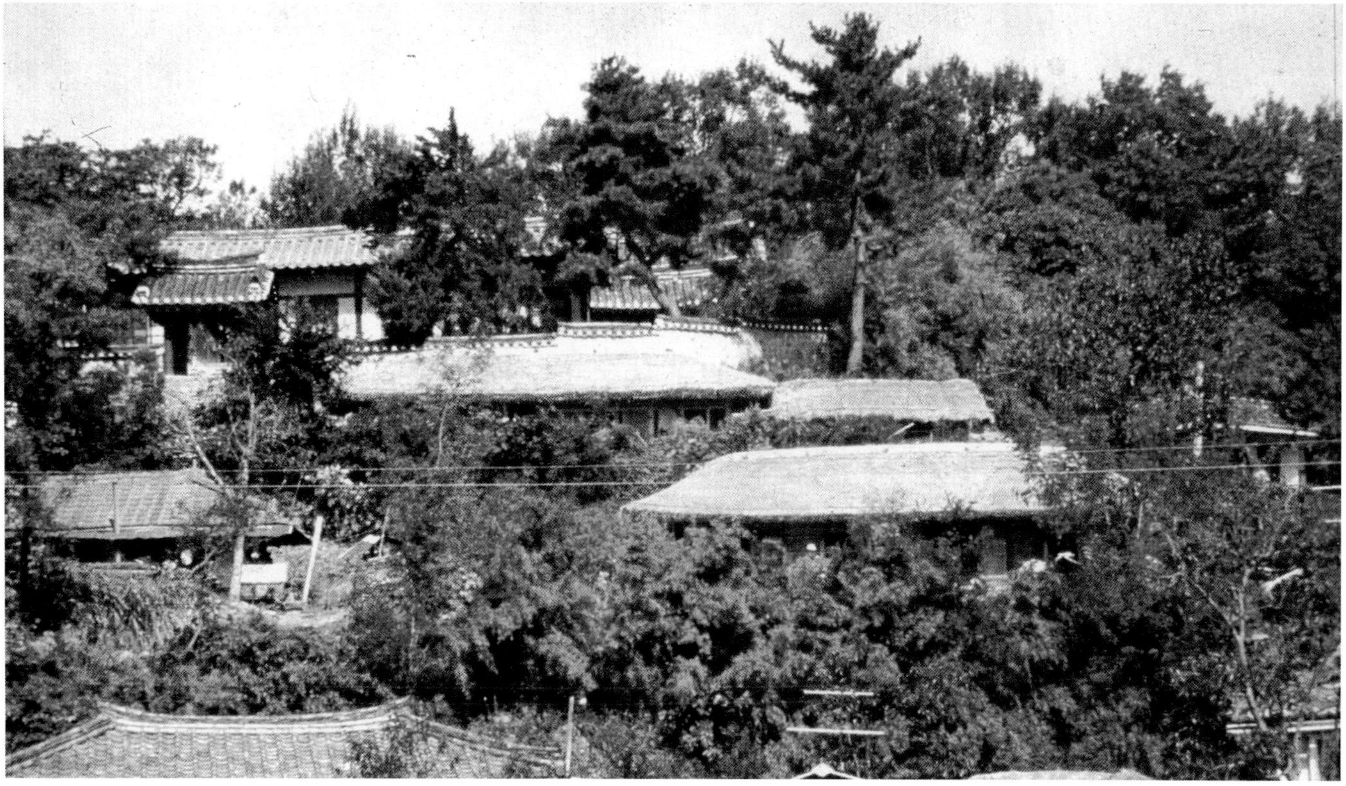

82 A rural village (Yangdong, Wŏlsŏng district).

sunny southern slopes is a recurring theme in traditional Korean poetry (Figure 82).

The Forbidden City in Beijing was built on a broad plain against a man-made mountain backdrop. The buildings are laid out on a straight axis that starts at the Gate of Divine Prowess in the north and continues through the Hall of Earthly Peace, the Hall of Union and Peace, the Palace of Heavenly Purity, the Hall of Protective Harmony, the Hall of Medium Harmony, and the Hall of Supreme Harmony, and then even beyond the great square outside the Gate of Supreme Harmony, across the man-made Jin-shui Channel, all the way to the Meridian Gate. A large expanse of flat land, extending one kilometer from north to south, has been artificially reshaped on a majestic scale.

The terrain of Seoul, the capital of South Korea, on the other hand, is completely different. Seoul is a city of hills and slopes. Kyŏngbok Palace, located at the center of the city, stands against the soaring backdrop of Mount Pukak to the north and overlooks the broad Han River to the south—with the mountain behind and river in front fulfilling the conditions for *myŏngdang* land, or choice sites (Figure 83). Both Beijing and Seoul represent the ideal of a city that faces south with a "mountain behind and river in front," but the former was achieved artificially, while the latter was built on land carefully selected for its natural features.

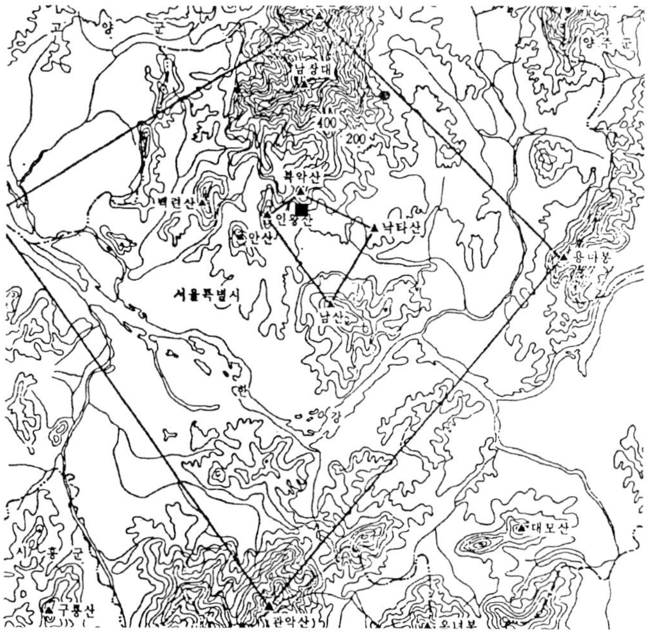

83 Topographical map of the Seoul area, with Kyŏngbok Palace at its center.

The theory behind the selection of "mountain behind, river in front" locations as suitable residential sites, and other favorable and unfavorable land characteristics, is based on geomancy, known as "*p'ungsu*" in Korea, and "*feng shui*" in China, where the term originates. *P'alyŏkchi* (Record of eight districts) describes the six requisite factors that comprise a positive dwelling site: water source, vital force of the land, shape of the mountains, color of the soil, hydrography, and balanced prospect over water

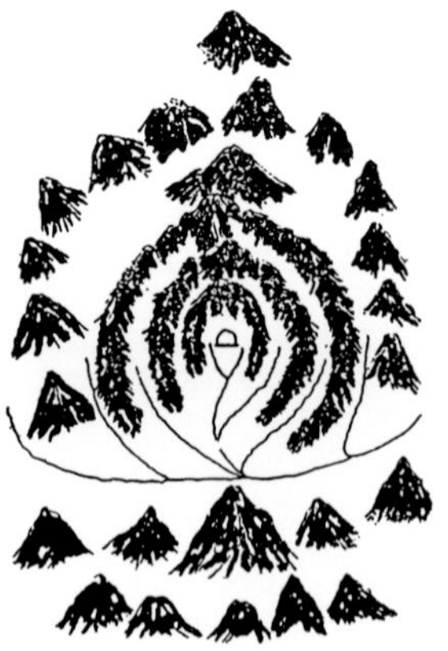

84.1 Favorable topographical conditions according to *p'ungsu.*

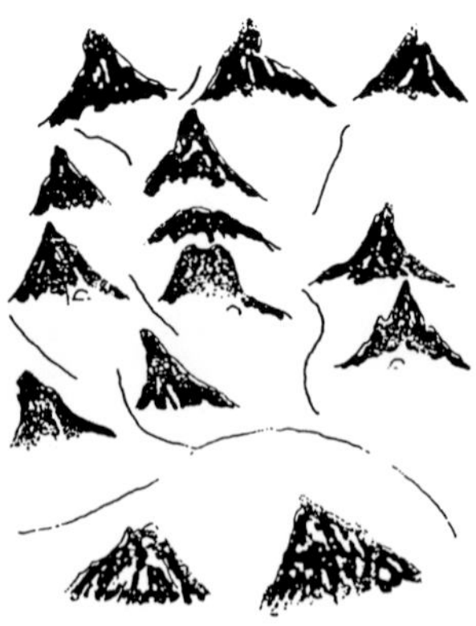

84.2 Unfavorable topographical conditions.

and mountains.[3] The characteristics that define a positive site are actually based on extensive real experience and on extremely straightforward, practical considerations of what constitutes a comfortable place to live (Figures 84.1–84.2).

The principles of *p'ungsu,* it is said, "developed under the influence of the ancient theories of yin and yang and the five basic elements, dating back thousands of years in China, took root in Korea during the Koryŏ period (A.D. 935–1392) and spread widely among the common people during the Chosŏn period."[4] In fact, beliefs about what, according to the principles of *p'ungsu,* makes a dwelling site suitable, became more influential in Korea than they had ever been in China; they became a fundamental factor in the composition of all Korean homes and gardens. This probably occurred because the distinctive topographical character of the Korean landscape was so well suited to the adoption of these principles.

The sites of such principal cities as Seoul and Kaesŏng were selected in accordance with the principles of *p'ungsu,* as were the sites and layouts of rural villages and even individual homes. Accordingly, most Korean towns and cities were built on southern slopes, surrounded by mountains or hills, and bounded on the south by rivers. The same was true of smaller communities as well. Private residences of wealthier Koreans were also constructed on southern slopes. A series of stone steps generally led up northward to the main gate, which faced south, as did the *taech'ŏng,* or the central living room of the main building. Moreover, the rear garden, which was exclusively for the family's private use, stood at the northern end of the compound and sloped toward the south, very often in a series of terraces. Finally, at the site's northernmost and highest point was a mortuary shrine dedicated to the family ancestors (Figures 85.1–85.2).

Selection of a favorable location according to the principles of *p'ungsu* typically provided a setting which "naturally" dictated both the position of the dwelling and the layout of the compound. *P'ungsu* is therefore one of the fundamental factors underlying the composition of Korean homes and gardens.

Social Status: Factors Based on the Traditional Hierarchical Class System

The village of Yangdong in the Wŏlsŏng district, about four kilometers (2.5 miles) south of Kyŏngju, is a treasure trove of traditional rural dwellings. Farmers' homes are scattered among low pine trees on the southern side of a medium-sized hill. Looming over all, near the summit of the hill and surrounded by a wall, is a particularly impressive estate, which is home to a *yangban* (civil or military official).

In order to clarify the importance of social status in the composition of traditional Korean homes and gardens, it is necessary here to examine the class system that set the *yangban* above all their neighbors, as well as the relationship of that class system to the Confucian ideas that served to maintain order in traditional Korean society.

The Centralized Feudal System

Chosŏn, as the kingdom was called, was a highly centralized feudal state, in which noble families and Buddhist temples were forbidden to own large parcels of land. Instead, agricultural land was distributed under a unique system codified in the *kwanjŏnpŏp* (rank land) law.

This law decreed that all land belonged to the state and was to be meted out to individual farming families by

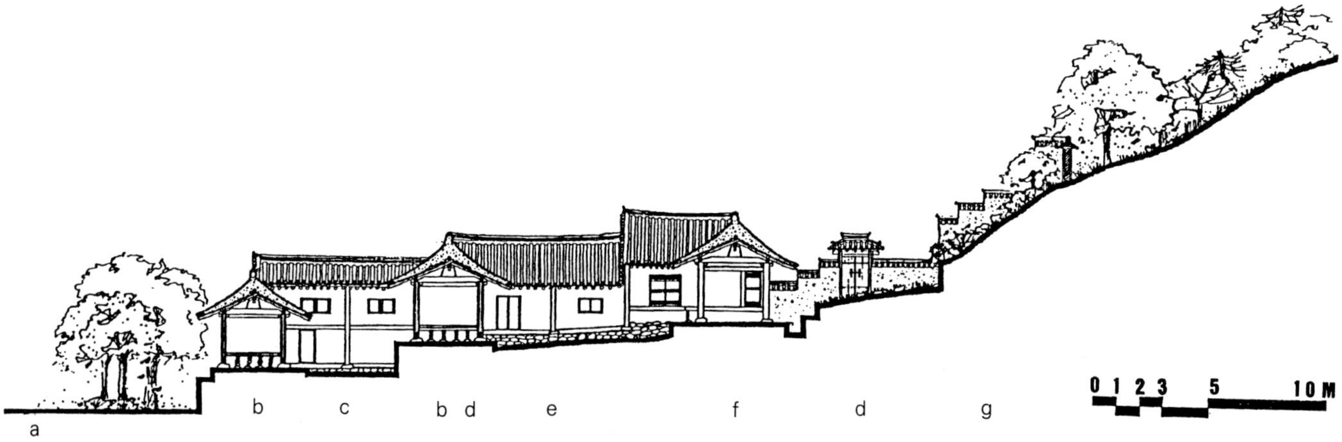

85.1 Section view of a *yangban* estate on a south-sloping site (Imch'ŏnggak, Andong).
a. main gate. b. *haengnagch'ae.* c. *haengnag madang.* d. inner gate. e. *sarang madang.* f. *sarang taech'ŏng.* g. *twitmadang.*

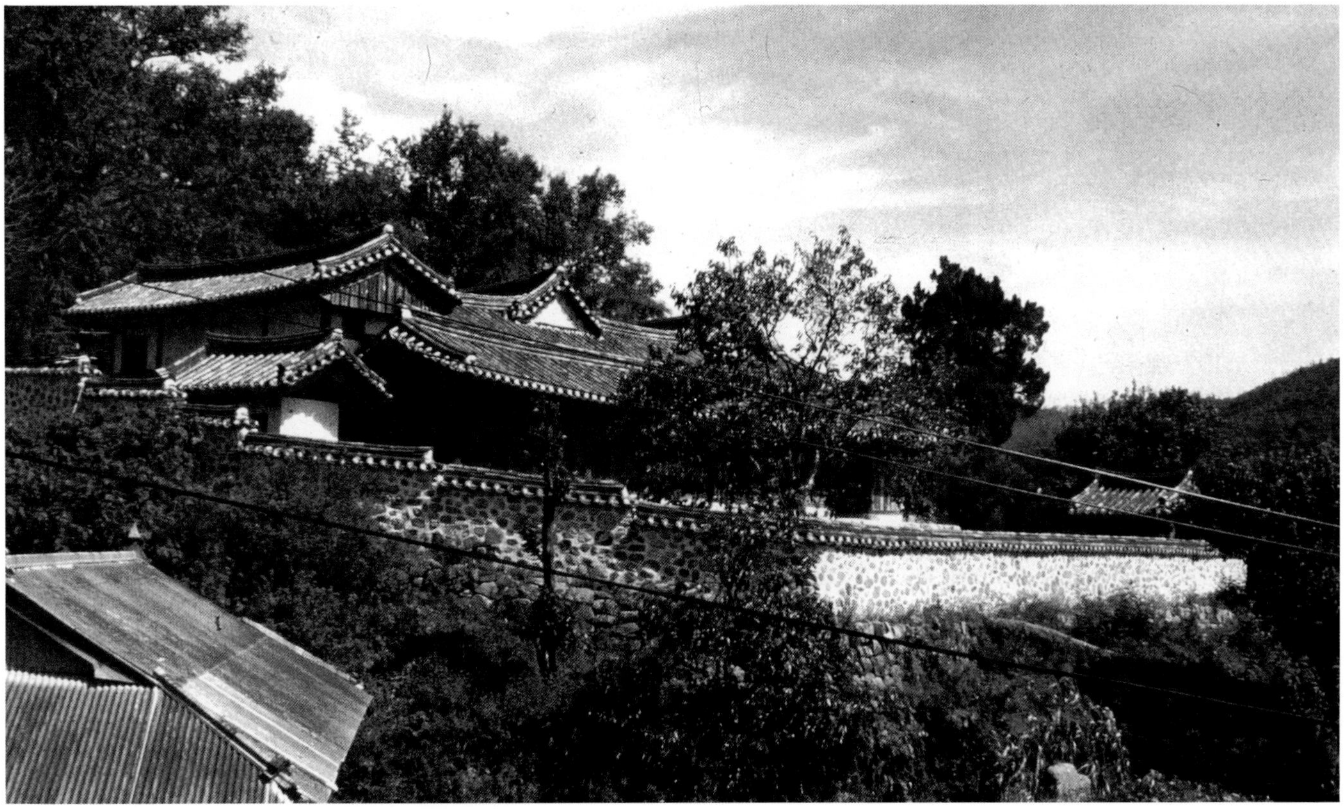

85.2 An upper-class estate (Hyangdan, Yangdong).

government officials. Title to the land was hereditary, but it was also subject to an inheritance tax. The relationship between landlord and tenant was also governed by this law, which stipulated, for example, that landlords were prohibited from taking land back from a tenant. The government officials responsible for this system's implementation were the *yangban*, who formed a privileged class and were paid for their official duties with land and the power to levy taxes.

Adherence to this strict hierarchical social order enabled the Chosŏn dynasty to prevent the development of a powerful land-owning aristocracy and to maintain its own direct control over ordinary farming people. There were five broad social classes in Chosŏn, of which *yangban* were the highest:

Yangban—Scholar/civil officials, military officials (whose status was lower than that of scholar/civil officials), and the descendents of each. In principle, members of *yangban* families were expected to marry within their own class.

Chungin—Skilled professionals, such as lawyers, doctors, and accountants, including low-level government officials.

Sangmin—Traders, artisans, farming families that tilled the fields administered by the *yangban*, and others. These were the common people, who made up the vast majority of the population.

Nobi—Slaves of the state administration and slaves of wealthier families. (At the beginning of the Chosŏn dynasty, since slavery was hereditary, nearly half the population was slaves.)

Ch'ŏnmin—Buddhist monks, actors, dancers, musicians, young men with no particular occupation, and other groups generally held in contempt by members of the other four classes.

In most cases, it might seem that the only way to control a nation of small farmers who enjoy a high degree of independence in the running of their farms would be to rely on military strength, which would then lead to the creation of a decentralized feudalism. The Chosŏn dynasty, however, had good reason to maintain a highly centralized feudal system, in the ever-present dual threats of foreign invasion and of interference from the powerful Ming dynasty in neighboring China. Had the Chosŏn dynasty resorted to a decentralized form of feudalism based on military power, it is extremely likely that this would have provoked the intervention of China or some other powerful neighbor.

While it did concentrate power in relatively few hands, centralized land administration by the *yangban* also provided the machinery for the control of the farming population.

The Introduction of Neo-Confucianism

Neo-Confucianism was a philosophy based on the concept of moral duty. It decreed that each person, from the king down to the lowliest servant, must observe the moral principles appropriate to his or her social class. This philosophy served as the intellectual foundation for the continuation of the class system that gave the *yangban* their authority. Thus, neo-Confucianism, with its emphasis on duty, took on the status of a state religion, and Buddhism was harshly suppressed. Buddhist monks were outcasts relegated to the lowest rung of society—called the *ch'ŏnmin*—and the precepts of neo-Confucianism came to be accepted by the entire population, including Buddhist monks.

From the *yangban*'s point of view, the common people were not only responsible for the maintenance of production, they were also pupils to be tutored in the principles of neo-Confucianism. Moral duty, as stipulated by this belief system, dictated which virtues were appropriate to each class, to the common people as well as to their rulers. It demanded that individuals must submit to authority, and that family loyalty, with its emphasis on respect for one's ancestors, should be sacrosanct. Under this system, a complex code of etiquette, including rituals of mourning the dead and various ceremonies that enhanced the authority of the elders and helped to preserve order in the villages, was conscientiously observed.

The importance of family names in modern Korea and the *chokbo* (genealogy book) that people consult before deciding upon a marriage partner are just two examples of how this tradition of maintaining distinct social classes lives on today.

Thus the prevalence of neo-Confucian ideas of moral duty provided a basis and support for the social class system and for the strict system of regulations governing the size of the parcels of land and the homes that each class was permitted to have. These detailed regulations even extended to what kind of rooms a dwelling was to have, and how they were to be decorated.

The village of Yangdong provides a perfect example of the ubiquity of symbols of social status as they are represented in architecture.

Social Mores: Factors Based on Confucian Principles

Social status, as described above, was an important factor in the composition of every traditional Korean dwelling, but the Confucian principles underpinning the hierarchical social system also had an influence on the basic design and layout of homes in other, much more direct, ways.

Once neo-Confucianism, with its emphasis on moral duty, was established as the dominant philosophy in the land, ancestor worship became the core practice of the people's spiritual life. The basic unit of society was not the individual, but the family. Several generations of an extended family lived together under the charge of the family patriarch.

Order was maintained within the extended family, as within the broader community, by Confucian principles. Accordingly, the separation of men from women and of superior from inferior, and the need for an ancestral shrine became fundamental elements in the composition of the traditional Korean residence.

The Composition of a Yangban *Estate*

The residence of a *yangban* can be broadly divided into an *anch'ae*, a *sarangch'ae*, and a *haengrangch'ae*, each having its own inner garden. The *anch'ae* also typically has a rear garden, and there is a *sadang*, or ancestral shrine, at the northern end of the compound (Figures 86.1–86.2).

Anch'ae

The *anch'ae* is the family's living quarters. Intended primarily for use by the women of the household, it is connected to the *puŏk*, or kitchen. It consists mainly of a number of rooms with *ondol* floor heating (*pang*) and a number of wooden-floored rooms (*maru*), the principal one of which is called a *taech'ŏng*. (The *taech'ŏng* within the *anch'ae* family living quarters is distinct from the

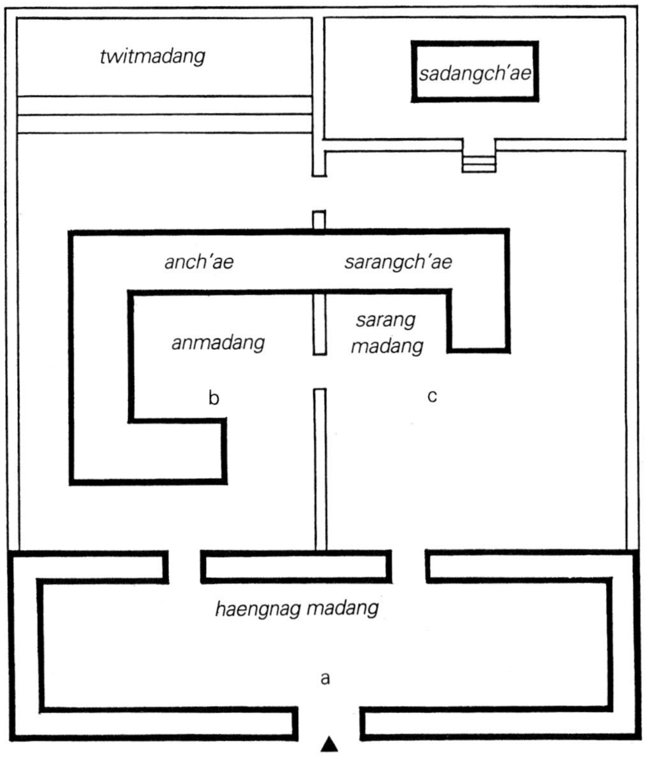

86. 1 Schematic layout of a *yangban* estate.
a. work area. b. family area. c. master/guest area.

taech'ŏng within the *sarangch'ae* master's quarters, and is thus referred to as the *andaech'ŏng*.) The northern side of the *taech'ŏng* is enclosed, by two sliding wooden doors, but the southern side is open to the elements—without walls, doors, or windows—and contiguous with the *anmadang* (inner garden). It has an exposed beam ceiling and a floor constructed of wooden boards laid across long horizontal beams. The *taech'ŏng*, with its open southern aspect, is a place for various ceremonial occasions and religious observances connected with Confucianism (Figures 87.1–87.2).

A rice storage chest is commonly kept in the middle of the *taech'ŏng*, against the northern wall. This is a large and sturdy wooden chest with four legs, the grain contained in which represents the family ancestors. It is kept in the *taech'ŏng*, where the many ceremonies of homage to the ancestors are held.

Anmadang

The *anmadang* is the garden on the south side of the *anch'ae*. On ceremonial occasions, a *ch'a'il*, or awning, is erected to turn the *anmadang* into an extension of the *taech'ŏng*.

In principle, the *anmadang* is a "white" garden (area of bare earth), but sometimes a fruit tree or two—usually a pomegranate, apricot, peach, or Chinese date tree—and

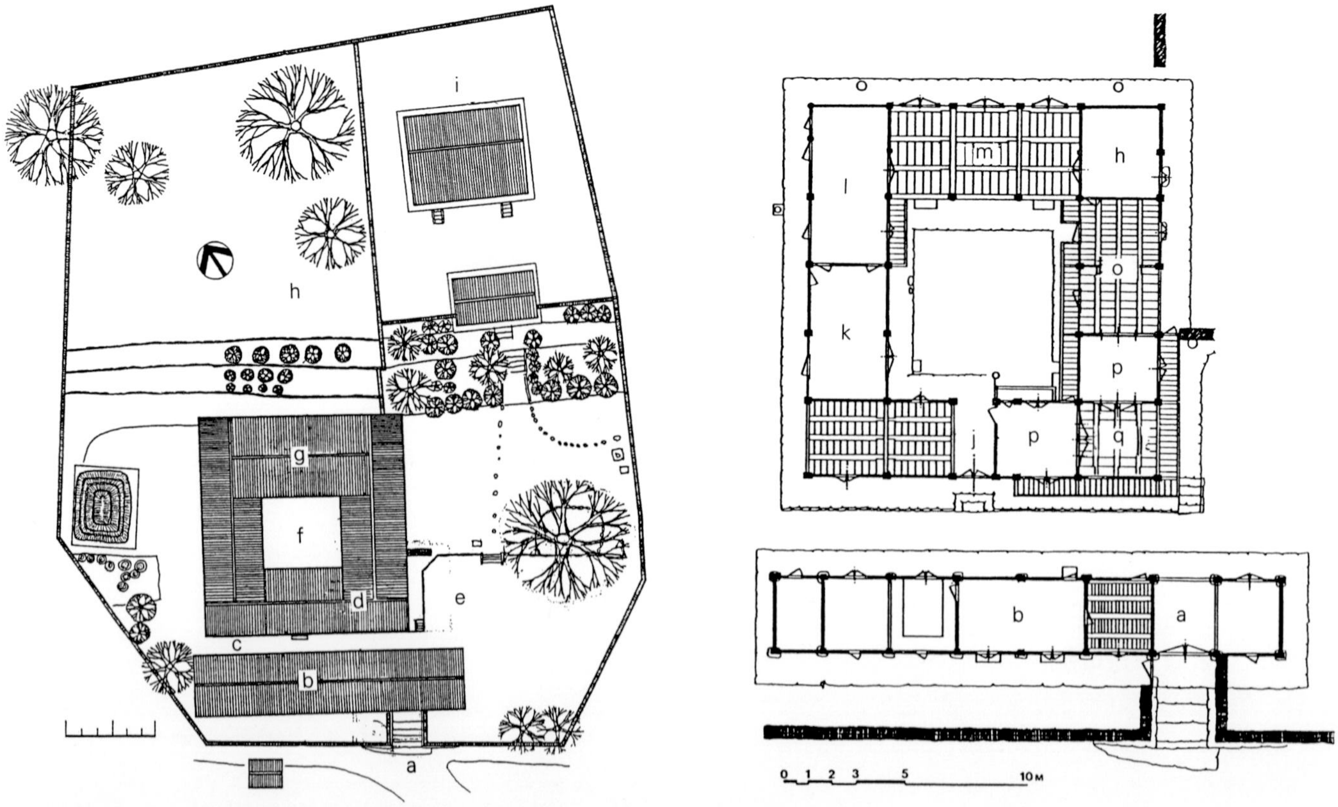

86.2 Site plan and plan view drawings of the Son Tongman residence (Wŏlsŏng).
a. main gate. b. *haengnagch'ae.* c. *haengnag madang.* d. *sarangch'ae.* e. *sarang madang.* f. *anmadang.* g. *anch'ae.* h. *twitmadang.* i. *sadangch'ae.* j. inner gate. k. *puŏk.* l. *anbang.* m. *andaech'ŏng.* n. *kŏnnŏbang.* o. *maru.* p. *pang.* q. *numaru.*

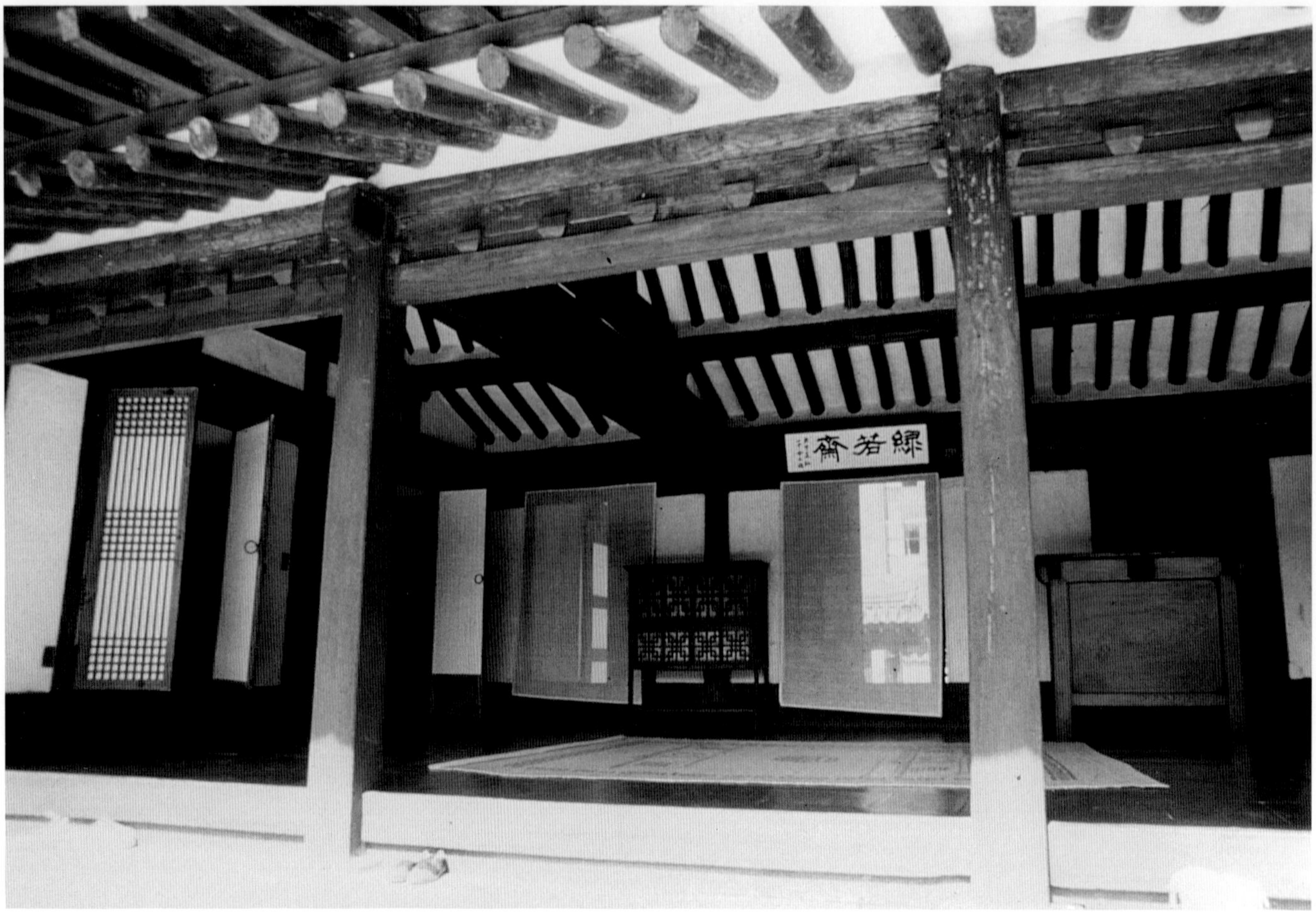

87.1 *Andaech'ŏng*, Kungmin University, Folk Museum (Seoul).

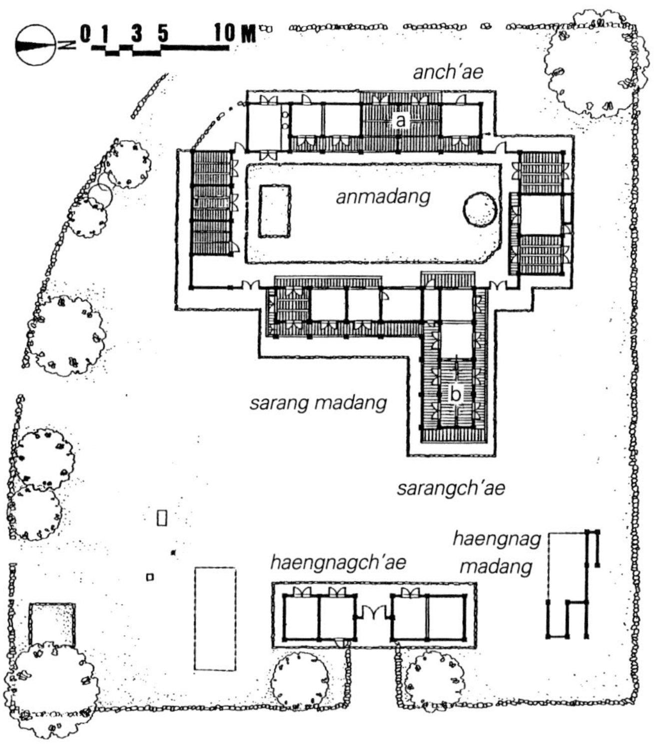

87. 2 Site plan of the Chŏng residence (Yŏngch'ŏn).

a. *andaech'ŏng.*

b. *sarang taech'ŏng.*

perhaps some flowers, such as peonies, are planted there. Nevertheless, it is not an ornamental garden intended to be admired from the *anch'ae.*

Sarangch'ae

The *sarangch'ae* is the private quarters for the master of the house as well as the space in which he receives visitors. It is frequently a free-standing structure, but may occasionally be connected to the *anch'ae* to form single building. When the *sarangch'ae* is separate, it is usually surrounded by a wall or corridor. When it is linked to the *anch'ae,* there is still a clear division between the two wings, since male visitors were not traditionally permitted to enter, and the women of the family were not traditionally allowed to leave, the *anch'ae.*

Like the *anch'ae,* the *sarangch'ae* consists of a number of *pang* (rooms with *ondol* floor heating), a *taech'ŏng* (in this case, the *sarang taech'ŏng*), and possibly a number of other *maru* (wooden-floored rooms). In houses owned by a man of particularly high status, the *maru* may include a *numaru* (Figures 88.1–88.2).

A *numaru* is a room for entertaining and receiving visitors, adjacent to the *taech'ŏng.* Its wooden floor is constructed a step higher than that of all the other rooms, with the sub-floor space left open for ventilation, and the walls on three sides consisting of doors that swing up, leaving the room open to the outside.

The garden in front of the *sarangch'ae* is called the *sarang madang* and, like the *anmadang,* it is generally a "white" garden, with little or no vegetation.

Haengnagch'ae

The *haengnagch'ae* is a long, narrow building only 1 *k'an* in width.[5] It is traditionally used to accommodate lesser family members and servants.

It also contains storage rooms and the compound's main entrance; its outer wall is connected to the outer wall of the compound. The inner garden of the *haengnagch'ae,* called a *haengnag madang,* is used as a work space (Figures 89.1–89.2).

Sadangch'ae

The *sadangch'ae,* or ancestral shrine, is usually located in an elevated area at the northern end of the residential compound, facing south and overlooking the other buildings. It is dedicated to the four previous generations of ancestors. The area around the *sadangch'ae* is also generally walled off from the rest of the compound (Figures 90.1–90.2).

Twitmadang

The *twitmadang,* or rear garden, lies to the north of the *anch'ae* on a southern slope, or as the uppermost of a series of terraces, in accordance with the principles of *p'ungsu.*

This was traditionally a private space used mainly by women and children, both of whom were forbidden to leave the compound without good reason. Like the *anch'ae* proper, it was off limits to any man not belonging to the family.

Unlike the inner gardens mentioned above, all of which are nearly bare of vegetation, the rear garden features grass and shrubs as well as fruit trees. Nevertheless, the art of garden making is not traditionally involved, giving the

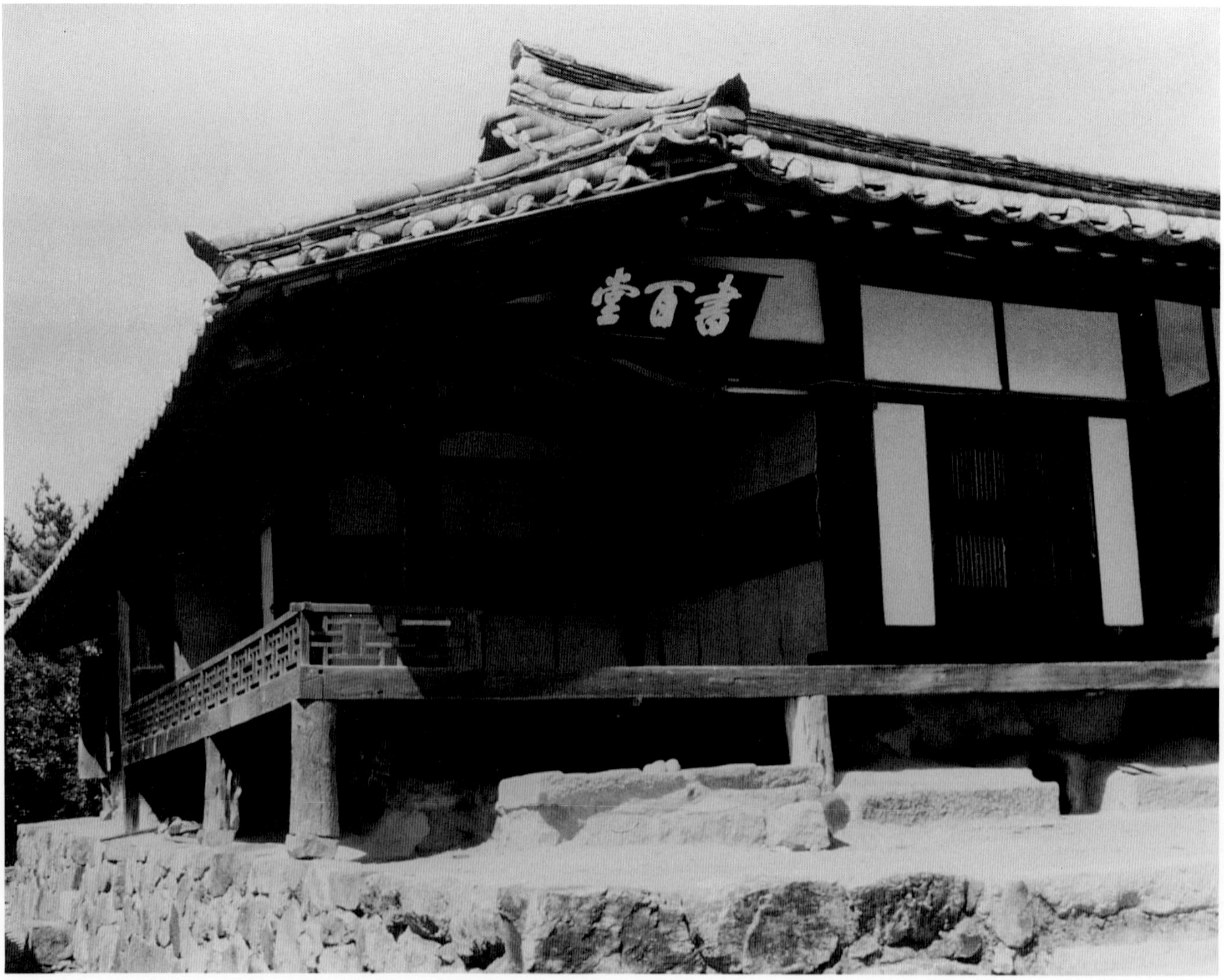

88.1 *Sarangch'ae numaru* of the Son Tongman residence (Wŏlsŏng).

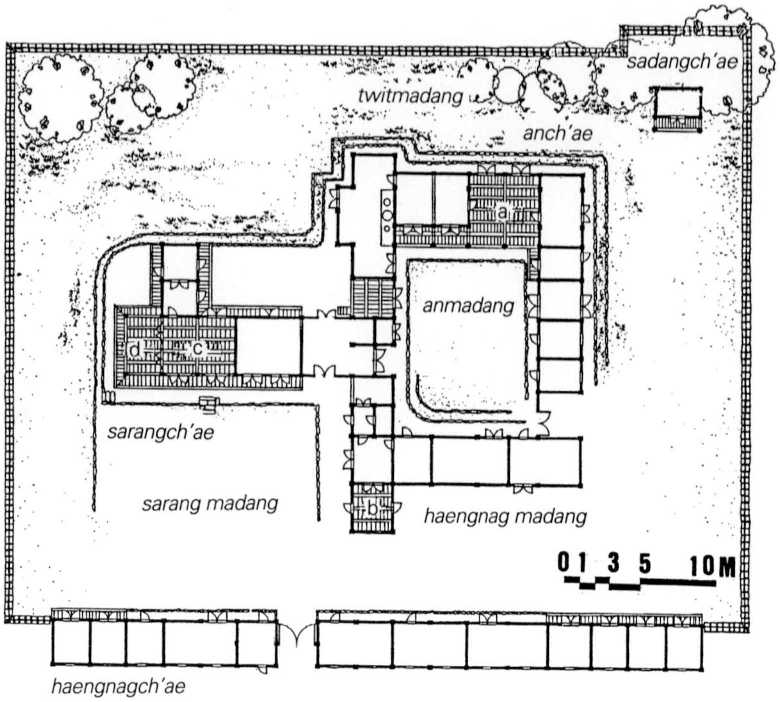

88.2 Site plan of Unjoru (Kurye).

a. *andaech'ŏng.*
b. *maru.*
c. *sarang taech'ŏng.*
d. *numaru.*

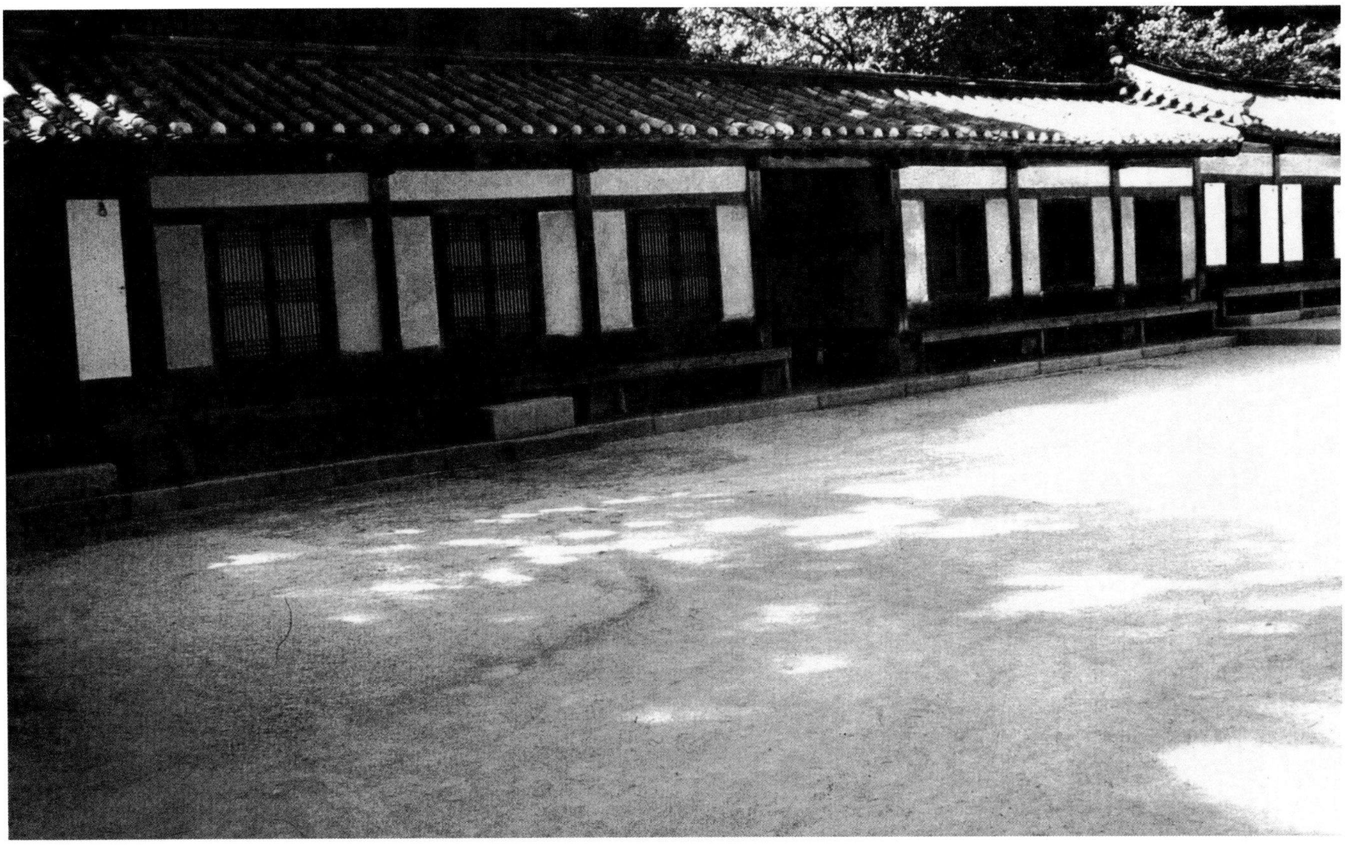

89.1 *Haengnagch'ae* Yŏn'gyŏngdang (Piwŏn).

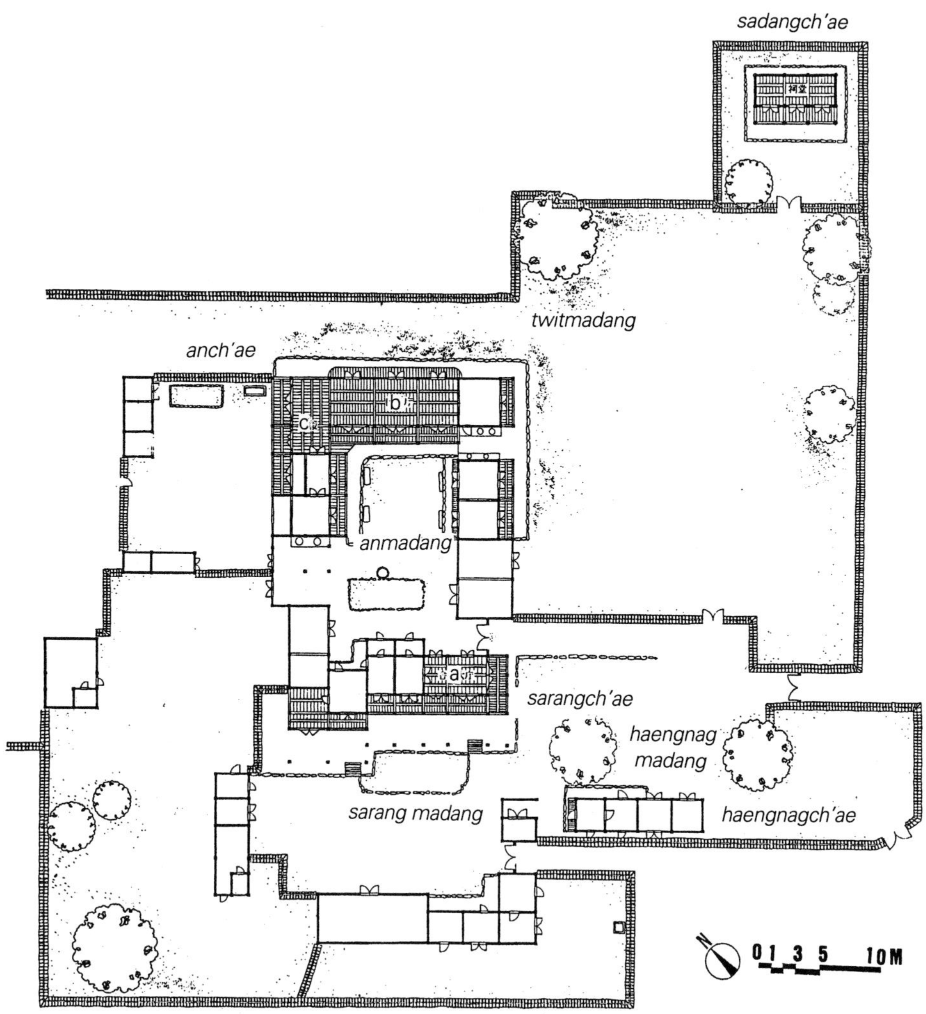

89.2 The original residence of Yun Kosan (1587–1675), a famous poet of Chosŏn (Ingosan).

a. *sarang taech'ŏng*. b. *andaech'ŏng*. c. *maru*.

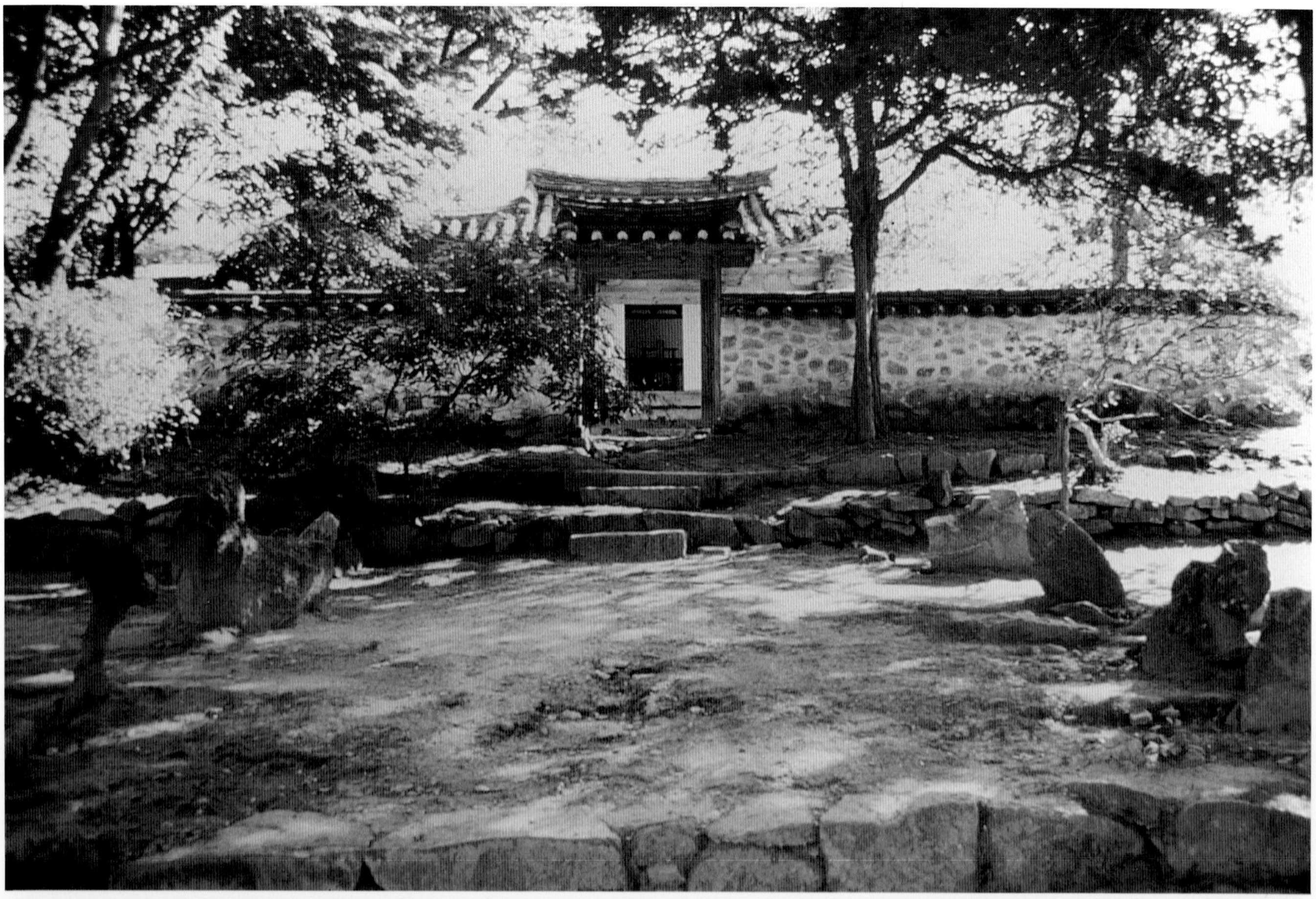

90.1 *Sadangch'ae* of the Maeng residence (Asan).

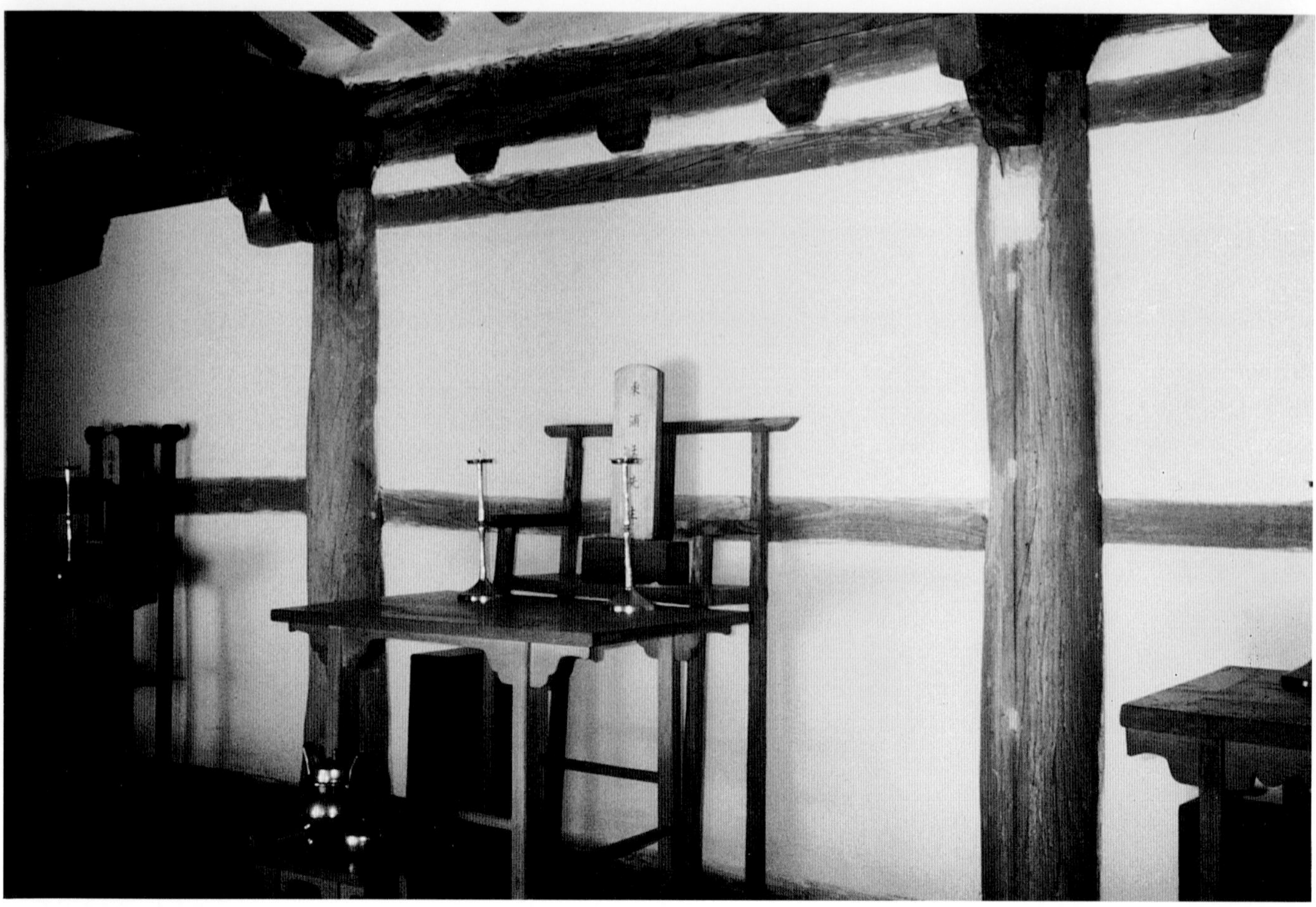

90.2 *Sadangch'ae* interior.

91 Site plan of an extended family residential compound (The Kim residence, Koch'ang).

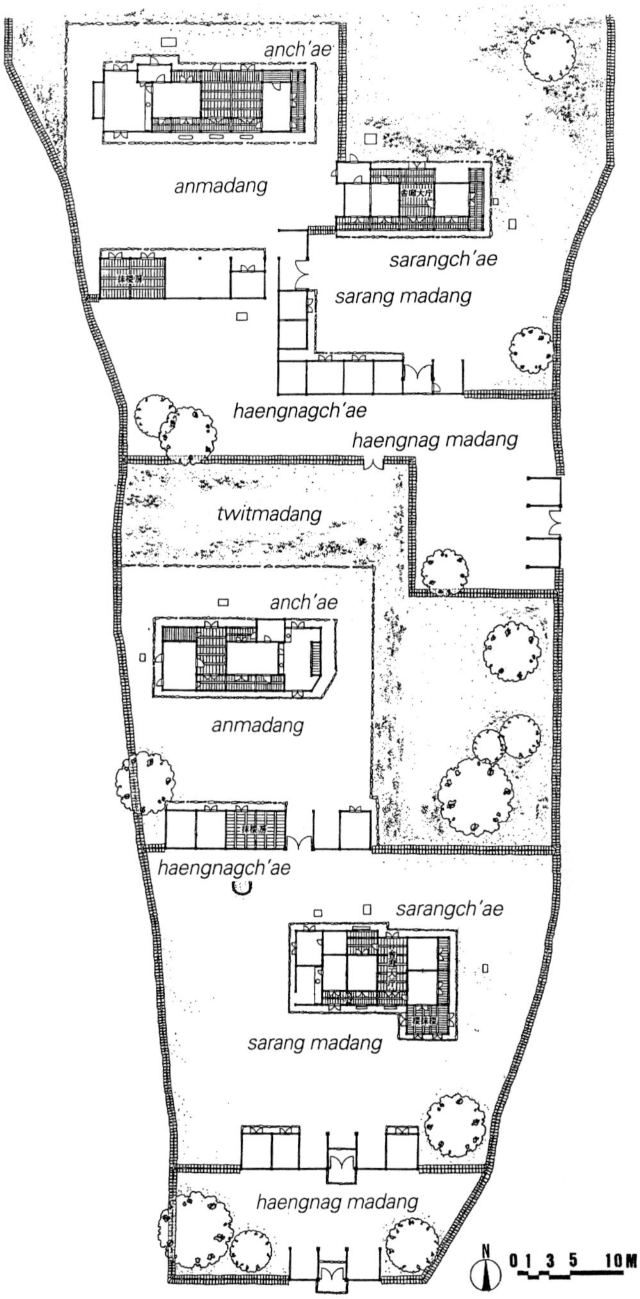

area a rough, natural look. The rear garden is also surrounded by a wall, which follows the natural contours of the land (see Figures 113.1–113.4).

As all these elements would suggest, the composition of a *yangban*'s estate is determined first and foremost by the guiding principles of Confucianism. The provision of separate buildings and gardens with distinct uses maintained the obligatory distance between male and female, as well as senior and junior, family members, while preserving the authority of the patriarch and allowing for proper respect to be shown the ancestors. No examination of traditional Korean residences can afford to overlook these vital factors.

The Family Village and School

In many cases, villages in Korea formed naturally as single extended families grew larger. It was not unusual for a village to develop, with a number of neighboring compounds housing branches of the same family (Figure 91).

Family villages of this kind, centered on a head family, provided a network of support for the related households. A typical example is the village of Hahoe near Andong. Such traditional villages often contained schools (*sŏwŏn*)—some of which are extant today—and these schools together constituted a kind of national education system during the Chosŏn period for the children of the *yangban* scholars (*yusaeng*).[6] They also provided an opportunity for social contact.

Sŏwŏn schools were centered around the *Kongjamyo* (Confucian shrine). There were also book-storage areas and print rooms, where printing blocks were stored and books were printed and bound. These schools were given a prime location, on the edge of the village, on sites of particular scenic beauty. In later days, children of humbler origins were allowed to attend, and some went on to become respected intellectuals.

While these *sŏwŏn* schools represented a kind of national education system, Confucian-based private educational facilities called *chŏngsa* served as centers of spiritual retreat and occupied sites of special beauty. *Chŏngsa* are discussed at greater length in Chapter 8.

Function: Factors Based on the *Ondol* System of Heating

The constraints imposed by the *ondol* system of floor heating were a major factor in the interior layout of traditional Korean homes.

Confucian philosophy was central to the division of the

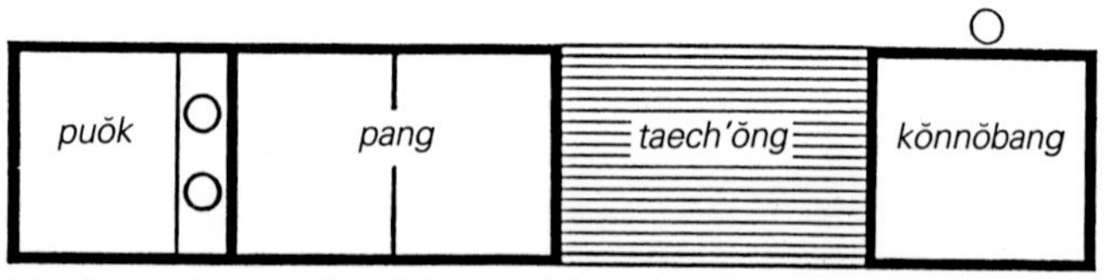

92 Typical layout of *ondol*-heated *(pang)* and wooden-floor (*maru*) rooms.

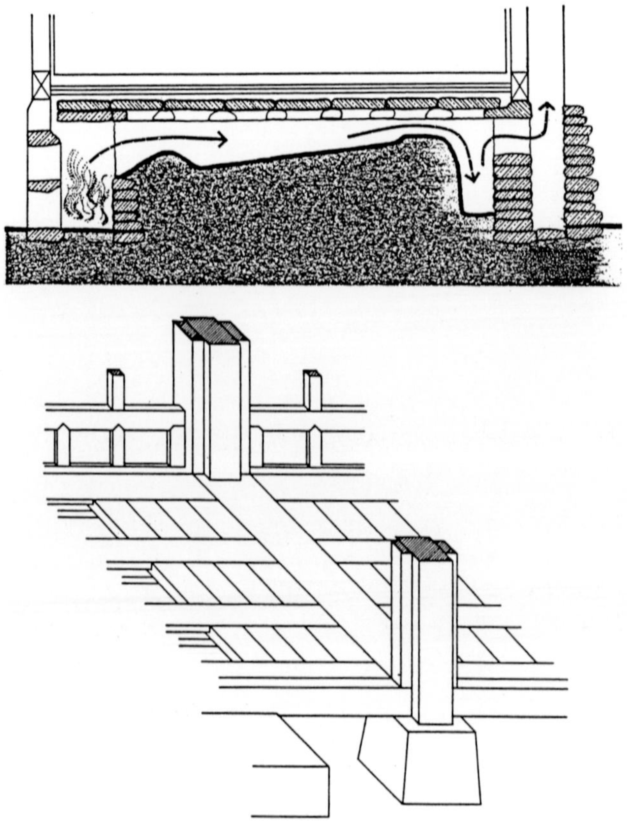

93 Section and perspective views of the *ondol* heating system and wooden floor structures.

dwelling into the *anch'ae*, *sarangch'ae*, and *haengnagch'ae*, but the composition of rooms within each of those buildings was based on a distinction between rooms with floor heating (*pang*) and those without (*maru*). Furthermore, the size of each *pang* and the number of *pang* connected to the same heating system were determined by the physical limitations of the *ondol*'s effectiveness.

Thus, each of the three areas of a *yangban*'s estate was made up of rooms small enough to be heated effectively by the *ondol* (the number of *pang* dependent on a single furnace was similarly limited), as well as a number of rooms without any heating devices that had no such size limitations (Figure 92). The former were traditionally used as private apartments, and the latter as ceremonial spaces.

The Structure of the Ondol

The *ondol* system utilizes the heat of smoke from an enclosed furnace. Excess heat from the furnace passes through flues located beneath the floor to a chimney at the other end of the room or rooms. The furnace is most commonly located in the *puŏk* (kitchen), and the rooms it heats are called *pang*. Once smoke has passed through the flues to heat the *pang*, it is ventilated through an external chimney.

The floors of the heated rooms, or *pang*, were traditionally constructed of a layer of thin *ondol* stone slabs laid upon *kudul* stone risers, covered with a thick layer of clay and a top layer of varnished *ondol* paper.

The *ondol* was designed in such a way that flues distributed heat evenly throughout the room. It was traditionally fueled by wood, but anthracite coal and even porous briquettes may have been used on occasion, when forestry management considerations required alternative fuels (Figure 93).

Ondol, Kang, *and* Pao

The *ondol* of Korea is similar to the heating system known as *kang* which is used widely in homes across northern China and Manchuria, but there are essential differences. The *kang* heating system in China is designed for use in homes in which people sit on chairs, so it is installed only in the bed platforms of the sleeping quarters (Figure 94). The Mongolians also use floor heating in their *pao* (semi-permanent dwellings); this shares features in common with both the *kang* of China and the *ondol* of Korea and can therefore be assumed to have some connection with both.

While the Chinese custom of sitting on chairs inside the home meant that floor heating was used only in sleeping areas and its potential benefits were never fully utilized, the use of the *ondol* heating system was so well matched to the Korean people's custom of sitting on the floor that it has become a basic identifying feature of the Korean way of life.

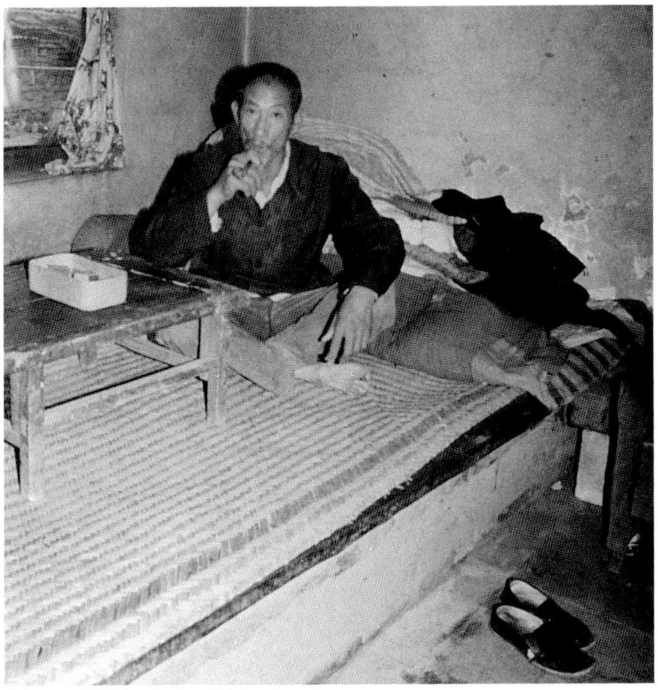

94 A Chinese *kang* brick sleeping platform with internal flues (near Beijing).

The Combination of Ondol *and* Taech'ŏng

Stone wares are habitually used even today among the common people of Korea for cooking, keeping foods warm, and serving food at mealtimes. Similarly, the *ondol* heating system is still found throughout the peninsula. Among the reasons that it became so ubiquitous are that it is simply constructed from granite and high-quality clay readily available throughout the country, it is fueled by wood, which is a plentiful resource in heavily forested Korea, and it is best suited to prevailing climatic conditions.

Nomura Takafumi explains in *Chosen no minka* (Traditional Korean dwellings) that the *ondol* heating system was probably introduced to the ruling classes by provincial officials who traveled to the capital under the highly-centralized bureaucracy of the Chosŏn-dynasty government:

> There are many differing theories as to the origin of *ondol*. The most plausible of these, given the evidence we have to date, appears to be that it was first developed in Koguryŏ, which was the northern part of Korea during the Three Kingdoms period [37 B.C.–A.D. 668] … It does seem safe to say that floor heating was used in Koguryŏ long before it was known in China … Even when the *ondol* system came into widespread use during the Koryŏ period, it seems to have been popular only in rural areas among the common people, and not among the upper classes or in the major cities, where people generally slept on raised beds instead of on quilted mats on the floor. The first appearance of *ondol* in the homes of the upper classes was during the Chosŏn dynasty, when the floors of *ondol*-heated rooms [*pang*] were covered with oiled paper … It is likely that this custom was introduced to the capital and other cities by government officials and warriors based in the provinces … It is common for customs and habits of the upper classes to filter down to the middle and lower classes, but the *ondol* heating system appears to have been a rare example of the opposite: a lower-class custom filtering up to the elite.[7]

By contrast, the wooden-floored *taech'ŏng*, which was essentially a ceremonial space, was an architectural element that spread from the central aristocracy to the residences of the *yangban* in the provinces, and from there to residences of the common people, as the principles of Confucianism gained wider acceptance in Korean society. As a result, if we now compare the traditional homes extant in Seoul to those in the provinces, we can observe two different modes of development: one centered on the *taech'ŏng*, and the other centered on *puŏk* and *pang*. Therefore, from this point, these two patterns will be referred to as urban and rural residential forms of composition. In both cases, however, *ondol*-heated rooms are seen side-by-side with unheated wooden-floored rooms, and it is this combination which is the single most remarkable characteristic of traditional Korean residences in general.

Architectural Constraints Dictated by Ondol, *and Functions of* Ondol*-Heated Rooms*

A traditional *ondol* is only effective when used with a flue structure of limited length, and this inevitably limits the size of the rooms in which it can serve as a sufficient heat source.

The basic unit of measure for *pang* is one *k'an* (a square

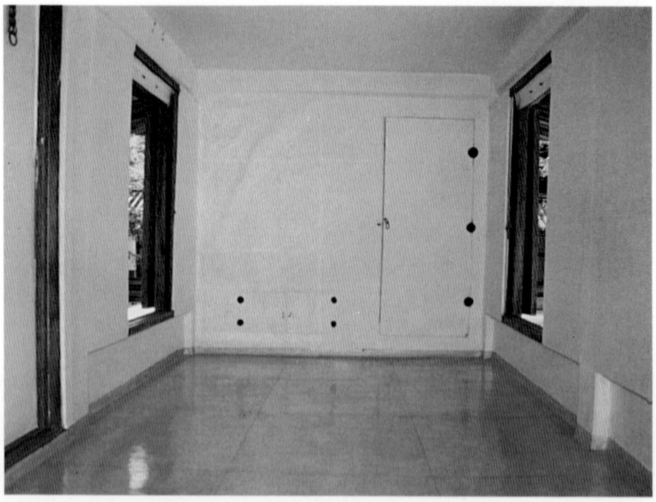

95 Paper covering all interior surfaces of the *pang*.

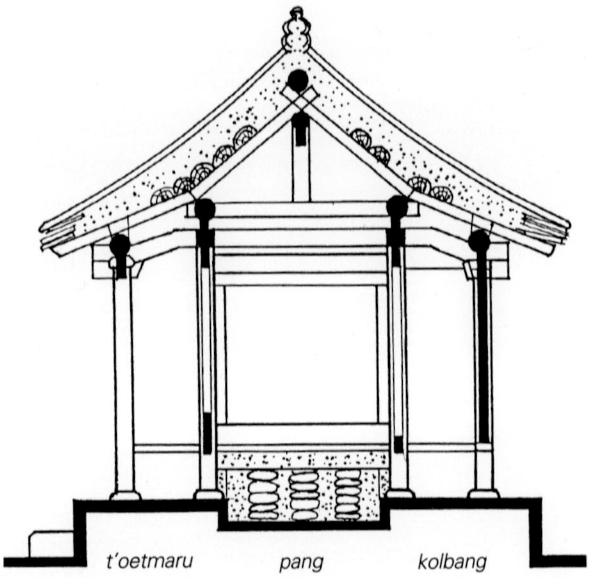

96.1 Section view of the *t'oetmaru* (corridor), *pang*, and *kolbang* (closet space) spatial structure.

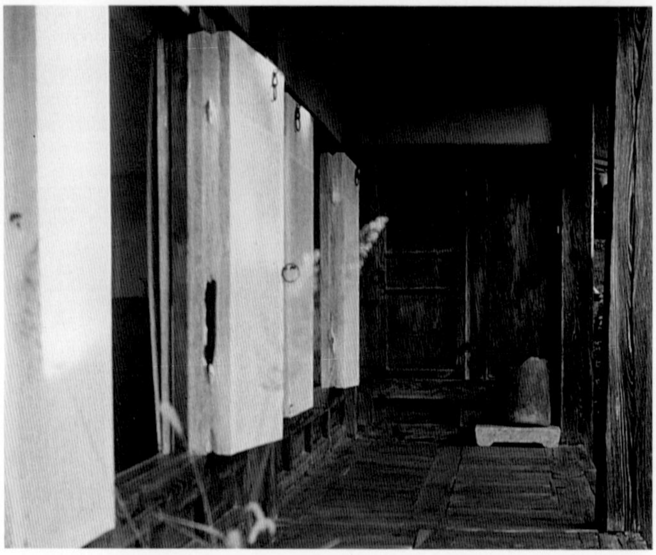

96.2 View of the *pang* and *t'oetmaru*.

measure each side of which is equal to the width of the span between columns).[8] Occasionally a *pang* may be one-and-a-half *k'an* (i.e., having two one-span walls and two one-and-a-half–span walls).

Generally, two of these *pang* are served by a single *ondol* furnace/flue system, and the entire length of the heated area is never more than three *kan*, which is the largest area that an *ondol* can effectively heat. The *pang* located closer to the furnace is called an *anbang* (inner *pang*), while the other is called an *utpang* (outer *pang*).

The floor of the *pang* is traditionally covered with varnished paper, giving it an amber cast. The walls, the ceiling, and the inside surface of all the windows and doors are covered in translucent white paper, thus the room is, as a rule, predominantly white (Figure 95). The *pang* is flanked on either side by a space one-half–*k'an* in width; one, called the *kolbang*, is used as a walk-in closet, while the other, the *t'oetmaru*, serves as a corridor (Figures 96.1–96.2).

Anbang

The *anbang* is the heart of the home, a private space with a wide variety of uses including sleeping, eating, and other daily activities.

The side of the room closest to the *ondol* furnace—the

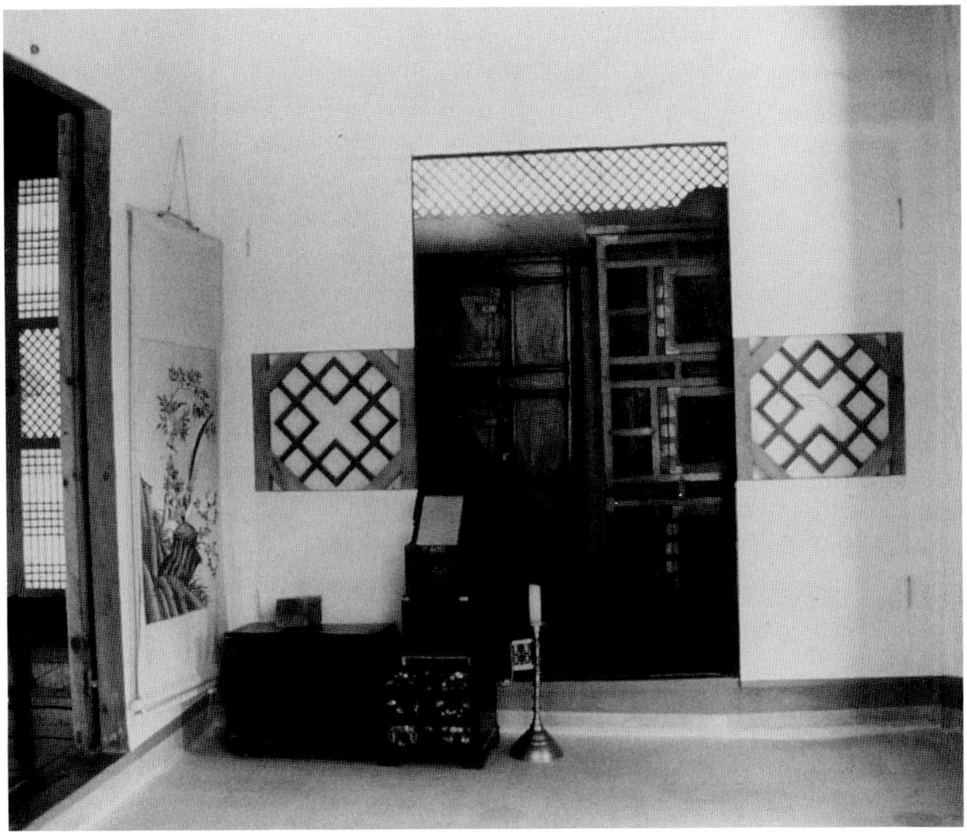

97 A view of a *pang* and *kolbang*.

warmest and hence regarded as the seat of honor—is traditionally reserved for family elders, and the *ansŏk* back cushion and other privileged seats are invariably placed along that wall. The adjacent *puŏk*, or kitchen, is entered through a sliding door built into the same wall; the entire wall is normally hidden by a decorative folding screen (see Figure 105.2).

Utpang

The *utpang* is secondary to the *anbang*, since its heating is inferior. It is used mainly for storage, as an additional sleeping area, or as a study, but in situations in which a large family must share a limited number of rooms, it often becomes as multipurpose as the *anbang*.

Anbang and *utpang* may be completely separate. In other cases, the wall between them may be removed to create a single larger room, or they may be partitioned by removable sliding doors. The latter of these is the most common arrangement. Whatever the preferred arrangement, there are traditionally never more than two *pang* to a single *ondol* furnace, and any interior partitioning of the maximum three-*k'an* space occurs between the *anbang* and *utpang*.

Kolbang

The *kolbang* is an adjunct to the *pang*, usually separated from it by doors that slide into a reveal in the wall. Its main use is as a repository for large pieces of furniture, such as chests of drawers. When not in use, bedding is folded and stored on top of this furniture (Figure 97).

In homes with no *kolbang*, bedding is stored on top of furniture within the *pang*, and clothes are hung on special racks.

Kŏnnŏbang

Kŏnnŏbang is the name used for an *ondol*-heated room located just beyond the *taech'ŏng*, on the side furthest from the *puŏk* (kitchen). The *kŏnnŏbang* has its own furnace and is used as part of the women and children's quarters, or as a study (Figure 98).

Sarangbang

The *sarangbang* is an *ondol*-heated room within the *sarang-ch'ae*. It is traditionally used by the master of the house for receiving visitors, or as a study.

Puŏk

The *puŏk*, or kitchen, is located adjacent to the *anbang*, and contains a stove built along the wall separating the two spaces. This stove also acts as the furnace for the *ondol*. Since the furnace needs to be set at a height below the

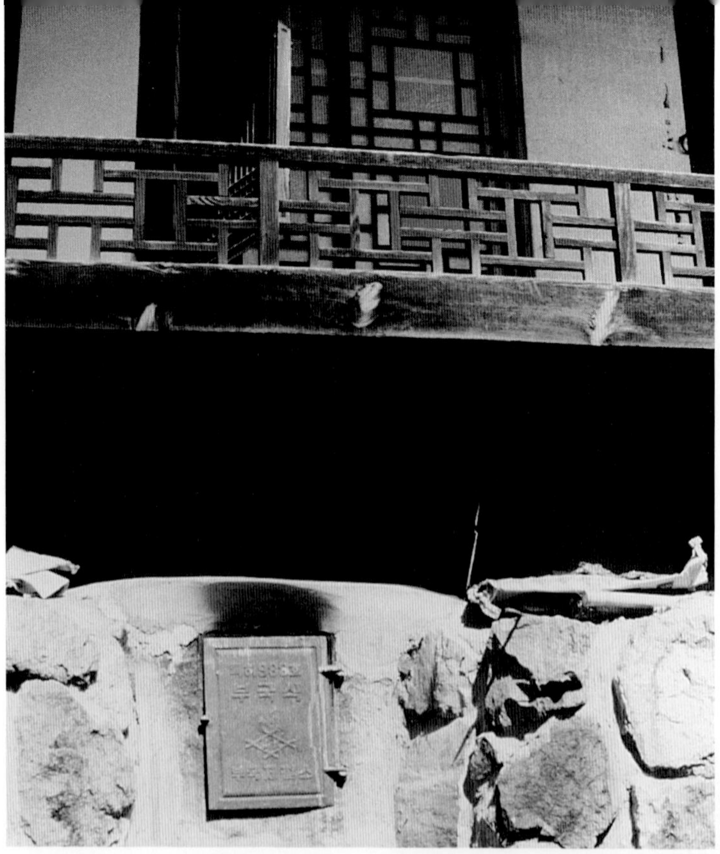

98 A view of a *kŏnnŏbang* exterior and its independant furnace.

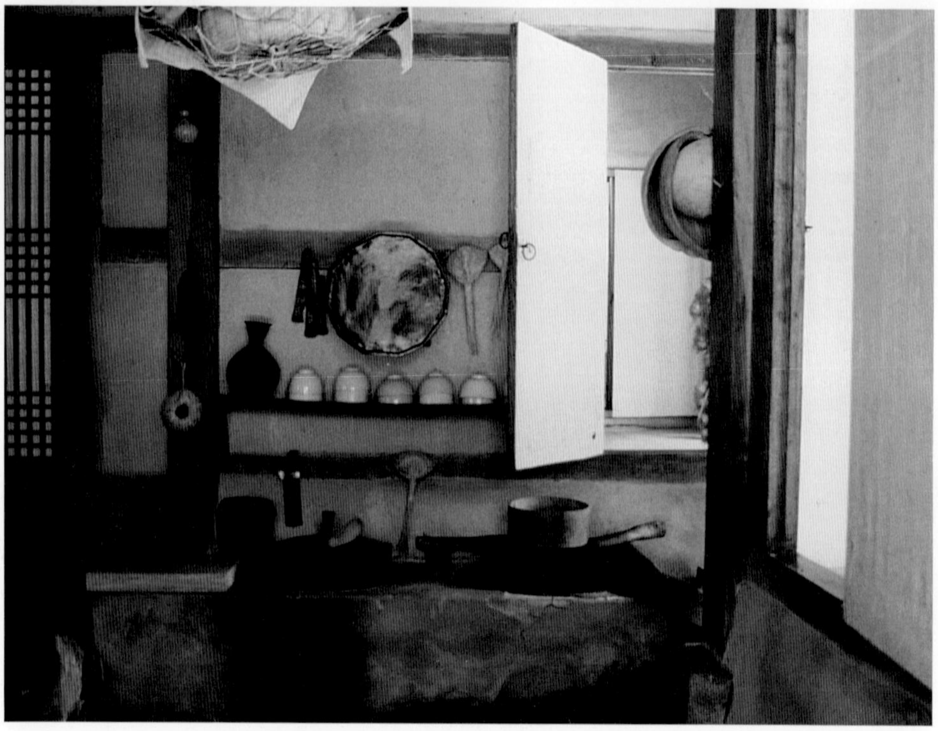

99 A view of a *puŏk* (kitchen) and *pang* showing a combination stove/*ondol* furnace.

floor of the rooms which it heats, the pounded earth floor of the *puŏk* is generally two steps lower than the floor of the *pang* (Figure 99).

With the resulting excess ceiling height, a mezzanine is frequently built above the kitchen for use as storage space, called the *tarak*, which is accessed through sliding doors from the adjacent *anbang*.

A serving area, or *ch'an'ggan*, is usually built alongside the *puŏk*. A typical Korean meal consists of rice, soup, and a number of side dishes served in individual portions on *papsang* (short-legged tables) that are carried to each member of the family or guest seated in the *pang* or the *taech'ŏng*. The *ch'an'ggan*, like the larger *ch'anbbang*, or pantry, is used both for serving meals and for storage.

As we can see from the above, the compositional charac-

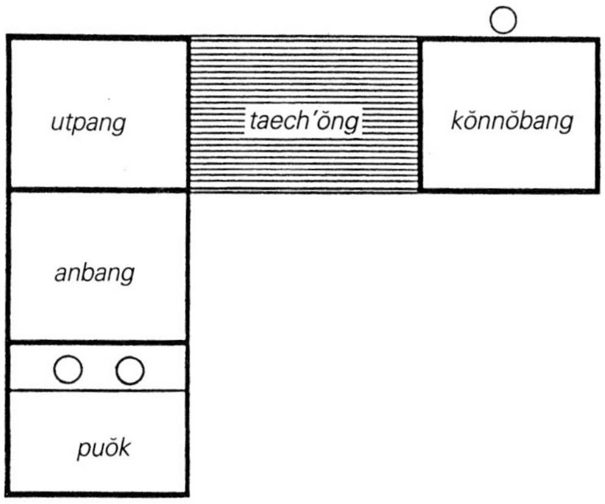

100 Schematic of a rural residence centered on the *puŏk* (kitchen).

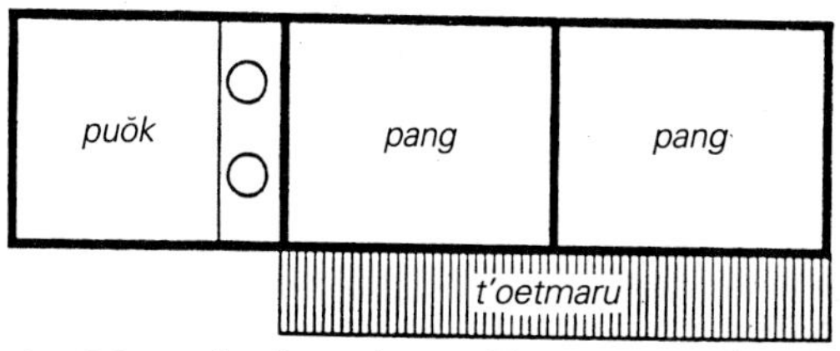

101 Schematic of an urban residence centered on the *taech'ŏng*.

teristics of the traditional Korean residence dictated by existence of the *ondol* heating system starts with the *puŏk*, or kitchen, almost invariably located alongside the *anbang*, or the inner of two heated rooms, with the *utpang*, or outer *pang*, located next to the *anbang*. There may also be a third heated room (*kŏnnŏbang*) with an independent exterior furnace, located at the far end of the *taech'ŏng*. Thus the residence is composed of a series of small *ondol*-heated rooms one *k'an* in width flanked by narrow wooden-floored spaces, and open wooden-floored rooms the width of the combined *ondol* and adjunct spaces. Accordingly, since the *ondol* is an indispensable part of Korean life, there are traditionally no multiple-story dwellings.

The several factors listed here—the combination of *ondol*-heated and wooden-floor rooms, the requirements of Confucian morals, the use of divination according to the theories of yin and yang, and the design considerations dictated by *p'ungsu* geomancy—combined in different situations, in both urban and rural settings, to produce homes that were L-shaped, U-shaped, oblong, or square with an inner garden.

Locality: Factors Related to the Dwelling's Locale (Urban Versus Rural)

The Convergence of Ondol- *and* Maru-*Based Structures*

The spread of the *ondol*-heated *pang* from the homes of the rural masses to the upper classes and the cities, and the spread of the wooden-floor *taech'ŏng* and *maru* in the other direction, together contributed to the distinctive composition of traditional Korean dwellings.

The major difference between traditional homes in rural areas and those that have survived in Seoul is that the rural home is the built around the *puŏk* and *pang*, which make up the majority of its interior space, and the wooden-floored rooms appear somewhat secondary (Figure 100). In the urban dwelling, on the other hand, the *taech'ŏng* and the other *maru* form the core of the home, while the *puŏk* and *pang* appear to be rather secondary; the *puŏk* is often located at the southwestern or southeastern end of the building (Figure 101). This contrast highlights the historical origins and formative process of the composition of traditional Korean dwellings.

In traditional urban residences, the inner gardens resemble the *yuanzi* of Beijing *siheyuan* residential quadrangles, or the *tianjing* of a traditional common dwelling in Huizhou province. But the composition of rooms and courtyards in Chinese urban dwellings was based on and preserved bilateral symmetry, while in Korea, urban dwellings—whose main determining factor was that the *taech'ŏng* must face south and have a private garden space behind it—let the shape of the site determine the layout of the other rooms and their corresponding rectangular gardens. For this reason, the composition of Korean dwellings was irregular and exhibited a freedom to adapt to the particular conditions of a site (Figures 102.1–102.2). The design and significance of Korean gardens was fundamentally very different, therefore, from the *yuanzi* and *tianjing* designed to complement the symmetrical layout of Chinese homes.

The Walled Compound

One characteristic common to both urban and rural versions of the traditional Korean residence is that the entire site, including the rear garden, is always completely surrounded by a wall. In rural areas, the wall is usually made of mud, stone, or ceramic tiles, or some mixture of those materials, while the wall around upper-class urban dwellings

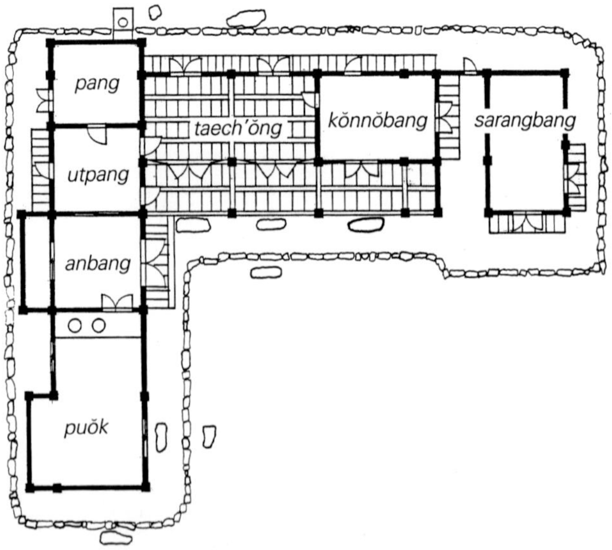

102.1 A typical plan of the *anch'ae* of a *yangban* residence (Hahoe).

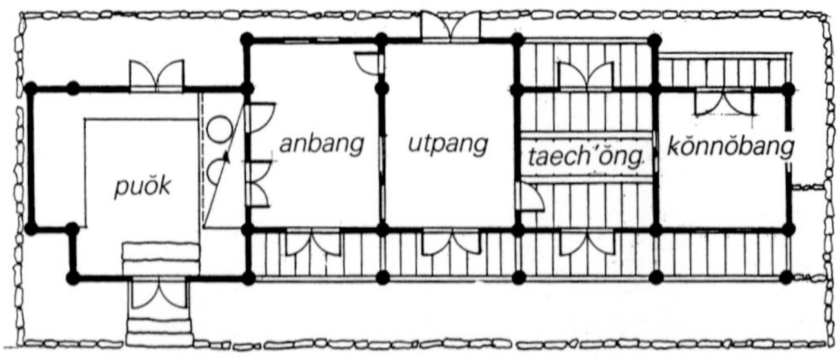

102.2 A typical plan of a common farming family dwelling (Hahoe).

is more likely to be of brick. Hedges and rough-woven fences can be found in some rural areas but are never seen in the cities. In every case, the top of the wall or fence is lower than the eaves of the house. This feature is intended to preserve the view from inside the rooms and to create a sense of intimacy with the surrounding landscape. In order to make the walls more secure in the cities, however, a woven bamboo mesh is inserted between the top of the wall and the eaves of the house, creating a distinctive cityscape (Figures 103.1–103.2).

Ch'ae and *Madang*: Combined Interior and Exterior Spaces

Any consideration of the Korean home and lifestyle must first take into account the fact that Koreans do not habitually use chairs, but sit on the floor, a custom central to the *ondol* method of heating.

Perhaps the most distinctive feature of the plan of the dwelling is the versatility and multipurpose nature of nearly all the rooms. Rooms tend not to have a single, set function. This feature pervades all Korean domestic architecture.

Even in the estates of the elite *yangban*, all gardens other than the rear garden were an integral part of the family's daily living space and an essential part of the residential composition. Accordingly, they should be considered as much a part of the dwelling as are the interior spaces.

For purposes of this discussion, different parts of the residence will be analyzed not in terms of their functions, but in terms of interior and exterior space, or *ch'ae* and *madang*. Interior and exterior space can be identified as follows:

> Interior space (*ch'ae*)=enclosed interior spaces (*pang*) + open interior spaces (*taech'ŏng* and *maru*).

> Exterior space (*madang*)=open interior spaces (*taech'ŏng* and *maru*) + exterior spaces (gardens).

Interior Space (Ch'ae)*: Repetitive Juxtaposition of Enclosed and Open Spaces*

The traditional Korean home comprises three *ch'ae*, or wings—the *anch'ae*, *sarangch'ae*, and *haengnagch'ae*. The distinction between these three wings of the home was founded on the Confucian sense of order; however, compositionally, each wing repeats the same pattern of *pang* (enclosed spaces) alongside *taech'ŏng* or *maru* (open spaces). The juxtaposition of enclosed and open spaces is simultaneously a juxtaposition of elements that are intricate and rough, white and brown, and warm and cold (Figure 104).

Pang are multipurpose, enclosed rooms of predominantly white hue. In the *anch'ae*, which was traditionally the wife's domain, the *anbang* (inner *pang*) was furnished and decorated for the use of the female members of the family. Conversely, the *sarangch'ae* was a social area for the master of the house, so the *sarangbang* was furnished and decorated for use by men (Figures 105.1–105.2).

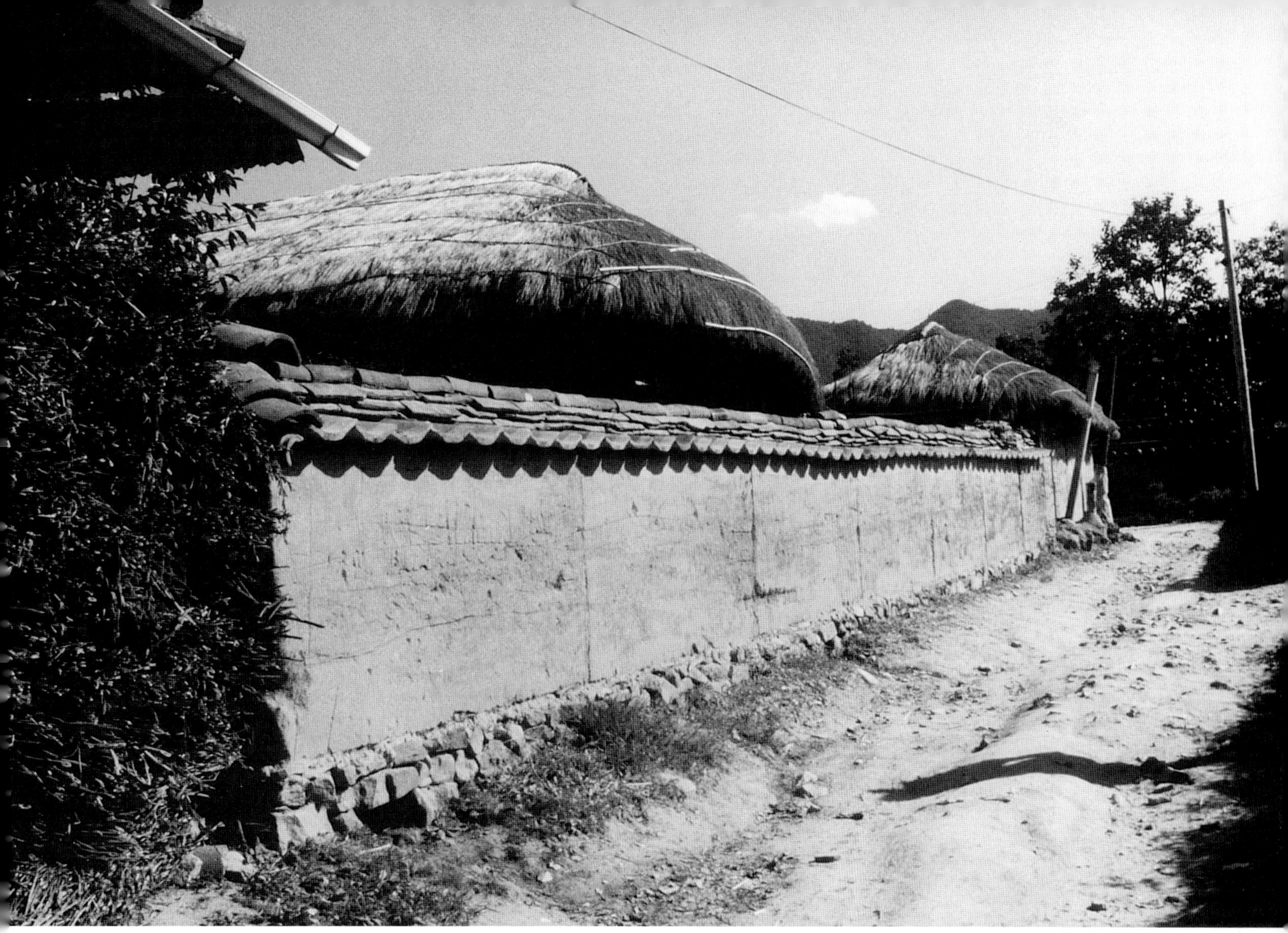

103.1 Exterior view and site plan of a rural village compound (Hahoe).

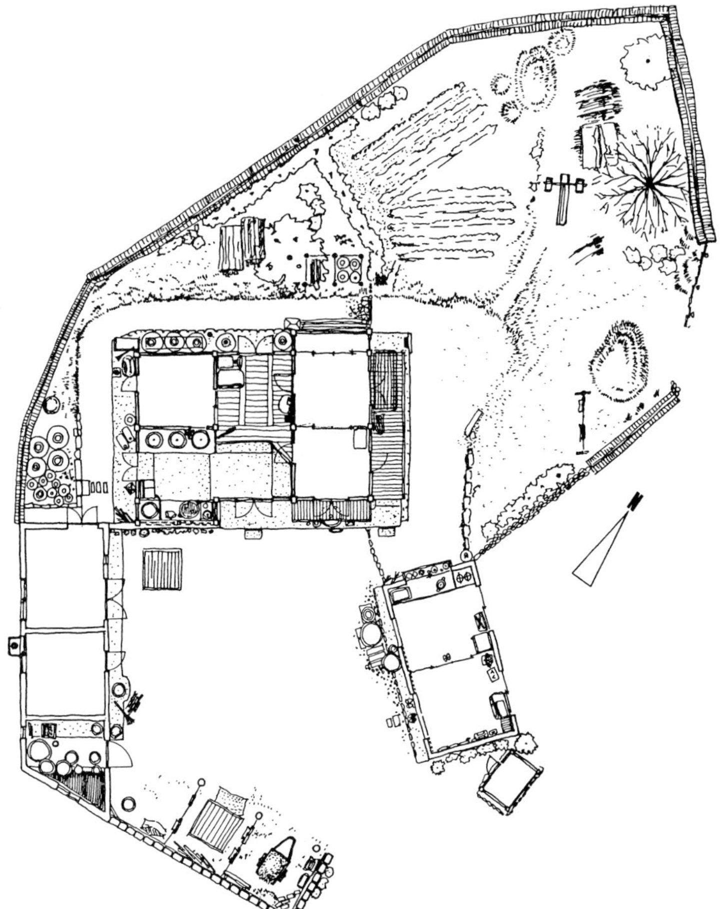

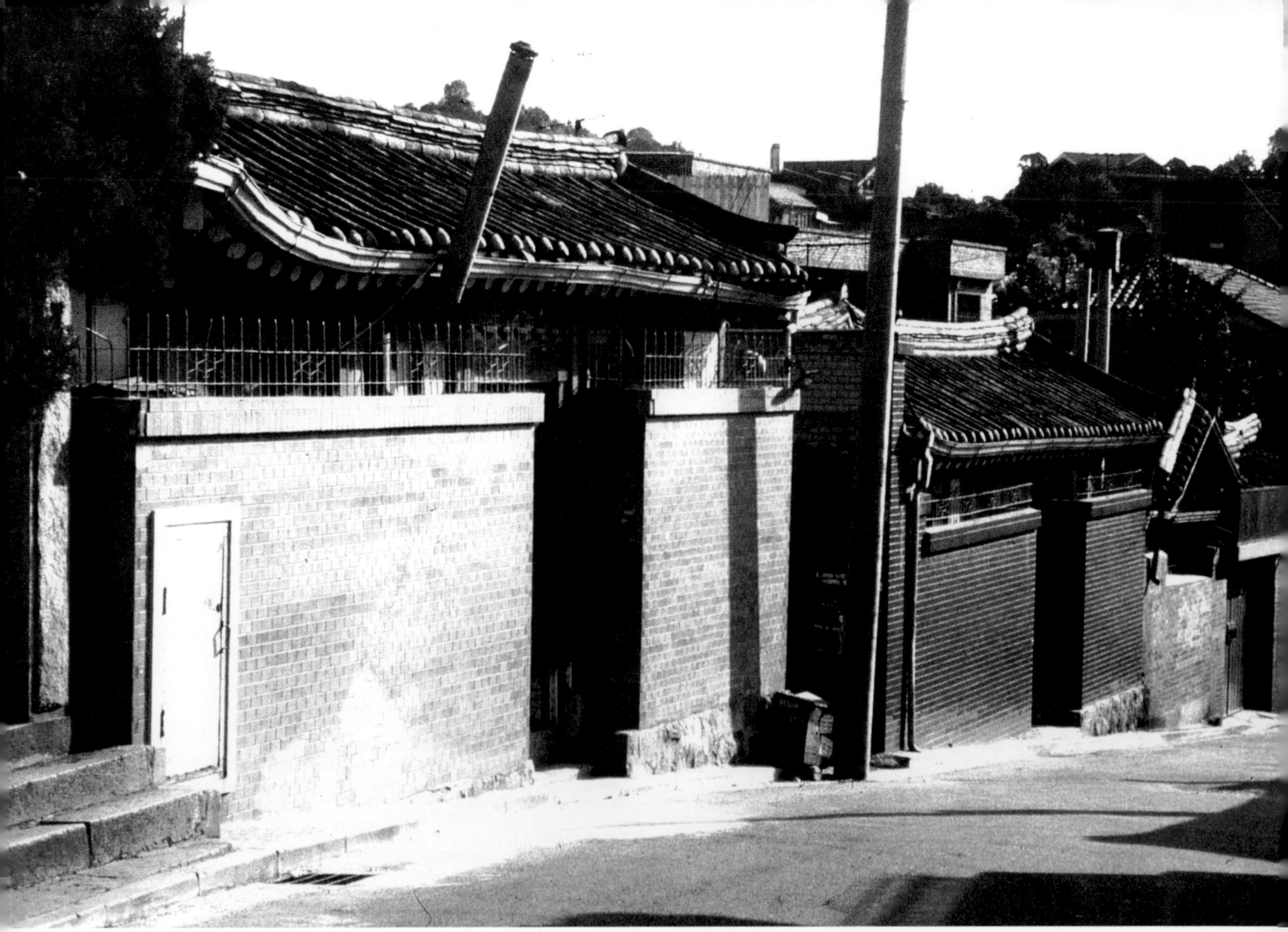

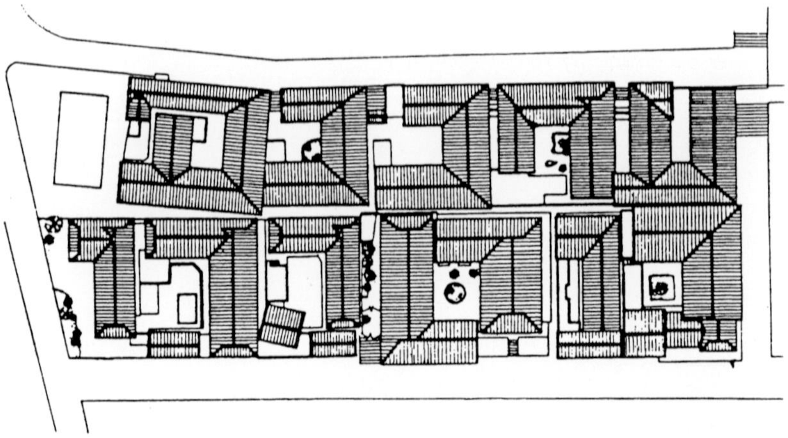

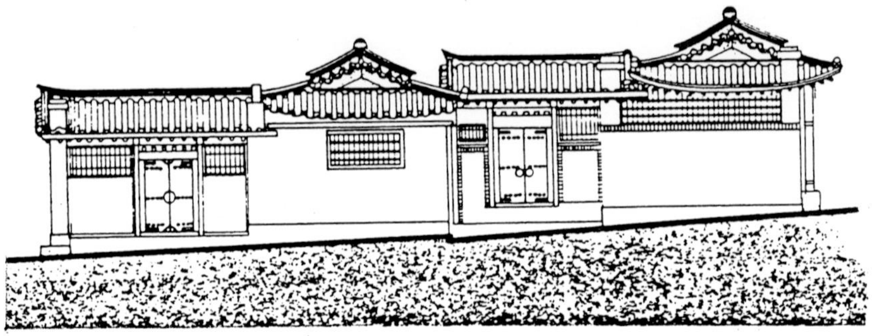

103.2 Exterior view, elevation, and ground plan of a traditional urban residential block (Seoul).

Pang do not have any built-in shelves or cupboards; the only furniture in the room consists of moveable chests and shelves for ornaments. As people sit on the floor, lines of sight are low, so any larger pieces of furniture are kept in either the *kolbang* or the *utpang*. All furniture in the *anbang*, therefore, tends to be ornamental, low, and relatively small, and—since the walls and ceiling of the room are plain white—brightly decorated, frequently with inlaid mother-of-pearl, and colored lacquer.

To derive the maximum benefit from the floor heating, bedding is rather thin; thus it can be folded and stored on top of a chest of drawers when not in use. This means that it is always likely to be in view, and so tends also to be brightly and decoratively colored.

Meals are usually eaten in the *ondol*-heated rooms, carried from the kitchen on individual low tables (*papsang*). In summer, however, meals are often eaten in the nearby *taech'ŏng*.

Pang are highly versatile rooms with a wide range of uses. They are extremely concentrated spaces, in terms of both size and decor. By contrast, the adjacent *taech'ŏng* and *maru* are very simple—almost rustic—and have somewhat loose spatial definition.

The *taech'ŏng* has bare wooden floors, mud or wooden walls, and an exposed beam ceiling. Its northern wall is enclosed by large wooden doors, but its southern side is completely open to the elements (Figure 106). Although its original function was as a ceremonial space, the need for the chilly *taech'ŏng* is difficult to understand, even if it does occasionally provide a cooler alternative to the adjoining *ondol*-heated rooms. Nevertheless, the *pang* and *taech'ŏng* do exist side by side, in stark contrast to one another, and this pattern is repeated throughout the dwelling.

Exterior Space (Madang)*: Repetitive Juxtaposition of Exterior and Open Interior Spaces*

Each *ch'ae* has its own *madang*, or garden: *anmadang*, *sarang madang*, and *haengnang madang*. As with the *ch'ae*, the reason for this distinction can be found in the Confucian sense of order. If we look past their particular classifications, however, we can see that all three of these gardens are fundamentally similar in that they are "white" gardens (areas of bare ground with little or no vegetation). The role of these singularly unornamental "gardens" becomes clear if we consider them in terms of their essential unity with the open interior spaces (i.e. the *taech'ŏng*) of the *ch'ae* interior space to which they correspond.

The floor of the *taech'ŏng* is usually constructed of thick boards laid on supports 60–70 centimeters (23.5–27.5 inches) in height. These are set on a solid earthen base built up 50–60 centimeters (about 19.5–23.5 inches) above the level of its adjoining *madang* garden. The space beneath the floorboards is left open for ventilation. This means that the *madang* garden is about 120 centimeters (47 inches) lower than the level of the *taech'ŏng* floor (Figure 107). In homes that have a *numaru*, or special reception room, the floor level of this room is raised an additional 40 centimeters (15.75 inches) above that of the *taech'ŏng*.

The height of the fences or hedges is kept to 130–140 centimeters (51–55 inches), so as not to restrict the view from these rooms. On its northern side, the *taech'ŏng* has doors that open out onto the greenery of the rear garden, but its southern side is permanently open to the elements, linking the room to the *madang* garden. The open and extremely simple *taech'ŏng* maintains a link to the enclosed *ondol*-heated *pang* that usually adjoin its eastern and/or western sides, while it simultaneously correlates to the gardens it faces to the north and south (Figures 108.1–108.4).

In *yangban* estates built near the top of a hill's south face, the *taech'ŏng* is raised high enough to command a panoramic view—beyond the *madang* garden and the outer wall—which encompasses the lower hillside, forest, plains, and usually a river. The wide doors on the

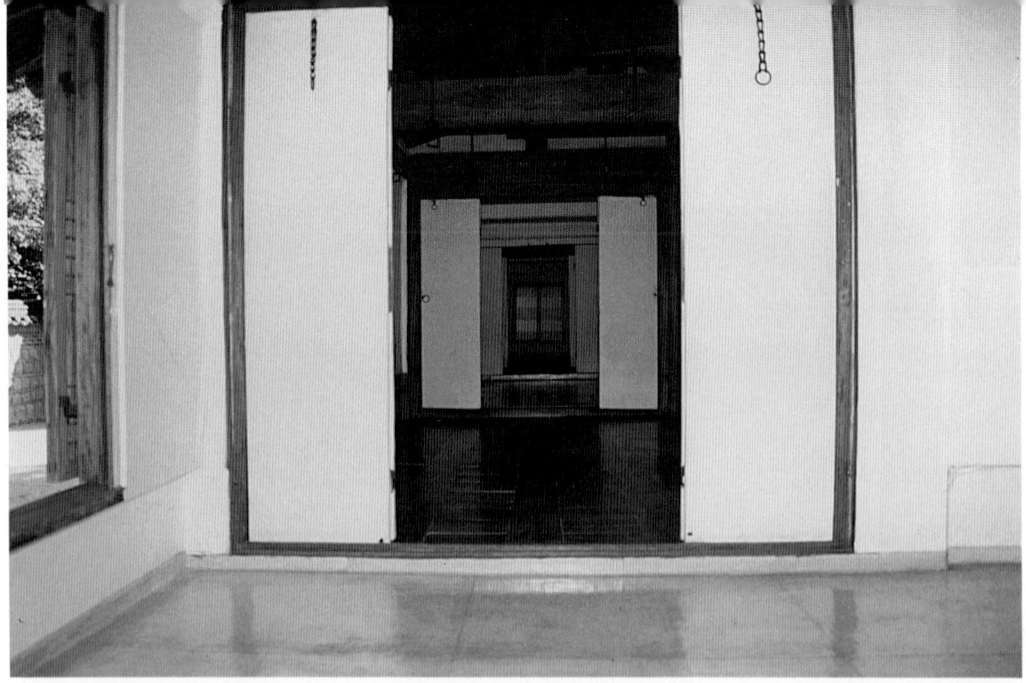

104 The repeated juxtaposition of enclosed spaces and open interior spaces.

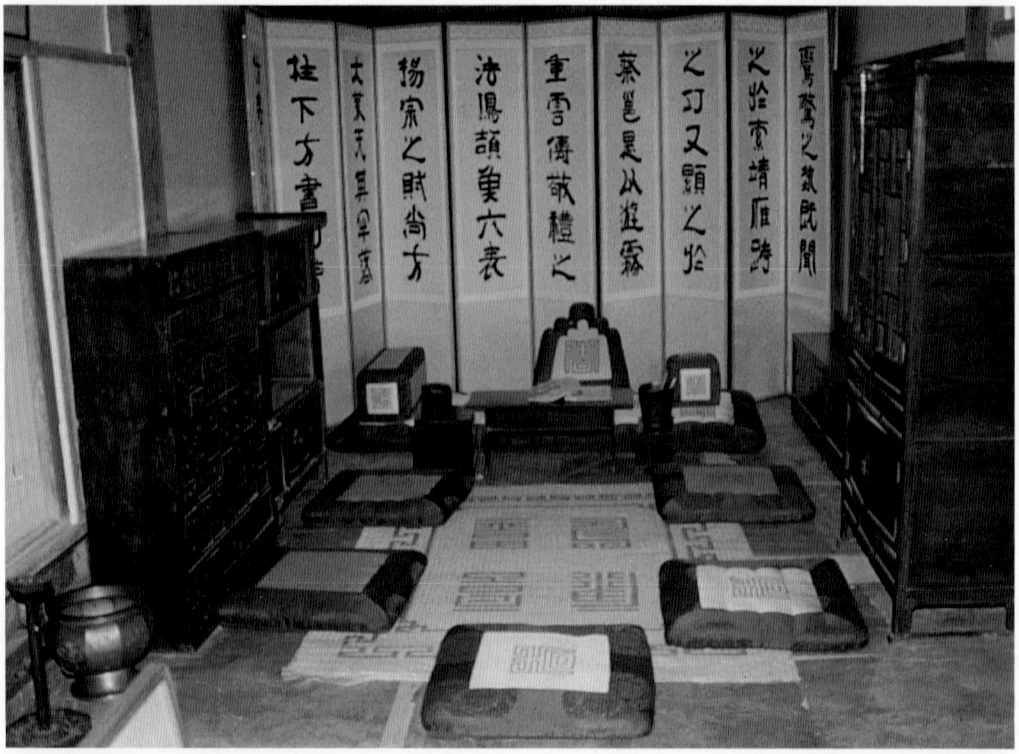

105.1 Male *sarangbang* furnishings in a *sarangch'ae*.

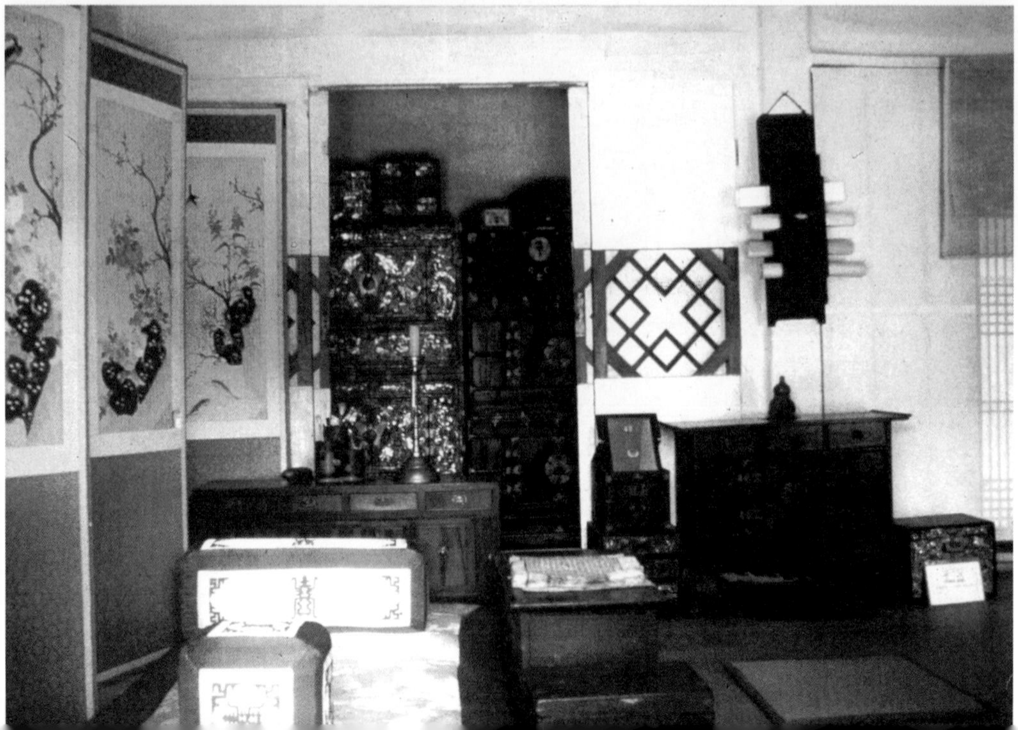

105.2 Female *anbang* furnishings in an *anch'ae*.

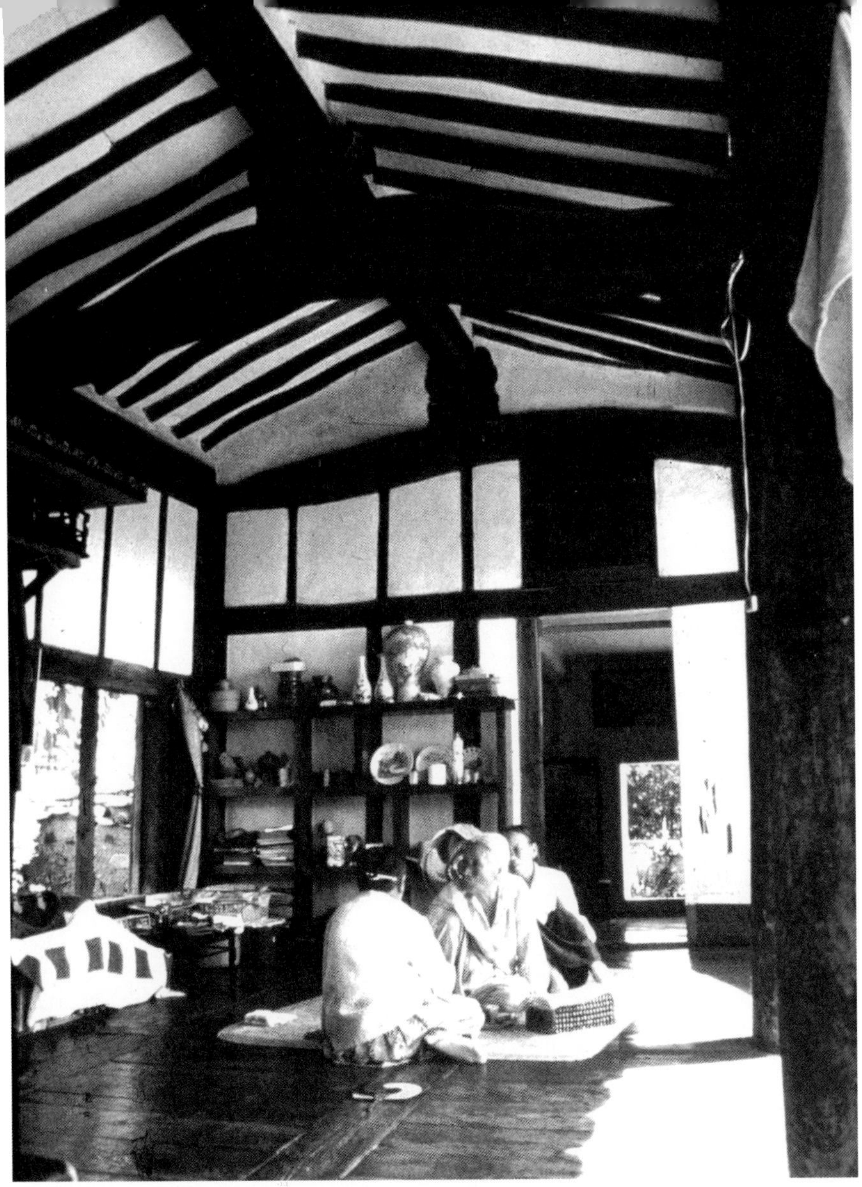

106 A view of the *andaech'ŏng* interior and lifestyle.

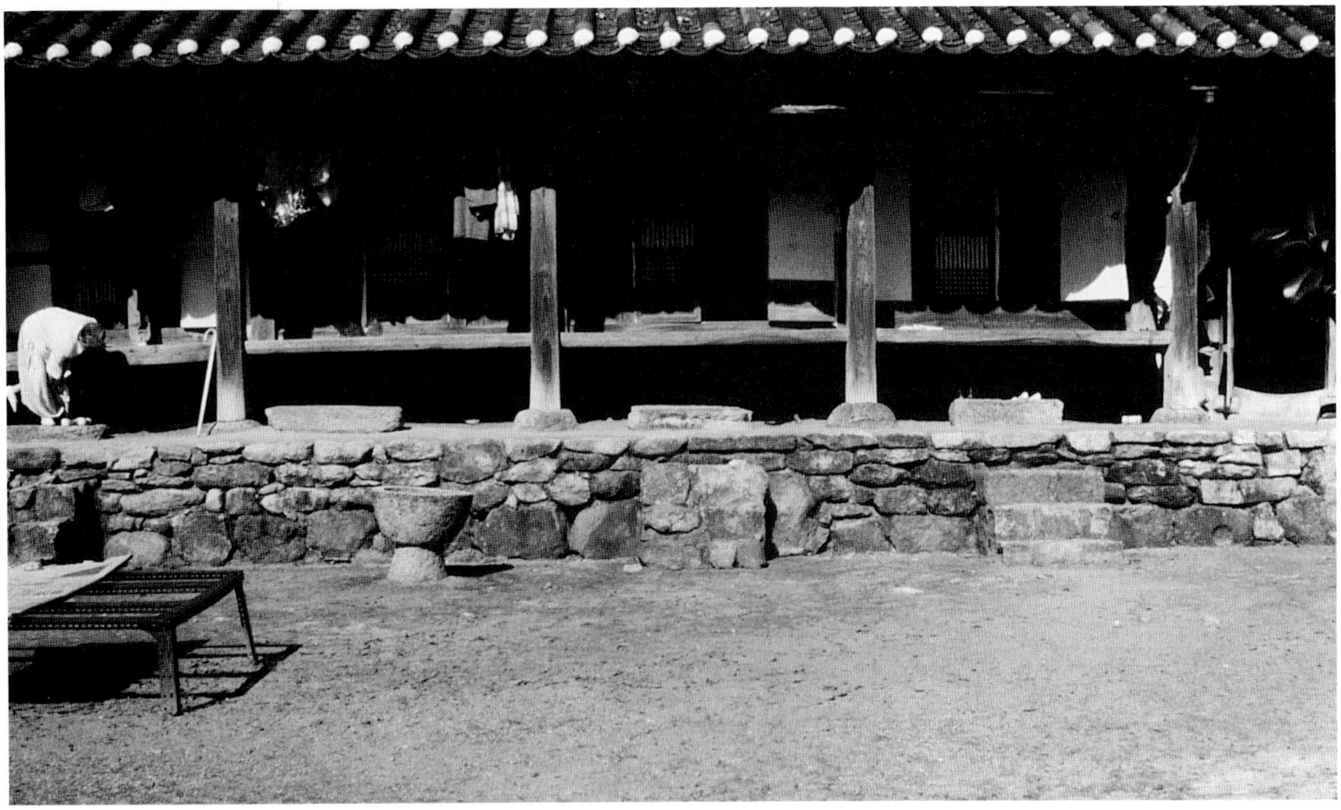

107 A view of the *anmadang* and the raised floor structure of the *taech'ŏng*.

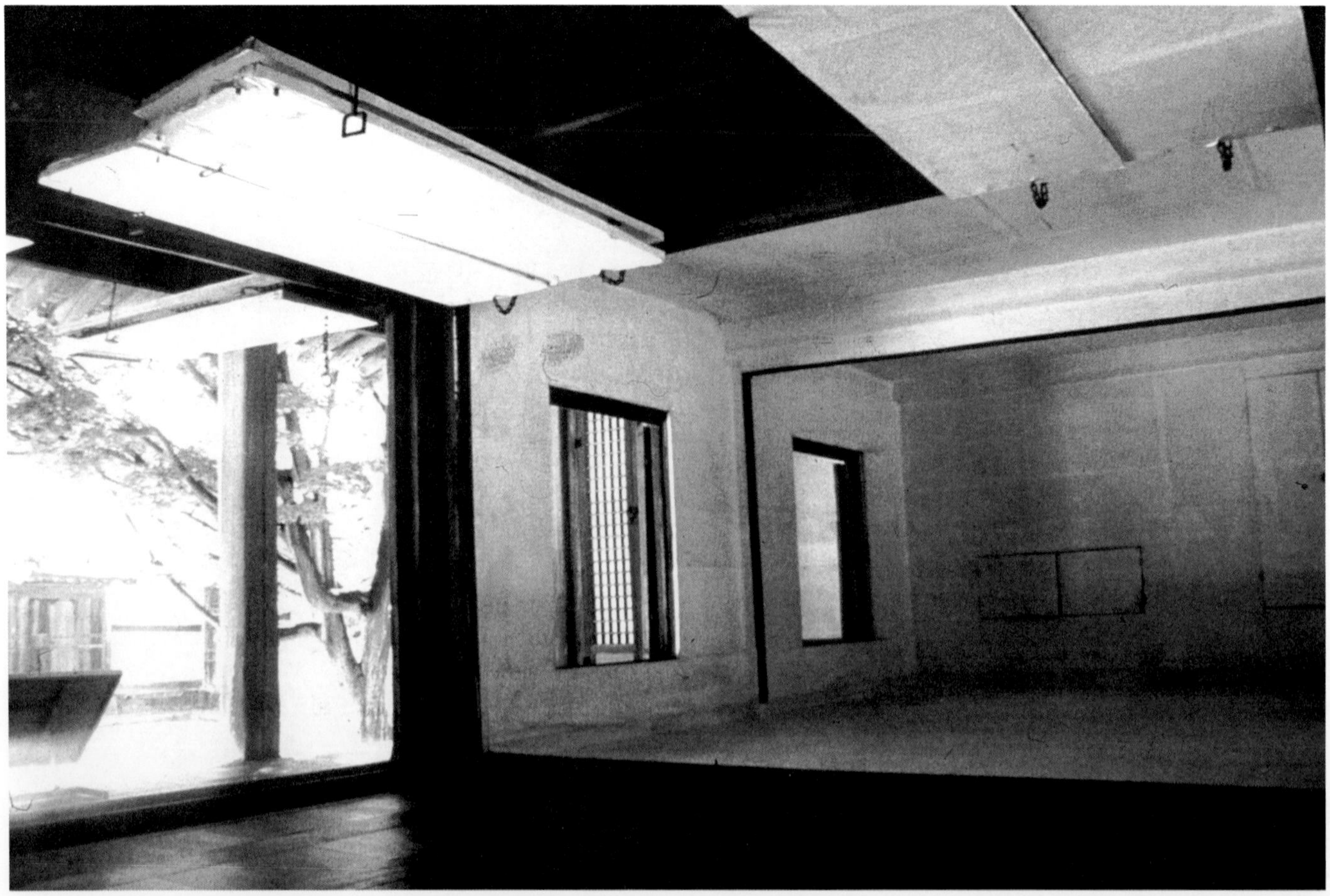

108.1 A view showing the threshold between closed (*pang*) and open (*taech'ŏng*) spaces.

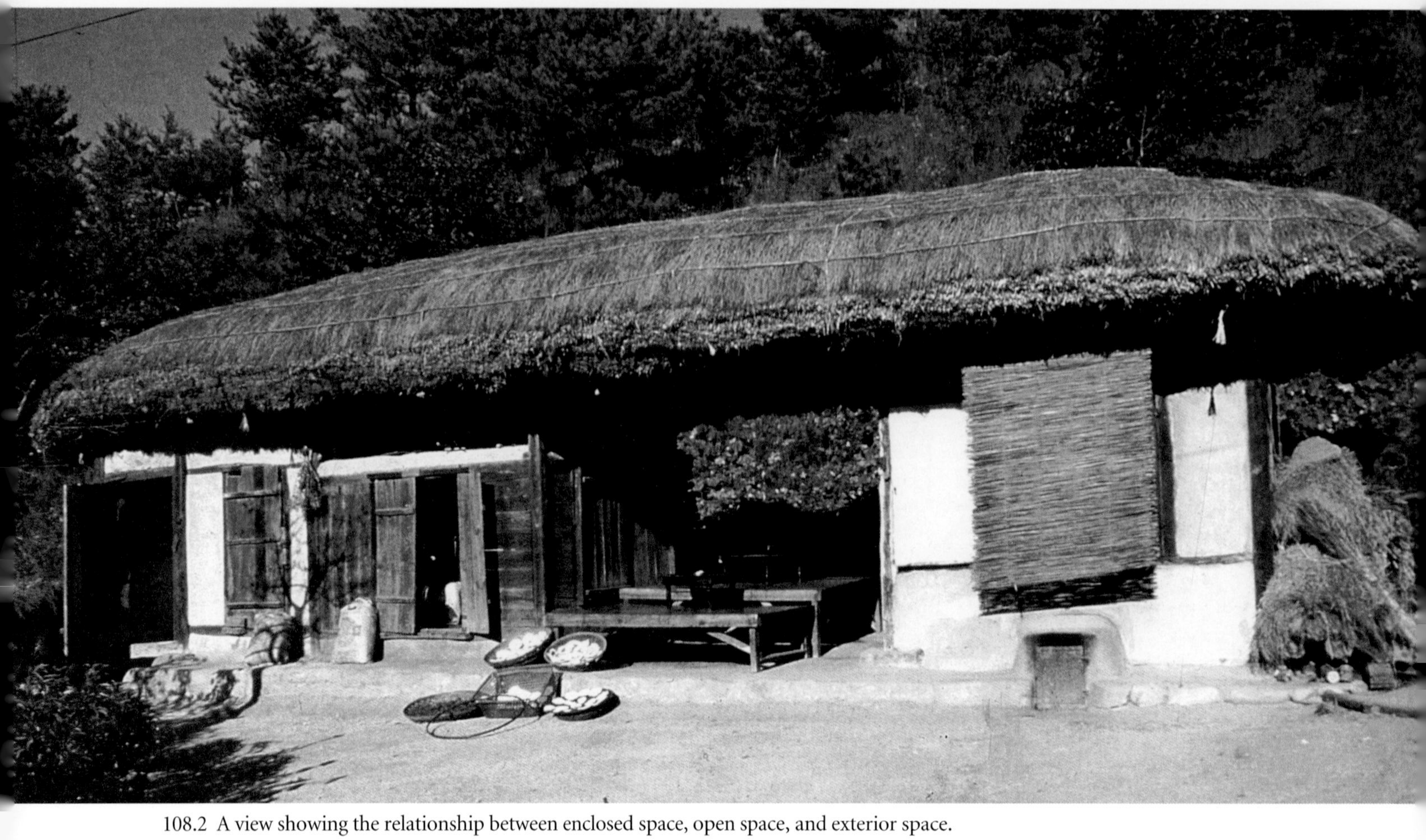

108.2 A view showing the relationship between enclosed space, open space, and exterior space.

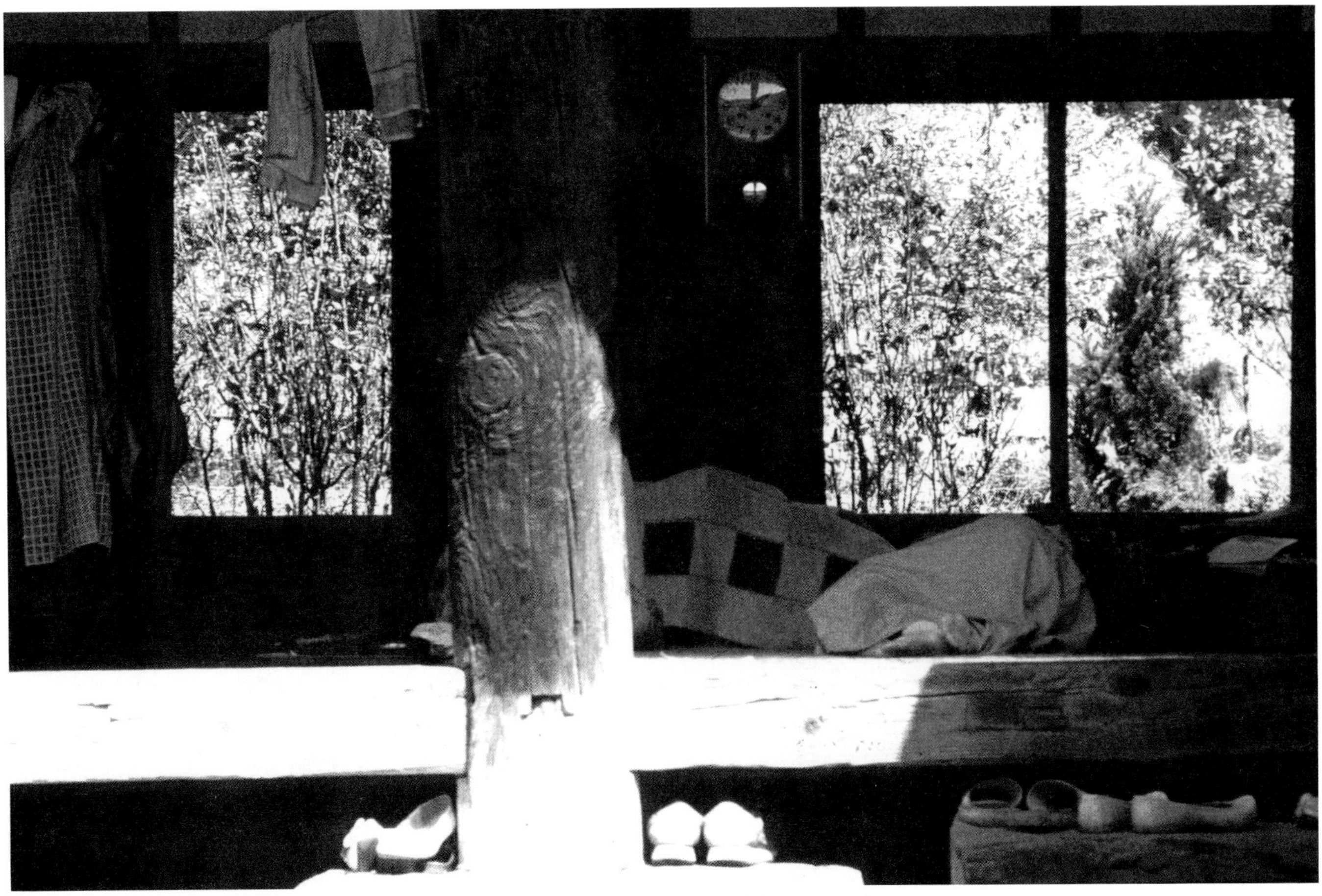

108.3 A view showing the relationship between the interior of a *taech'ŏng* and the rear garden.

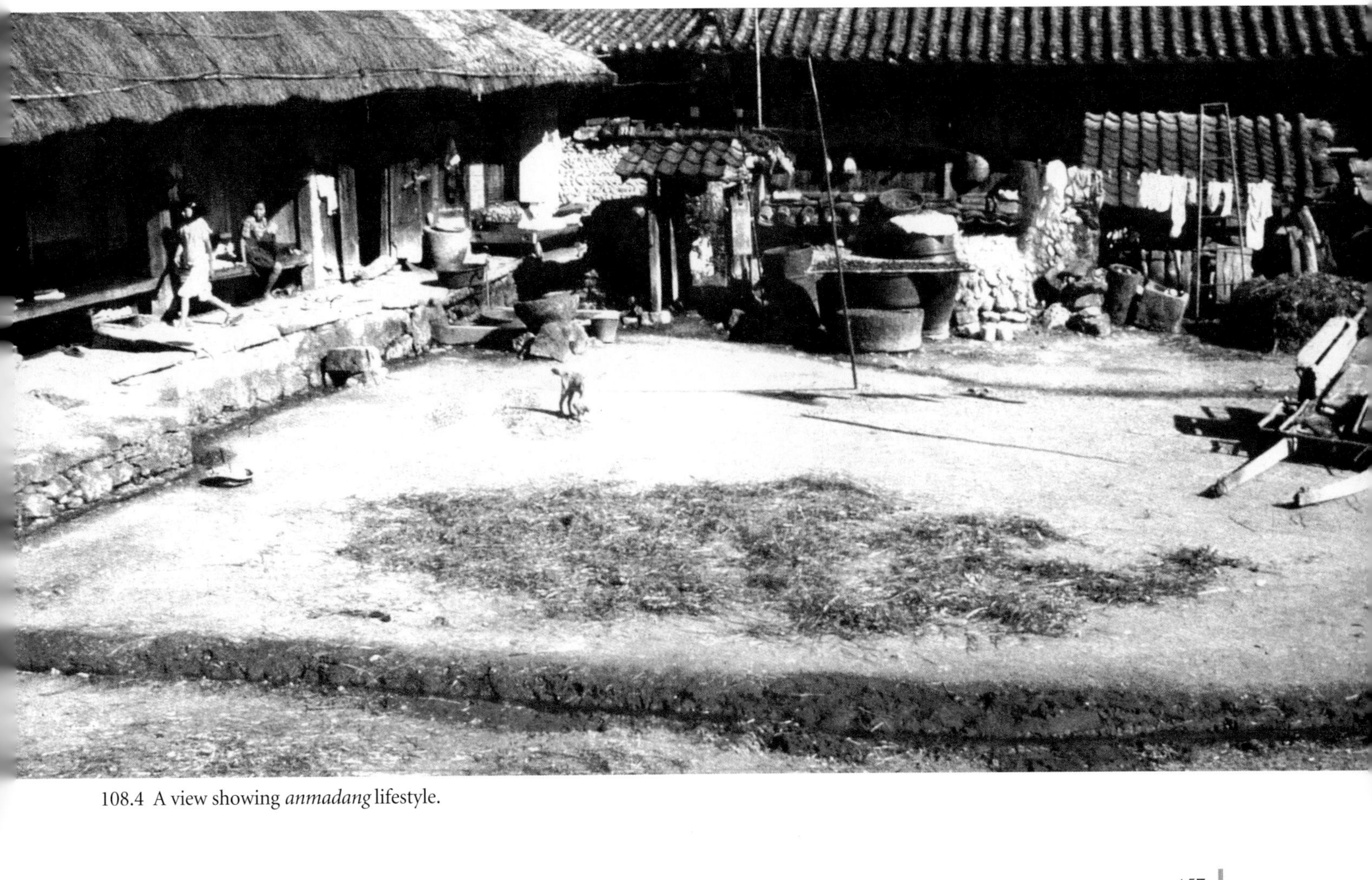

108.4 A view showing *anmadang* lifestyle.

taech'ŏng's northern side frame a view of the green upper slope of the rear garden. The *numaru* (reception room), raised higher still, has the optimal view.

Comparison of Korean with Chinese and Japanese Residences

The composition of the *ch'ae* interior space and *madang* garden of traditional Korean dwellings corresponds fairly closely to the hall and courtyard composition in traditional Chinese residences.

In the same way as a Korean *ch'ae* consists of *pang* and *taech'ŏng* (or *maru*), with the *taech'ŏng* open to the *madang* garden, the halls of Chinese dwellings are composed of private rooms and communal living rooms, or *tang*, which open onto the *yuanzi* or *tianjing* courtyard. In other words, in both Korea and China, the courtyard "garden" serves as an outdoor extension of the adjoining room, and is in no way an ornamental garden for viewing from indoors.

The *tang* of a Beijing *siheyuan* has doors on its southern facade, with several steps leading down to the *yuanzi*. Throughout southern China, on the other hand, the living room is quite similar to a Korean *taech'ŏng*, in that it has an exposed beam ceiling and wooden walls on the northern, eastern, and western sides, and is completely open to the south, where the courtyard lies. The main difference is that the floor of the *tang* is on the same level, and covered in the same material—stone or brick—as the *tianjing* courtyard outside. It is even more closely linked physically to the courtyard than is the *taech'ŏng* of a Korean dwelling, since the *taech'ŏng* is not only raised above the level of the adjoining *madang*, but may be entered only after footwear is removed. Nevertheless, the openness and simplicity of the *taech'ŏng* creates a visual link with the *madang* that reflects their essential unity. The Chinese arrangement gives priority to function, while the Korean endures a certain inconvenience in order to enjoy an unobstructed view.

The *woshi* of a traditional Chinese dwelling and the *pang* of a traditional Korean dwelling are also similar, in that both are enclosed spaces. They are also of a similar size, the Chinese *woshi* usually being 3 meters by 6 meters (9.8 feet by 19.6 feet) and the Korean *pang* ranging from 2.4 meters by 4.8 meters (7.9 feet by 15.7 feet) to 3 meters by 6 meters. The main points of divergence are that the Chinese use chairs and beds while Koreans sit and sleep on the floor, and the fact that in Chinese dwellings private rooms are used exclusively for sleeping. Because they are completely private spaces, Chinese *woshi* are decorated in accord with the individual occupant's taste, while the *pang* of a traditional Korean home are multipurpose rooms, each used by a number of people and as a result, Korean *pangs* are decorated in keeping not with individual preference, but with function and custom.

The rooms of traditional Korean and Japanese residences are similar in that they are multiplepurpose. But whereas a wide variety of movable furniture is used for decoration and storage in the Korean *pang*, one basic characteristic of the Japanese *zashiki* (reception room with *tatami*-mat flooring) is that decoration and storage are built-in. Such integral ornaments includes the *tokonoma* (ornamental alcove), *chigaidana* (staggered shelves), and *tsukeshoin* (desk alcove), while storage spaces include auxiliary rooms (*tsugi no ma*), built-in closets (*oshi-ire*), small storerooms (*nando*), and storehouses (*kura*). The latter were used for a kind of rotational storage, with different items being stored away or taken out seasonally, at three- or six-month intervals. Moreover, many of the items used in a traditional Japanese home can be folded, rolled up, or stowed away for convenient storage when not in use. The long-term rotational storing of items in storehouses, however, is something that does not occur in either China or Korea.

One other distinctive feature of a traditional Japanese dwelling is the intimate relationship between a room's character and the items used in it. That a room has a distinctive character is a factor of the building in of decorative accoutrements, such as the *tokonoma* and *tsukeshoin*, but since the beginning of the Edo period, mansions were composed of a combination of rooms built in distinctly different styles—the formal *shoin*, semiformal *sukiya*, and rustic *sōan*. Each of these specialized spaces has its own set of appropriate furnishings and utensils, which are also changed periodically to fit the season or the occasion (i.e., celebratory or somber), and which through their combination create a vast range of decorative settings.

This essential relationship between a space and the items used in it survives in the multipurpose rooms of today's Japanese homes. It is a feature unique to Japan, seen in neither Korea nor China.

8

The "Uncultivated" Garden

The closest Korean equivalent to the type of residence in China that would have its own *ting yuan* or *yuanlin* is the estate of a *yangban* (civil or military official), and the factors governing the composition of a *yangban* residence have been examined in the previous chapter.

Although the traditional Chinese residence and the *yangban* residence differ in layout and form, the hall and courtyard composition of the former is much the same as, and corresponds to, the *ch'ae* and *madang* of the latter.

The Korean *madang* is an outdoor extension of the adjacent *taech'ŏng* in the same way that a Chinese *ting* (courtyard) is an extension of the adjacent *tang* (central living room). The *madang* and *ting* both serve as functional work spaces, and as places where ceremonies are performed. Neither is designed as a decorative garden to be admired from the interior space. There is, however, nothing within the Korean residential complex that is equivalent to the Chinese "unworldly" gardens—the *ting yuan* (contemplative landscape garden) or the *yuanlin* (landscape park garden).

The *ting yuan* or the *yuanlin* of a traditional Chinese residence is an "extraordinary" space adjacent to the everyday living space but sufficiently separated from it to remain untouched by the mundane. The only possible equivalent in the Korean tradition would be the outer garden centered around a lotus pond, beyond the main gate, or the garden around a *pyŏldang* (a sanctuary used exclusively by the master of the household; Figure 109). Both these gardens, however, are rooted in the tradition of the hermit priests of the Unified Silla (A.D. 668–935) and Koryŏ kingdoms, which is quite distinct from the philosophical foundation of the Chinese *yuanlin*.

At the same time in which Confucian thought—with its tremendous influence on people's lifestyle—was incorporated directly into Chosŏn society, the *yuanlin* gardening techniques of Ming- and Qing-dynasty–China were also transplanted. It was originally believed that Chosŏn-dynasty *wŏnlin* (*yuanlin*) were the product of the combination of this influence with older Korean traditions. It is conceivable that there was a native gardening tradition with a place in the history of Korean gardening parallel to that of Koryŏ celadon in ceramics. Yet the only gardens now extant are better compared with Chosŏn-dynasty white porcelain. Unfortunately, there are no Chosŏn *wŏnlin* in existence today.

Defining the Korean Approach to Garden Making

The most straightforward of motivations for making a garden is the desire to recreate nature as realistically as

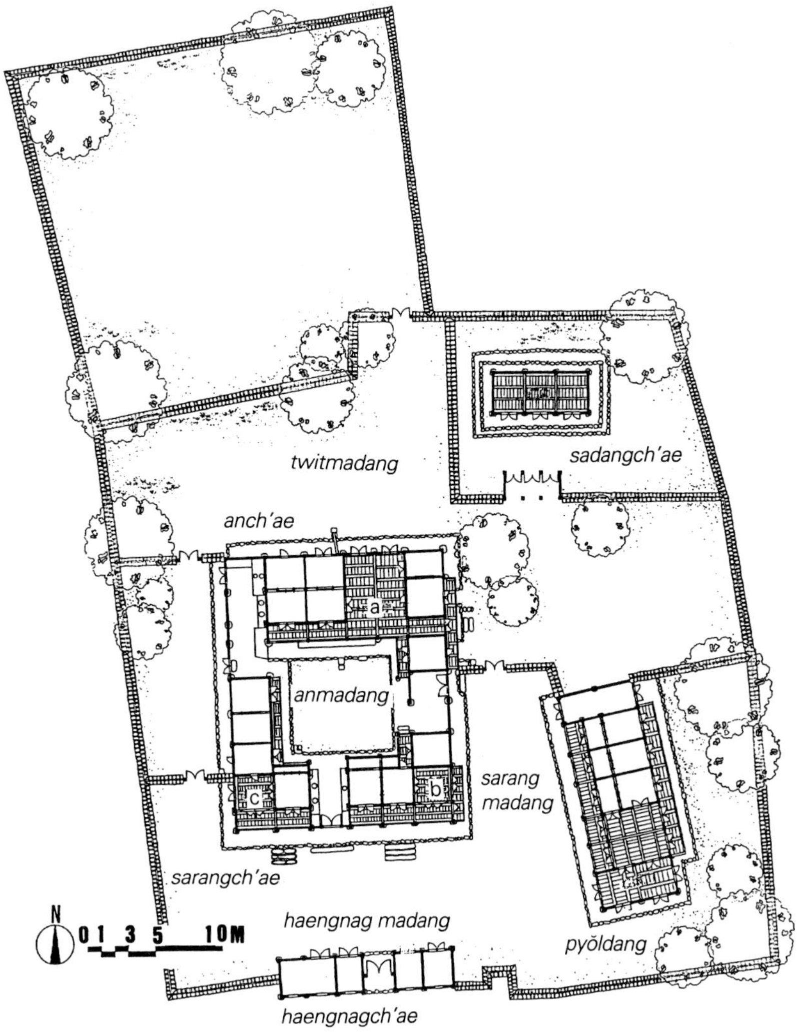

109 Site plan of the Pukch'on residence (Hahoe).
a. *andaech'ŏng.* b. *sarang taech'ŏng.* c. *maru.*

possible within the particular limitations and conditions of a given space.

In the opinion of architect and historian Horiguchi Sutemi, "Only when the expression of a garden is such that it encompasses the space does the structure of the garden take on true expression. 'Encompassing the space' means going beyond 'raw nature'—both the nature within and surrounding the garden—to create a 'nature' that everyone can see and enjoy."[1]

To some extent, gardens have always been viewed by this measure alone. In the case of Japanese gardens, *Sakuteiki* specifies "recalling your memories of how nature presented itself for each feature," and a similar principle is applied to Chinese gardens as well, despite huge differences in scale and methods.

A consideration of whether the *yuanlin* gardening techniques of Ming- and Qing-dynasty–China were relevant to the climate and customs which shaped the composition of *yangban* estates in Korea should help to clarify any areas of Chinese influence, just as it is evident that the form of traditional homes of the Chinese upper classes exerted an influence on the configuration of *yangban* dwellings. This should make it easier to appreciate the special characteristics of traditional Korean gardens as they exist today.

How then are the five aspects of *yuanlin* garden making outlined in the late-Ming–dynasty gardening manual *Yuan ye* related to Korean gardens?

Situation (Xiang-di)

Xiang-di is the factor that dictated the design approach used in creating the Chinese *yuanlin.* A sense of harmony with the surrounding landscape was preserved by building high points up higher, and digging low-lying areas deeper—in China these techniques served to accentuate the natural contours of the land. This was the principal method used to create a *yuanlin* on the basically flat land of the Jiangnan region, where conditions were fundamentally very different from those in Korea. In Korea, of course, the natural topography provided an abundance of favorable sites with mountains behind and rivers in front.

Layout of Buildings (Li-ji Wu-yu)

Li-ji wu-yu refers to the way in which buildings are to be laid out on the site, and how they are to be constructed. As is indicated by the stipulation "1. Buildings, 2. Flowers and trees, 3. Water and rocks," the location and position of the various buildings is given highest priority.

In Korea, on the other hand, the first step is selecting a site with suitable natural features, after which the layout of the buildings is determined so as to provide the best possible prospect (*chomang*) and borrowed scenery (*ch'agyŏng*).

The layout of buildings in a Chinese *yuanlin* seeks to achieve a reciprocal relationship between each building, creating mutual and intersecting views, whereas in Korea views from one building to another are deliberately avoided.

Screens (Ge) *and Curves* (Qu)

Ge and *qu* refer to the artificial means used to create different scenic areas on multiple levels in a large *yuanlin,* the principle behind which is expressed by the terms *bu-yi jing-yi* ("changing step, changing view") and *bie you dong tian* ("another world"). Devices for segmenting the garden space and creating these multiple levels are walls, caves, gates, and covered walkways.

In large Korean rear gardens such as Piwŏn (Secret Garden), a number of scenic areas are laid out, one leading into another, to be enjoyed while meandering through the environment. However, these areas are bound together not by artifice, but by nature, thus they are better described as landscapes for strolling than as gardens in the traditional Chinese sense. The natural distribution of trees is the primary means of linking one scenic area to another. Gates, walls, and other man-made additions form demarcations of "territory" in keeping with Confucian principles, and are not used for the purpose of delineating a shift from one scenic area to another.

Raising Mountains (Duo Shan) *and Selecting Rocks* (Xuan Shi)

Duo shan and *xuan shi* are the factors that determine the forms of artificial mountains—the main scenic features in the Chinese *yuanlin*—and the types of stones selected as the materials for those mountains. Since the *yuanlin* is usually laid out on flat terrain, great emphasis is placed on layering and piling up rocks to create vertical contrast as a means of expressing images such as "strange and steep peaks" and "waterfalls dropping from steep cliffs." Pavilions are built on top of piled rocks to afford a "high climb, distant view," and caves are cut into layered rocks to provide spaces to "think meditatively and ponder in silence." The importance accorded these focal points in the garden means that stones with particularly striking shapes are prized highly—in fact so highly that Chinese scholars have compiled lists of the most fantastic and most famous stones.

In Korea, artificial hills called *tongsan* are sometimes featured in rear gardens or outer gardens, but they are always gentle, grass-covered slopes quite different from the mountains of the Chinese *yuanlin.* In some Korean gardens we can see vestiges of a tradition introduced from China of admiring distinctive stones, known in Korea as *sŏkkasan* (literally, "pseudo rock mountains") which are displayed singly or in simple arrangements.

Borrowed Scenery (Jiejing)

In traditional Chinese gardening, there are four types of borrowed scenery: *yuanjie* (scenery in the distance), *linjie* (scenery nearby), *yangjie* (scenery above), and *fujie* (scenery below). These generally refer to views obtained from buildings or the tops of artificial mountains. The object of all these techniques is to create a connection and a sense of harmony between the *yuanlin*—which is surrounded by a wall—and the scenery beyond that wall.

In Korea, on the other hand, the location of the site—known as *sanji*, or discernment of favorable land from the unfavorable—is itself key to the view afforded, and buildings are configured in such a way as to reap the full benefit of the views provided by the site. Thus borrowed scenery (*ch'agyŏng*) is the only one of the five principles outlined in *Yuan ye* that truly applies to traditional Korean gardens.

It is clear then that the character of the inner garden of a traditional Korean dwelling is determined primarily by its prospect, (*chomang*) and that it is fundamentally very different from the character of a Japanese garden or a Chinese *yuanlin*.

Borrowed Scenery Versus Prospect

Borrowed scenery is, by Japanese standards, a natural element that forms the background of a picture plane in which the actual garden forms the foreground. In other words, borrowed scenery refers to the intentional incorporation of a distant scenic element—the actual focal point of the garden—against which a garden scene is created in the foreground to complement the greater effect. It is a technique whereby a garden of limited area is set against a feature of a distant natural scene, such as a mountain, to draw a sense of the infinite into a finite environment.

Take the garden of Jikō-in, near Nara, in which a panoramic scene is framed by the eaves and the veranda of the temple. It is composed of a shallow garden of clipped bushes in the foreground, and the Yamato mountains shrouded in mist in the background, across the broad sweep of the Nara Basin. The Jikō-in garden is made limitless by this composition.

"Prospect," meanwhile, refers to a panoramic vista unobstructed by an artificial framing element—or the type of view, for example, which would be afforded someone standing in the far corner of the foreground garden at Jikō-in, looking out toward the mountains of Yamato. It is as though one has stepped through the picture frame into a landscape painting. This is where we can draw the line—delicate though it may be—between the artifice of a cultivated garden and the beauty of nature, or between viewing nature as part of a composed scene and merely viewing nature.

It is only when the interior of the building and the view of the outside are completely balanced, as they are in architectural forms specifically designed to provide panoramic views, that prospect qualifies as a category of gardening methodology.

The gardener's art creates a composed picture by capturing the beauty of nature in the frame formed by the building's eaves or lintels, pillars, and door sill or floor line. What makes it the "art" of gardening is that the human hand has, in some way or another, enhanced nature as it exists.

On the whole, the garden-making approach used in traditional Korean residences falls somewhere between "prospect" and "borrowed scenery," and represents a view of garden making that came into prominence in Korea during the Chosŏn period. The gardens of Chosŏn Korea developed from two traditions: the first is this approach to gardening that lies somewhere between prospect and borrowed scenery, and the second is that handed down from the older kingdoms of Unified Silla and Koryŏ. The former may be called an introverted approach (not intended for display), and the latter, extroverted. Indeed, the extroverted approach produced highly symbolic garden compositions, such as the Kyŏnghoeru Pond of Kyŏngbokkung and the ponds in the outer gardens of *yangban* estates. The introverted approach, on the other

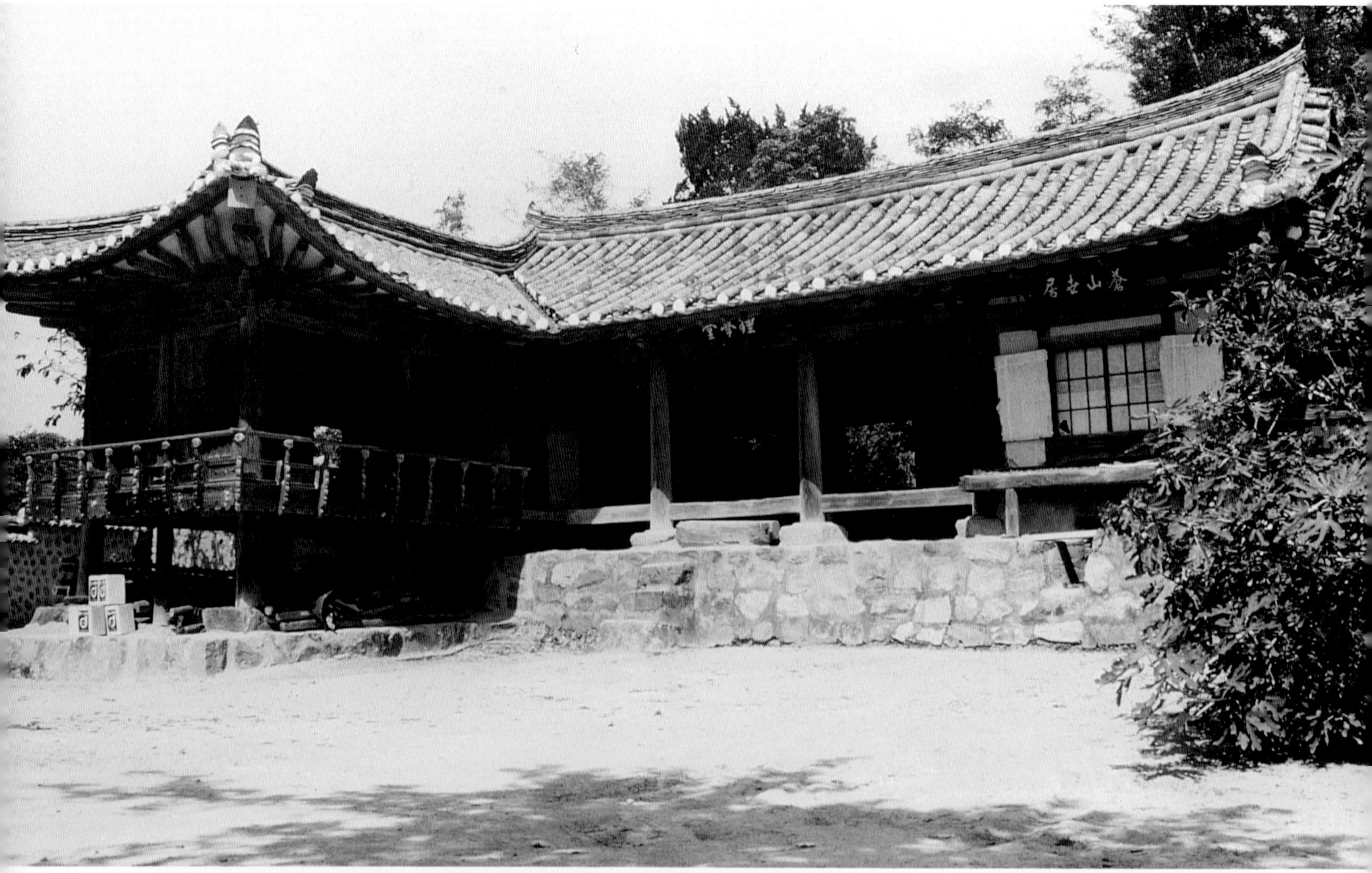

110.1 A *sarangch'ae* composed of (from left to right) a *numaru, sarang taech'ŏng,* and *sarangbang* (Mugongdang, Wŏlsŏng).

hand, is characteristic of the Chosŏn period, and closely related to everyday household activities. However, the introverted approach also includes another garden form—the creation in Korea of environments for the *pyŏlsŏ* (retreats) of Confucian scholars—which are very similar in their ideological background to Chinese *yuanlin.*

Prospect and Borrowed Scenery in the Composition of Residences

In Korea it was traditionally believed that the majority of the design decisions involved in laying out a residence could be resolved simply by selecting a suitable site according to the geomantic principles of *p'ungsu.* The most desirable sites, known as *myŏngdang* land, were on southern slopes, as was mentioned earlier, with mountains behind them and rivers in front.

The *taech'ŏng,* with its open southern facade, is always built on an elevated base with a raised wooden floor, and if there is a drawing room, or *numaru,* it is raised even higher. There are no fixed standards for how high above the ground each of these rooms should be. Perhaps the only criterion is that the floor should be set high enough for people sitting on it to enjoy the benefit of the view (Figure 110.1–110.3). Prospect provides the basis on which to build a raised-floor structure to create borrowed scenery.

This structure is open wide to the south, and has roof beams that are totally exposed, and no obstructing doors or walls that cannot easily be removed or slid out of the way. In this way, prospect becomes borrowed scenery. Unlike the wall around a Chinese *yuanlin,* the outer wall of the residential compound is not so high that it shuts out the scenery on the other side. Viewers inside can enjoy the panorama over the top of the wall, which has been kept to just the right height to permit a clear view. The optimal view is afforded from a seated position on the floor of the *taech'ŏng.* A person sitting in the *taech'ŏng*

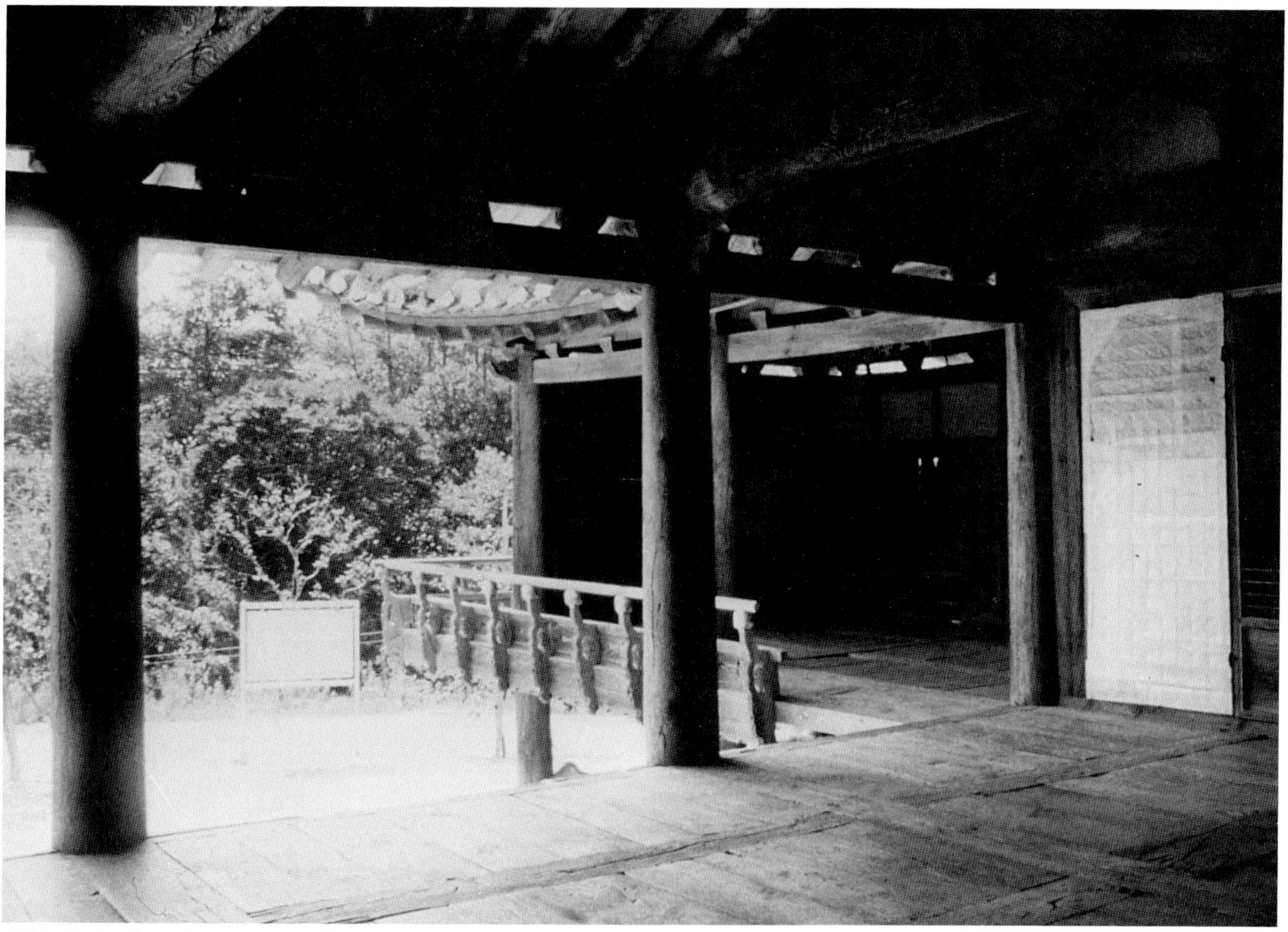

110.2 A view from the *sarang taech'ŏng* to the *numaru*.

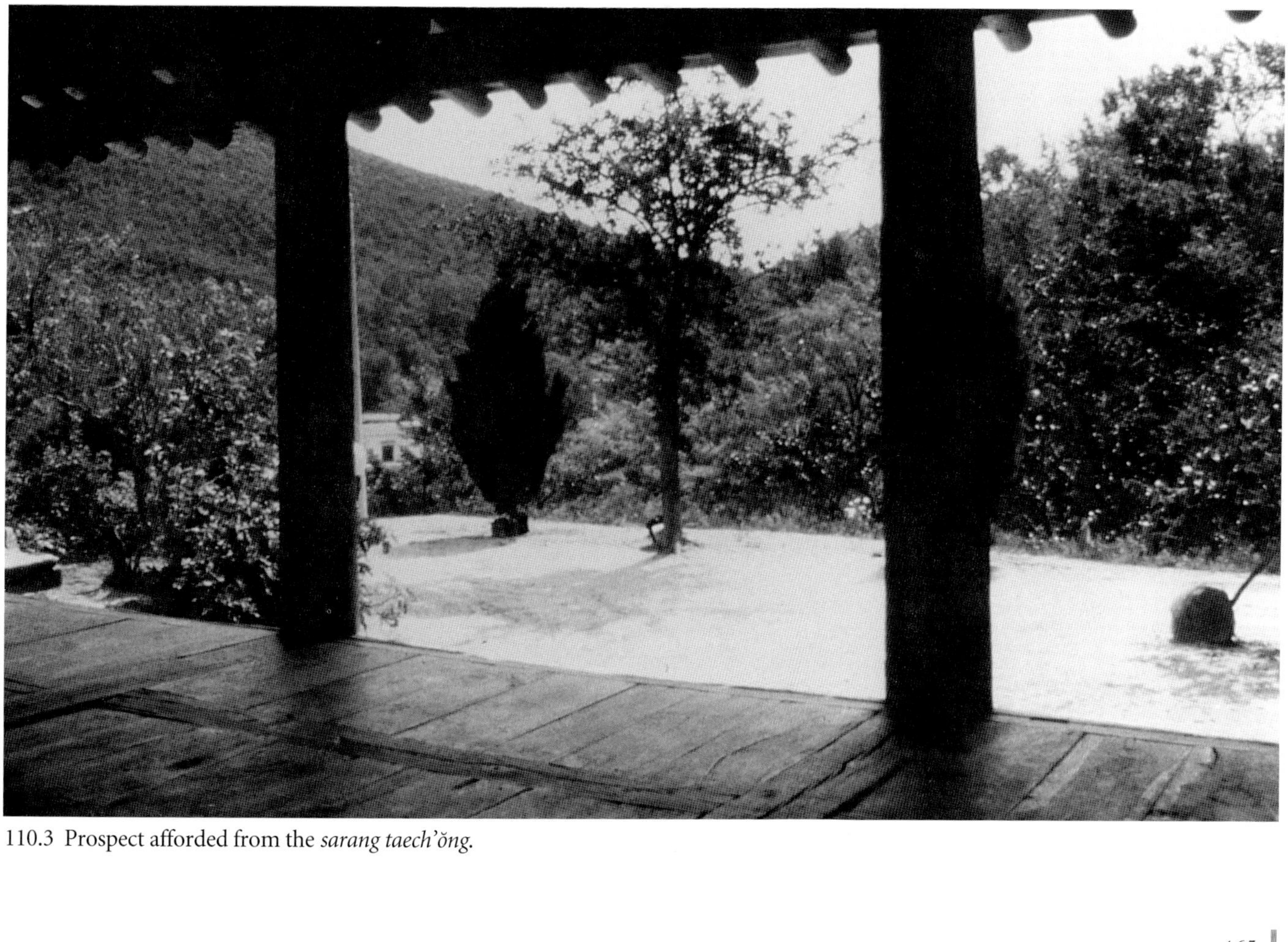

110.3 Prospect afforded from the *sarang taech'ŏng*.

can also look out through the frame of the sliding doors in the wall at the greenery of the rear garden to the north (Figures 111.1–111.5).

The Korean approach to creating a garden starts from the point of "building a house in keeping with prospect," where the entire southern slope of the hill is spread out before the viewer's eyes (Figures 112.1–112.3).

Twitmadang (Rear Garden)—A Private Exterior Space

The area of open ground on the slope behind and north of the *anch'ae* is called the *twitmadang*, or the rear garden. It is sometimes located at the top of a series of stepped terraces.

The significance of this rear garden lies in its role as an exterior space for the leisure activities of the women and children of the household, who traditionally lived in the *anch'ae* and were forbidden to leave the residential compound without good reason. It was a very private space, which men—particularly men from outside the household—were not permitted to enter.

In contrast to the inner gardens, which are essentially bare of vegetation, the *twitmadang* may contain grass, shrubs, flowering trees, and fruit trees. In a corner is sometimes a large ornamental stone, and it is not unusual for a pavilion to be built in very spacious rear gardens. In many cases, though, the rear garden is no more than an area of open grass with a cluster of unruly trees. Since prospect is the chief objective in planning, the garden itself is not thought to require any particular attention (Figures 113.1–113.4).

Thus, the rear garden is part of the family's living space, closely linked with the *anch'ae*; in this sense its *raison d'etre* is completely different from that of a Chinese *ting yuan* or *yuanlin*. If a garden is defined as a place to be viewed and admired by owner and guests, a *twitmadang* does not qualify as a true garden.

There are two ancient palaces in Seoul—Kyŏngbokkung and Ch'angdŏkkung—both of which are great royal palaces preserving something of the glory of Chosŏn Korea amid the rush and bustle of the modern capital. During the Chosŏn period, however, Kyŏngbokkung was the seat of government, where visitors were granted audience or entertained, while Ch'angdŏkkung was home to the royal family. One particular feature of Ch'angdŏkkung is the huge Piwŏn (Secret Garden), which sprawls over 27,000 square meters (6.66 acres) behind the palace buildings.

The Secret Garden was the rear garden of Ch'angdŏkkung, and it played the same role in the Imperial residence as did the *twitmadang* of any *yangban* estate. Just as the women and children who lived in the *anch'ae* of a *yangban* mansion were able to stroll around their walled rear garden, so too were the queen, princesses, and young princes able to enjoy the private, open space of the Secret Garden behind their palace home. Piwŏn spreads out over a gentle slope and contains many trees—102 different species in all. Quarried-stone–lined ponds, halls, and pavilions are scattered strategically around the garden, belvederes are set amid lawns, and paths run through the woods linking these features one to another. Piwŏn is submerged in nature. The importance of prospect and borrowed scenery in the composition of the buildings applies here just as much as it does in other gardens (Figures 114.1–114.3).

The *twitmadang* of a *yangban* estate and the huge park-like grounds of the royal palace were essentially the same kind of space, rooted in the same traditions. Piwŏn was a very private place; it was never used for entertaining visitors from outside the royal family.

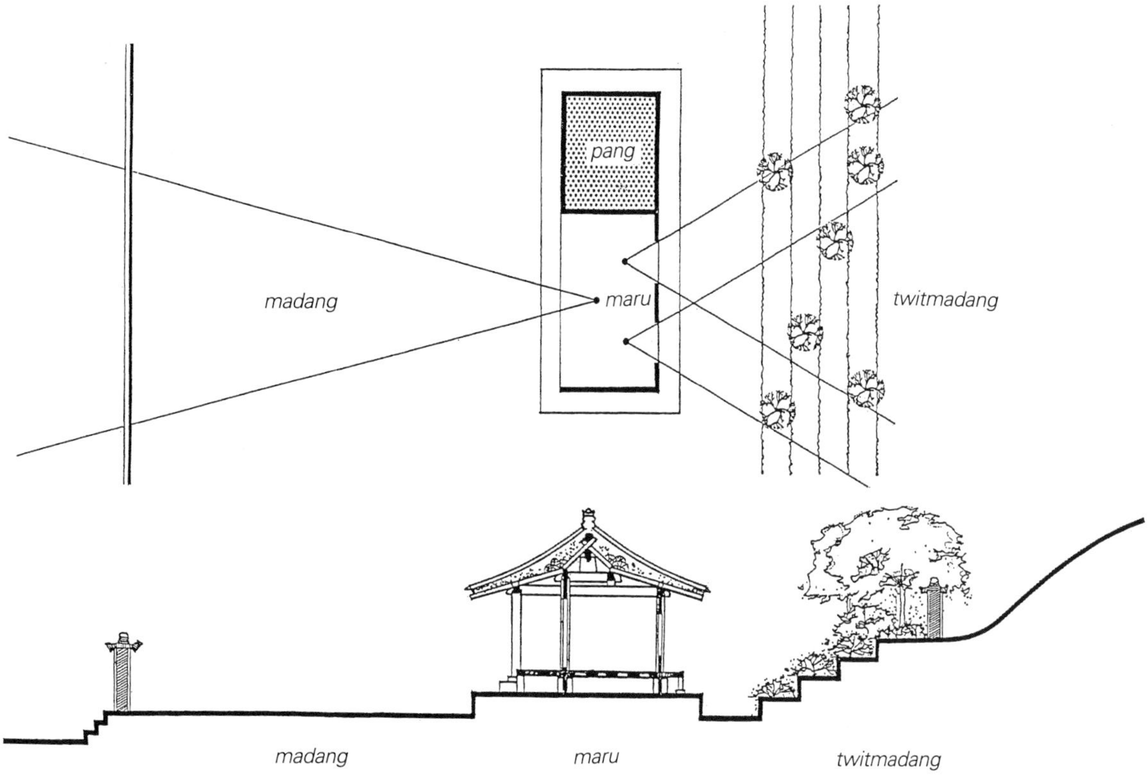

111.1 Ground plan and section schematics showing the location and structure of buildings on the site composed to afford optimal views.

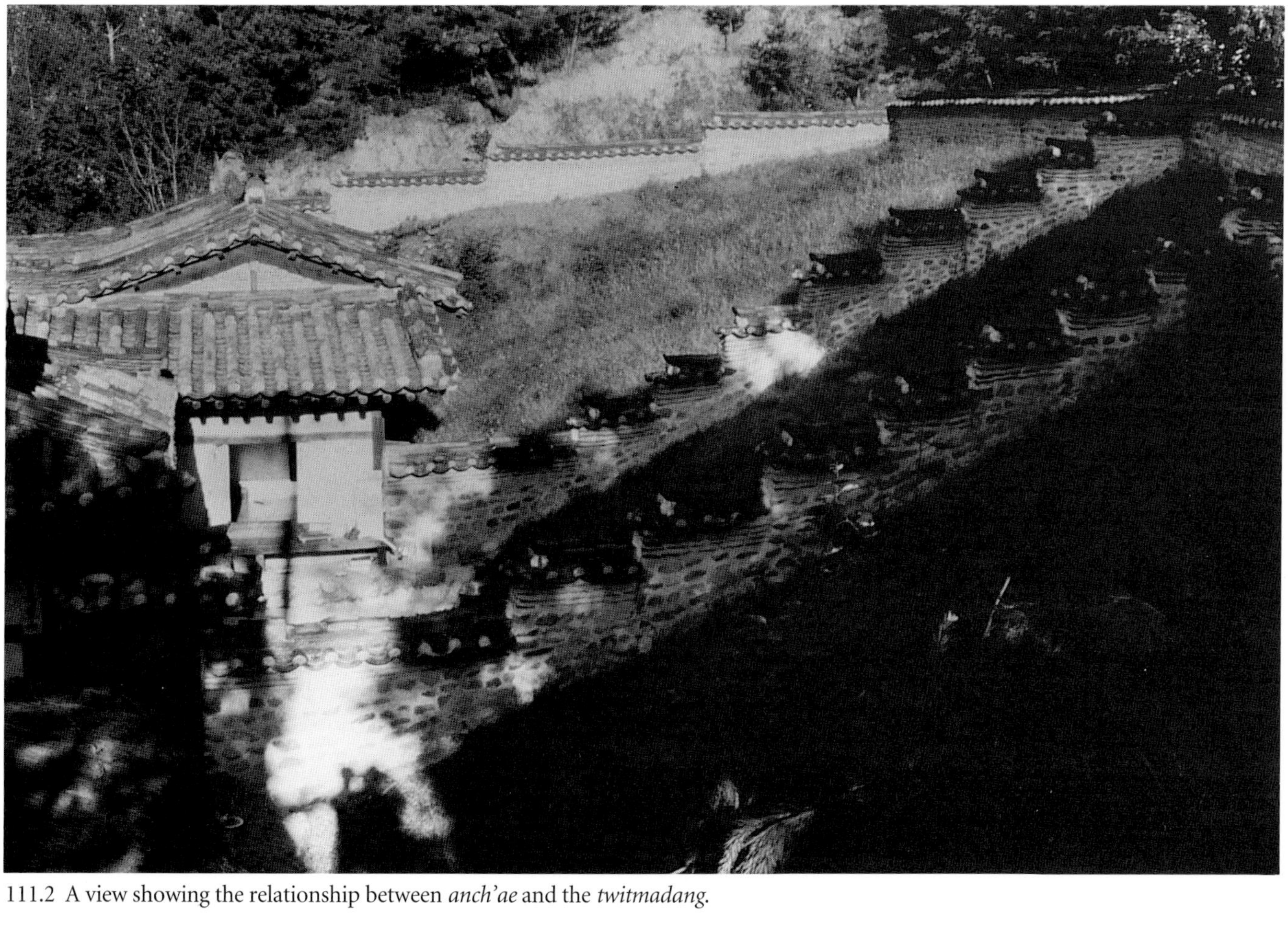

111.2 A view showing the relationship between *anch'ae* and the *twitmadang*.

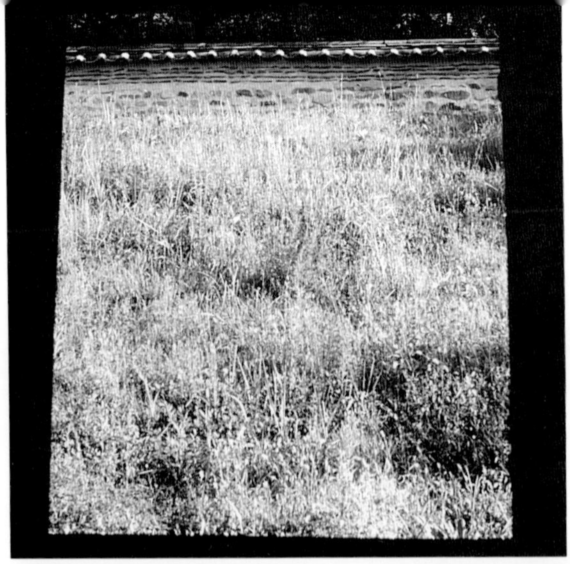

111.3 A view through the *taech'ŏng* north wall window of the *twitmadang*.

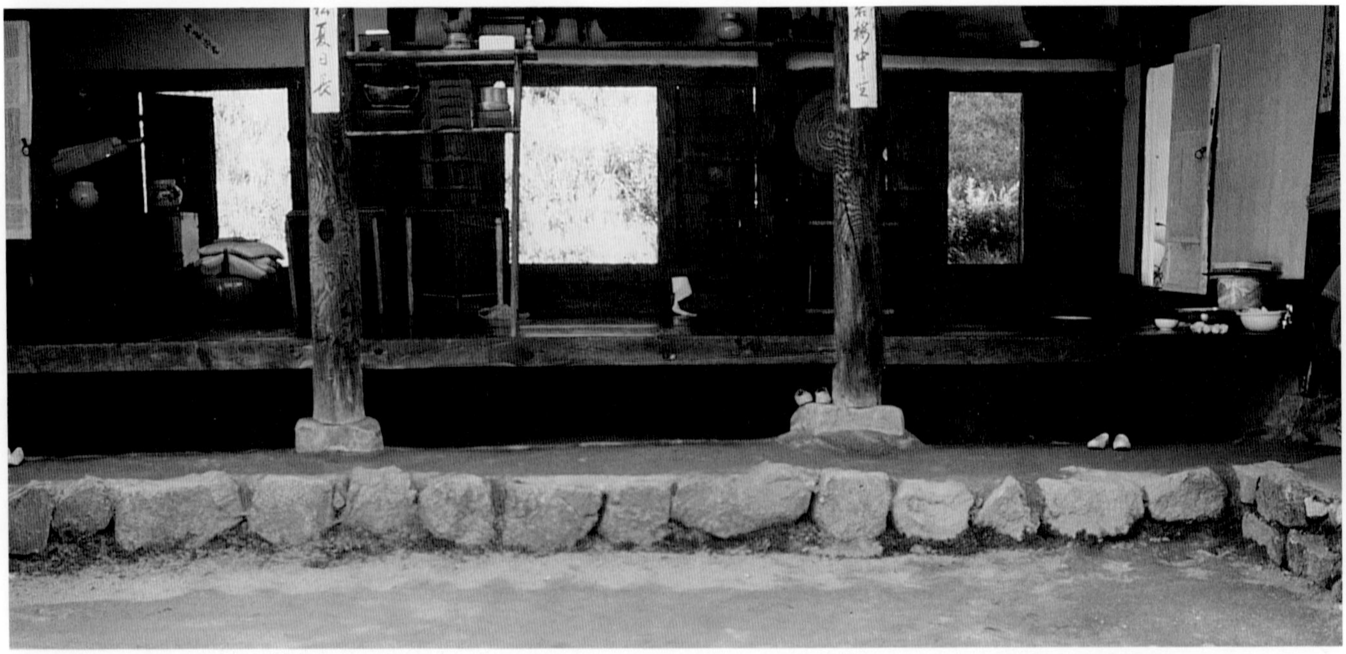

111.4 A view showing the relationship between the *taech'ŏng* interior and the *anmadang* in front and *twitmadang* behind.

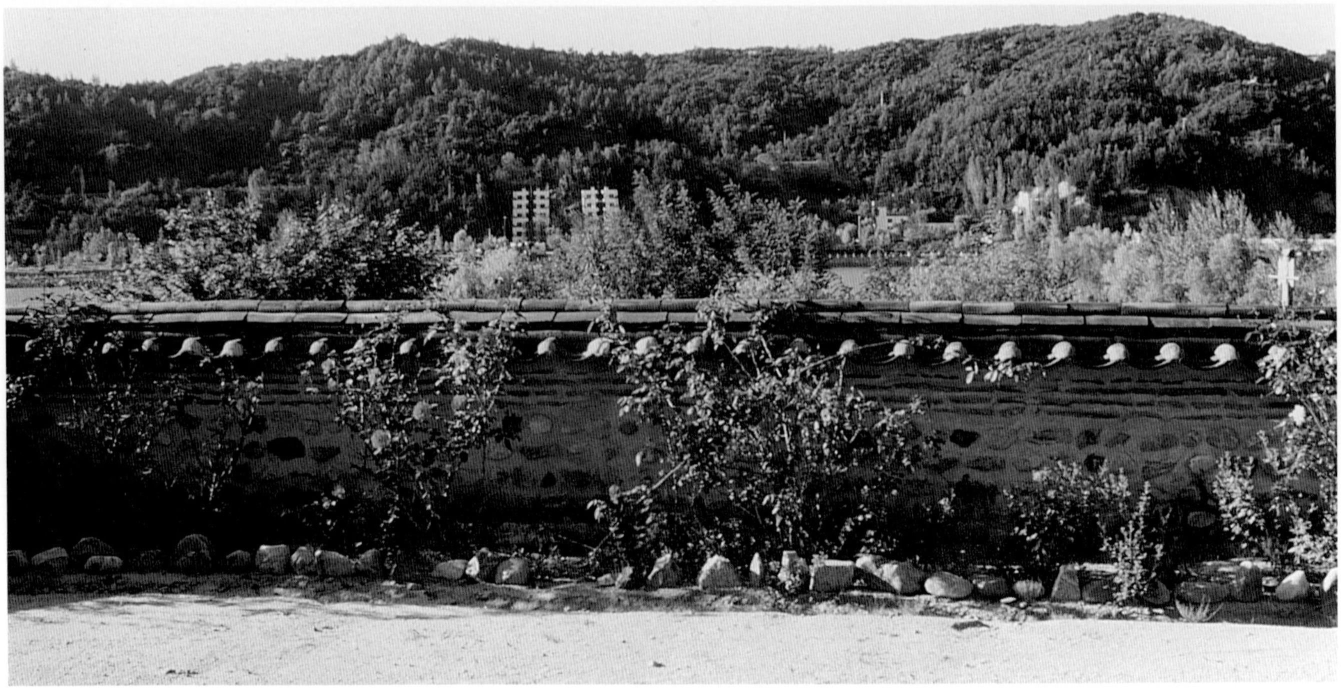

111.5 A view of the *anmadang* outer wall and the scenery beyond.

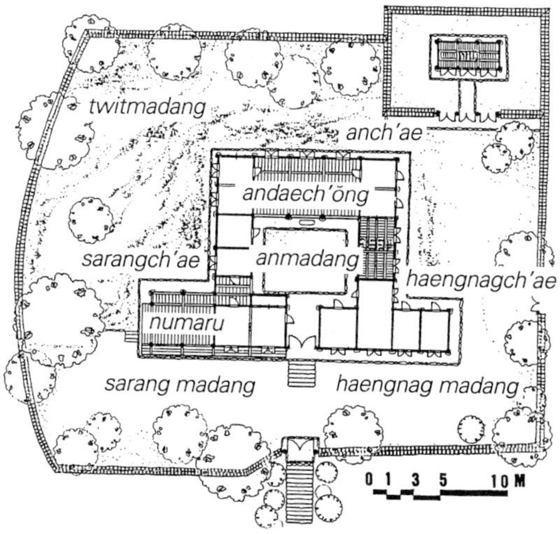

112.1 Site plan of Kwan'gajong (Wŏlsŏng).

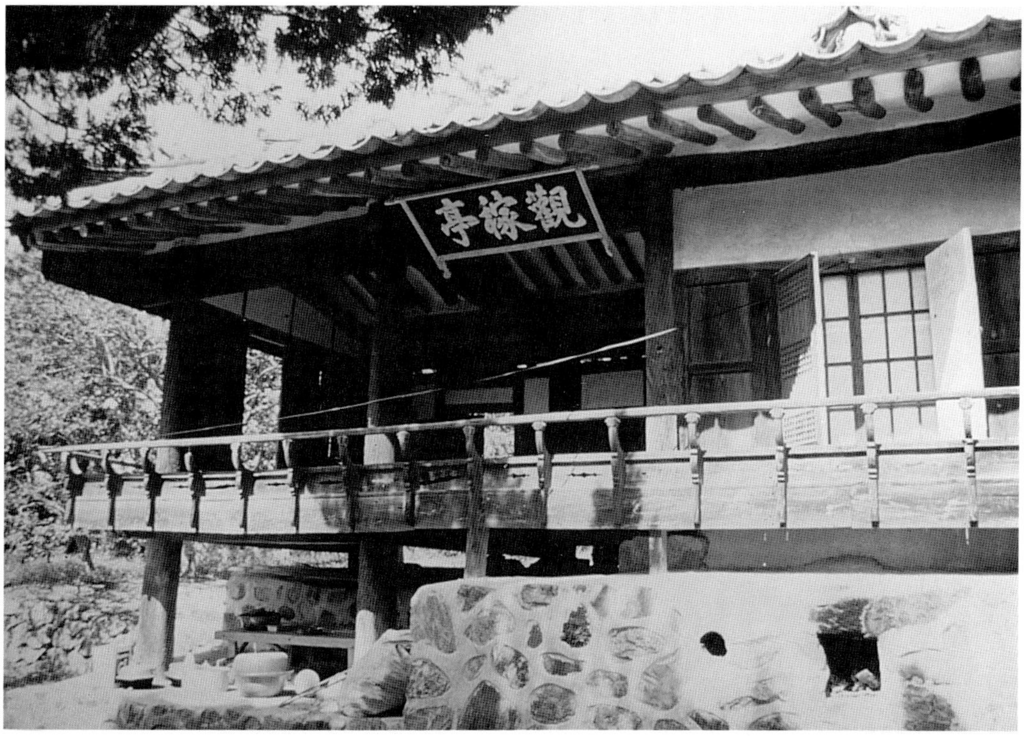

112.2 The *sarangch'ae numaru* and adjacent *sarangbang.*

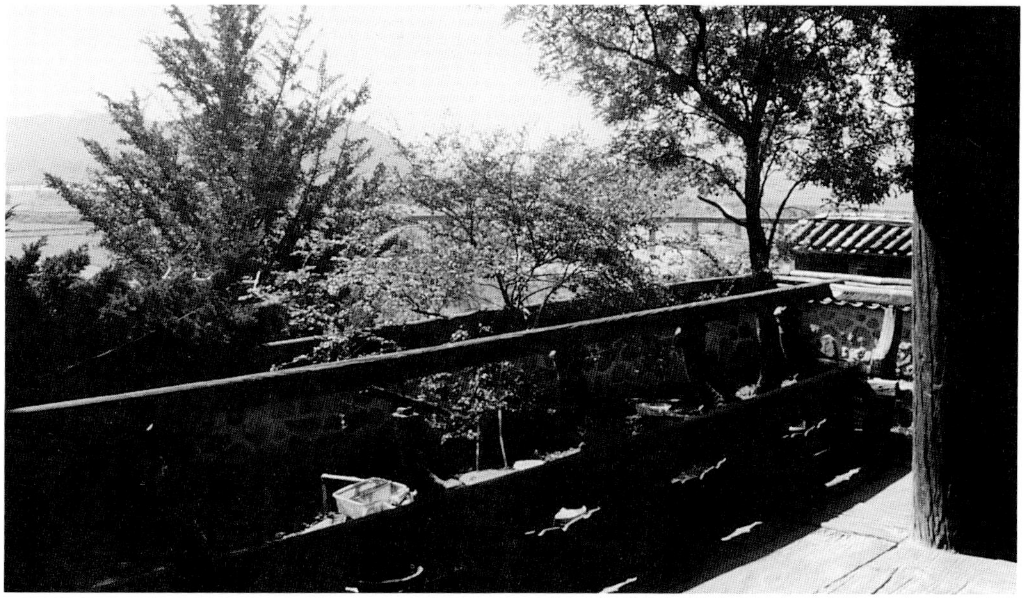

112.3 The prospect afforded from the *numaru.*

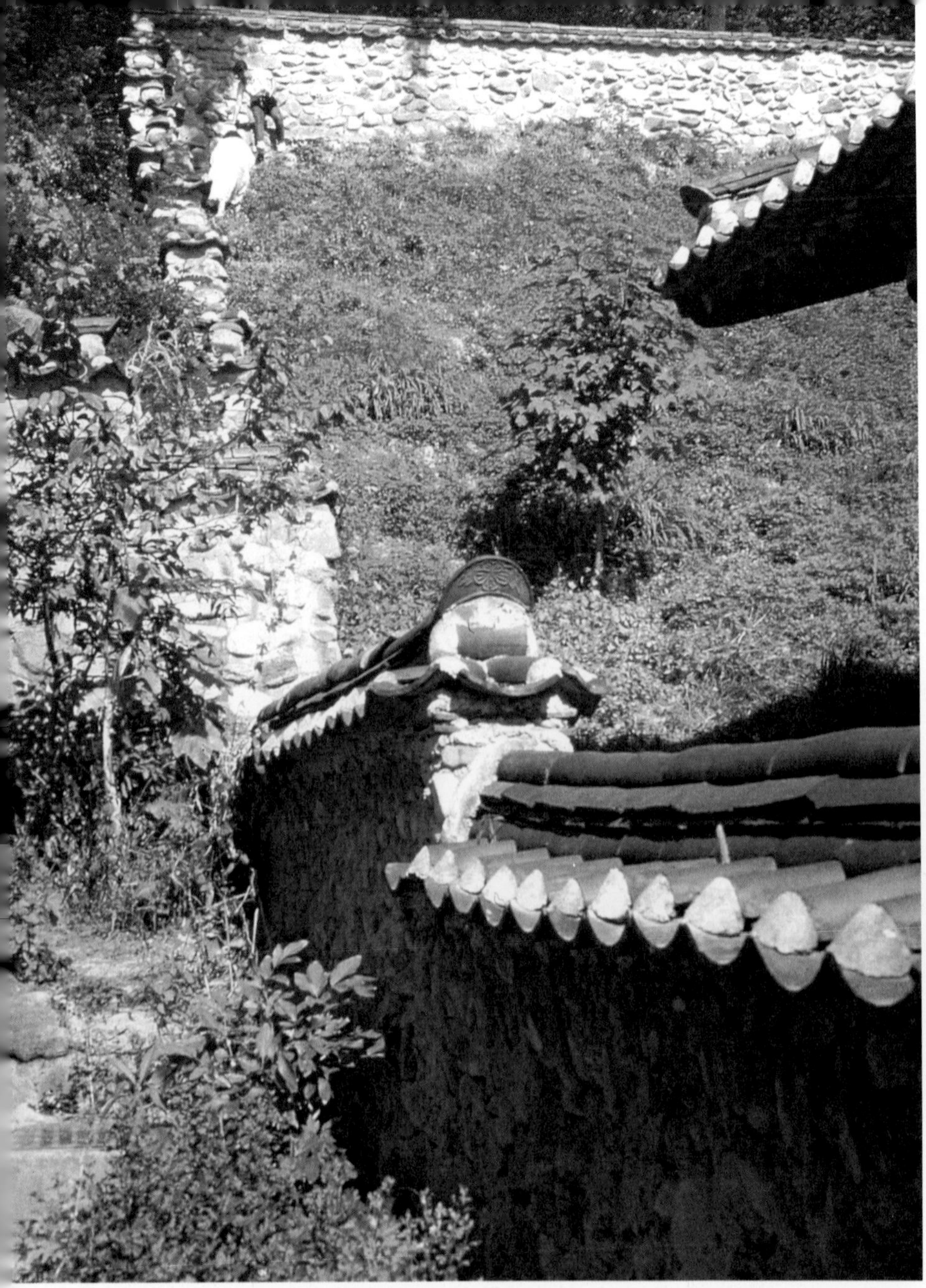

113.1 View of the rear garden of a *yangban* estate (Imch'ŏnggak, Andong).

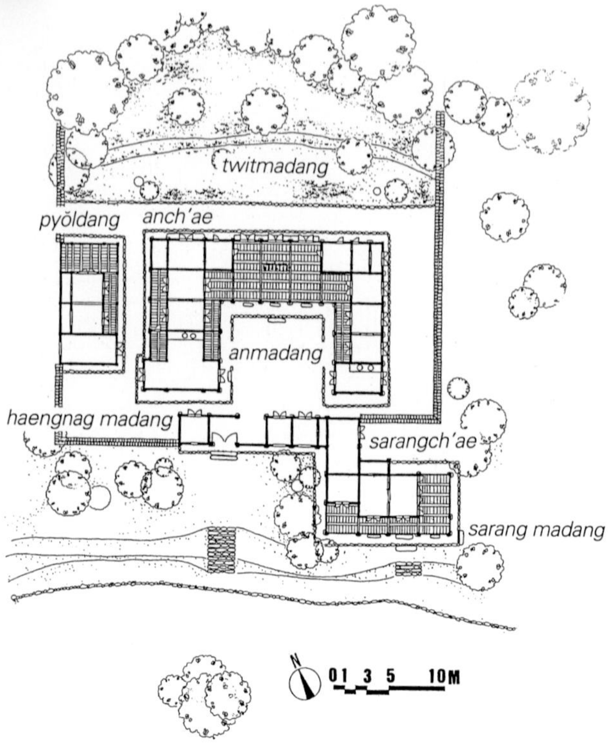

113.2 Site plan of the original residence of Yun Chŭng (1629-1714), a famous scholar official of Chosŏn.

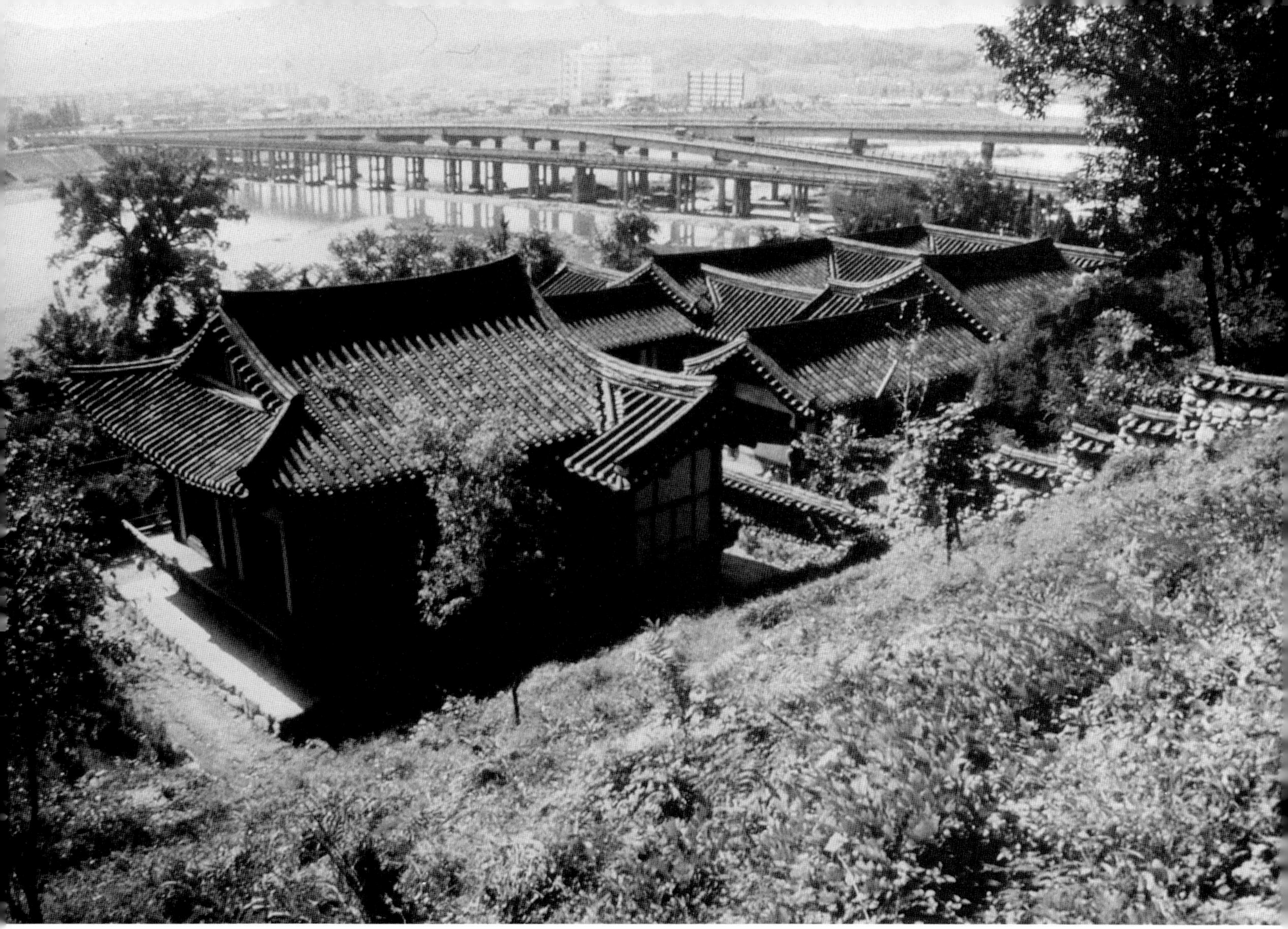

113.3 View from the rear garden of a *yangban* estate (Imch'ŏnggak, Andong).

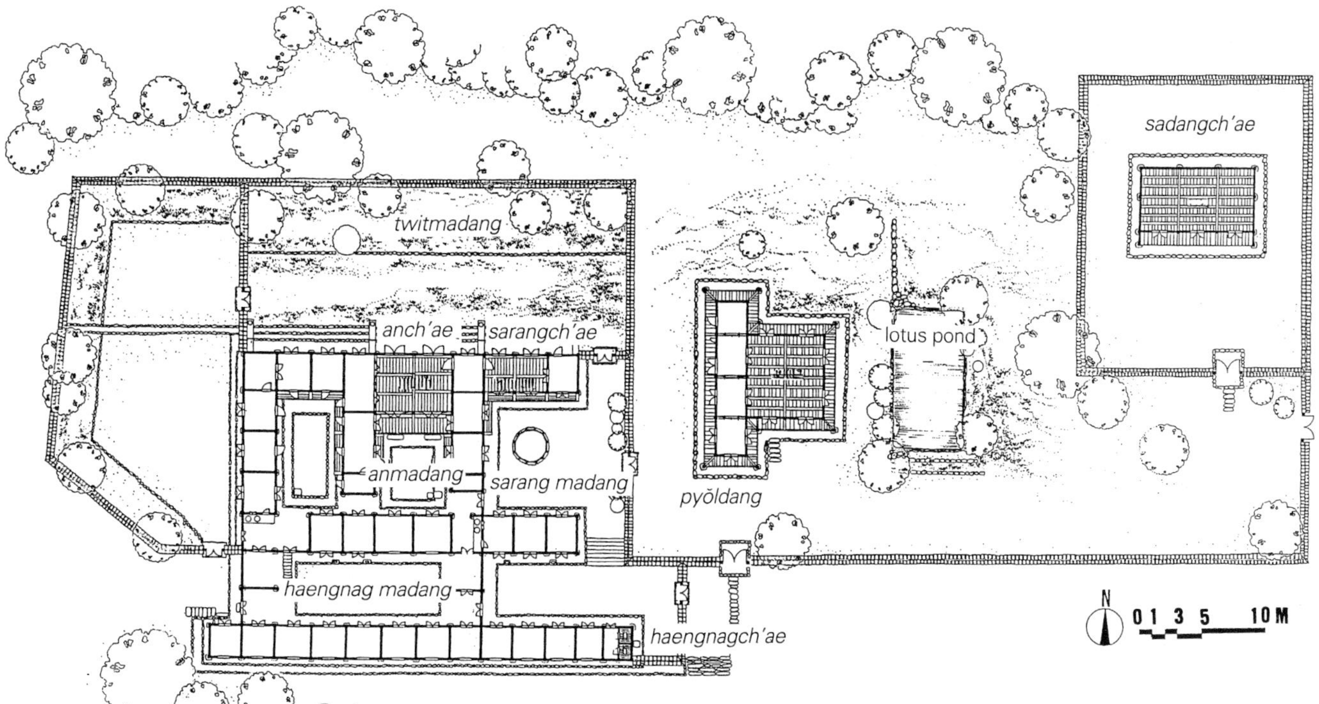

113.4 Site plan of the *yangban* estate.

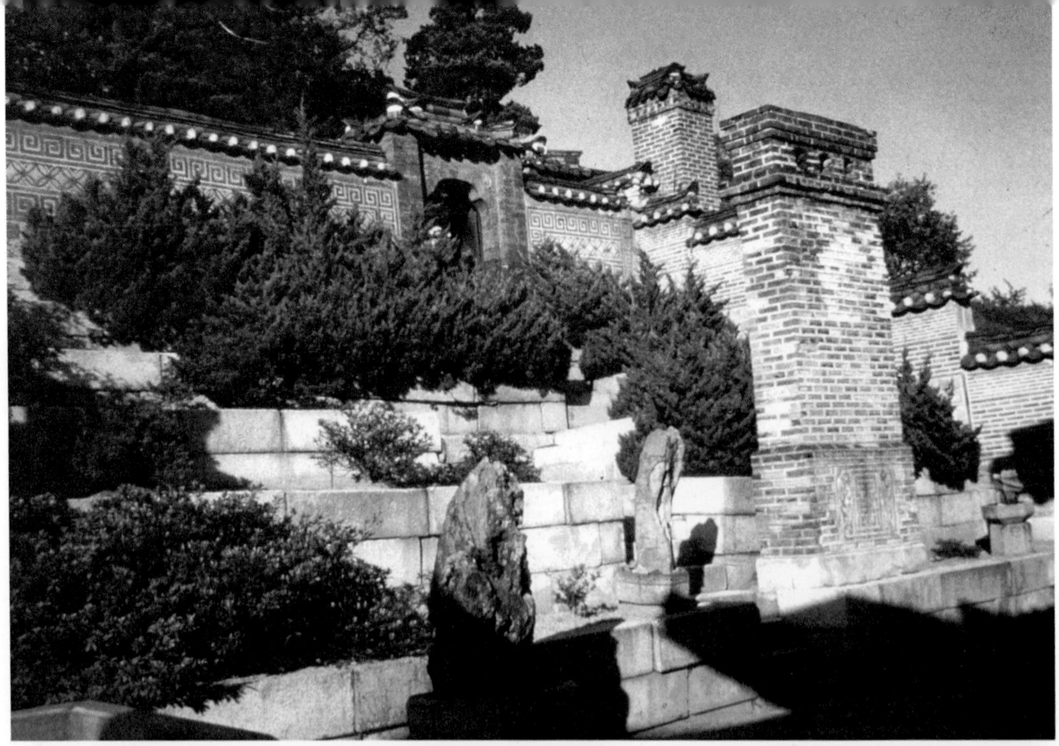

114.1 The terraced entry to the rear garden of a royal palace (Naksŏnjae, Seoul).

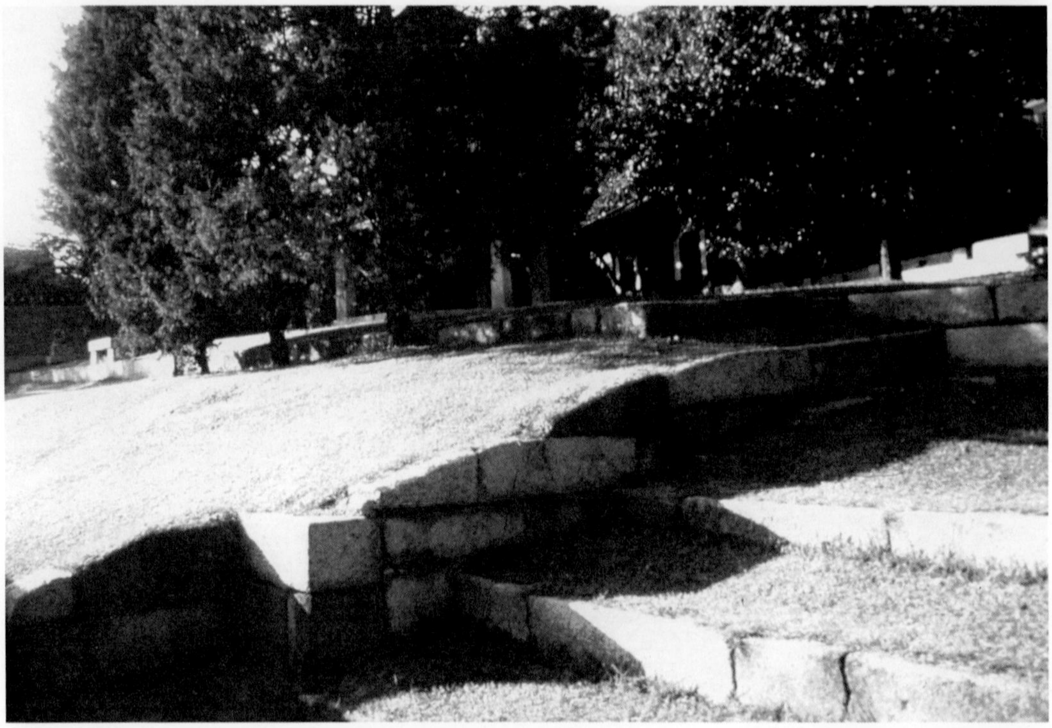

114.2 A rear garden scene.

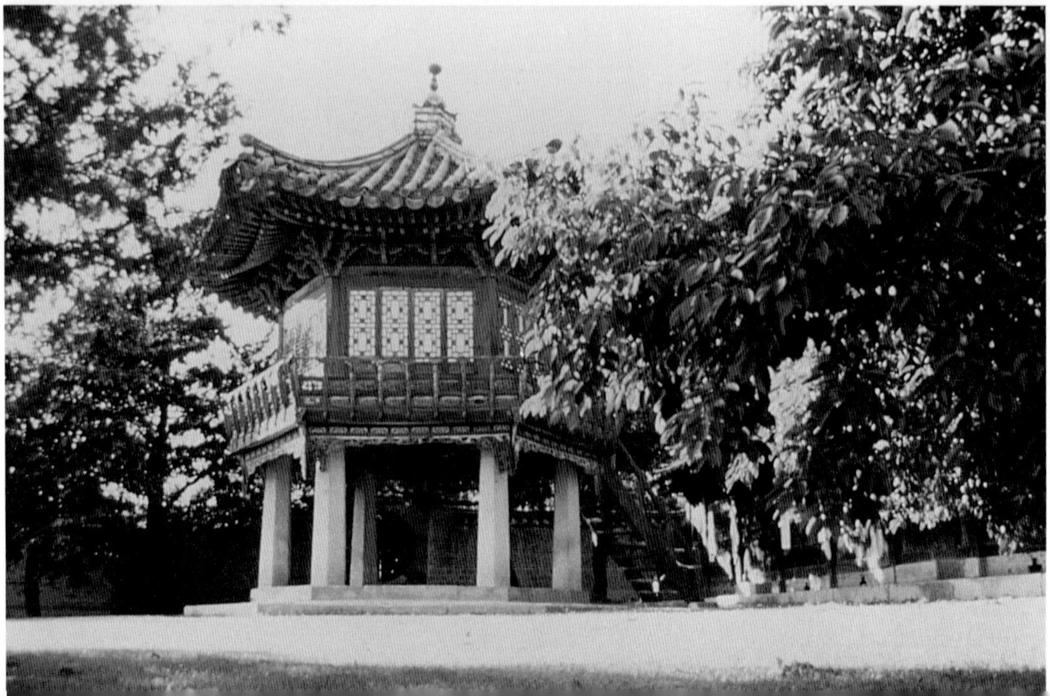

114.3 A rear garden pavilion.

Outer Gardens—The Traditional Form Presented to the Outside World

Sŏn'gyojang in Kangnŭng City, Kangwŏn Province, is a typical example of the *yangban* homes built in the provinces toward the end of the Chosŏn period (in this case, A.D. 1816). In floor plan composition, it contains all the elements symbolic of the Korean upper classes at the time. Its outer garden, consisting of a lotus pond and a pavilion, lies outside the main gate on flat ground to the southwest of the outer wall of the residential compound, which is formed by the *haengnagch'ae* (Figures 115.1–115.3).

The lotus pond in Sŏn'gyojang's outer garden is square in shape and its walls are lined with quarried stone. The pavilion, called Hwallaejŏng, consists of an *ondol*-heated wing and a wooden-floored wing, which cantilevers out over the pond. Directly in front of the pavilion, a circular island, also with quarried stone embankments, is set exactly in the center of the pond, and features a few pine trees. This is a classical Korean outer garden.

The outer garden—usually an area of flat land near the main gate and outside the wall of the residential compound—is generally laid out in straight lines and geometric forms, with particular attention paid to symmetrical balance. Islands set in decorative ponds are most often round, and are usually planted with a few pine trees. In principle, there should be no bridge connecting the island to the shore. In many cases, the corner stones and the water outlet of the pond's quarried-stone wall are carved into the shapes of mythical animals or monsters. Thus, the overall effect contrasts sharply with the natural simplicity of the gardens inside the residential compound (Figures 116.1–116.3).

Sometimes an outer garden was laid out around a *pyŏldang*, or an annex where the master of the household could spend time reading in private, but more often its purpose was to catch the eye of visitors passing through the main gate to the *sarangch'ae.* Rather than serving any particular functional purpose, its main role was as a formal symbol of the *yangban* household (Figure 117).

The design elements of the lotus pond and the island are rooted in the prayers for long life and perennial youth of ancient hermit wizardry. These gardens are believed to have been first built in the sixth-century Paekche palaces and can be seen in the pond of Anapchi (A.D. 671) in Kyŏngju, among remains discovered from the Silla Kingdom. If we look at this pond, which is still undergoing restoration, we can see that its embankments at the eastern end, closest to the original palace building, are perpendicular lines, while the western end is composed of more free-form curves. The entire pond, however, is lined with quarried stone, behind which groupings of *sŏkkasan* stones are displayed on the slope (Figures 118.1–118.2). The treatment of the pond's edge is stylistically completely different from that of a Japanese garden—designed to express a seascape—where the ground would slope gently down into the pond and stone groupings would extend into the water.

The composition of the pond's edge in a Japanese garden is designed to create a sense of unity between the pond and surrounding garden, but in Korea straight lines and quarried stone are used to create a sense of separateness between the viewer and the surface of the pond. This sense of separateness is heightened by the construction of a pavilion or belvedere cantilevered over the water. In Chosŏn-period gardens all sides of these ponds are straight lines, the regularity and formalization of which differs markedly with the freedom demonstrated in the smooth curves at one end of the much older Anapchi.

As mentioned above, Kyŏngbokkung in Seoul was not only a royal palace but also the seat of government and a place for important ceremonies and the granting of audiences. Northwest of the main administrative apartments

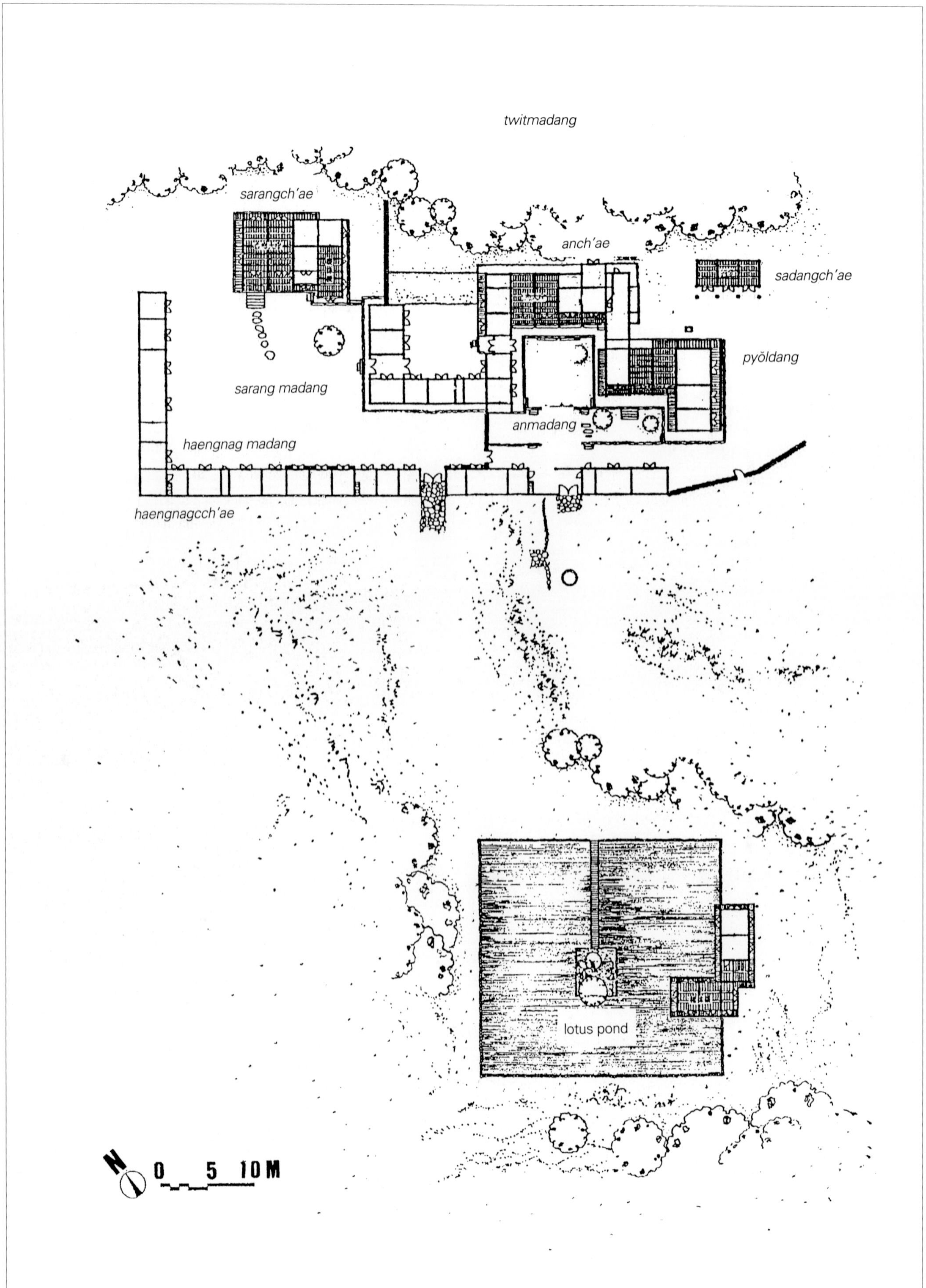

115.1 Site plan of a *yangban* estate with an outer garden (Sŏn'gyojang, Kangnŭng).

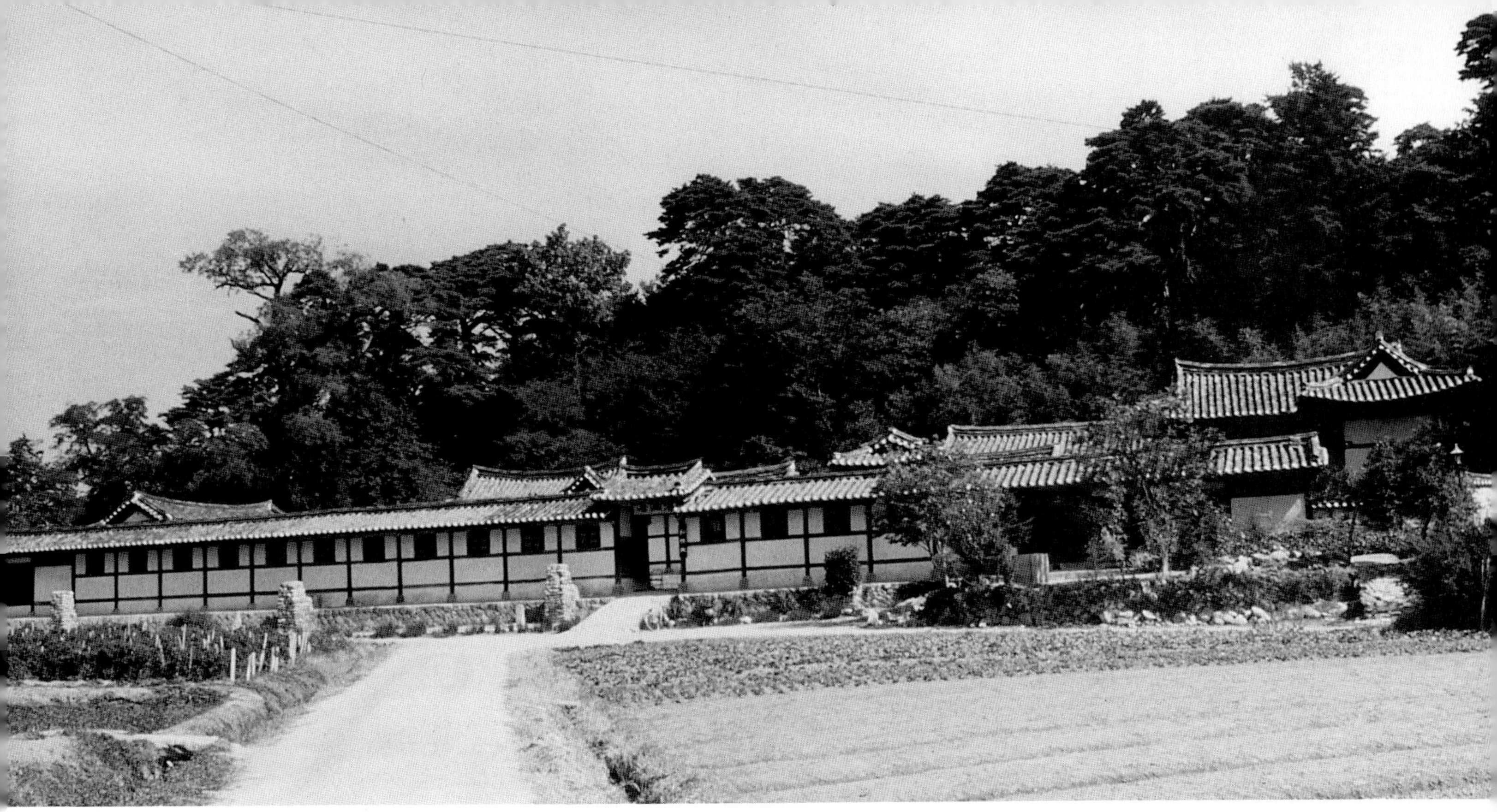

115.2 The Sŏn'gyojang exterior facade.

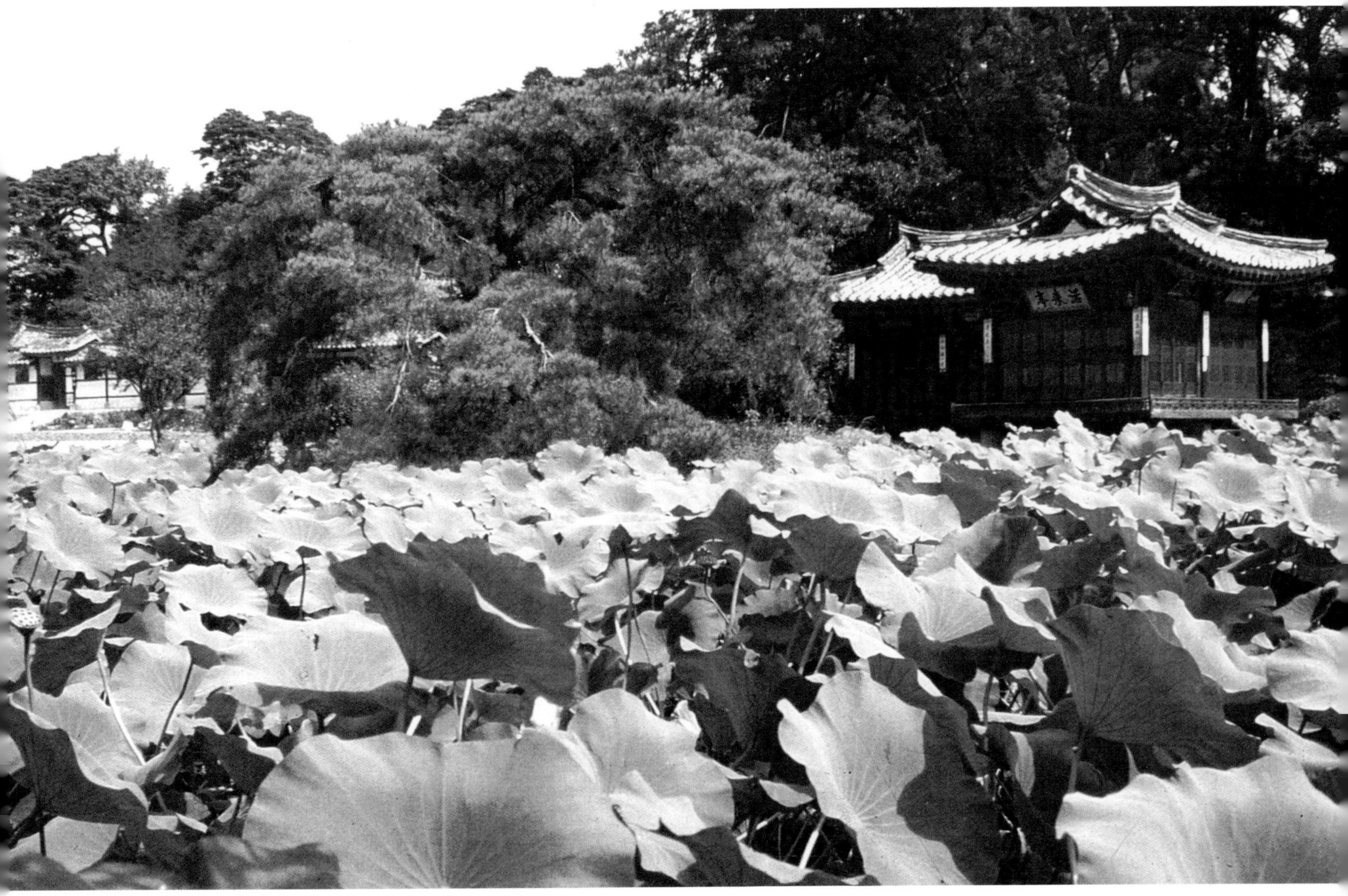

115.3 Hwallaejong pavilion and lotus pond.

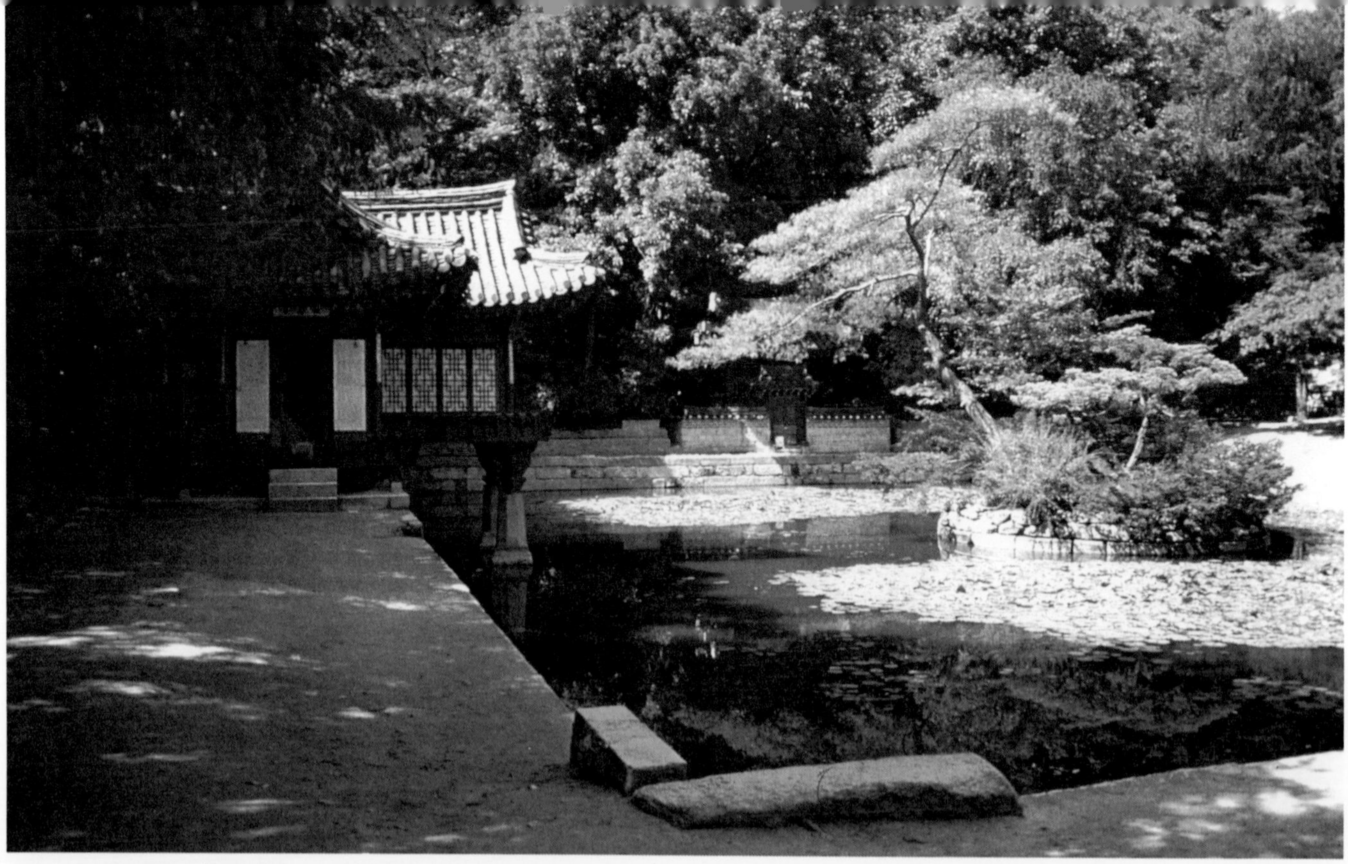

116.1 Puyong Pond (Piwŏn).

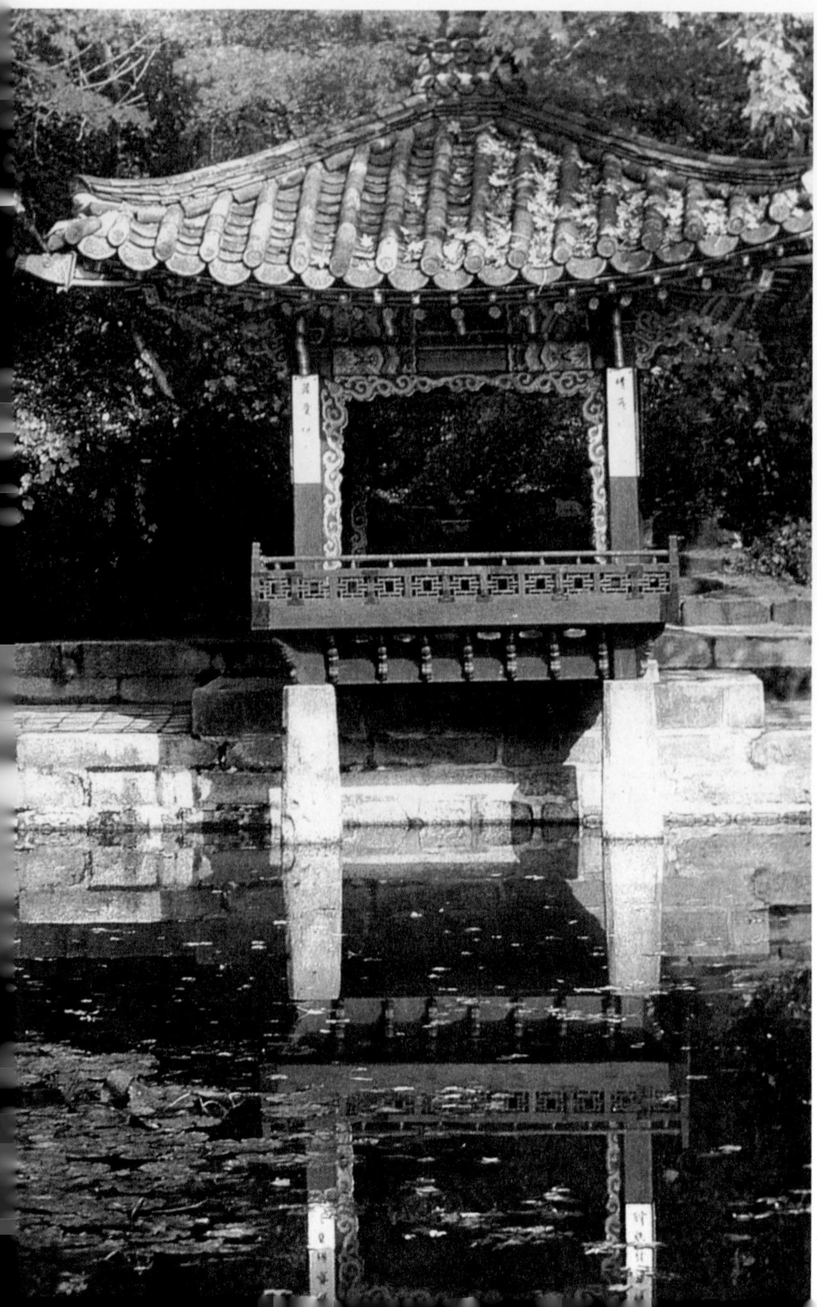

116.2 The Yŏn'gyŏngdang pond.

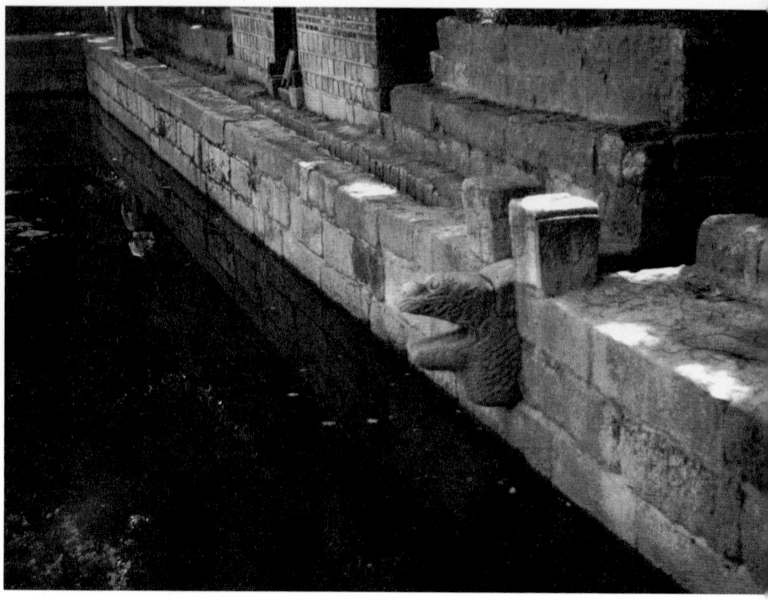

116.3 Mythical figures in the Puyong Pond wall.

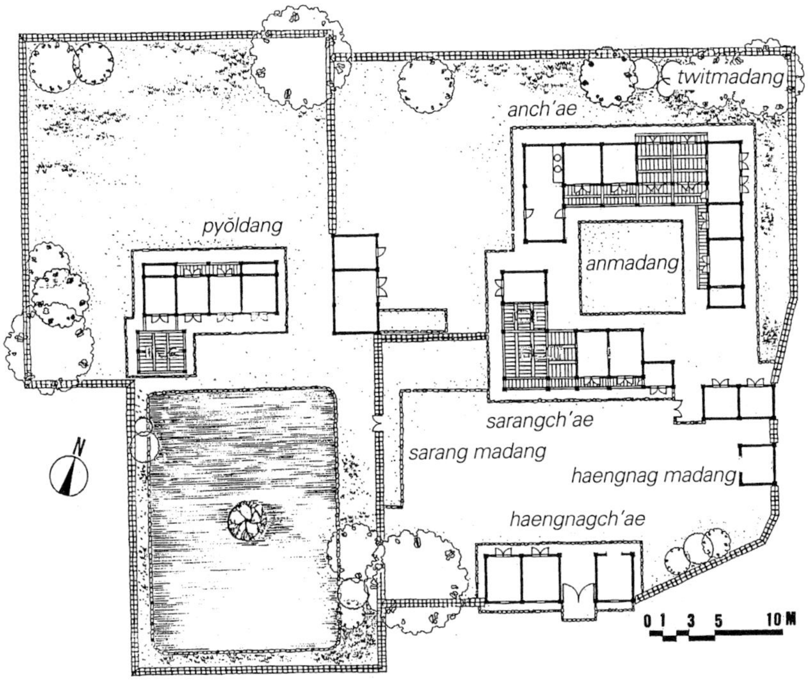

117 Site plan of the Pak Residence (Talsŏng).

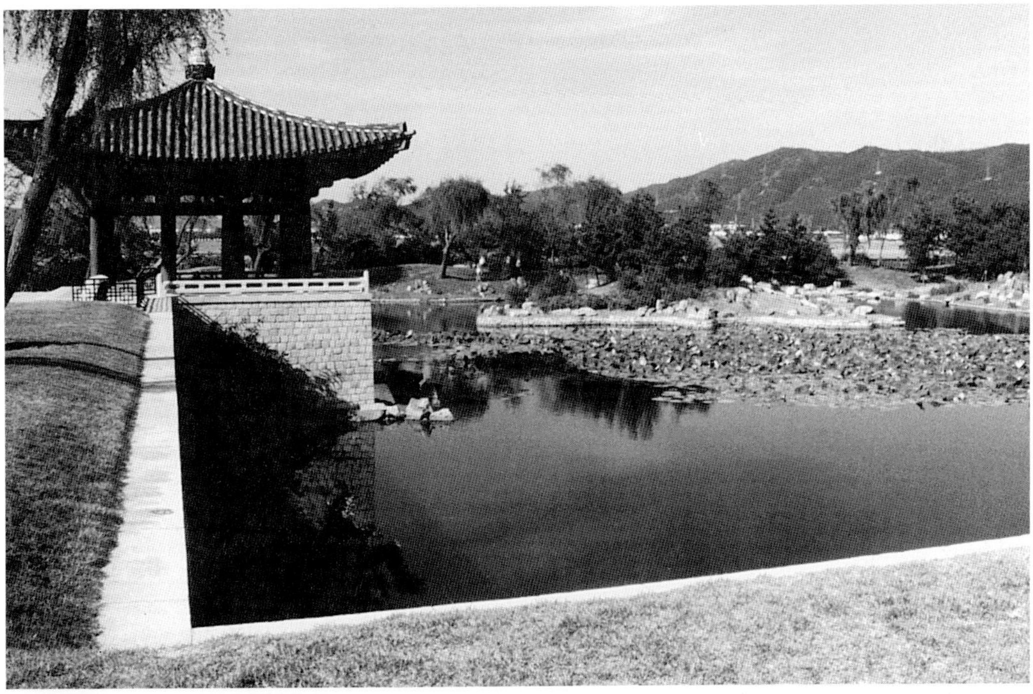

118.1 Linear and curvilinear walls of the Anapchi Pond.

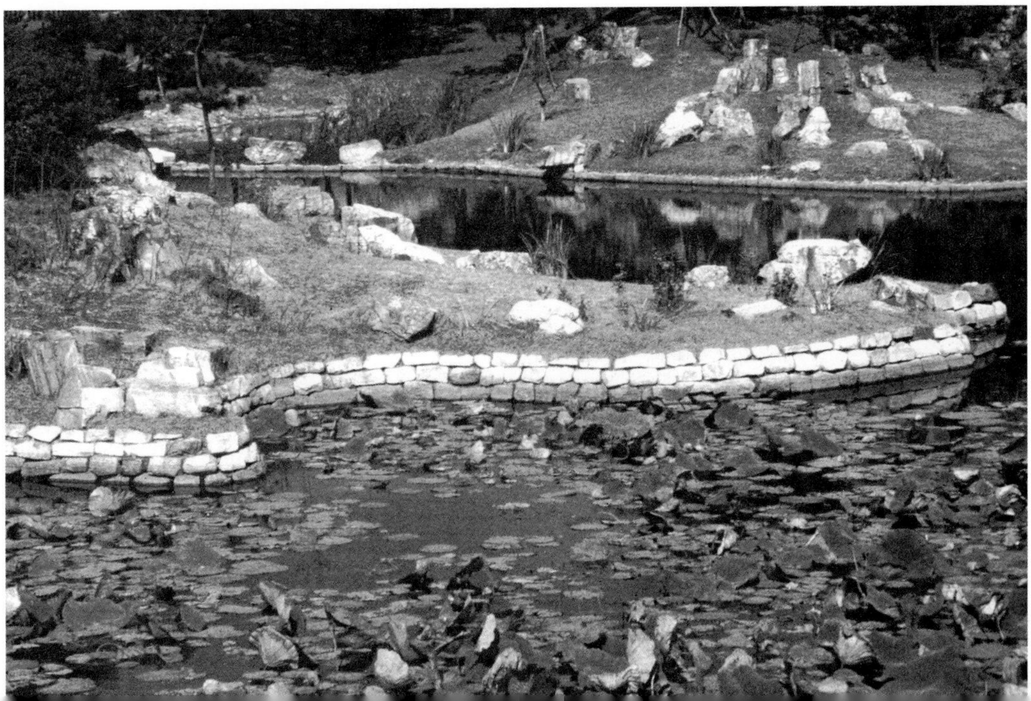

118.2 Anapchi Pond curvilinear walls and *sŏkkasan* stones.

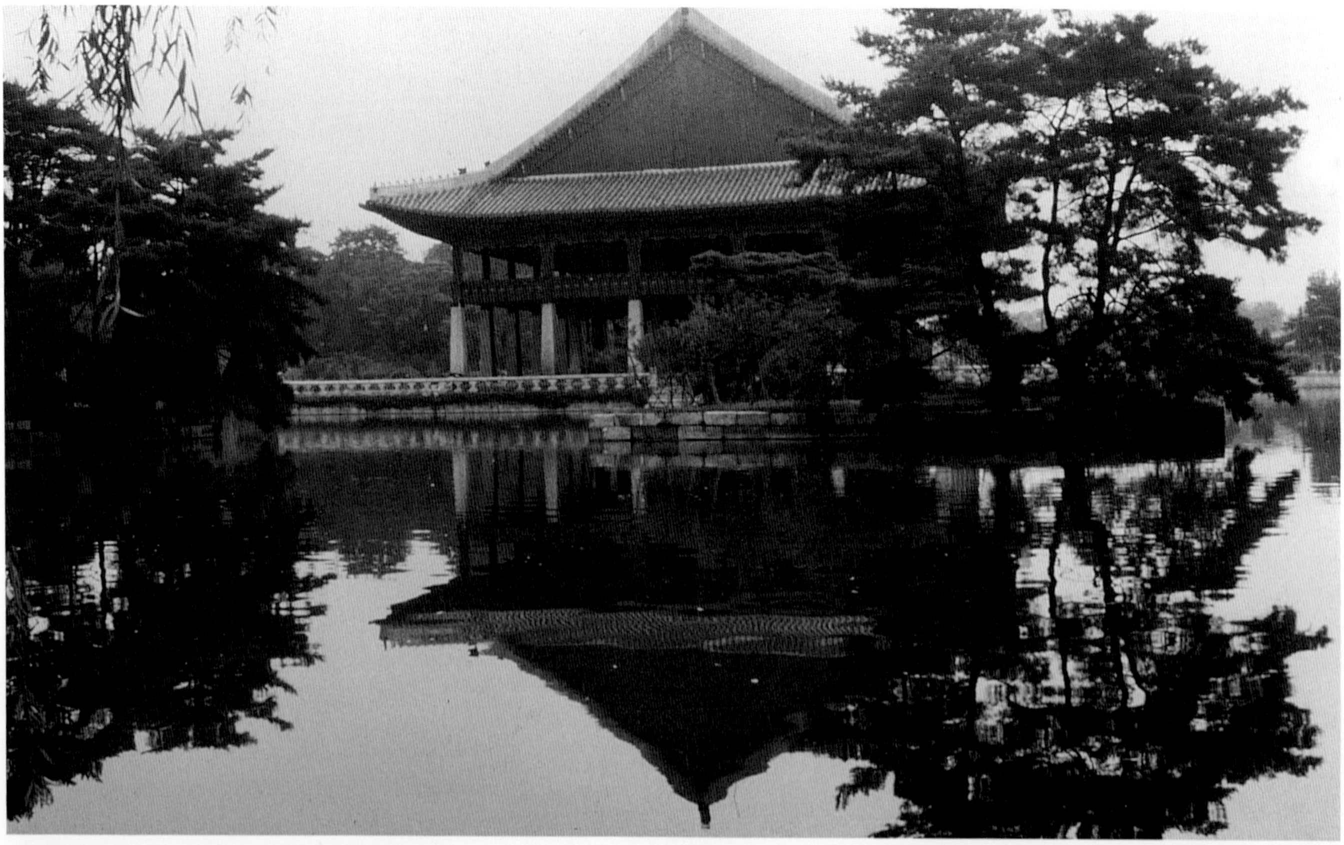

119 Kyŏnghoeru and pond (Kyŏngbokkung).

is the enormous Kyŏnghoeru standing on a plaza of stone pilotis, which was used as a place for greeting and entertaining visitors. The pond alongside this building is a rectangular expanse of water 113 meters (370 feet) from north to south and 128 meters (420 feet) from east to west. It features two long, narrow islands planted with pine trees. The sides of the pond are perfectly straight and lined with quarried stone. The Kyŏnghoeru pond is one of the best extant examples of Chosŏn-period design, but its form owes much to the traditions passed down from the creators of Anapchi (Figure 119).

The outer gardens of *yangban* estates also share with the royal palaces the same traditional forms handed down from the days of the Unified Silla and Koryŏ kingdoms. In the royal palaces, the outer gardens are characterized by straight lines and geometric patterns while the private rear gardens retain a high degree of naturalism. The same contrast between a highly ordered and a natural approach is seen in the outer gardens and rear gardens of *yangban* estates. Following the forms inherited from royal palace gardens, the *yangban* outer gardens—so unique among all the gardens of traditional Korean residences—acquired the same authoritative and symbolic qualities.

Interestingly, a form similar to these outer garden rectangular ponds and embankments of quarried stone appears as a garden-making method during the early Edo period in Japan. It can be seen in the section of the Nijōjō pond known as Ikejirifunadamari, the pond in front of the moon-viewing platform, and the Shōiken *funatsukiba* (boat mooring inlet) at Katsura Rikyū, all of which are attributed to designer Kobori Enshū. Many such linear compositions, which disappeared from Japan, also appear in the drawings entitled *Kan'eido sentō nyoin gosho sashizu.* This has given rise to a great deal of speculation about whether it might be a direct sign of an exchange of gardening techniques between Korea and Japan.

The *Pyŏlsŏ* Environment

As we have seen, the composition of residences in Chosŏn Korea was directly influenced by Chinese Confucianist political thought, and we can safely conclude that the kind of garden often depicted in Chinese landscape paintings and based in the tradition of retirement from society, was not part of the *yangban* domestic environment. The only similar garden in the Korean tradition to these Chinese gardens was the *pyŏlsŏ* environments surrounding the hermitages of the

Confucian scholars who lived in the mountains and forests.

Confucian scholars were men whose profession it was to read books. One fundamental precept of neo-Confucianism was that a person could achieve a higher level of virtue through reading and could thereby qualify for a role in government. Such study was an absolute prerequisite for all government officials. Since neo-Confucian thought held character and virtue in higher esteem than any other qualities, some individual *yangban* living in the provinces who already enjoyed a tranquil, untroubled existence eschewed official rank completely and devoted their lives to study. These men were highly respected in traditional Korean society, and were renowned as *ilmin*, or "hermit scholars."

Ilmin hermit scholars built places of retreat at locations of exceptional natural beauty, far from the villages where their families and neighbors lived, and operated schools called *chŏngsa*, which offered the only form of education available other than the *sŏwŏn* national system attended by children of the upper classes. These schools were usually named after the locale, some particular characteristic of the local scenery, or even the pen name of the teacher himself. The *chŏngsa* played an important role, alongside the *sŏwŏn*, in Confucianism's spread among the common people and its establishment as the national religion of Korea (Figure 120).

If the hermitage and *chŏngsa* were a form of inner garden, the surrounding natural environment was the outer garden. "*Pyŏlsŏ*" was used to denote the environments created by *ilmin* hermit scholars through the construction of belvederes, halls and pavilions amid valleys, waterfalls, springs, and artificial hills which were ensconced in nature. The composition of this natural scenery was based on concepts and methods that are free and uninhibited, which would never be found in the grounds of a *yangban* mansion, yet are just as much an integral part of Korean gardening tradition. Soswaewŏn is a prime example of this garden style (Figures 121.1–121.6).

Soswaewŏn is a garden of approximately 5,000 square meters (1.25 acres) set deep among the mountains of South Chŏlla Province. It was the *pyŏlsŏ* garden belonging to a great noble in the mid-Chosŏn period (around A.D. 1530), and has recently been restored by the Office of Cultural Properties.

A nearby valley with its fast-running stream and surrounding mountains were skillfully utilized to create this beautiful garden. The front garden (or approach), the low-walled garden, and the slope garden, all of which overlook the central valley garden, are circled to reach the Chewŏldang. This hall stands on a high point affording a view of the entire garden and consists of a single *ondol*-heated room (*pang*) of one *k'an* and a wooden-floored room (*maru*) of two *kan*, which has a rear garden. Behind a stone wall set back from the far side of the Chewŏldang are the gardens of the Koam *chŏngsa* and Puhwŏndang, which have not yet been restored.

An earthen bridge crosses the lower end of the valley stream and leads from the approach directly to the inner gardens. The valley garden is located at the heart of Sŏswaewŏn and features a single building, the Kwang-p'unggak, a pavilion consisting of an *ondol*-heated room of one *k'an* surrounded on all sides by wooden-floored rooms. This open-sided pavilion looks out over the fast-running stream and a waterfall.

Soswaewŏn's composition is expressive of retirement and seclusion—the very same realm as is expressed in the landscape painting traditions in which poetry and painting are regarded as one. *Pyŏlsŏ* garden composition involves concepts not applied to any garden of the *yangban* estate, even in a more artificial or stylized form. These *pyŏlsŏ* gardens evoke, rather, forms predicated on the philosophy behind Chinese *yuanlin*.

Yet there are fundamental differences in Chinese and Korean thought about the design of their respective gardens. *P'ungsu*, or *feng shui*, is the art of divining features

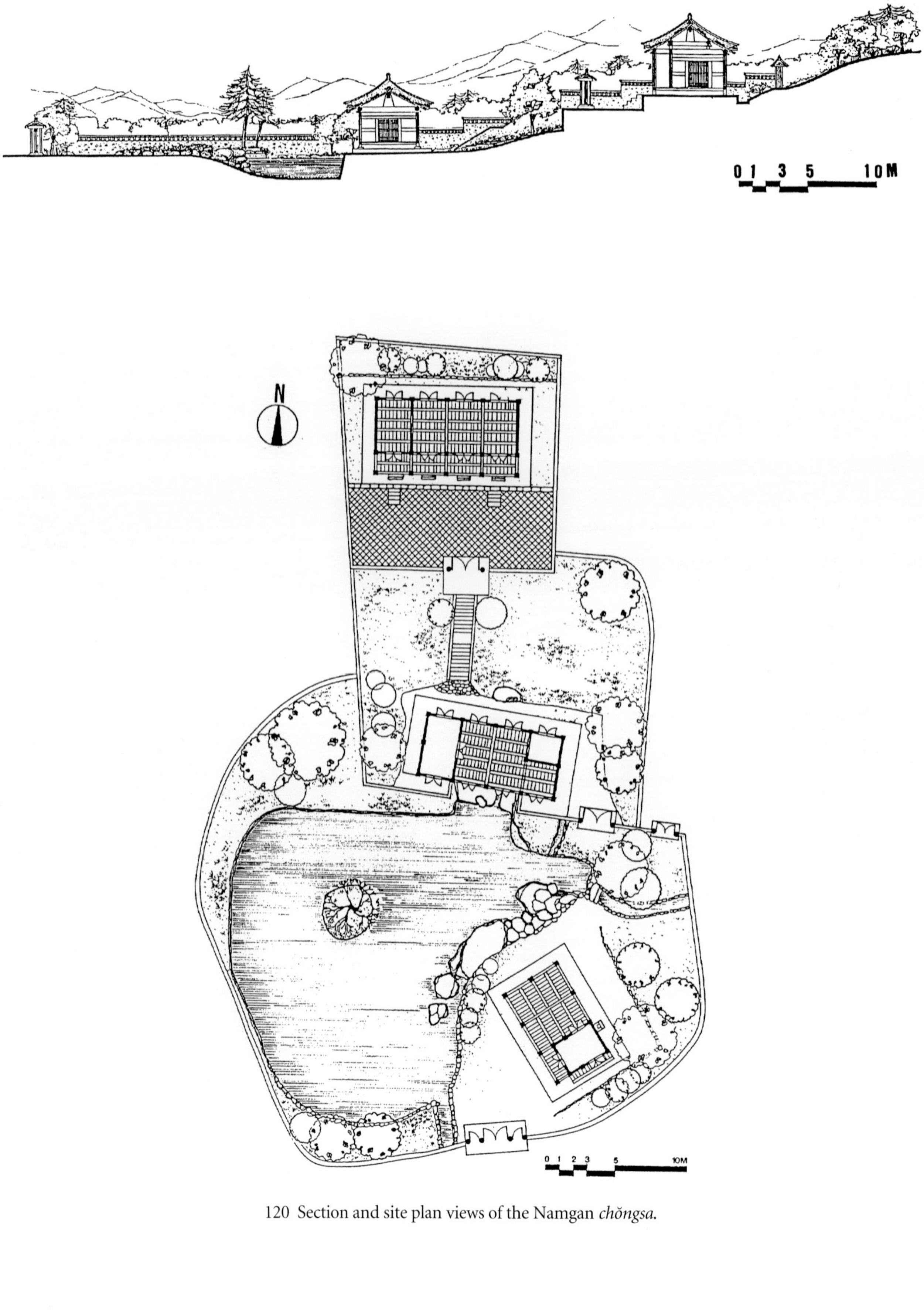

120 Section and site plan views of the Namgan *chŏngsa*.

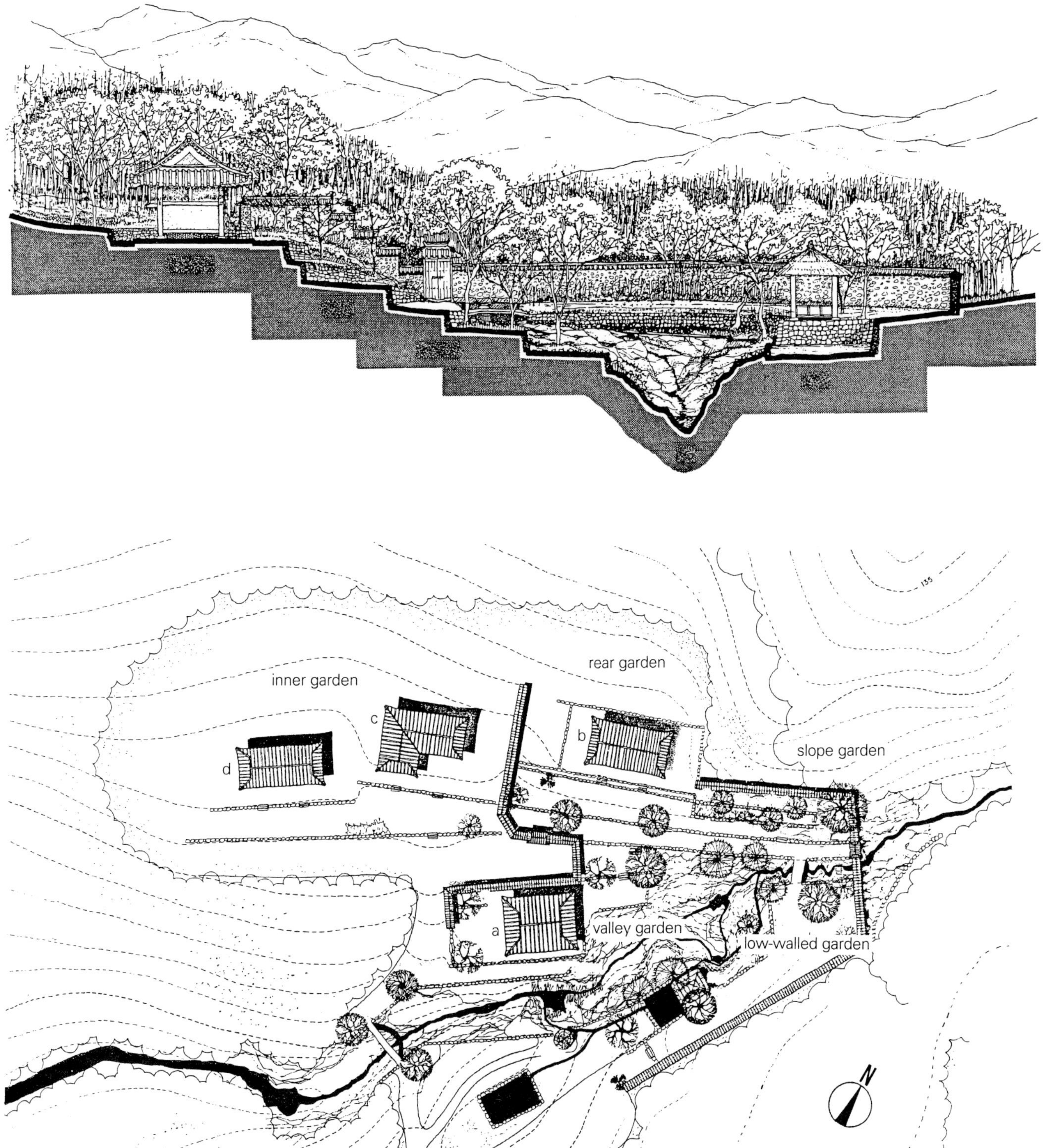

121.1 Section and site plan views of the *pyŏlsŏ* of a Confucian scholar (Soswaewŏn, Tamyang).

a. Kwangp'unggak. b. Chewŏldang. c. Koam *chŏngsa.* d. Puhwŏndang.

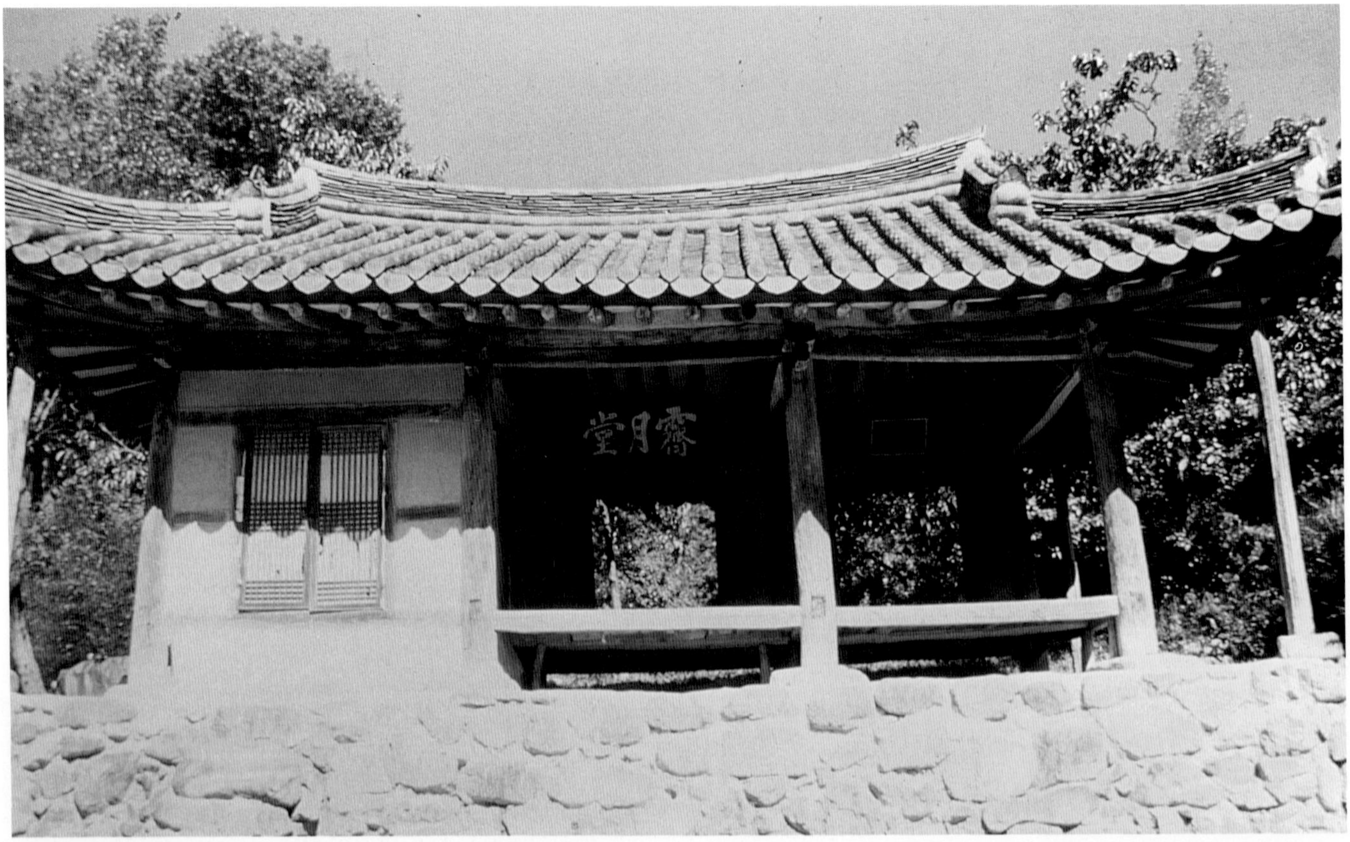

121.2 Chewŏldang.

associated with good and bad fortune in any site—whether for a city, a village, a single home, or a grave. This point is common to both China and Korea, but whereas the Chinese set about to construct landscapes which would fulfill the conditions for good *feng shui*, Koreans selected sites whose natural characteristics already met those same requirements and therefore needed no modification.

The Forbidden City in Beijing was built on a broad plain, which meant that the "mountain behind, river in front" condition for favorable *feng shui* needed to be created artificially, and thus a man-made mountain was erected as backdrop to the palace buildings and an artificial river, the Jin-shui Channel, was dug to the south of the complex. The site of Kyŏngbokkung in Seoul was selected because it was *myŏngdang*, or choice land—overlooking the wide Han River to the south, and with Mount Pukak standing behind it to the north.

As we have seen, the Chinese garden treatise *Yuan ye* defines the primary method of site preparation as *yin-di zhi-xuan*, or accentuation of the natural lay of the land by raising high points and deepening low points. By contrast, the selection of a site that offered all the requisite natural features was foremost in Korea. The reason for this difference in approach lies in the two countries' differing topographies. Whereas the two regions central to Chinese culture under the Ming and Qing dynasties—the political and administrative center around Beijing and the commercial/economic center of Jiangnan—were both flat, broad plains, Korea is a land of undulating hills and mountains. These geographical factors seem to have helped shape the divergent senses of beauty in the two cultures.

Although the composition of traditional dwellings in China and Korea alike was based on the principles of Confucianism, garden styles in the two countries differed. In China, gardens were symbols of the elite, independent from but contiguous to dwellings, and reminiscent of the Chinese *shanshui* landscape paintings that gave visual form to the precepts of Taoism. In Korea, gardens were incorporated into the residence in accordance with the Confucian sense of order, and any Taoist expression was effected within the highly natural environment of the hermit scholar's *pyŏlsŏ*. These differences also stem from the fact that the concept of retirement in Ming- and Qing-dynasty China—where retired officials could return to their posts—became largely symbolic and lost much of its true meaning. The seclusion of Korea's *ilmin* hermit scholars was permanent. The *ilmin* gained the respect of the common people by renouncing the mundane world and any chance of one day returning to it. Nevertheless,

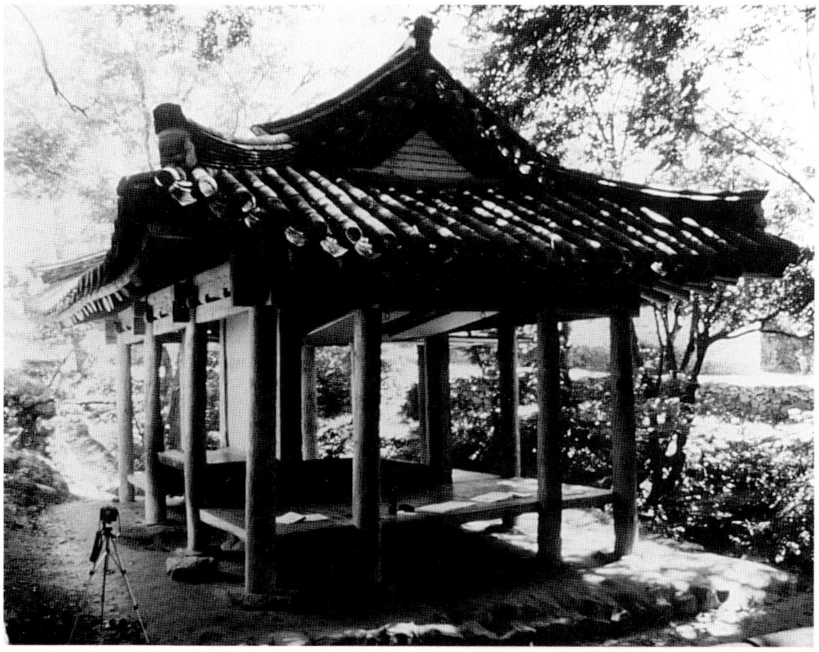

121.3 Kwangp'unggak.

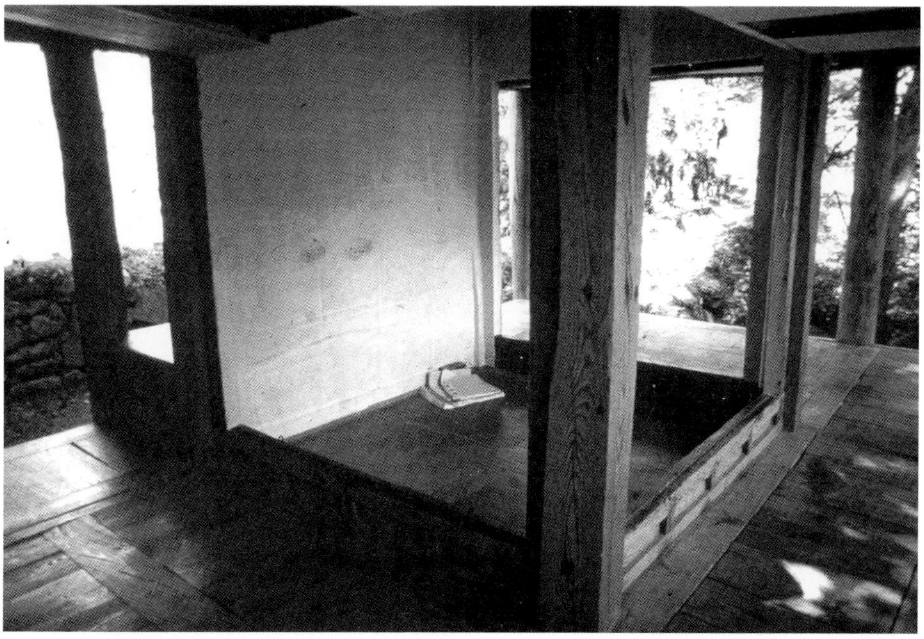

121.4 Kwangp'unggak *pang* and *maru.*

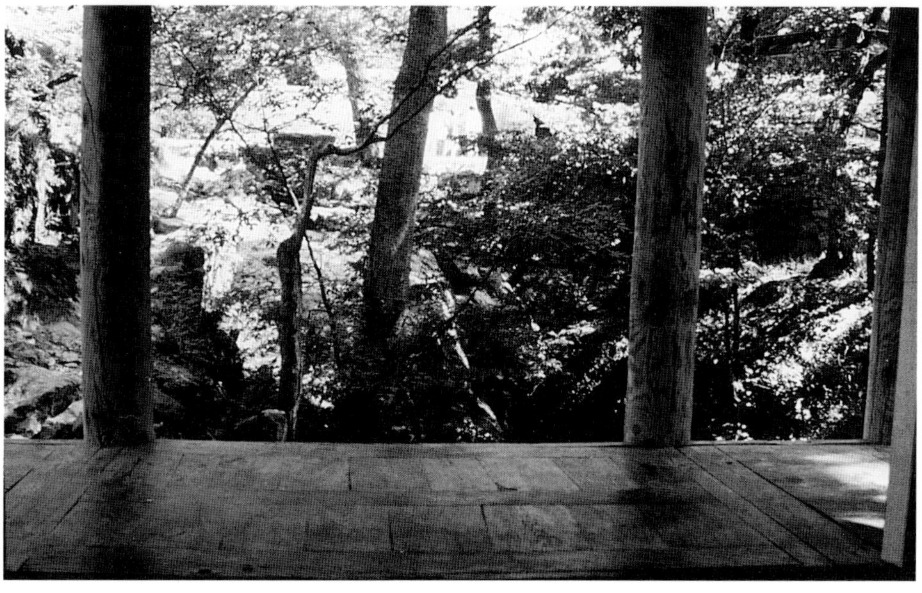

121.5 Kwangp'unggak and the valley garden.

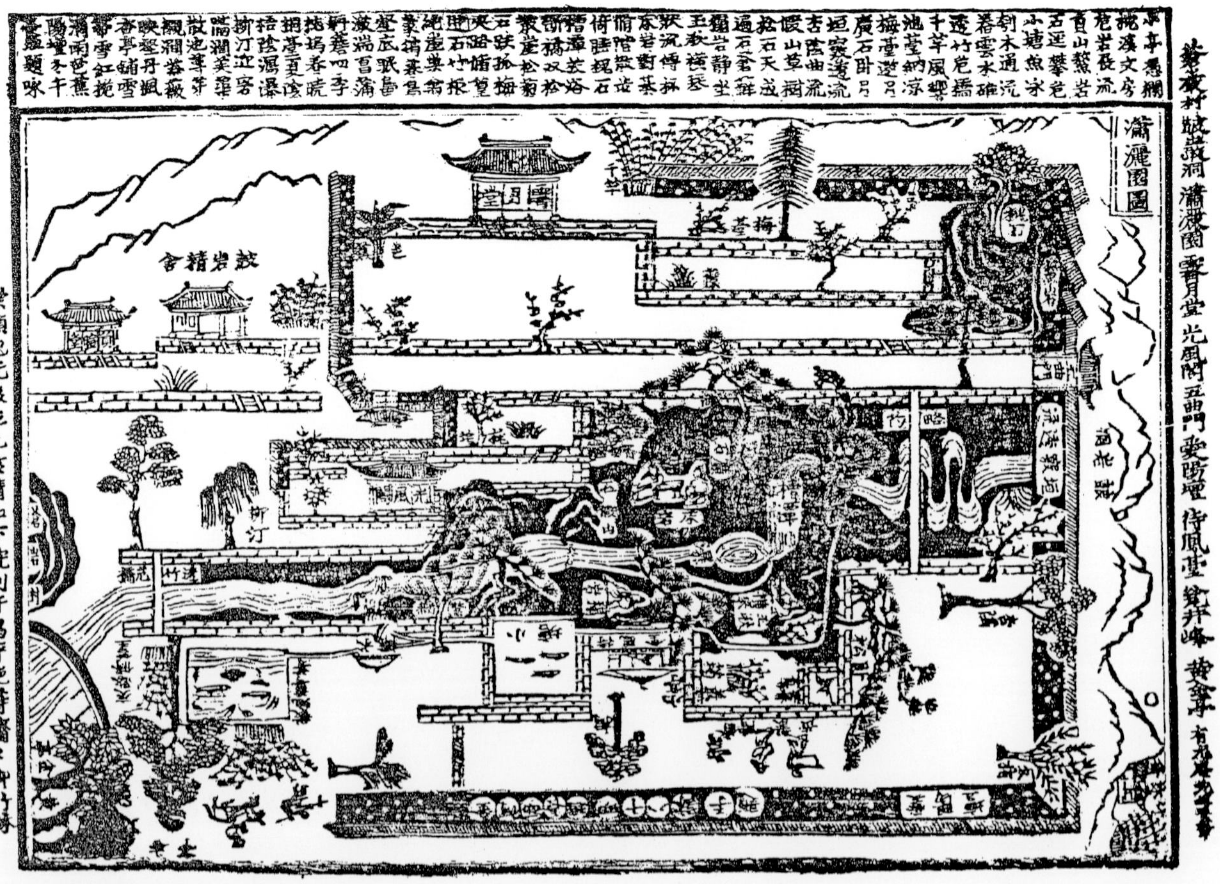

121.6 Historical map of Soswaewŏn.

the prototype for each was the expression of the concept of retirement as embodied in Chinese landscape paintings and landscape painting theory in which poetry and painting were perceived as one.

Korean Garden Forms

As previously mentioned, if the standards for a traditional Japanese garden or Chinese *yuanlin* are applied to the Korean residential setting, no garden form as such exists. Thus it is clearly necessary to adopt a completely different standard by which to define the gardens of Korea, and this standard might be termed the "uncultivated" garden. Based on this standard, traditional Korean gardens can be summarized as follows:

Inner Gardens Within the Residence

Prospect and borrowed scenery are the foundation upon which inner gardens (*madang*) are composed and have traditionally served as essential prerequisites in the selection of residential sites, though more as underlying factors than openly recognized conditions.

In the composition of the traditional Korean residence, open interior spaces such as the *taech'ŏng* and *numaru* are located at points of connection and intersection between the adjoining *madang*, *twitmadang*, and surrounding scenery outside the residential compound. An attempt is made to link them all through prospect and borrowed scenery. This leads to the supposition that residences were built to match the prospect.

Rear Garden Within the Residential Compound

The rear garden (*twitmadang*) of a *yangban* estate is essentially a private outdoor space for the family, and forms an integral part of the living space of the *anch'ae*. It is related to the parklike rear gardens of royal palaces, which also fall into this category of private garden spaces where prospect is again the chief consideration.

Outer Garden Beyond the Residential Compound

The composition of the outer garden, based as it is on the philosophy of the hermit wizards, is completely different stylistically from the garden spaces within the residential complex. These outer gardens do not qualify as "uncultivated." Their angular configuration and abundant use of quarried stone, with buildings looking directly onto the surface of a pond, makes them highly symbolic, and places them within the same tradition as the outer gardens of royal palaces.

Pyŏlsŏ

It is at first difficult to understand why there was no garden even remotely similar to the Chinese *yuanlin* in the *yangban* estates of Chosŏn Korea despite the direct influence of Chinese Confucianism on Korean society in that period. However, this phenomenon appears to be related to the fact that the true meaning of "retirement" was very different in Chosŏn—a small and homogenous nation-state where the Yi family held centralized power for a very long time—and the vast, multiethnic state of China, where local chieftains vied constantly for influence.

In Korea, the *ilmin* hermit scholars had no desire for entry or reinstatement to political life, so perhaps their "retirement" would be better termed a "retreat." The isolated environments which they created deep in the mountains ensconced in nature, stand as another form of traditional Korean garden.

Unfortunately, as Soswaewŏn is the only example of an extant *pyŏlsŏ* garden, material for research is limited. The destruction and loss of these special environments is a great pity, but it is heartening to note that they are currently the object of study by the Graduate School of Environmental Studies at Seoul National University.

The Aesthetics of the "Uncultivated" Garden

Late Professor Kim Wŏn-yong of Seoul National University described the sense of aesthetics that dominated the Korea of the Three Kingdoms period as "the development of Korean naturalism," and characterized Unified Silla as having the "aesthetics of refinement and harmony," Kŏryŏ the "originality of nonartificiality," and Chosŏn "a world of thoroughgoing ordinariness." Throughout all the ages, he emphasized, "nature and self-effacement remained constant aesthetic ideals."

Yanagi Sōetsu defines the Korean aesthetic in the Buddhist terms "just as it is," and Tanaka Toyotaro terms it "something born, not created."

As we can see from all of the above, the word "nature" is crucial to any understanding of the Korean sense of aesthetics. Indeed, works of art can be summarized into the single expression "an offspring of nature." However, the meanings of these words may be difficult to grasp, as they are sometimes taken to mean no more than the unaware, immature efforts that precede true art. For this reason, a comprehensive consideration based on the interrelationship between the structure of space and the structure of lifestyle, and on the historical roots and social background of Korea, is essential to the questions of what constitutes the Korean sense of aesthetics and how it has taken form.

Notes

JAPAN

1: Early Prototypes and Interpretive Approaches

1. Tachibana no Toshitsuna [?], *Sakuteiki: The Book of Garden* (Sakuteiki). Translated by Shigemaru Shimoyama. Tokyo: Tokyo Town & City Planners, 1976, pp. 23–24.
2. Tsuyoshi Tamura, *Sakuteiki.* Tokyo: Sagami Shobō, 1977, p. 5.
3. Toyojirō Tamaki, *Nihon toshi seiritsushi* (The historical formation of Japanese cities). Tokyo: Rikōgakusha, 1974, pp. 142, 144.
4. Ibid, pp. 137, 142.
5. Ibid, pp. 73–74.
6. *Asahi Shinbun*, 30 July, 1979.
7. Tachibana no Toshitsuna, *Sakuteiki*, p. 2.
8. Ibid.
9. Ibid.
10. Ibid.
11. Nadari Sawada. *Kaoku zakkō* (A miscellany of reflections on architecture). Tokyo: Yoshikawa Kōbunkan, vol. 1.
12. Ibid.
13. Hirōtarō Ōta, *Shoin-zukuri* (The *shoin* style). Tokyo: Tōkyō Daigaku Shuppankai, 1996, pp. 14–16.
14. Ibid., p. 107.
15. Tachibana no Toshitsuna, *Sakuteiki*, p. 1.
16. Ibid.
17. Ibid., p. 32.
18. Ibid., p. 1.
19. Ibid.
20. James Cahill, "The Six Laws and How to Read Them," *Ars Orientalis* 4 (1961), p. 380.
21. Tachibana no Toshitsuna, *Sakuteiki*, p. 2.
22. Ibid., p. 9.
23. Ibid., p. 6.
24. Ibid.
25. Ibid., p. 9.
26. Ibid., p. 2.
27. Ibid., p. 19.
28. Ibid., p. 21.
29. Ibid., p. 14.
30. Tamura, pp. 290, 302.
31. Tachibana no Toshitsuna, *Sakuteiki*, p. 5.
32. Ibid.
33. Ibid., p. 6.
34. Ibid., pp. 8–9.
35. Ibid., p. 9.
36. Ibid.
37. Ibid., p. 14.
38. Ibid., p. 13.
39. Ibid., p. 22.
40. Ibid., p. 25.
41. Ibid., p. 6.
42. Ibid., p. 14.
43. Ibid., p. 15.
44. Ibid.
45. Ibid., p. 21.
46. Ibid., pp. 8–9.
47. Ibid., p. 32.
48. Ibid., p. 37.
49. Ibid., p. 9.
50. Ibid., p. 6.
51. Ibid., pp. 2–3.
52. Ibid., pp. 22–23.
53. Ibid., p. 5.
54. Ibid., p. 3.
55. Ibid.
56. Ibid., p. 27.
57. Ibid., p. 28.
58. Ibid., p. 9.
59. Ibid., p. 10.
60. Ibid., p. 13.
61. Ibid., p. 21.
62. Ibid., p. 24.

2: *Shinden-Zukuri* As Prototype, and Two Divergent Interpretations

1. Donald Keene, trans., *Essays in Idleness: The Tsurezuregusa of Kenkō.* Rutland, Vt. and Tokyo: Charles E. Tuttle Co., 1981, p. 101.
2. Matsuo Bashō, *The Narrow Road to the Deep North and Other Travel Sketches.* Translated by Nobuyuki Yuasa. Harmondsworth, Eng.: Penguin Books, 1966, p. 71.
3. Masaaki Tachihara, *Nihon no niwa* (Japanese gardens). Tokyo: Shinkōsha, 1977.
4. *Tatami* mats are standardized by region, and are used as a unit of measure for Japanese-style rooms. One *tatami* mat generally measures 1.91 by 0.95 meters (6.3 by 3.1 feet) in the Kyoto area, 1.82 by

0.91 meters (6 by 3 feet) in the Nagoya area, and 1.76 by 0.88 meters (5.8 by 2.9 feet) in the Tokyo area. [—TRANS.]

3: Kinetic, Multifaceted Gardens and *Miegakure*

1. Harumichi Kitao, *Roji*. Suzuki Shoten, 1943, p. 59.
2. D. T. Suzuki, *Zen and Japanese Culture*. Princeton, N.J.: Princeton University Press, 1970, p. 322.
3. Shimoyama, *Sakuteiki*, p. 29.
4. A. L. Sadler. *Cha-no-yu: The Japanese Tea Ceremony*. Rutland, Vt. and Tokyo: Charles E. Tuttle Co., 1962, p. 20.
5. Dennis Hirota, "Memoranda of the Words of Rikyū: *Nanpōroku* Book 1," *Chanoyu Quarterly* 25, 1980, p. 42.
6. Adapted from Paul Varley, *Tea in Japan: Essays on the History of Chanoyu*. Edited Paul Varley, and Isao Kumakura. Honolulu: University of Hawaii Press, 1989. (From the *Yama no Sōji ki* [Records of Yama no Sōji]).

CHINA

4: Coexisting "Unworldly" and "Mundane" Worlds

1. Yūzō Sugimura, *Chūgoku no niwa* (Chinese gardens). Tokyo: Kyūryūdō, 1986.

5: Spatial Composition of the Unworldly

1. Yūzō Sugimura, *Chūgoku no niwa*. Tokyo: Kyūryūdō, 1986.
2. Adapted from Cheng Ji. *The Craft of Gardens*. Translated by Alison Hardie. New Haven, Ct. and London: Yale University Press, 1988, pp. 5–6.
3. Ji, *The Craft of Gardens*, p. 54.

6: Ideology and Prototypes

1. Ji, *The Craft of Gardens*, p. 43.
2. Cong-zhou Chen, *Shuo yuan* (On gardens). Tongji Daxue Chubanshe, 1984, pp. 2–3.
3. Huai-qi An. *Zhang guo yuanlin yishu* (The art of the Chinese *yuanlin* [garden]). Shanghai: Shanghai Kexue Jigei Chupanhui, 1986, p. 51.
4. Susan Bush and Hsio-yen Shih, eds. and comps., *Early Chinese Texts on Painting*. Cambridge, Mass. and London: Harvard University Press, 1985, p. 49.
5. Bush and Shih, *Early Chinese Texts on Painting*, pp. 50–51.
6. Adapted from Hironobu Kohara. *Garon* (Painting theory). Tokyo: Meitoku Shuppansha, 1988, p. 10.
7. Bush and Shih, *Early Chinese Texts on Painting*, p. 150.
8. Ibid., p. 203.
9. Ibid., pp. 150–151.
10. Hironobu Kohara. *Garon*, p. 12.
11. Adapted from Kōichi Obi, *Chūgoku no inton shisō* (The philosophy of seclusion in China). Tokyo: Chūōkōronsha, 1988, pp. 2-11.
12. Ichitada Miyazaki. *Kakyo* (The Chinese *keju* examination system). Tokyo: Chūōkōronsha, 1987.

KOREA

7: Traditional Korean Residences and Their Gardens

1. Wŏn-yong Kim, *Han'guk mi ŭi t'amgu* (A study of Korean beauty). Sŏnggap Sŏbang, 1982.
2. Sunu Ch'oe, *Han'guk ŭi p'ung'a* (The elegance of Korea). Sŏnggap Sŏbang, 1981.
3. Toyang No, *T'angniji* (Records on site selection for villages). Chinmyŏng Ch'ulp'ansa, 1987, p. 69.
4. Adapted from Takafumi Nomura, *Chosen no minka* (Traditional Korean dwellings). Tokyo: Gakugei Shuppansha, 1981, pp. 95–101.
5. A *k'an* is a unit of area measure equal to the span between columns squared. A two-span by three-span room is a six-*k'an* room. However, the span between columns is not constant, varying from as little as 6.5 *shaku* (1 *shaku*, a traditional Japanese unit of measure, is marginally less than 1 foot, or .28 meters) to 10 *shaku*. Nevertheless, a measurement of 8 *shaku* (8 feet or 2.25 meters) is a reasonable standard for our purposes. [—TRANS.]
6. Members of the *yangban* class who pursued Confucian studies including history and literature not necessarily to prepare themselves for civil service examinations but who chose instead to devote their lives to study were known as *yusaeng*. Such people were held in high regard in Korean society. [—TRANS.]
7. Adapted from Takafumi Nomura, *Chosen no minka*, pp. 52-54.
8. See note 5 above.

8: The "Uncultivated" Garden

1. 1. Sutemi Horiguchi, *Niwa to kūkan kōsei no dentō* (Traditions of gardens and spatial composition). Tokyo: Kajima Shuppankai, 1977, p. 5.

Chronology of Historical Periods in Japan, China, and Korea

	JAPAN	CHINA	KOREA
	10000 Jōmon		
		1766 Shang	
		1122 Zhou	
		770 Spring and Autumn Period	
500 BC		476 Warring States Period	
	300 Yayoi		
		221 Qin	
		206 Han	Three Kingdoms Period
			57 BC – 668 Early Silla
			37 BC – 668 Koguryŏ
0		9 Xin	18 BC – 663 Paekche
		25 Later Han	
		220 Three Kingdoms	
	250 Kofun	265 Jin	
		420 Northern and Southern Dynasties	
AD 500	552 Asuka	581 Sui	
		618 Tang	
	710 Nara		668 Unified Silla
			698 Parhae
	794 Heian		
		907 Five Dynasties and Ten Kingdoms	935 Kŏryŏ
1000		960 Northern Song	
	1185 Kamakura	1127 Southern Song	
		1280 Yuan	
	1333 Muromachi	1368 Ming	1392 Chosŏn
1500	1568 Azuchi-Momoyama		
	1603 Edo	1644 Qing	
	1868 Meiji		
	1912 Taishō	1911 Republic	1910 Republic
	1926 Shōwa		
	1989 Heisei		

Glossary

Words in bold type indicate separate glossary listings

A

akarishōji (明り障子) Sliding screens that face exterior walls, constructed of opaque white paper pasted to a latticed frame; more commonly referred to as *shōji.*

amado (雨戸) Wooden doors that slide in a single track, and are installed beyond the outer row of pillars of the *hiro-en.*

Amida Nyorai (阿弥陀如来) The Buddha Amitabha, who presides over Western Paradise, where souls of the faithful are welcomed after death.

anbang (内房) The inner ***pang*** located closer to the furnace, when two adjacent *pang* are served by one furnace in a traditional Korean dwelling, as opposed to the *utpang* (上房), or outer *pang.*

anch'ae (主屋棟) The wing or building of a traditional Korean residence used as the family's living quarters.

anmadang (主屋庭) A "white" garden (area of bare earth) on the south side of the ***anch'ae*** family's living quarters in a traditional Korean residence.

azuma-zukuri (四阿造り) An antiquated Japanese term for buildings with hipped roofs, more commonly known today as *yosemune.*

B

bie you dong tian (别有洞天) An ideal expressed in a Chinese ***yuanlin*** garden related to creating an utopian realm; literally, "another world of the Taoist Immortals."

birō (尾廊) The roofed corridor attached to the rear of the Hōōdō of the Byōdō-in; literally "tail corridor."

bu (歩) An ancient Chinese unit of measure, one *bu* being equal to approximately 1.5 meters, or 4.9 feet.

buke (武家) A Japanese feudal warrior's residence.

butsuden (仏殿) Buddha hall.

bu-yi jing-yi (步移景異) A principle of Chinese ***yuanlin*** garden making related to providing contrast and variety; literally, "changing step, changing view."

C

chafang (茶房) A drawing room; one of the halls in a Chinese ***ting yuan*** garden.

ch'agyŏngi (借景) Borrowed scenery, which by Korean garden-making standards relates to selecting a site and positioning and constructing the buildings on that site so as to enjoy the prospect. See also *chomang.*

Changan (長安) The capital of China during the Tang dynasty (618–907); present-day Xian.

chanoyu (茶の湯) The practice of tea ceremony; literally "hot water for tea."

chigaidana (違い棚) A pair of staggered, open shelves built into an alcove. One of the definitive decorative features of a ***shoin-zukuri*** reception room.

chiriana (塵穴) A small "dust pit" used originally to collect fallen leaves and other debris; now symbolic of leaving behind the cares of this world before entering the tearoom.

chō (町) The basic unit of subdivision in the Heian-kyō grid plan; one *chō* being equivalent to approximately 120 meters, or 394 feet, square.

chōdaigamae (帳台構) Decorative set of four doors on the inner wall of the ***jōdan zashiki*** in ***shoin-zukuri.*** Originally the entrance to a sleeping or storage area, these eventually became purely ornamental and nonopening.

chomang (眺望) Prospect, or panoramic view; one of the criteria that defines a choice residential building site by traditional Korean standards, and for positioning and constructing the buildings and gardens on that site. The principal garden-making approach applied to inner and rear gardens.

chŏngsa (精舍) Schools built and run by Korean *ilmin* hermit scholars within their mountain retreats, which offered the only form of education available other than the *sŏwŏn* national system attended by children of the upper classes.

chōnin (町人) Townspeople; particularly the Edo-period merchant class, who sparked the development of a popular culture including Kabuki theatre, *ukiyoe* wood-block prints, and haiku poetry.

ch'onmin (賎民) The lowest of five classes of **Chosŏn** Korean society, which included Buddhist monks, actors, dancers, musicians, young men with no particular occupation, and other groups generally held in contempt by members of the other four classes.

Chosŏn (朝鮮) Korea as the kingdom was known for the six-hundred year period from A.D. 1392 to 1910.

chuan feng lu (串風路) A long, narrow alleyway built between walled portions of a traditional Chinese residence for ventilation.

chufang (厨房) Cooking area or kitchen in Chinese residences.

chūmon (中門) An inner gate of a ***shinden-zukuri*** residence located at the center of the *chūmonrō*, or ***sukirō*** corridors that extend south from the east and west ***tainoya*** or, in their absence, directly from the ***shinden***.

chungin (中人) The second of five classes of **Chosŏn** Korean society, which included skilled professionals such as lawyers, doctors, and accountants as well as low-level government officials.

D

daimyō (大名) Landholding military lords in feudal Japan.

denshō (伝承) Traditions related to the Japanese arts transmitted from master to disciple.

duiting (対庁) Opposing halls; two halls constructed as the focal point of the main view from one to another respectively.

F

feng shui (風水) Chinese geomancy; literally, "wind and water."

fukinuki-yatai (吹抜屋台) A compositional technique used in ***yamato-e*** painting, in which roofs and ceilings of buildings are omitted to show interior scenes from a bird's-eye view.

fūryū (風流) An aesthetic ideal that refers to the refined manners of an urbane person and all things regarded as elegant, tasteful or artistic; also used in reference to the more ostentatious beauty seen in popular arts.

G

gankōkei (雁行型) A Japanese architectural arrangement of buildings or wings in a zigzag, or stepped, pattern; literally, "geese-in-flight form."

gedan (下段) A room in a feudal reception hall with a floor level lower than the adjoining *chūdan* and ***jōdan***; the seating area, during audiences, for persons of lower rank.

H

haengnag madang (行廊庭) A "white" garden, with no vegetation, located in front of the ***haengnagch'ae*** servant's quarters in a traditional Korean residence. Used as a work space.

haengnagch'ae (行廊棟) A long, narrow building of a traditional Korean residence used to accommodate lesser family members and servants.

haiden (排殿) The worship hall of a ***Shintō*** shrine, usually separate from the *honden* (本殿) or main sanctuary.

hajitomi (半蔀) The upper shutter of a pair of ***shitomido*** shutters, sometimes used alone.

hare (晴) The formal ceremonial space usually occupying the south side of a feudal reception hall; literally, "clear skies." Used to characterize places, objects, and occasions that are formal and public, as opposed to ***ke***.

Heian-kyō (平安京) The capital of Japan from 794–1185, thereafter known as Kyoto.

Heijō-kyō (平城京) The capital of Japan from 710–794; present-day Nara.

hiden (秘伝) Esoteric traditions passed on in the form of secret transmissions, usually texts, that are accessible only to the initiated.

hiro-en (広縁) A wide veranda built beyond the *shōji* but covered by the eaves.

hisashi (庇) An aisle one bay deep added to the sides of the core building (***moya***).

hōjō (方丈) The abbot's quarters in a Zen monastery; usually comprising two rows of three rooms each, the center rear room containing an alter, and the corner room adjacent to it used as the abbot's private study.

hu zhong you hu (湖中有湖) An ideal of ***yuanlin*** garden composition; literally, "lake within a lake."

huating (花庁) A banquet hall; the main hall of a Chinese ***ting yuan*** or ***yuanlin*** garden.

I

iki (粋) Urbane chic with undertones of sensuality; an aesthetic ideal which developed with Edo-period popular culture.

ilmin (逸民) Hermit scholars who were highly respected in Chosŏn Korean society for renouncing the mundane world and any chance of one day returning to it.

irikawa (入側) An enclosed veranda with *tatami*-mat flooring.

iwakura (磐座) Boulders believed to be inhabited by ***kami***, or divine spirit.

J

jiejing, (借景) Generic term for borrowed scenery in Chinese *yuanlin* garden making of which there are four types: *yuanjie* (遠景), or "scenery in the distance"; *linjie* (隣景), or "scenery nearby"; *yangjie* (仰景), or "scenery above"; and *fujie* (俯景), or "scenery below."

jin (進) A single family unit, i.e., hall/courtyard and two *woshi*, in traditional residential architecture of eastern central China.

jōdan (上段) A room in a feudal reception hall with a floor level higher than the adjoining *chūdan* and ***gedan***; used by the highest-ranking person(s) at audiences. Also features a ***tokonoma***, ***chigaidana***, ***tsukeshoin***, and, in many cases, coved and coffered ceilings.

Jōdo (浄土) The term used to describe the Western Paradise of the Buddha Amida; literally, "Pure Land."

jōdo hensō (浄土変相) Paintings that serve as visual "transformations" of Western Paradise as described in sutras.

jōza (上座) A privileged seat in the ***jōdan*** during audiences in feudal Japan, as opposed to *chūza* (middle-ranking seat) or *geza* (lower-ranking seat).

K

kabeshiro (壁代) A heavy drape hung between the ***moya*** and ***hisashi*** in ***shinden-zukuri*** to guard against cold in winter; literally "wall substitute."

kaiyūshiki-teien (回遊式庭園) A Japanese stroll garden; literally, "touring garden." A garden style that developed in the Edo period composed of a series of thematically-based sub-gardens arranged around a central pond.

kami (神) Shintō deities or spirit.

k'an (間) A square measure each side of which is equal to the width of the span between columns, which varies in length from 1.8 meters (6 feet) to 2.8 meters (10 feet). It is the basic unit of measure used in traditional Korean dwellings.

Kanō-*ha* (狩野派) The Kanō school of painting, founded by Kanō Masanobu (1434–1530). The principal school of academic court painters for over 400 years in Japan.

kanshō niwa (観賞庭) Contemplation garden. A garden form that developed during the Japanese medieval period; this was not physically entered, but was viewed from an adjacent room or veranda.

kasaneirome (襲色目) The color combinations shown at the sleeves, neckline, and hem of the many layers of robes worn by court ladies during the Heian period.

kata (型) A definitive form or style.

ke (褻) The private, everyday quarters in residences of the late Heian through the Kamakura and Muromachi periods, usually located on the north side of the building; as opposed to ***hare***.

keju (科挙) A system of civil service examinations established during the Tang dynasty, which served as the means of selection of the nation's officials until 1904.

ken (間) Bay or span between pillars.

kichō (几帳) A free-standing textile screen with a T-shaped frame, used in ***shinden-zukuri*** residences, a standard 3 or 4 ***shaku*** (90 or 120 centimeters; 3 or 4 feet) in height.

kōan (公案) A Zen Buddhist conundrum which frees the mind from conceptualizing.

kolbang (傍房) A space one-half–***k'an*** in width attached to the side of a ***pang***, used as a walk-in closet.

konnobang (越房) An *ondol*-heated room located just beyond the ***taech'ong***, on the side furthest from the ***puŏk*** (kitchen), which has its own furnace and is used as part of the women and children's quarters, or as a study.

koshikake machiai (腰掛け待合) A covered bench in tea gardens where guests wait to be called to the teahouse.

kuden (口伝) Verbally transmitted insights or techniques about any of the traditional Japanese arts.

kumo-gasumi (雲霞) A compositional technique used in ***yamato-e*** painting, in which mist and clouds are used to separate different scenes on a single picture plane.

kyakuden (客殿) A room or hall for receiving guests in warrior and temple residences of the Japanese medieval period.

M

ma (間) An interval in time or space; a void that by its very absence (whether of sound or of form) asserts its existence, adding to the articulation of the overall space.

madang (庭) Generic term for inner gardens, usually bare of vegetation, in a traditional Korean residence.

mairado (舞良戸) A sliding wooden door faced with thin, closely spaced wooden strips. This was installed in early ***shoin-zukuri*** architecture as a set of two wooden doors and one paper screen (***akarishōji***) per bay that slid horizontally in a three-track gutter.

manabi (学び) Learning, which includes simulation and modeling after.

maru (抹楼) Rooms in a traditional Korean dwelling which have wooden floors and are completely open to the elements on at least one side.

men (面) Side of the *moya* to which *hisashi* is attached.

miegakure (見え隠れ) A method of garden composition employing a variety of techniques to fully or partially obscure buildings and garden scenes, hiding and revealing them in turn as the viewer moves through the space; literally, "reveal-and-hide."

misu (御簾) A roll-up blind of finely split bamboo stems connected by thread.

miyabi (雅び) Refined beauty, elegance; an aesthetic ideal associated with the Heian court.

mono no aware (物の哀れ) An aesthetic ideal that relates to the capacity to be emotionally moved by "things"; a heightened sensitivity to the ephemeral beauty embodied in nature and human life, thus tinged with an element of sadness.

moya (母屋) The core or central portion of a building.

munewakedo (棟分け戸) An interior partition constructed directly below the roof ridge in ***shinden-zukuri*** residences.

myŏngdang (明堂) Choice land or sites as defined by the standards of Korean geomancy.

N

nijiriguchi (躙口) The low sliding-door entrance to the teahouse.

nobi (奴稗) The fourth of five classes of **Chosŏn** Korean society, which were the slaves of the state administration and of wealthier families. (At the beginning of the Chosŏn dynasty, since slavery was hereditary, nearly half the population was slaves.)

numaru (楼抹楼) A special reception room in the ***sarangch'ae*** master's quarters in a traditional Korean residence, the floor level of which is raised approximately 40 centimeters (15.75 inches) above that of the other rooms in the dwelling, to enjoy the benefit of the view.

O

ochi-en (落縁) A veranda built outside and one step lower than the main floor or broad veranda.

ondol (温突) The traditional Korean system of floor heating, which utilizes the heat of smoke from an enclosed furnace forced through flues located beneath the floor to a chimney at the other end of the room or rooms.

oriage-gōtenjō (折上げ格天井) A ceiling in which the central portion is raised higher than the surrounding flat area through the use of curved timbers. A decorative feature of the ***shoin-zukuri jōdan zashiki.***

oshi-ita (押板) An early form of the ***tokonoma*** alcove, of shallow depth and with a thick, single plank floorboard.

P

pang (房) Food preparation area or kitchen in a traditional Korean dwelling.

puŏk (釜屋) Enclosed rooms with floor heating in a traditional Korean dwelling.

p'ungsu (風水) Korean geomancy; a system of principles which defines favorable and unfavorable land characteristics, based on ancient Chinese theories of yin and yang and the five basic elements.

pyŏldang (別堂) A sanctuary-like annex of a traditional Korean residence, where the master of the household spent time reading in private.

pyŏlsŏ (別墅) Environments created by Korean ***ilmin*** hermit scholars who lived in the mountains and forests, through the construction of belvederes, halls and pavilions amid valleys, waterfalls, springs, and hills.

R

roji (露地) A tea garden; originally the path (and its surrounds) leading to the teahouse; literally "dewy ground."

rōkaku (楼閣) Multistoried pavilions, often constructed over the corners of the side corridors in Hōōdō-style temple architecture.

S

sabi (寂) An aesthetic ideal related to tea culture; appreciation of the patina of use and age.

sadangch'ae (祠堂棟) An ancestral shrine located in an elevated area at the northern end of the compound of a traditional Korean residence, facing south and overlooking the other buildings. It is dedicated to the four previous generations of ancestors.

Sakuteiki (作庭記) (Notes on garden making), an eleventh century Japanese gardening text attributed to Tachibana no Toshitsuna, the son of a Fujiwara nobleman and renowned garden maker.

sangmin (常民) The third of five classes of **Chosŏn** Korean society, which included traders, artisans, farming families that tilled the fields administered by the ***yangban***, and others. These were the common people who made up the vast majority of the population.

sanzonseki (三尊石) A triangular arrangement of three stones representing a Buddhist trinity; literally, "Buddhist triad rocks."

sarang madang (舍廊庭) A "white" garden, with little or no vegetation, located in front of the ***sarangch'ae*** master's quarters in a traditional Korean residence.

sarangbang (舍廊房) An ***ondol***-heated, enclosed room within the ***sarangch'ae***.

sarangch'ae (舍廊棟) The wing or building of a traditional Korean residence used by the master of the house as his private quarters and for receiving guests.

seiden (正殿) Another term for the main hall of a ***shinden-zukuri*** residence. See *shinden.*

shaichang (晒場) An enclosed area of a traditional Chinese residence containing the laundry area, clotheslines, well, and frequently vegetable gardens, livestock pens, and toilet; literally, "drying area."

shakkei (借景) Borrowed scenery; a garden-making method in which a feature of a distant view is incorporated into the garden as an integral element. The garden site proper comprises the foreground, and the distant feature the background. The middle ground is composed to frame the "borrowed" feature, which foreshortens the distant view and draws it into the garden, extending the perceived scale of the garden far beyond the boundaries of the site.

shaku (尺) A traditional Japanese unit of measurement; one *shaku* being marginally less that one foot, or .28 meters.

shanshui (山水) Chinese term for landscape; literally, "mountains and water."

shinden (寝殿) The central hall, or main structure of a ***shinden-zukuri*** residence, in which the master resided.

shinden-zukuri (寝殿造り) A style of aristocratic residence that developed in the Heian period. In its unabbreviated form, consists of a central hall (***shinden***) surrounded by annexes (***tainoya***) on the north, east, and west sides which are interconnected by covered walkways, and faces a garden to the south.

Shintō (神道) Japanese indigenous animistic religion.

shiroroji (白路地) A garden form composed purely of coarse white sand which developed in Zen temples during the Japanese medieval period.

shitomido (蔀戸) Latticed shutters backed with wooden panels that swing outward and upward on a horizontal pivotal axis set between the outer row of pillars in ***shinden-zukuri*** architecture.

shōheiga (障屏画) Screen and wall paintings, used in architectural decoration, executed on walls, ceilings, pillars, and *fusuma* sliding screens.

shoin-zukuri (書院造り) A style of residential architecture that developed during the Kamakura and Muromachi periods, used in warrior residences and Zen temple abbot's quarters. It is divided into rooms with fixed walls and sliding doors, has *tatami*-mat flooring and square posts. In its most elaborate form it is decorated with a ***tokonoma*** alcove, ***chigaidana*** staggered shelves, a ***tsukeshoin*** built-in desk, coved and coffered ceilings, and a ***jōdan*** raised-floor area.

shufang (書房) A study; one of the halls in a Chinese ***ting yuan*** garden.

siheyuan (四合院) The style of traditional residential architecture typical of Beijing; composed of four halls facing a central courtyard.

simianting (四面庁) A type of ***huating*** hall comprised of an open interior space surrounded by latticework doors and open walkways on all four sides; literally, "four-sided hall."

sōan (草庵) A tiny, rustic teahouse as used in the ***wabi*** form of tea ceremony in the early Momoyama period; literally a "thatched hut."

sŏkkasan (石仮山) Rocks which are displayed singly or in simple arrangements in Korean rear gardens or outer gardens; literally, "pseudo–rock mountains."

sŏwŏn (書院) Schools for the children of the ***yangban*** scholars, which constituted a kind of national education system in **Chosŏn** Korea.

suki (数寄) An Edo-period aesthetic ideal referring to artistic taste and connoisseurship.

sukirō (透廊) Roofed, open-structure corridors forming the passageways between buildings in a ***shinden-zukuri*** residence.

sukiya (数寄屋) A large tearoom (*hiroma*); or a building in the *sukiya* style.

sukiya-zukuri (数寄屋造り) An architectural style that blends elements of the formal *shoin* style and rustic ***sōan*** teahouse, characteristics of which include columns with unbeveled corners (*menkawabashira*), earthen walls (*tsuchikabe*), and understated, delicate decoration.

T

taech'ŏng (大庁) The central living room in a traditional Korean dwelling. The northern side is enclosed by two sliding wooden doors, but the southern side is completely open to the elements. (The *taech'ŏng* within the *anch'ae* family living quarters is distinct from the *taech'ŏng* within the *sarangch'ae* master's quarters, and is thus referred to as the *andaech'ŏng*).

tainoya (対屋) An annex of a ***shinden-zukuri*** residence built to the north, east or west of the central main hall (***shinden***).

tang (堂) The central living room in traditional Chinese dwellings.

tatami (畳) Rectangular straw mats covered in woven rush laid side-by-side as flooring in Japanese-style rooms; slightly less than one by two meters in size (although dimensions vary regionally); the size of a room is generally indicated by the number of *tatami* mats it accommodates.

tianjing (天 井) A deep narrow courtyard typical of traditional dwellings in eastern central China; literally, "skywell."

ting (庭) Generic term meaning "courtyard" in Chinese.

ting yuan (庭院) A small, walled landscape garden built adjacent to, but separated from, the living area of a traditional Chinese residence; contains one or two halls and garden scenes composed to be contemplated from inside these halls. Unlike Japanese contemplation gardens, however, the garden is walked through to enter these halls.

t'oetmaru (槵抹楼) A space one-half–***k'an*** in width attached to the side of a ***pang***, which serves as a corridor.

tokonoma (床の間) An ornamental alcove in a Japanese ***zashiki*** with a raised floor and lowered lintel, used to display a hanging scroll or flowers.

tongsan (東山) Artificial hills sometimes featured in Korean rear gardens or outer gardens, which are formed as gentle, grass-covered slopes.

torii (鳥居) A gatelike structure marking the threshold of a sacred (***Shintō***) space.

tsuboniwa (坪庭) A small garden enclosed by buildings, corridors, or walls in ***shinden-zukuri***, temple and *machiya* (townhouse) Japanese architecture.

tsukeshoin (付け書院) A built-in desk alcove; one of the definitive decorative features of a ***shoin-zukuri*** reception room.

tsukubai (蹲踞) A stone water basin used for ritual rinsing of the hands and mouth in the tea garden; also refers to an arrangement of stones, including the water basin.

tsumado (妻戸) Swinging paneled doors, usually paired, placed at the four corners of a ***shinden-zukuri*** building.

twitmadang (後庭) The rear garden, which lies to the north of the ***anch'ae*** in a traditional Korean residence on a southern slope, or as the uppermost of a series of terraces. This was a private space used mainly by women and children. It features grass and shrubs as well as fruit trees and is surrounded by a wall that traces the natural contours of the land.

W

wabi (わび) An aesthetic ideal related to the way of tea; utter simplicity, or the appreciation of a higher beauty amid apparent lack of beauty.

woshi (臥) Private, sleeping quarters in traditional Chinese dwellings.

woyou (臥遊) "Travel by imagination"; derived from stories—possibly apocryphal—told about the painter Zong Bing (373/75–443), who was known for wandering through the countryside and so enjoying the scenery that he sometimes forgot to return home. It is said that when he was old, infirm, and bedridden, he was able to paint landscapes on his walls from memories of his wanderings.

Y

yamato-e (大和絵) An indigenous style of painting which depicted Japanese scenes mostly on doors and screens in the late Heian and early Kamakura periods.

yangban (両班) The highest of five classes of **Chosŏn** Korean society, this includes scholar/civil officials, military officials (whose status was lower than that of scholar/civil officials), and the descendents of each.

yin-di zhi-xuan (因地製宣) A principle of Chinese ***yuanlin*** garden making; literally, "follow the natural lay of the land."

yō (様) Form or shape; a definitive style; appearance, air or state.

yokurō (翼廊) A roofed corridor that extends from the side of a main hall; literally, "wing corridors."

yuanlin (園林) A small landscape park composed of multiple scenes designed for viewing both from inside the various buildings and while strolling along the paths linking these buildings.

Yuan ye (園冶) A Ming-dynasty Chinese gardening text (Craft of gardens) written by Ji Cheng, a renowned garden maker, poet, and painter of the Jiangnan region.

yuan zhong you yuan (園中有園) An ideal of ***yuanlin*** garden composition; literally, "garden within a garden."

yuanzi (院子) The central courtyard of a residential quadrangle (***siheyuan***) typical of Beijing.

yūgen (幽玄) Mystery and depth; the leading aesthetic ideal of the Japanese middle ages concerned with the true nature hidden behind the illusory aspects of the world.

Z

zansan jōsui (残山剰水) A compositional style of ink-wash landscape painting in which large areas of unarticulated space suggest mountains and water receding into the "mist" between landscape scenes.

zashiki (座敷) A reception room with ***tatami***-mat flooring which developed in the Japanese medieval period with ***shoin-zukuri***.

zazen (座禅) Seated meditation practiced in Zen Buddhism.

zeshō (軟障) Thin curtains hung behind ***misu*** blinds from rods that fit between the pillars in ***shinden-zukuri*** residences.

zhuan (磚) Fired brick; used both for load-bearing and curtain wall construction and courtyard flooring along with tamped earth and adobe bricks in traditional Chinese residential architecture.

zutang (祖堂) Ancestral room; the most formally decorated room in a traditional Chinese dwelling, where ancestors are worshipped.

Selected References

Adams, Edward B. *Palaces of Seoul.* Seoul: Seoul International Publishing House, 1972.

An Huai-qi. *Zhang guo yuanlin yishu* (The art of the Chinese *yuanlin* [garden]). Shanghai: Shanghai Kexue Jigei Chupanhui, 1986.

Bring, Mitchell, and Wayembergh, Josse. *Japanese Gardens: Design and Meaning.* New York: McGraw-Hill, 1981.

Bush, Susan, and Shih, Hsio-yen, comp. and ed. *Early Chinese Texts on Painting.* Cambridge, Mass. and London: Harvard University Press, 1985.

Chen Cong-zhou. *Shuo yuan* (On gardens). Tongji Daxue Chubanshe, 1984.

Chen Cong-zhou. *Setsu en* (Shuo yuan; On gardens). Translated by Kawahara Taketoshi. Tokyo: Nihon Zōen Shūkei Kyōkai, 1986.

Ch'oe, Sunu. *Han'guk ŭi p'ung'a* (The elegance of Korea). Sŏnggap Sŏbang, 1981.

Doi, Tsugiyoshi. *Momoyama Decorative Painting* (Momoyama no shōheigi). Heibonsha Survey of Japanese Art Series, vol. 14. New York and Tokyo: Weatherhill/ Heibonsha, 1976.

Fukuyama, Toshio. *Heian Temples: Byodo-in and Chuson-ji.* (Byōdō-in to Chūsonji). Translated by Ronald K. Jones. New York and Tokyo: Weatherhill/Heibonsha, 1976.

Hashimoto, Fumio. *Architecture in the Shoin Style* (Shoin-zukuri). Translated and adapted by H. Mack Horton. Tokyo: Kodansha International, 1981.

Hayakawa, Masao. *The Garden of Japan.* Translated by Richard L Gage. Tokyo: Weatherhill/Heibonsha, 1973.

Hirota, Dennis. "Memoranda of the Words of Rikyū: *Nampōroku* Book 1," *Chanoyu Quarterly* 25. Kyoto: 1980.

Hisamatsu, Shin'ichi. "The Way of Tea and Buddhism." Translated by Robert F. Rhodes. *Chanoyu Quarterly* 74. Kyoto: 1993.

Horiguchi, Sutemi. *Niwa to kūkan kōsei no dentō* (Traditions of gardens and spatial composition). Tokyo: Kajima Shuppankai, 1977.

——. *Rikyū to chashitsu* (Rikyū and tearooms). Tokyo: Kajima Shuppankai, 1977.

Inaji, Toshirō. *Kankyō dezain no rekishi tenbō* (Historical perspectives on environmental design in Japan). Tokyo: Sanseidō, 1991.

Inaji, Toshirō, Katayama, Kazutoshi and Mogi, Keiichirō. *Chūgoku minkyo no kūkan wo saguru* (An exploration of space in Chinese dwellings). Tokyo: Kenchiku Shiryō Kenkyūsha, 1991.

Inoue, Mitsuo. *Space in Japanese Architecture* (Nihon kenchiku no kūkan). Translated by Hiroshi Watanabe. New York and Tokyo: Weatherhill, 1985.

Itoh, Teiji. *Kekkai no bi* (The beauty of boundaries). Kyoto: Tankōshinsha, 1966.

——. *Space and Illusion in the Japanese Garden* (Shakkei to tsuboniwa). Translated and adapted by Ralph Friedrich and Masajiro Shimamura. New York, Tokyo and Kyoto: Weatherhill/Tankōsha, 1973.

——. *The Gardens of Japan.* Tokyo: Kodansha International, 1984.

——. *Traditional Domestic Architecture of Japan* (Minka). Translated by Richard L. Gage. New York and Tokyo: Weatherhill/Heibonsha, 1972.

Itoh, Teiji, Tanaka Ikkō and Sesoko Tsune, ed. *Wabi, Sabi, Suki.* Hiroshima: Mazda Corporation, 1993.

Japan: An Illustrated Encyclopedia. Tokyo: Kodansha, 1993.

Ji, Cheng. *The Craft of Gardens* (Yuan ye). Translated by Alison Hardie. New Haven: Yale University Press, 1988.

Keene, Donald, trans. *Essays in Idleness, The Tsurezuregusa of Kenkō.* Rutland, Vt. and Tokyo: Charles E. Tuttle Co., 1981.

Kenchiku dai jiten (Encyclopedia of architecture). Tokyo: Shōkokusha, 1978.

Keswick, Maggie. *The Chinese Garden; History, Art & Architecture.* 2d ed., rev. London: Academy Editions, 1978 and New York: St. Martin's Press, 1986.

Kim, Bong Yeol. *Kankoku no kenchiku* (Korean architecture). Translated by Nishigaki Yasuhiko. Tokyo: Gakugei Shuppansha, 1943.

Kim, Wŏn-yong. *Han'guk mi ŭi t'amgu* (A study of Korean beauty). Sŏnggap Sŏbang, 1982.

Kitao, Harumichi. *Roji.* Suzuki Shoten, 1943.

Knapp, Ronald G. *China's Traditional Rural Architecture.* Honolulu: University of Hawaii Press, 1991.

——. *China's Vernacular Architecture.* Honolulu: University of Hawaii Press, 1989.

Kohara, Hironobu. *Garon* (Painting theory). Tokyo: Meitoku Shuppansha, 1988.

Kuck, Loraine. *The World of the Japanese Garden: from Chinese Origins to Modern Landscape Art.* Tokyo: Walker/Weatherhill, 1968.

Kundaikansōchōki. In *Kodai chūsei geijitsuron* (Art theories of the ancient and medieval periods). Edited by Tatsusaburō Hayashiya. *Nihon shisō taikei* (Compendium of Japanese thought), vol. 23. Tokyo: Iwanami Shoten, 1975.

Matsuo Bashō. *Bashō: The Road to the Deep North and Other Travel Sketches.* Translated by Noboyuki Yuasa. Harmondsworth, England: Penguin Books, 1966.

Miyazaki, Ichisada. *Kakyo* (The Chinese *keju* examination system). Tokyo: Chūōkōronsha, 1987.

Mori, Osamu. *Nihon no teien* (Japanese gardens). Tokyo: Kōbunsha, 1964.

Morris, Edwin T. *The Gardens of China: History, Art, and Meanings.* New York: Scribners, 1983.

Murasaki Shikibu. *The Tale of Genji* (Genji monogatari). Translated by Edward Seidensticker. New York: Alfred A. Knopf, 1986.

Nihon kenchiku-shi zushū (History of Japanese architecture through selected illustrations). Compiled by Nihon Kenchiku Gakkai. Tokyo: Shōkokusha, 1980.

Nihon no toshi kūkan (Urban space in Japan). Toshi Dezain Kenkyūtai. Tokyo: Shōkokusha, 1978.

Nishi, Kazuo, and Hozumi, Kazuo. *What is Japanese Architecture?* (Nihon kenchiku no katachi: seikatsu to kenchiku zōkei no rekishi). Translated by H. Mack Horton. Tokyo: Kodansha International, 1983.

Nishizawa, Fumitaka. *Teien ron 1–3* (Theory on gardens, vols. 1–3). Tokyo: Sagami Shobō, 1975.

No, Toyang. *T'angniji* (Records on site selection for villages). Chinmyŏng Ch'ulp'ansa, 1987.

Nomura, Takafumi. *Chosen no minka* (Traditional Korean dwellings). Tokyo: Gakugei Shuppansha, 1981.

Obi, Kōichi. *Chūgoku no inton shisō* (The philosophy of seclusion in China). Tokyo: Chūōkōronsha, 1988.

Ōchō emaki—kisoku no sekai (Heian-period painted scrolls: the noble's world). Tokyo: Mainichi Shinbunsha, 1990.

Okawa, Naomi. *Edo Architecture: Katsura and Nikko* (Katsura to Nikkō). Translated by Alan Woodhull and Akito Miyamoto. New York and Tokyo: Weatherhill/ Heibonsha, 1975.

Okazaki, Jōji. *Pure Land Buddhist Painting* (Jōdo kyōga). Translated and adapted by Elizabeth ten Grotenhuis. Tokyo: Kodansha International, 1977.

Ōta, Hirotarō. *Shoin-zukuri* (The shoin style). Tokyo: Tōkyō Daigaku Shuppankai, 1966.

Parent, Mary Neighbour. *The Roof in Japanese Architecture.* New York and Tokyo: Weatherhill/Kajima, 1983.

Sadler, A. L. *Cha-no-yu: the Japanese Tea Ceremony.* Rutland, Vt. and Tokyo: Charles E. Tuttle Co., 1962.

Saitō, Katsuo. *Zukai Sakuteiki* (The illustrated *Sakuteiki*). Tokyo: Gihōdō, 1964.

Sawada, Nadari. *Kaoku zakkō.* (A miscellany of reflections on architecture). Tokyo: Yoshikawa Kōbunkan, vol. 1.

Slawson, David. *Secret Teachings in the Art of Japanese Gardens.* Tokyo: Kodansha International, 1987.

Sugimura, Yūzō. *Chūgoku no niwa* (Chinese gardens). Tokyo: Kyūryūdō, 1986.

Suzuki, D. T. *Zen and Japanese Culture.* Bollingen Series, vol. 64. Princeton, NJ: Princeton University Press, 1959.

Tachibana no Toshitsuna [?]. *Sakuteiki* (Notes on garden making). In *Kodai chūsei geijitsuron* (Art theories of the ancient and medieval periods), edited by Tatsusaburō Hayashiya. *Nihon shisō taikei* (Compendium of Japanese thought), vol. 23. Tokyo: Iwanami Shoten, 1975.

Tachibana no Toshitsuna [?]. *Sakuteiki: The Book of Garden* (Sakuteiki). Translated by Shigemaru Shimoyama. Tokyo: Town and City Planners, 1976.

Tachihara, Masaaki. *Nihon no niwa* (Japanese gardens). Tokyo: Shinkōsha, 1977.

Takeda, Tsuneo. *Kanō Eitoku.* Translated and adapted by H. Mack Horton and Catherine Kaputa. Tokyo: Kodansha International, 1977.

Tamaki, Toyojirō. *Nihon toshi seiritsushi* (The historical formation of Japanese cities). Tokyo: Rikōgakusha, 1974.

Tamura, Tsuyoshi. *Sakuteiki.* Tokyo: Sagami Shobō, 1977.

Tanaka, Ichimatsu. *Japanese Ink Painting: Shūbun to Sesshū.* Tokyo: Weatherhill/Heibonsha, 1972.

Tanaka, Seidai. *Nihon no teien* (Japanese gardens). Tokyo: Kajima Shuppankai, 1977.

Treib, Marc, and Herman, Ron. *A Guide to the Gardens of Kyoto.* Tokyo: Shufunotomo, 1980.

Ueda, Atsushi. *The Inner Harmony of the Japanese House* (Nihonjin to sumai). Tokyo: Kodansha International, 1990.

Uehara, Keiji, ed. *Tsukiyama teizō den* (Artificial mountain garden-making traditions). Tokyo: Kajima Shoten, 1976.

——, ed. *Tsukiyama sansui den/Sagaryū niwa kohō hiden no koto* (Traditions on artificial hill and mountain and water landscapes; Secret teachings on ancient gardening techniques of the Saga school). Tokyo: Kajima Shoten, 1976.

Varley, Paul. *Japanese Culture: A Short History.* Rutland, Vt. and Tokyo: Charles E. Tuttle Co., 1973.

——. *Tea in Japan: Essays on the History of Chanoyu.* Edited by Paul Varley and Isao Kumakura. Honolulu: University of Hawaii Press, 1989.

Yanagi, Sōetsu. *Chosen wo omou* (Thoughts on Korea). Tokyo: Chikuma Shoten, 1984.

Acknowledgments

Permission was received from the following to reproduce the illustrations indicated:

Byōdō-in: *Figure 7.2*
Chishaku-in: *Figures 35.2, 35., 35.4*
Daichiji: *Figure 11*
Daisen'in, Daitokuji: *Figures 18.1, 18.3*
Funda-in, Tōfukuji: *Figure 19.33*
Hōsen'in: *Figure 37*
Jōeiji: *Figure 25.2*
Suizenji Kōen: *Figure 45.5*
Kanchi-in, Tōji: *Figure 32.1*
Katsura Rikyū: *Figures 9.2, 41.1–41.4*
Keishun'in, Myōshinji: *Figures 24.1–24.3*
Kinkakuji: *Figure 10.3*
Kitano Shrine: *Figure 10.4*
Kohō-an, Daitokuji: *Figures 44.1–44.4, 44.6*
Koishikawa Kōrakuen: *Figures 45.3, 45.4*
Kōjō-in, Onjōji: *Figures 34.1–34.2*
Kōtō-in, Daitokuji: *Figure 22.3*
Kuboso Memorial Museum of Arts (Izumi): *Figure 5*
Kyoto National Museum: *Figure 9.3*
Manpukuji: *Figure 10.1*
Manshu-in: *Figures 43.2–43.5*
Mohri Museum: *Figure 20.2*
Mōtsūji:* *Figures 10.2, 12*
Murin'an (Kyoto-shi Kanri Meishō Murin'an): *Figure 13*
Myōki-an: *Figure 38.2*
Nanzen'in: *Figure 10.6*
Nijōjō: *Figure 30*
Nin'naji: *Figures 10.5, 14.1*
Omote Senke: *Figure 39*
Onjōji: *Figures 2.1–2.3*
Rikugien: *Figure 45.2*
Ryōanji: *Figures 22.1, 26.2*
Ryōgen'in, Daitokuji: *Figures 14.2, 19.2*
Shinju-an, Daitokuji: *Figure 20.1*
Shōdenji: *Figure 22.2*
Tenryūji: *Figure 28.2*
The Palace Museum (Beijing): *Figure 48*
The Seikado Bunko Art Museum: *Figure 78*
Tōkai-an, Myōshinji: *Figure 21*
Tokyo National University of Fine Arts and Music: *Figures 57.1–57.4, 58.1, 58.2, 59.2, 59.4–59.6, 60, 65.2*
Yonezawa City, Yamagata Prefecture: *Figure 15*

Photographer Haruzo Ohashi: *Figures 7.2, 9.1–9.2, 18.1, 22.2, 26.2, 39, 44.1*

*Mōtsūji was photographed prior to major renovations.

Index

A

abbreviation 13, 26–27, 34, 38, 41

abstract interpretations 17, 27, 37, 40–43, *Figures 21–26*, 49, *Figure 29.1*. *See also* abstraction.

abstraction 17, 24, 27, 34

adopting and assimilating 4

aesthetic ideals, Korean 185. *See also fūryū, miyabi, mono no aware, wabi, yūgen.*

amado sliding doors 59–60, *Figure 36.3*

Amanohashidate 14, *Figure 9.1–9.3*, 16, 17

Anapchi 173, *Figures 118.1–118.2*, 178

ancestral: form of Japanese gardens 3; room (*zutang*) 84, 91, 93; shrine (*citang*) 127; shrine (*sadangch'ae*) 137, 139, *Figures 90.1–90.2*

anch'ae (family living quarters) 137, 139, 144, 150, 166

anmadang (inner garden) 137, 139, 153, *Figures 108.4, 111.4–111.5*

artificial hills: in Japanese garden design 8–9, 17, *Figures 10.1*, 25, 27, 41, 55, *Figures 45.4–45.5*, 110, 116; in Korean gardens 162, *Figure 118.2*. *See also* artificial mountains.

artificial mountains: in Chinese garden design 109, 110, *Figure 72.3*, 116; *Figure 75.1, 76*, 162. *See also* artificial hills.

asymmetry, in abbreviated interpretations 11, *Figures 6, 8*, 13, 29, 34. *See also* symmetry.

attention, manipulation and focusing of 62, 63, 66, 67

azuma-zukuri 10

B

Bashō. *See* Matsuo Bashō.

Beijing 83, 85, 90, 107, 116, 132–133, 182

blinds and curtains 29

bonsai 93, 96, 98, 102

borrowed scenery: in Japanese garden design 41, *Figure 22.2*, 43, 163; in Chinese garden design 109, 112, 116, 118, *Figures 77.1– 77.2*; in Korean gardens 162–164, 166, 184

bridges 10, 27–28, 37, 73, 173, 179

Buddhism: Pure Land 12; Zen 34; in Korea 136

buildings: as garden features 80, *Figure 47.1*, 103, 109–112, 116, 118, 120, *Figure 72.3*; layout of in *yuanlin* 109–111, *Figure 71*, 162

buke. *See* warrior residences.

Byōdō-in 13, *Figure 7.2*, 80

C

caves 109, 115–116, *Figure 75.2*, 162

ceremonial area 8–9, 19, 27, 34, 40, 137, 160, 173

ch'ae (interior space) 150, 153; and Chinese hall/courtyard composition 158, 160. *See also madang.*

chafang (drawing room). *See shufang* (study).

Changan 5–6, *Figure 3.1*

chanoyu (way of tea) 62, 66–67

chŏngsa schools 143, 179, *Figures 120, 121.1*

city plan 6, *Figures 3.1–3.2*, 9, 32, 85, *Figure 65.1*

civil service examinations (*keju*) 119–120, 127–128

climatic influences 90–91, *Figure 56*, 98, 100, 145

collective residential complexes 91, *Figures 57–59*, 93, 143, *Figure 91*

communal space 91, 93, 96, *Figures 56.3, 60*, 98,100, 127, 158

conceptual prototype *ix*, 5

condensed interpretations 17, 43, *Figures 29.2, 34.1–34.2, 35.1–35.6*, 55, 67, 108, 110. *See also* abstract interpretations.

Confucian: social structure 119–120, 136; influence on painting 122, 124–128; spatial composition of homes 93, 100, 127–128, 136–137, 143, 145, 150, 153, 182; hermit scholars (*ilmin*) 179, 182, 185. *See also* Neo-Confucianism.

connoisseurship 49, 67

contemplative gardens (Japanese *kanshō niwa*) 38, 43, 48, 60. *See also ting yuan.*

continental (Chinese) cultural influence *x*, 4–5, 10, 32, 49, 134, 160–1, 178

contrast and change, as a Chinese garden ideal 112, 115–116, 162

corridors, *sukirō* open 7–8, 10, 29, 34; *yokurō* "wing" and *birō* "tail" 13; *ochi-en* (lower veranda) 58–59; external 68; roofed 78; *t'oetmaru* 146

courtyards, *ting*, 83, 93, 100, 102–104, 160; *yuanzi* 83–84, 90, 93, 98, *Figure 62.2*, 102, 149, 158; *tianjing* 83–84, 90–91, *Figure 56*, 96, 98, 100, 102, 149, 158

creativity, and individuality *viii, xi*, 14, 24, 25

D

Daitokuji: Daisen'in 37, *Figures 18.1–18.3*, 43; Kōtō-in 41, *Figure 22.3*; Kohō-an 71, *Figures 44.1–44.6*, 74, 80

Daichiji 22, *Figure 11*

design process *viii*, 22, 24, 25

dry landscape (*kare sansui*) 22, 27, 40, 68, *Figure 43.4*

duiting (opposing buildings, or *dui-ge*) 110, 112, *Figure 72.3*

E

Edo 78

elitist symbols, gardens as 104, 106, 108, 119–120, 124, 182

essence, portraying/expressing 13, 17, 19, 24, 25, 34, 62, 120

F

feng shui. *See* geomancy.

feudal society, Japanese 34, 49, 74–76; Chinese 119, 127; Korean 134–136

filial piety 93, 127

fishing pavilion (*tsuridono*) 10, 34

Forbidden City. *See* palaces.

furnishings/furniture, 29, 61, 84 *Figure 50.2*, 93, *Figures 61.1–61.3*, 99, 147, 150, 153, 158–159

fūryū 67, 78

G

garden stream 17, 19 *Figure 10.4*, 26, *Figure 13*, 27, 29, 37, 55

garden-making approaches, defining 131–132, 160–161, 163, 166, 184

"geese-in-flight" form (*gankōkei*) 11, 13, *Figures 6, 8*, 68, *Figures 42, 43.1*, 71, *Figure 44.5*

geomancy, and taboos 19; Chinese (*feng shui*) 111, 133, 179, 182; Korean (*p'ungsu*) 132–134, *Figures 84.1–84.2*, 139, 149, 164, 179

H

haengnagch'ae (servant's quarters) 139, *Figures 89.1–89.2*, 173, *Figures 115.1–115.2*

Hakka dwellings 93, *Figures 59.1–59.6*

hall/courtyard units 83–84, *Figures 49, 51, 57–58*

hare (formal) space 34, *Figure 17*, 38, 43, 53, 55, 58

Hasedera 78, *Figure 46.1*

heating, *kang* 84, *Figure 50.1*, 144, *Figure 94*; portable 99, *Figures 64.1–64.2*; *ondol* floor 143–149, *Figures 92–93, 98–99*, 150

Heian-kyō 5–7, *Figure 3.2*, 8–11

hierarchy, spatial representation of: in Japan 49, 52, 74, 76; in China 91, 93, 127; in Korea 134–136

hill island style 17, 22, 28, 41

hillside fields 19, 27–29

hiroma (large tearoom) 67

hōjō (abbot's quarters) 34, *Figures 18.2–18.3*, 40, 41, 43, *Figures 25.1–25.2, 26.1–26.2*, 71, 74

huating 80, 103–104, 106, *Figures 66, 67.1–67.2, 68.2–68.3*, 110–112, 116, 118–119

Huizhou popular dwellings (*minju*) 83–85, *Figures 51–57*, 90–91, 93, 98–100, 103, 127

I

ideals of Chinese garden design 107, 109

illusion, of depth 28; spatial 27

ilmin hermit scholars. *See* Confucian scholars and retreats.

Imperial gardens 106–107

intrinsic quality 17

islands: in Japanese gardens 9–10, 16, *Figure 9.2*, 17, *Figure 10.3*, 22, 26–28, 40, 41, 55, 68; in Chinese gardens 80, 107; in Korean outer gardens 173, 178

iwakura 3, *Figure 2.1*

J

Ji Cheng 108

jōdan zashiki, arrangement of 49; decorative style of, *Figure 30*, 52, 55

Jōeiji 43, *Figures 25.1–25.2*

K

kasaneirome 29

Katsura Rikyū *Figures 9.2, 41.1–41.4*, 74, 178

ke (informal) space 34, *Figure 17*, 43, 53, 55, 58

kitchen, *chufang* 98–99, 100; *puŏk* 144, 147–149, *Figures 99–100*

Kiyomizudera 78, *Figure 46.2*

Kobori Enshū 74, 178

koma (small tearoom) 66–67

koshikake machiai (waiting bench) 61, 63, 74, *Figure 44.6*

kumogasumi (cloud and mist) technique 29, *Figure 15*, 38

kyakuden (guest hall) 34, *Figures 32.1–32.2, 33.1–33.2*, 53, *Figures 34.1–34.2*, 55

L

latticework: windows and doors 104, 109, 111–112, *Figures* 70, 72.1, 115, 118

layering and piling 116, *Figures 75.1–75.2, 76*, 162

limitlessness, creating 13, 28, 163

Lushan *Figure 45.4*, 112, *Figure 77.1*

M

ma 38

madang (inner gardens) 150, 153, 184; and Chinese courtyards 158, 160. *See also ch'ae.*

mairado sliding doors 37, *Figures 19.1–19.3*, 43, 55, 59–60, *Figure 36.2*

Mandarin Duck *huating*/hall 106, *Figure 68.3*, 111–112

Manshu-in 68, *Figures 43.1–43.5*, 71, 74, 80

matou bi (horse's head wall) 85, *Figure 54*

Matsuo Bashō 34

metaphor 14, 16

miegakure 61–63, *Figures 40, 41.1–41.4*, 66, 68, *Figures 42, 43.2, 44.6*, 74–75, 78, 80, *Figures 47.2*, 115

miyabi 14, 29

mono no aware 29

"modeling after" 14, 16–17, 22–25, *Figures 9.1–9.3*

mountain locale 62, 67

multipurpose rooms 147, 150, 158–159

mundane world 62, 104, 125–128, 160, 182

myŏngdang land 133, 164, 182

Myōshinji: Taizō-in 37; Tōkai-an 40, *Figure 21*, 43; Keishun'in *Figures 24.1–24.3*

N

natural landscape: as prototype 14, 16–17, 22, 29, 62, 75, 107; –style gardens 14, 80, 112

neo-Confucianism 136–137, 179. *See also* Confucian.

north garden: in Japanese feudal residences 34, *Figures 18.1–18.2*, 37–38, *Figures 19.1–19.3, 20.1*, 43, 61; and ink-wash painting techniques 37–38, *Figures 20.1–20.2*; and *mairado* fixtures 37, *Figures 19.1–19.3. See also* south garden.

numaru (special reception room) 139, *Figures 88.1–88.2*, 153, 158, 164, *Figures 110.1–110.2, 112.1–112.3*

O

ocean style 9, 17, *Figure 10.2*, 22, 23, *Figure 12*, 40

Onjōji Kōjō-in 34, 53, *Figures 33.1–33.2, 34.1–34.2*, 55

outer gardens 160, 162–163, 173, *Figures 115–119*, 178, 184–185

P

painting, Japanese (*yamato-e*) 29, 38; (ink-wash) 37–38, *Figure 20.2*; (Kanō school screen and wall) *Figure 30*, 52, 55, *Figure 35.4*, 58, 71; (*rakuchū rakugai-zu*) 32, *Figure 15*; Chinese (import and display of) 32, 49, 93; (landscape, as a prototype for gardens) 104, 106, 116, 120, *Figures 78–79*, 122, 124; (theory and gardens) 120, 122, 124, 127; (as a didactic tool) 120, 122, 124; (Xie He's Six Laws [*liu-fa*] of)16, 18, 120. *See also* poetry and painting as one.

palaces, Japanese, (Higashisanjō) *Figure 3.2*, 9–11, *Figure 6*; (Nijōjō) *Figure 30*, 178; Chinese (as prototypes for Heian architecture) 10, *Figure 7.1*, 13; (E-fang) 107; (Forbidden City) 133, 182; Korean, (Ch'angdŏkkung) 166; (Ch'ilgung) 131; (Kyŏngbok[kung]) 133, *Figure 83*, 163, 166, *Figure 119*, 173, 182. *See also shinden-zukuri.*

pang enclosed, heated rooms 144–150, *Figures 95–99*, 153, *Figures 104–105, 108.1–108.2*, 158

paradise, Pure Land (Western) 12–13, 78, 80; of the Taoist Immortals 107, 116, 122. *See also* utopia.

past masters 14, 17

pavements *Figure 38.2*, 63, *Figures 41.2, 44.6*, 74, 109. *See also* stepping-stones.

picture plane 29, 38, 41, 55, 58, 163

pilgrimage 76, 78

Piwŏn (Secret Garden) 162, 166, *Figures 116.1–116.3. See also* rear gardens.

pleasure gardens 75–76, 78, 80, 104, 106

poetry: and gardens 14, 29, 120; and painting as one 122, 12. *See also* painting, Chinese.

ponds: in Japanese gardens 9–10, 13, 14, 16, 17, *Figures 10.2–10.3*, 22–27, *Figure 12–13*, 40, 43, 55, 75, 80; and lakes in Chinese gardens 106, 107, 109–110, 115–116, *Figure 74.2*; in Korean outer gardens 160, 163, 166, *Figure 113.3*, 173, *Figures 115–120*, 178, 185

prospect 133; as a garden-making approach 162–164, *Figure 110.3*, 166, *Figures 111.5, 112.3*, 184. *See also* vista.

p'ungsu. See geomancy.

Pure Land: Buddhism 12; villa-temples 13 *Figure 7.2*; temple precinct gardens 74, 76, 78, *Figures 46.1–46.2*

pyŏldang (annex sanctuary) 160, *Figure 109*, 173, *Figure 117*

pyŏlsŏ (Confucian scholars' retreats) 164, 178–179, *Figures 121.1–121.6*, 182, 185

Q

quarried-stone embankments 166, 173, *Figures 116–119*, 178, 185

R

rapids 19, *Figure 18.1*, 37

rear gardens: in *yangban* estates (*twitmadang*) 131, 134, 137, 139,

143, 149, 150, 153, *Figure 108.3*, 158, 166, *Figures 111.1–111.3, 113.1–113.4*, 178, 184; in Imperial residences 162, 166, *Figures 114.1–114.3. See also* Piwŏn.

retirement. *See* seclusion.

Rikyū. *See* Sen no Rikyū.

rocks, fantastic/strange/unusual, as garden features 103, 109, 111, 112, *Figures 72.2–72.3, 73.1*, 116, *Figures 75–76*, 131, 162; table 93, 98, 102. *See also* stones.

roji 61–63, *Figure 38–40*, 66–68, *Figures 43.5, 44.1*, 74, 80

rural settings, as garden ideals 122; features of Korean dwellings in 145, 149–150, *Figures 100, 102.2, 103.1. See also* urban settings.

Ryōanji 41, *Figure 22.1*, 43, *Figure 26.1–26.2*

S

Sakuteiki 4; garden requirements in 8–9; influences on later gardens 38, 41, 61, 62, 66, 75; on addressing spatial constraints 25–28; on setting stones 3, 19, 22; on trees and shrubs 19, 22; overall principles in 13–14, 16–17; six compositional elements and 17, 19; and stylized forms (*yō*) 22–25; and Xie He's Six Laws of painting 16–17

sarangch'ae (master's quarters) 137, 139, *Figures 88.1–88.2*, 144, 147, 150

scale 5, 9, 13, 24, 27, 32, 55, 93, 106, 109, 116, 133, 161; human 13, 116, 120; perceived 41; reduction of 6, 12–13, 34, 161, 120

scenic space cells 115, *Figures 73.1–73.2, 74.1–74.2*

screen and curves 112, 115–116, *Figures 73.1–73.2, 74.1–74.2*, 162

seascape and seashore scenes 17, 24, *Figure 12*, 173

seclusion (retirement): in China 123–128, 182, 184; gardens as an expression of 179; in Korea 179, 182, 184–185

secret teachings/transmissions (*hiden*) 25, 43. *See also* transmitted traditions.

Sen no Rikyū 34, 62, 66–68

shinden-zukuri: architecture 7–8, *Figure 4.1–4.2*, 10–11, 13, 29, 37; gardens *Figure 5*, 9, 13–14, 25–29; vestiges of, in medieval architecture 32, *Figures 15–16*, 34, 43. *See also* palaces, Japanese.

shin-gyō-sō 68

Shintō 3

shitomido shutters 29, 34, 37, 43, *Figures 32.1, 33.1*, 55, 58–60, *Figure 36.1*

Shōdenji 41, *Figure 22.2*

shoin/sukiya/sōan structures 68, *Figures 42–44*, 74, 75

shoin-zukuri: architecture 32; transitional 32, *Figures 16–17*, 34, 43, 53, *Figures 32–34*, 55, 59, 93; mature, 49, *Figure 30*, 52, 55, *Figure 35.1*; gardens. *See* south garden in warrior residences.

shufang (study) 103–104, 106, *Figures 67.3, 68.1*, 119, 132

siheyuan residential quadrangles 83–85, *Figure 49*, 90–91, *Figures 58.1–58.2*, 93, 98, *Figures 62.1–62.2*, 100, *Figure 66*, 127

simianting (four-sided hall) 111, *Figures 70, 72*

single-family dwellings 100

site: conditions, adapting to 10–13, 19, 25, 27–28, 32, 34, 49, 118, 149; selection and excavation of 109, 110, 162, 182, 184; layout of buildings on the 134, 149, 162–164; characteristics, favorable. *See also* geomancy, *myŏngdang* land.

skylights 85 99, *Figure 63.1*

sōan (thatched, rustic tearoom) 62, 66, 68

social status, architectural representations of 134–137

Soswaewŏn 179, *Figures 121.1–121.6*, 185

south garden: in *shinden-zukuri* 8–9, *Figure 5*, 25–29; white sand, 17, *Figure 10.5*, 25; simplification of 38; in feudal Zen temples 40–41, 43, *Figures 21–26, 29.1*; in warrior residences 43, *Figures 27, 28.1–28.2, 29.2*, 49, *Figures 34.1–34.2*, 55, *Figures 35.1–35.5. See also* north garden.

sŏwŏn schools 143, 179

sukiya-zukuri 67–68, 74

stepping-stones 63, *Figure 39*, 68, *Figure 43.5*, 74, 76. *See also* pavements.

stones: as the structural elements of gardens 22–23, 27; as garden features 3, 14, 17, 19, 22, 24, 27–28, 41, 43, 110, 162, 166, 173; *sŏkkasan* 162, 173. *See also* rocks.

storage, space 93, 139, 143, 147, 148, 158; rotational 158

stroll gardens, Japanese *kaiyūshiki teien* 61, 66, 74–76, *Figures 45.1–45.5*, 78, 80, 111; Chinese *yuanlin* 112, 116, 132; Korean rear gardens 162, 166, *Figure 47.2*

stylized forms (*yō*) 22–26, 49

sub-gardens 68, *Figures 43.1–43.5*, 75 *Figures 45.1–45.5*

symmetry: as prototype 10–11; abandonment of 10–11, 13, 34; in Korean outer gardens 173. *See also* asymmetry.

T

Tachibana no Toshitsuna 4, 9, 14, 17, 30

taech'ŏng (central living room) 137, *Figures 87.1–87.2*, 139, 145, 149, 150, 153, *Figures 106–108*, 158, 164, 184

tang (central living room) 84–85, 91, 93, 96, *Figures 60–61*, 98, 100, 102, 158, 160

Taoism, and painting theory 120, 123–124, 128; and seclusion in nature 125–127; and gardens 124, 127–128, 182

tatami-mat flooring 32, 59

tea ceremony. See *chanoyu.*

tearoom (teahouse) 61–63, *Figures 38.1, 41.1, 41.4,* 66–68, 71, *Figures 44.1, 44.5,* 74–75

Tenryūji *Figures 28.1–28.2,* 49

terraces 40, 109, 111; stepped 134, 139, 166, *Figures 111.1, 114.1*

themes, in Japanese gardens 14, 37, 62, 75–76, *Figures 45.1–45.5*; in Chinese gardens 112, 116

threshold, interior/exterior 58–60

tianjing. See courtyards.

ting. See courtyards.

ting yuan 100, 103–104, *Figures 66–68,* 106, 118, 120, 124, 128, 132

Tōji Kanchi-in 53, *Figures 32.1–32.2,* 55

tokonoma alcove 32, 93, 158–159

Tokugawa shogunate 67, 74–76

topography, and site excavation 110, 133, 161, 182; of cities and towns 132–133, 182; and site selection 134, 162

torii gate 3, *Figure 1*

transmitted traditions (*denshō*) 24–25, 26. *See also* secret teachings.

trees and shrubs, as structural elements 22, *Figure 11,* 41, *Figure 22.3*; restricted planting of 27; as screening devices in *miegakure* 61, *Figures 41.1–41.4, 43.2,* 68, 71, *Figure 44.6,* 75; blossoming, linked with faith 78; in Chinese courtyards 98, *Figure 62.2*; in Chinese *yuanlin* 110–111, 118, 120; in Korean gardens 139, 162, 166, 173. *See also Sakuteiki,* on trees and shrubs.

tsuboniwa 29, *Figures 14.1–2*

tsukubai (ritual washbasin) 62, 63, *Figure 44.1*

twitmadang. See rear garden.

U

unworldly realm 122, 127–128, 160

urban settings, and *yuanlin* 106–108, 110; features of Korean dwellings in 145, 149–150, *Figures 101, 103.2. See also* rural settings.

urban merchants (*chōmin*), and popular culture 67; pleasure "gardens" of 74–76, 78, *Figures 46.1–46.2,* 80

utopia, gardens as an expression of 104, 106, 108, 112. *See also* paradise.

V

vantage point, fixed 37; moving 37, 75; multiple 80; high, 116

views, static and seated, 25, 27, 37, 43, *Figure 23,* 52, 55, 60, 61, 116, 164; unidirectional and frontally composed 25–29, 43, *Figure 27,* 49, 52, 61, 78; panoramic 29, 37–38, 58, 153, 163–164; parallel 52–53, *Figure 31.2*; framed or cropped 37, *Figure 19.1,* 41, 59, 158, 163; kinetic and ambulatory 66, 67; foreshortened 41, 55, 58; obscured or blocked 61, 66, 68, 71, 74, 75; sequential 61; mutual and intersecting *Figures 71, 72.3,* 110–112, 116, 162

vista 66, 110, 112, 123, 163. *See also* prospect.

W

wabi 66, 67

walkways, covered 109, 111–112, *Figure 73.2,* 115; open 111

walls, retaining or surrounding 83, 85, *Figure 54,* 90, 96, 98–100, 103, *Figure 67.1,* 106, 118, 139, 143, 149–150, *Figures 103.1–103.2*; garden 109–110, 131, 162–164

warrior residences (*buke*) *Figures 15–16,* 43, 55. *See also* south garden, in warrior residences.

waterfalls 3, 17, 19, *Figure 10.6,* 22, 23, *Figure 18.1,* 37, 55, 68, 109, 116, *Figure* 81, 169, 179

West Lake *Figures 45.1, 45.3,* 107, *Figure 74.2,* 116

woshi private/sleeping quarters 84, 85, *Figure 50.1–50.2,* 91, 93, 100, 158

woyou (travel by imagination) 122–124, 127–128

Y

yin/yang 66, 134, 149, *Figure 57.4*

yangban estates, composition of 137, *Figure 86.1–86.2,* 139, 143–145, 153, 160, 173; and social class 134–137

yō. See stylized forms.

Yuan ye 108–110, 116, 161, 163, 182

yuanlin 100, 103, 106–112, *Figures 69, 71,* 115–116, *Figure 76,* 118, 120, 122, 124, 127–128, 132, 160–164, 179

yuanzi. See courtyards.

yūgen 34

Z

zansan jōsui (lingering mountains and water) technique 37–38, *Figure 20.2*

Zen, Buddhism 34; sub-temple architecture 34; practice, gardens for 40–41, 43, 78; *kōan* 40, 41; and tea 66–67, 78. *See also* south gardens, in feudal Zen temples.

其上近年方丈回禄しけれハむかしを惜ミ慕ひ侍る

一庭空曠白砂平
頑石誰鋪形勢成
宛似昔時渡渓虎
分蹄両子泛波行

皆川愿

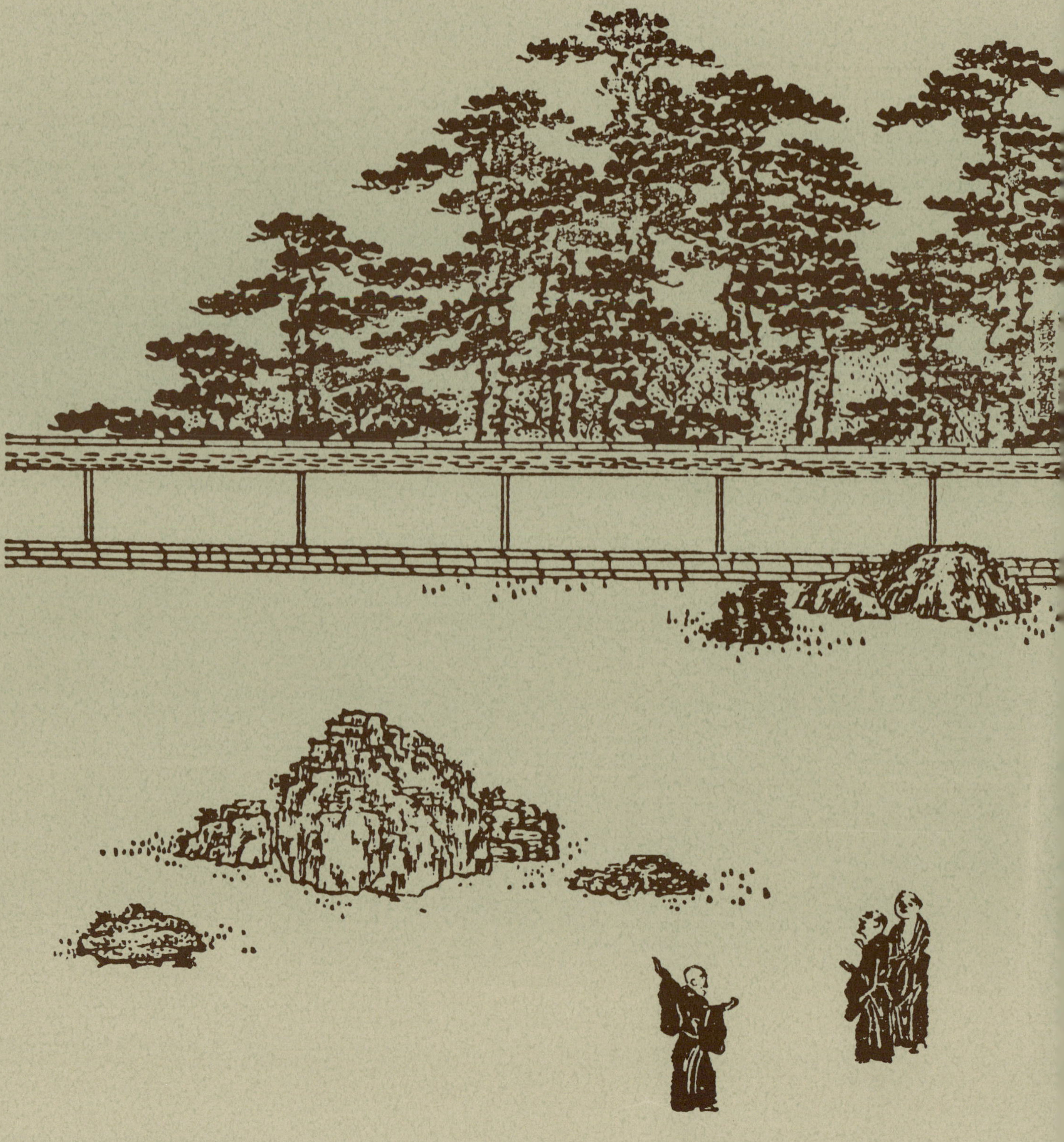